Principles of
Laboratory Instruments

Principles of Laboratory Instruments

Larry E. Schoeff, M.S., MT (ASCP)
Director and Associate Professor
Medical Technology Program
Department of Pathology
University of Utah School of Medicine

Education Director
Associated Regional and University Pathologists, Inc. (ARUP)
Salt Lake City, Utah

Robert H. Williams, Ph.D., MT (ASCP)
Director, Section of General Chemistry/Toxicology
University of Illinois Hospital
Division of Clinical Pathology
Department of Pathology, College of Medicine
University of Illinois at Chicago
Chicago, Illinois

*with **315** illustrations*

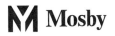 Mosby

St. Louis Baltimore Boston Chicago London Philadelphia Sydney Toronto

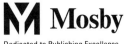

Editor: Stephanie Manning
Assistant Editor: Jane Petrash
Project Manager: John A. Rogers
Senior Production Editor: Shauna Burnett Sticht
Designer: David Zielinski

Printed in the United States of America

Mosby–Year Book, Inc.
11830 Westline Industrial Drive
St. Louis, Missouri 63146

Library of Congress Cataloging in Publication Data
Principles of laboratory instruments / [edited by] Larry E. Schoeff,
  Robert H. Williams.
        p.   cm.
    Includes bibliographical references and index.
    ISBN 0-8016-7489-1
    1. Diagnosis, Laboratory—Instruments.   2. Medical laboratories
—Instruments.   I. Schoeff, Larry E.   II. Williams, Robert H.
(Robert Henry),
    [DNLM: 1. Equipment and Supplies.   2. Laboratories.
3. Technology, Medical—instrumentation.   W 26 P957]
RB36.2.P75   1992
610′.28—dc20
DNLM/DLC
for Library of Congress   92-49752
                                                            CIP

93 94 95 96 97 UG/MY 9 8 7 6 5 4 3 2 1

Contributors

Lemuel Bowie, Ph.D., DABCC
Clinical Chemistry Laboratory
Evanston Hospital
Evanston, Illinois

John M. Brewer, Ph.D.
Department of Biochemistry
University of Georgia
Athens, Georgia

I-Wen Chen, Ph.D.
Department of Radiobiology Laboratory
University of Cincinnati Medical Center
Cincinnati, Ohio

Mary Ann Dotson, MT (ASCP), CLS (NCA)
Duke University Medical Center
Durham, North Carolina

David Hage, Ph.D.
University of Nebraska
Lincoln, Nebraska

Debra Hoppensteadt, MS, MT (ASCP)
Department of Pathology
Loyola University Medical Center
Maywood, Illinois

Barbara Lewis, MS, SM (ASCP)
Management and Microbiology Consultant
Batavia, Illinois

Sherwood C. Lewis, Ph.D., DABCC
Department of Pathology and Laboratory
  Medicine
St. Francis Hospital and Medical Center
Hartford, Connecticut
Department of Laboratory Medicine
University of Connecticut School of Medicine
Farmington, Connecticut

Jack Maggiore, MS, MT (ASCP)
University of Illinois Hospital
Chicago, Illinois

Andrew Maturen, Ph.D., DABCC, MT (ASCP)
OCLS Clinical Chemistry
Rush Presbyterian St. Luke's Medical Center
Chicago, Illinois

Anthony O. Okorodudu, Ph.D., DABCC
Clinical Chemistry Division
Department of Pathology
University of Texas Medical Branch
Galveston, Texas

Marguerite Quale, M.S., MT (ASCP)
Ravenswood Hospital Medical Center
Chicago, Illinois

Kathy Ristow, MT (ASCP)
Clinical Microbiology Laboratory
University of Illinois Hospital
Chicago, Illinois

Jeanine Walenga, Ph.D., MT (ASCP)
Department of Pathology
Loyola University Medical Center
Maywood, Illinois

Robert Webster, Ph.D., DABCC
OCLS Clinical Chemistry
Rush Presbyterian St. Luke's Medical Center
Chicago, Illinois

Preface

The intended audience for **Principles of Laboratory Instruments** includes all clinical laboratorians who expect to operate laboratory instruments. In addition to students of clinical laboratory science, this may include pathology residents, medical students, and graduate students in the medical sciences. Much of the information provided in this text should also be invaluable to clinical chemists, pathologists, supervisory personnel in the clinical laboratory sciences, and others who may have a vested interest in laboratory medicine, such as instrument manufacturers.

No field in medicine has expanded as rapidly as laboratory medicine, especially in the area of laboratory automation. Understanding how an instrument operates is difficult because of the great variation in the complexity of instrumentation that exists, especially in today's marketplace where instrumentation has become highly computerized. It is paramount that individuals working in this field have a basic understanding of the function of electronic components and units used in the manufacturing of instruments, those principles applied to instruments that are inherent in their operation, and the concept of instrument subsystems and how they are integrated to form a functioning unit. In addition they should be knowledgeable about the instruments that are currently available in the marketplace, have a working knowledge of their unique characteristics, and be aware of their applications to patient testing in the clinical laboratory.

It is hoped that teaching the basic principles and theory of instrumental analysis as applied to the field of laboratory medicine will provide a working knowledge for instrument selection; an effective means of instruction for operators to make proper judgments during the operation of an instrument and to recognize the limitations, advantages, and disadvantages of each; a means of identifying instrumental problems; and common approaches to troubleshooting some of the problems that cause an instrument to malfunction.

The purpose of this text is twofold: to provide a foundation of knowledge in basic electronics and principles of instrumentation, and to apply the theoretic principles of electronics and instrumentation to the automated systems that are currently available in the marketplace. To accomplish these goals the text has been organized into three sections: **Basic Electricity and Electronic Components, Principles of Instrumentation, and Automation in the Clinical Laboratory.** The section on Basic Electricity and Electronic Components covers basic and intermediate principles of electronics and serves as a background for subsequent sections. The section on Principles of Instrumentation covers basic principles that are applied to instrumental analysis and addresses specific instruments that employ that particular mode of analysis. The last section, Automation in the Clinical Laboratory, contains information pertaining to automation in general and is divided according to subspecialty, describing in detail the principles of operation and unique features for many of the major instruments that are currently used in the clinical laboratory.

With the rapid advances and changes in instrumentation technology it is difficult for a book of this nature to remain up-to-date. What is "cutting edge" technology today, seen as concepts on design tables and prototypes in research and development laboratories, can become reality in clinical laboratories in a matter of months. Such "hot" topics as front-end automation (robotics); in vivo, noninvasive mobile analyzers; spectral mapping for simultaneous, multiple chemistries; artificial intelligence in analyzers; enhanced system integration and miniaturization; and other new concepts will likely appear in the clinical laboratory in the not too distant future. We hope to include these topics in the next edition of **Principles of Laboratory Instruments.**

Larry E. Schoeff
Robert H. Williams

Table of Contents

Principles of
Laboratory Instruments

BASIC ELECTRICITY AND ELECTRONIC COMPONENTS

CHAPTER 1

Fundamentals of Electricity

ROBERT H. WILLIAMS

Basic Concepts of Electricity
Sources of Electricity
Direct Current
Alternating Current

Clinical laboratory instruments contain complex electronic circuitry, and thus it is difficult to understand their principles of operation without some working knowledge of electricity and electronics. To comprehend the electronic principles that are used in the development and operation of laboratory instruments, it is also essential that clinical laboratory personnel develop a good electronics vocabulary. Only then can the laboratorian appreciate the complexity of the instrumentation found in today's clinical laboratory.

In this chapter the process of electron flow is discussed in terms of atomic structure and how it is related to the electron theory and the fluid (conventional) theory of electrical current. Electrical conductors and insulators are also described in terms of their atomic structure and how this structure is related to the flow of electricity. Electricity is defined in terms of the interrelated values of current, voltage, resistance, and power that are mathematically expressed by Ohm's and Joule's laws. The application of these fundamental laws is applied to important electronic concepts such as voltage drop, voltage division, and power. Applications of power are considered in the context of the clinical laboratory. Finally, the primary sources of electricity and the characteristics of direct and alternating current are briefly described.

The Atom. The basic building block of all matter is the atom, the ultimate particle of an element. All atoms of a single element are identical. The center of the atom is called the nucleus, which is composed of two different particles, the protons, carrying a positive charge, and the neutrons, considered to be electrically neutral. Elec-

trons orbit the nucleus and carry a negative charge. The simplest element is hydrogen, which has only one proton in the nucleus and one electron orbiting it. The other naturally occurring elements have neutrons along with an equal number of protons and orbital electrons. The positive charge of the proton is exactly equal to the negative charge of an electron. Because neutrons do not carry a charge, the net charge of a stable atom is neutral. It is possible, however, for an atom to lose or gain an electron. If an atom loses an electron, then it carries a positive charge and is called a positive ion. If the atom gains an electron, the atom carries a negative charge and is called a negative ion. Therefore positive ions are those that have a deficiency of electrons, whereas negative ions are those that have excess electrons.

Each element has a characteristic number of electrons and protons. The elements are arranged according to their atomic number, which is equal to the number of protons within the nucleus or the number of electrons revolving around the nucleus. Electrons have a great deal of energy and represent nearly the entire energy of the atom, but essentially they have no weight. The proton and neutron, unlike the electron, have measurable weight. Almost all the weight of an atom, called the atomic weight, is determined by the sum of the protons and neutrons within its nucleus.

Electrons revolve around the atom's nucleus in characteristic orbits, energy levels, or shells. These shells are designated as K, L, M, N, etc., lettering from the center outward. There is a maximum number of electrons that can be held by each shell (Fig. 1-1). The electron capacity of each shell must be satisfied before electrons will be found in the next shell.

As the temperature of the atom increases, the electrons move farther from the nucleus and the distance between atoms increases. When the

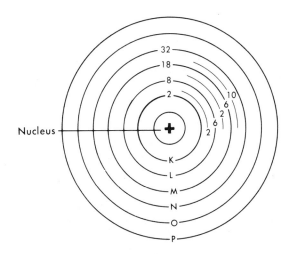

Fig. 1-1 Schematic representation of an atom, showing electron shells and their capacities. Note subshells of L and M.

atoms become far apart, the substance becomes a gas. If the atoms approach each other to the point where the distance between nuclei is about the same as the diameter of the atom, the substance will become a liquid. As the atoms get still closer together, their outer electron orbits begin to overlap and a solid forms. These outer electrons are called valence electrons.

In metals, many electrons are usually in the valence orbit. These valence electrons exist at high energy levels that are easily moved to free-electron status. Electrons in such a situation can be considered an electron cloud, or a sea of electrons in motion. Free charges moving about suggest electron flow or electricity. Thus the outermost shell of the atom is recognized as the most important orbit in electronics.

Electron Flow. Because most metals are made up of atoms with loosely bound valence electrons, they tend to move randomly from one atom to another. These electrons can be forced to move in one direction by placing an excess of electrons (negative charge) at one end of the wire and a deficiency of electrons (positive charge) at the other end. The loose electrons in the wire will be repelled by the extra electrons entering the

wire at the negative end and attracted to the positive charge at the other end. This electron flow is diagrammed in Fig. 1-2. This process is almost instantaneous, occurring at the speed of light or approximately 186,000 miles/second.

Conductors, Insulators, and Semiconductors. Materials that are composed of atoms with weakly bound electrons in the outer orbits make good pathways for electron flow. Such materials are called **conductors** because their electrons exist at higher energy levels and are easily moved to free-electron status. The more loosely bound the outer electrons of the atoms of the material, the better the material conducts electron flow (e.g., silver is the best conductor, followed by copper, and gold). Conductors are made up of materials having three or fewer valence electrons.

Substances that do not readily give up their electrons provide a high opposition to electron flow. These materials are considered nonconductors and may be called **insulators** (includes resistors and dielectrics). The valence electrons of nonconductors are held together in a tight bonding arrangement that does not allow them to be easily displaced. Hence, they are poor conductors of electricity. Examples of high resistance or insulating materials include air, glass, plastic, and rubber. Insulators are made up of materials having seven or eight valence electrons.

Semiconductors are neither good conductors nor good insulators. Silicon and germanium are the two elements most often used to make semiconductor devices. They are composed of materials that have four valence electrons.

Pure water is a relatively poor conductor, but nevertheless it does conduct electricity. If sodium chloride is added to pure water, the solution becomes a better conductor. When salt is dissolved, the sodium becomes a positively charged ion (Na^+) and the chloride becomes a negatively charged ion (Cl^-). These charges will conduct electricity through the solution. The numbers and types of ions present in the solution determine the conducting capacity, or conductivity, of that solution.

Electromotive Force. For electron flow to occur, a good conducting material must serve as

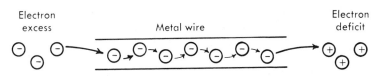

Fig. 1-2 Electron flow through a metal wire.

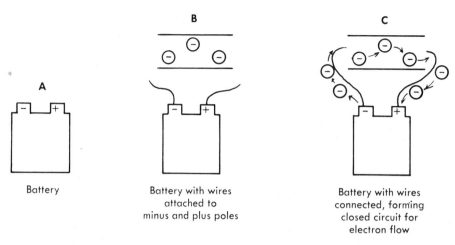

Fig. 1-3   Battery providing EMF for electron flow.

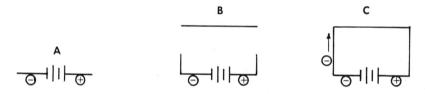

Fig. 1-4   Schematic representation of Fig. 1-3.

an unbroken pathway for electrons and a source having an electron excess and an electron deficit must be applied at opposite ends of the conducting pathway. As shown in Fig. 1-2, it appears that the excess electrons are pushing or forcing the free, or loose, electrons through the wire. This process is viewed as a force. Consequently, the force exerted by the excess electrons on the loose electrons in the conductor is called **electromotive force (EMF)**. The EMF is the force that causes electrons to move through a conductor from a negatively to a positively charged point. The unit of measure of EMF is the **volt (V)**.

Some type of battery or generator may be the source of the required EMF. A battery is a direct current (DC) voltage source consisting of cells that convert one form of energy (chemical, thermal, nuclear, or solar) to electrical energy. An alternating current (AC) generator is an alternating current voltage source consisting of a rotating mechanism that converts mechanical energy into electrical energy by a process called **induction.**

In general, batteries convert chemical energy to electrical energy. Through a chemical reaction, an electron excess is formed at one pole (negative pole), and an electron deficit is formed at the other pole (positive pole). As shown in in Fig. 1-3, if the positive and negative poles of a battery are connected with a conducting material, electrons will flow from the negative pole to the positive pole. The battery, therefore, provides the EMF required to move the electrons through the conductor. Fig. 1-4 is the same as Fig. 1-3 but is represented with electrical schematic symbols.

Current. In the past, experimentalists in electricity such as Benjamin Franklin advocated that work was performed by positive charges moving to a lower, or more negative level of potential. Such movement of positive charges in an electrical circuit is known as **conventional current flow** and has sometimes been referred to as the **Franklinian theory.** After the discovery of the atom, it was shown that the particle moving in an electrical circuit was the negatively charged electron, and thus the **electron theory** was developed. This theory states that electrons leave the negative pole of an electrical source, move through a closed loop, and then return to the source at its positive pole. The circuit illustrated in Fig. 1-5, *A*, represents the electron theory of current flow; the circuit illustrated in Fig. 1-5, *B*, represents the Franklinian theory of conventional current flow.

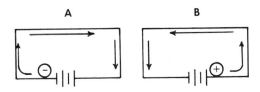

Fig. 1-5 Electrical current flow.

Though conventional current flow may still be found in older literature, the electron theory of current flow, being a more accurate description of the process, will be used in this text.

Each electron possesses energy called a charge (designated *Q*). The unit for measuring this charge is the **coulomb.** Each electron carries an approximate charge of 1.6×10^{-19} coulombs, therefore 1 coulomb would be equivalent to the charges of 6.24×10^{18} electrons added together. **Current (I)** is the rate at which a charge moves through a conductor (i.e., rate of electron flow). The unit of measure of current is the **ampere (A).** When 6.24×10^{18} electrons (1 coulomb) passes a point in a circuit every second, the circuit is said to be carrying a current of 1 A. The ampere is a rather large unit. In most cases, the current in circuits is in the milliampere (mA) or the microampere (μA) range. A milliampere equals one thousandth of an ampere; a microampere equals one millionth of an ampere.

Two factors that affect current or the rate of electron flow are the force, or **voltage,** that moves the electrons through the circuit and the ease with which the material in the circuit allows the electrons to pass (i.e., the **resistance** of the circuit to current flow).

Voltage. The force that moves electrons through a conductor is the electromotive force or **voltage (E).** The unit of measure of EMF is the volt (V). A force of 1 V is required to move 1 coulomb/second (1 A) through a resistance (R) of 1 ohm (Ω). Common units of voltage include the microvolt (μV), 0.000001 V; the millivolt (mV), 0.001 V; the kilovolt (kV), which equals 1000 V; and the megavolt (MV), 1,000,000 V.

EMF, voltage, and potential or potential difference are terms frequently used interchangeably; however, there are subtle differences. In Fig. 1-3, *B*, the circuit is not closed (i.e. electrons cannot move through the conductor) and thus no voltage develops. However, a potential for current flow does exist because there are two poles of different charges; it may be said that a potential difference exists between the two poles. In Fig. 1-

3, *C*, the circuit is closed and voltage or EMF forces a current to flow.

Resistance. If a material is a poor conductor of electricity, it will offer resistance to current flow in a circuit. **Resistance (R)** to current is measured in **ohms (Ω).** The kilohm (kΩ) is 1000 ohms; the megohm (MΩ) is 1 million ohms. *One ohm is the value of resistance through which 1 V maintains a current of 1 A.* The schematic symbol for resistance in a circuit is —⋀⋀—. If a fixed potential exists, such as in a battery, the amount of current that will flow in a closed circuit of conducting material depends on the ease with which electrons are allowed to move through the circuit. If the circuit has high resistance, electron flow will be difficult, and thus the amount of current will be small. However, with decreased or small resistance, electron flow will be high, and a large current will result.

Ohm's Law. The relationship of voltage, current, and resistance was determined by the German physicist George Simon Ohm (1787-1854) who stated that *"current in a circuit was directly proportional to the applied voltage, and inversely proportional to the resistance."* **Ohm's law** is expressed in the following formula:

$$I = E/R$$

where I = Current (amperes), E = Voltage (volts), and R = Resistance (ohms). Using this formula, if any two values are known, the third can be calculated. For example, if a device, having a resistance of 5 Ω, is placed in a circuit having a battery voltage of 12 V, then Ohm's law can be used to determine the total current (I_t) flowing in the circuit:

$$I_t = E_t/R_t \quad I_t = 12 \text{ V}/5 \text{ }\Omega \quad I_t = 2.4 \text{ A}$$

Transposition of Ohm's law results in the formulas:

$$E = I \times R \quad \text{and} \quad R = E/I$$

These three forms of Ohm's law can be seen in the triangular arrangement illustrated in Fig. 1-6. It can be used as a memory aid to help remember Ohm's law. To obtain the formula for an unknown, place a finger over the symbol for the required quantity; the formula is then revealed. Using this diagram it can be seen that any single value is equal to the other two in the relationship that they hold in the triangle. Thus, I = E/R, E = IR, and R = E/I. The proper units must be used with Ohm's law. For example, if the units in a problem are given as millivolts, microamperes, and kilohms, they must be converted to volts,

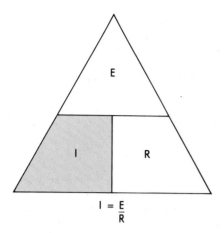

$$I = \frac{E}{R}$$

Fig. 1-6   Diagrammatic representation of Ohm's law.

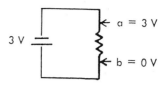

Fig. 1-7   Voltage drop.

amperes, and ohms, respectively, before they are used in any of the equations given above. The following example will help to illustrate this point. If a simple circuit contains a 10 mV battery and has a current flow of 200 μA, what is the total resistance of the circuit?

Solution:
1. Convert millivolts to volts: 100 mV = 0.1 V
2. Convert microamperes to amperes: 20 μA = 0.02 mA = 0.00002 A
3. Using Ohm's law, solve for the total resistance (R_t): $R_t = E/I$

$$R_t = 0.1 \text{ volt}/0.00002 \text{ A}$$
$$R_t = 5{,}000 \ \Omega \text{ or } 5 \text{ k}\Omega$$

A linear relationship between voltage and current will exist as long as resistance remains constant. Many circuits are composed of linear conductors (i.e., metals or alloys that maintain constant resistance), and therefore obey Ohm's law. However, some circuits contain materials that are known as nonlinear conductors (i.e., semiconductors, electrolytes, and ionized gases where the resistance can vary considerably), and therefore do not obey Ohm's law. Calculation of current, voltage, and resistance with these circuits becomes more complex.

Voltage Drop and Voltage Division. Voltage has been defined as the force required to push a current through a resistance. When the current goes through this resistance, energy is given off in the form of heat. This loss of energy can be regarded as a loss of voltage or as a **voltage drop.** Frequently, voltage drop is referred to as a *IR drop.* There is no difference in these terms because voltage (E) = I × R. In Fig. 1-7 the voltage at point *a* is 3 V, which is supplied by a 3 V battery. The voltage at point *b* is 0 V because 3 V were "dropped" or lost by passing through the resistor.

The concept of voltage drop may be used to obtain different voltages from one voltage source (i.e., divide a voltage source into smaller discrete sources). This process is called voltage division, and the circuit is called a **voltage divider**; refer to Fig. 1-8, *A.* The circuit shown has a 3 V battery and three 1 kΩ resistors. Three volts are dropped across three resistors of equal value. The voltage at point *a* is 3 V, and the voltage at point *d* is 0 V.

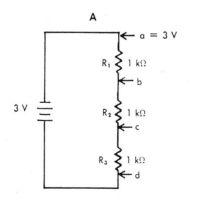
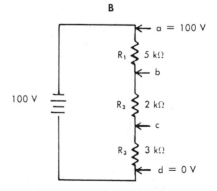

Fig. 1-8   Voltage division.

Because each of the three resistors will exert the same resistance to the flow of current, the voltage lost in each resistor will be the same. Thus 1 V is lost across each resistor.

Voltage may also be dropped across any number of different resistances. The amount of voltage lost across a particular resistor depends on the size of the resistor and can be calculated in two ways:

1. Multiply the total voltage by the fractional portion of a given resistance to the total resistance in the circuit (e.g., in Fig. 1-8, *B*, the voltage lost across each resistor can be calculated as follows):

Total resistance (R_t) = $R_1 + R_2 + R_3$
R_t = 5 kΩ + 2 kΩ + 3 kΩ = 10 kΩ

Voltage drop in R_1: IR_1 drop = 100 V $\times$ R_1/R_t
= 100 V $\times$ 5 kΩ/10 kΩ = 50 V

Voltage drop in R_2: IR_2 drop = 100 V $\times$ R_2/R_t
= 100 V $\times$ 2 kΩ/10 kΩ = 20 V

Voltage drop on R_3: IR_3 drop = 100 V $\times$ R_3/R_t
= 100 V $\times$ 3 kΩ/10 kΩ = 30 V

2. Multiply total current (in amperes) passing through the resistor by the value of the resistor (in ohms). For example, in Fig. 1-8, *B*, the voltage lost across each resistor would be:

Total current (I_t) = V/R_1 = 100 V/10 kΩ
= 10 mA or 0.01 A

Voltage drop in R_1 = IR_1 drop = I $\times$ R_1
= (0.01 A)(5,000 Ω) = 50 V

Voltage drop in R_2 = IR_2 drop = I $\times$ R_2
= (0.01 A)(2,000 Ω) = 20 V

Voltage drop in R_3 = IR_3 drop = I $\times$ R_3
= (0.01 A)(3,000 Ω) = 30V

The application of voltage division is seen frequently throughout the remainder of this text.

Power. In electronics, **power** is defined as the *rate* of doing work. When electrons are pushed through a circuit, work is done, and heat is generated as the electrons pass through resistive devices (i.e., motors, resistors, and other electronic components). The unit used to measure this work and the heat that is subsequently produced is called the **watt (W)**. One watt is the work done when 1 V moves 1 A (Joule's law):

Power = Voltage $\times$ Current or P = EI

Another expression of the power equation that is useful in electronics is P = IR^2. In these expressions:

P = Power in watts (W)

E = EMF in volts (V)

R = Resistance in ohms (Ω)

I = Current in amperes (A)

Power consumption or heat generation is an important consideration in determining whether a circuit component can withstand the amount of electricity to be passed through the circuit. The energy that a battery loses is converted to heat energy in the resistance components of a circuit. If these components are not constructed to dissipate the heat, the component will burn or melt. Resistors and other electronic components have a wattage rating that must be considered when a circuit is built or repaired. For example, if a 10 kΩ resistor is rated for 2 W, can it withstand a 10 mA current?

P = (I)(E) = (I)(IR) = (I)^2(R)
P = (0.01 A)^2 $\times$ (10,000 Ω)
P = 0.0001 $\times$ 10,000 Ω = 1 W

Ten mA of current passing through a 10 kΩ resistance generates only 1 W of energy, which can be easily dissipated by a resistor rated to dissipate twice that amount of heat.

Instruments used in the clinical laboratory are sophisticated and expensive, and thus contain circuits that are intricate and complex. To protect their circuitry, a simple device called a **fuse** is inserted into the path of current flow. Heat generation (expressed as I^{2}R in the power equation) is caused by the resistance exerted by the fuse as the current passes through. The fuse contains a resistive element, usually a filament of wire, that melts at a certain temperature, causing a gap or break in the circuit. This gap prevents further current conduction through the circuit. Fig. 1-9 illustrates examples of good and "blown" fuses. The schematic symbol for a fuse is ∿ .

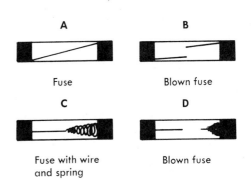

Fig. 1-9 Representation of good fuses and blown fuses.

Power is also an important consideration when determining if a series of clinical laboratory instruments can be connected to the same circuit without creating an overload. Every instrument has a power rating expressed in watts. The total power expended by all instruments on a given circuit should not exceed the power rating of that circuit line. For example, if a circuit, composed of a flame photometer (300 W), a blood gas analyzer (250 W), a Coulter counter (450 W), and an oven (600 W), were connected to a 120 volt line carrying a current of 15 A, would the load be exceeding the power rating capacity of this line?

Total carrying capacity of the power line is

$$P = IE$$
$$P = (15 \text{ A})(120 \text{ V})$$
$$P = 1800 \text{ W}$$

Total power consumed by the four instruments is

$$300 \text{ W} + 250 \text{ W} + 450 \text{ W} + 600 \text{ W} = 1650 \text{ W}$$

Because the total power expended by the instruments does not exceed the power rating of the line, the circuit is not overloaded. If the total power had been exceeded, then an overload would have occurred that would "trip" a device called a **circuit breaker.** The function of the circuit breaker is similar to that of a fuse except it protects the power line rather than an instrument or other device. Also, unlike a fuse, it can be reset after the overload is corrected. The schematic symbol for a circuit breaker is

Sources of Electricity

The primary sources of electricity are based on mechanical, chemical, photoelectric, thermoelectric, or piezoelectric generation. Electricity is produced mechanically in two ways, by **friction** or **induction.** When certain materials are rubbed together (i.e., glass rod rubbed with silk or a hard, rubber rod rubbed with fur), electrons are transferred by friction from one to the other and both materials become electrically charged. These charges are not in motion but reside statically on each substance. Therefore this type of electricity is known as **electrostatic,** or simply **static electricity.** Another way of producing electricity mechanically is by the relative motion of a conductor with respect to a magnetic field, a process known as **induction.** The interaction of electric and magnetic fields is studied in a branch of electricity called **electromagnetism.** A major portion of commercial electricity in the form of alternating current (AC) is produced by electromagnetic generators via induction.

Electricity can be generated chemically by inserting two dissimilar metals (i.e., zinc and copper or zinc and lead) into a conducting solution called an electrolyte. Each metal acts as an electrode. As a result of a chemical reaction at each electrode, a potential difference develops. This produces an electromotive force (EMF), or voltage, which can cause current to flow through an externally connected conducting circuit. Connecting a number of such chemical cells together can form a battery of any desired voltage that is capable of supplying a specific quantity of electricity. Electricity produced by chemical action is studied in the field known as **electrochemistry.**

Sunlight or artificial illumination falling on certain photosensitive materials, such as cesium or selenium, produces electricity by knocking out free electrons from the surface of the material. This process is known as photoelectric emission, or simply **photoelectricity,** and is commonly used as sources of electricity in various instruments containing light-sensitive devices such as photovoltaic cells or photomultiplier tubes.

When the junction of two dissimilar metals, such as an iron wire welded to a copper wire, is heated, an electromotive force appears between the free ends of the metals. Such a junction is called a thermocouple and the process is termed **thermoelectricity.** Thermocouples are primarily used in the clinical laboratory as temperature measuring devices, especially when a wide range of temperature measurements is required.

Electricity can also be generated by the mechanical compression, stretching, and twisting of certain crystals, such as quartz and Rochelle salts. When these crystals are subjected to mechanical pressure, a displacement of charges takes place on the crystal faces, resulting in a potential difference. The process by which materials generate an electromotive force by mechanical pressure is called **piezoelectricity.** In the medical field, the piezoelectric effect has found many applications including ultrasonic surgery.

Direct Current

Direct current (DC) is produced by batteries or power supplies that convert alternating current to direct current. The characteristics of DC and several types of batteries, as a source of direct current, are described below.

Characteristics. Direct current is characterized by unidirectional electron flow (i.e., it occurs in only one direction). Therefore the polarity of the voltage source remains unchanged. However, depending on its source, the voltage level can remain constant or vary over time. If a battery is used as the EMF source, the voltage level will remain constant. However, if a DC generator is used instead, the voltage will not remain constant, although the current remains unidirectional. This type of direct current is called variable DC or sometimes pulsating DC. The type of current that was discussed earlier in this chapter was unidirectional, and therefore was direct current. A source of voltage that gives rise to direct current is often abbreviated VDC, which indicates that the EMF source is Volts-DC or DC voltage.

Sources. Sources of direct current include batteries and electronic power supplies. The direct current needed in the circuits of a clinical laboratory instrument is generally provided by the power supply circuit of that instrument rather than a battery. The power supply circuit converts alternating current to direct current by a process called rectification. This section, however, will focus on the various types of batteries routinely encountered in the clinical laboratory and their application.

Some clinical laboratory instruments have a battery or batteries in their circuitry. These batteries are used either as a constant DC voltage source or as a voltage reference. Though batteries are common items, they usually do not receive adequate consideration from laboratory personnel who should be informed about the specifications, advantages, and disadvantages of the different types. A battery is a component of the circuit that laboratory personnel may be required to replace. Given the large variety of batteries that are available, it is essential that they are replaced with those that meet an instrument's specifications. If a battery of incorrect specifications is installed in a circuit, the circuit may be damaged and operate erratically or inaccurately.

Batteries as a DC Source of EMF. Basically, a battery consists of a potential difference developed as a result of a chemical reaction (Fig. 1-10). The various types of batteries discussed demonstrate that a potential can be generated by several different chemical reactions. The common feature shared by all batteries is that positive and negative charges are developed at two different electrodes or terminals, establishing a potential difference between them. Because a potential for current flow exists, batteries can act as a source of

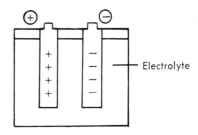

Fig. 1-10 Basic principle of a battery. Potential difference between the two electrodes develops as a result of a chemical reaction at each.

EMF. A multicell battery is symbolically designated ⊣⊢ or simply ⊣⊢ for a single cell battery. The longer vertical line represents the positive terminal **(anode)** and the shorter vertical line represents the negative terminal **(cathode)** of the battery. There are two general types of batteries, primary and secondary. A primary cell or battery cannot be recharged; once it is completely discharged (dead), it cannot be reenergized to produce current flow. However, a secondary cell or battery, after being discharged, may be recharged by reversing the current through the cell.

Primary Cells. Primary cells, such as the carbon-zinc, alkaline-manganese, and zinc-mercuric oxide dry cells, are generally used as sources of current. However, a special type of battery, called the cadmium sulfate cell or standard Weston cell, is used as a reference for voltage measurement rather than as a source of potential for current flow. The discussion of primary cells includes the characteristics of these various types of cells.

Cadmium Sulfate Cell (Standard Weston Cell). To measure an unknown voltage accurately, a comparison is made between the unknown voltage and a reference voltage or a standard voltage source. The standard voltage source, called the Weston cell, is kept at the National Bureau of Standards; it is composed of cadmium sulfate and is capable of producing a constant voltage for many years. The Weston reference cell can be saturated (Fig. 1-11) or unsaturated, with a potential of 1.0186 V or 1.019 V, respectively, at 20° C.

Carbon-Zinc Dry Cell (Flashlight-type Battery). An electrolyte may be absorbed by an inert material (e.g., paper) or may be mixed in a paste to be used in a battery's electrochemical reaction. When used in a voltage producing cell, that cell is called a dry cell. A simplified representation and

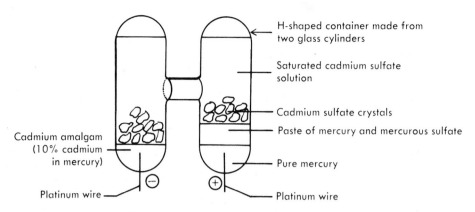

H-shaped container made from two glass cylinders

Saturated cadmium sulfate solution

Cadmium sulfate crystals

Paste of mercury and mercurous sulfate

Cadmium amalgam (10% cadmium in mercury)

Pure mercury

Platinum wire

Platinum wire

Fig. 1-11   Saturated standard Weston cell.

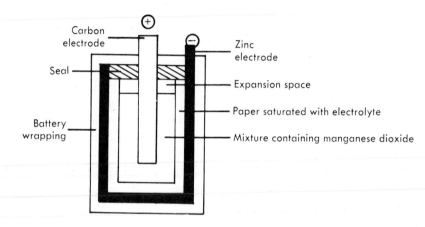

Carbon electrode

Zinc electrode

Seal

Expansion space

Paper saturated with electrolyte

Battery wrapping

Mixture containing manganese dioxide

Fig. 1-12   C-Zn dry cell.

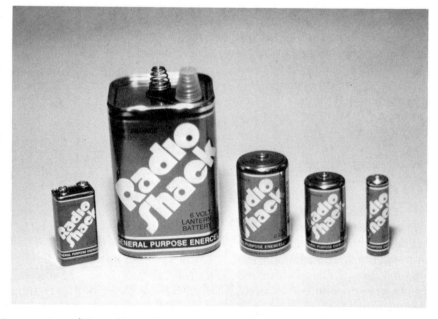

Fig. 1-13   Commonly used dry cell batteries. From left to right: 9 V, 6 V, 1.5 V (D size), 1.5 V (C size), 1.5 V (AA size). (Courtesy Radio Shack, a division of Tandy Corporation.)

a cutaway view of the construction of a carbon-zinc (C-Zn) dry cell are shown in Fig. 1-12. A chemical reaction occurs at each of the two electrodes, whereby the carbon electrode loses electrons while the zinc electrode gains electrons. This electrochemical reaction produces a potential difference of 1.5 to 1.6 V between the zinc cathode and the carbon anode. Dry cell batteries are generally made by alternately stacking a carbon plate, a layer of electrolyte paste, and a zinc plate as many times as necessary to give a desired voltage. Some of the more common battery sizes are shown in Fig. 1-13, although they can range from 1.5 to 90.0 V.

Several factors affect the storage and service life of dry cell batteries. For example, they are constantly discharging when they are not in use. An increase in temperature increases internal discharging thus decreasing storage life. At room temperature, the storage life of a C-Zn dry cell ranges from 6 months to 1 year; however, this can be prolonged if the battery is stored at low temperatures (2 to 8° C). The service life of C-Zn dry cell should be greater than 10 hours unless a heavy drain is placed on it. The potential of the C-Zn dry cell falls off continuously during use. Because the potential is not constant, this battery is of little value as a reference voltage source.

Because the zinc casing is the cathode, it tends to dissolve, thereby weakening the structure of the cell. Also, during discharge or storage, a pressure of evolved hydrogen gas builds up. This can lead to rupture of the zinc and leakage of the corrosive electrolyte into the instrument. Instruments using these dry cells should not be stored with the batteries installed.

Alkaline-Manganese Dry Cell (Alkaline Cell). The alkaline-manganese battery operates in a similar manner as the carbon-zinc dry cell but differs in respect to electrolyte and electrode composition. The alkaline cell consists of a zinc anode, a manganese oxide cathode, and a strong alkaline electrolyte of potassium hydroxide. The alkaline cell is 4 times the price of the C-Zn dry cell, but it provides the following advantages over the C-Zn cell: (1) the capacity (milliamperes per hour) is 3 to 5 times higher; (2) the capacity does not decrease under heavy drain; (3) the shelf life is about 2 years; (4) the internal resistance is lower, yielding higher current output; and (5) the operating temperature limit ($-40°$ C) is considerably lower. The battery is useful for applications requiring a relatively high current, which places a heavy drain on the battery. Considering its long shelf life and low operating temperature, it would be a good choice for an emergency power source.

Zinc-Mercuric Oxide Dry Cell (Mercury Cell). The mercury cell is composed of a zinc amalgam anode and a mercuric oxide-carbon cathode. The potential generated from this cell is 1.35 V, which is extremely reproducible from one cell to another. Mercury cells are available in voltages ranging from 1.35 to 42 V. The mercury cell is often used as a voltage reference in instruments because it has a very constant potential during discharge.

The mercury cell has several advantages over other batteries: a storage life of up to 2 years, service life 4 to 5 times that of the C-Zn dry cell, a very low internal resistance, and a greater capacity than the alkaline cell. The encasement of the mercury cell is also less likely to leak corrosives. Therefore mercury cells can be kept in instruments with relative safety. These batteries should be checked approximately every 6 months and corrosive materials cleaned off.

Laboratory personnel should be aware of those instruments in which mercury cells are used. The voltage of this battery is constant up to the time the battery is completely discharged. This means that an instrument that is working properly may suddenly malfunction. Simple replacement of the discharged mercury cell may remedy the problem.

Secondary Cells. Secondary cells are also known as electrolytic cells, wet cells, or rechargeable batteries. The nickel-cadmium battery is the secondary battery described below.

Nickel-Cadmium Battery. One type of rechargeable battery is the nickel-cadmium battery. This unit is completely sealed and requires no servicing other than recharging. The positive electrode is nickel hydroxide, and the negative electrode is cadmium. When the battery is discharging, the nickel hydroxide is converted to nickel, and the cadmium is oxidized. When it is recharging, the process is reversed. Each cell produces about 1.3 V and has a fairly high capacity. These batteries can be stored for long periods of time either charged or discharged. Though they are expensive, they are a practical source of constant current and are trouble free.

Alternating Current

Alternating current (AC) is generated commercially by electromagnetic generators or nuclear reactors. The alternating current produced from these sources is carried by means of power lines and eventually is supplied to the consumer via individual wall outlets. This section deals primarily with the descriptive aspects of alternating current, such as its characteristics and how they are related to direct current, rather than the mechanisms that are used to produce this type of current. The effects of alternating current on an electrically powered instrument and its different components or electronic units are included in subsequent chapters.

Direction of Alternating Current Flow. Unlike direct current, which is unidirectional, alternating current is bidirectional. It flows first in one direction and then in the opposite direction. For the current to change direction, the polarity of the voltage must also change. A voltage source that generates alternating current is often abbreviated VAC, which indicates that the EMF source is Volts-AC or AC voltage.

Voltage Variation over Time. There are seven basic AC waveforms that are common in electronics (Fig. 1-14); they all have the following characteristics:

1. The length of the horizontal axis of each waveform represents a period of time.
2. The height (amplitude) of a waveform represents change in either voltage or current over the period of time represented by the horizontal axis.
3. All waveforms have both positive and negative amplitude components.

To be alternating current, it must have all three characteristics. Reversal of voltage polarity is noted on the waveforms as amplitude above or amplitude below a center reference point. Voltage variation over time is very characteristic of alternating current. Except for polarity, waveforms are symmetric if their first and second halves are identical. In Fig. 1-14, all the waveforms except the rectangular waveform and one of the triangular waveforms are symmetrical.

The sine wave, or sinusoidal waveform, is the most common AC waveform and therefore this discussion will be limited to it. Because this waveform is so common, it is also used as the symbol for alternating current. The schematic symbol for an alternating current potential source or AC generator is ─◯─ . The sine wave shown in Fig. 1-15 starts at 0 V, increases over time to +10 V, then decreases to 0 V. From 0 V, the polarity is reversed, and the voltage goes to −10 V, then returns to 0 V again. One complete waveform is called a **cycle**.

Amplitude. The **amplitude** of the waveform is the peak value of the voltage or the peak amplitude (see Fig. 1-15). The total voltage in both directions (+ and −) from 0 V is called the peak-to-peak amplitude or **peak-to-peak voltage.** For example, in Fig. 1-15, the voltage reads 10 V in one direction and 10 V in the other direction. Therefore the total voltage, or peak-to-peak voltage, is 20 V. **Peak voltage** is voltage in one direction only (i.e., 10 V in Fig. 1-15).

Peak and peak-to-peak values are used for some electronic analysis, but the most valuable unit of AC voltage or current is the *effective value*. In the field of electronics it is often convenient to relate AC voltage to an equivalent amount of DC voltage. In fact, measuring devices such as the Volt-Ohm Milliammeter (VOM) read

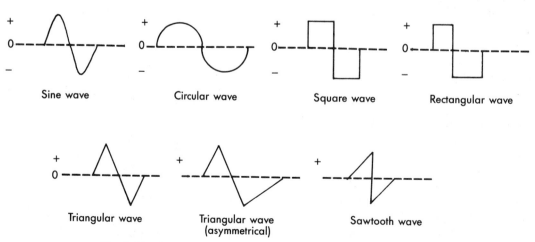

Fig. 1-14 Seven common waveforms encountered in electronics.

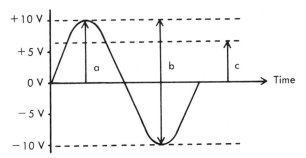

Fig. 1-15 Sinusoidal waveform and alternating current voltage: *a*, peak amplitude or peak voltage; *b*, peak-to-peak amplitude or peak-to-peak voltage; *c*, root mean square (rms) value of voltage (rms = peak voltage × 0.707).

AC voltage in values equivalent to DC voltage. This equivalent DC voltage, referred to as the **Root-Mean-Square (RMS) voltage,** is considered to be an average of the AC voltage (see Fig. 1-15) and is less than the peak voltage by a factor of 0.707. That is:

AC peak voltage × 0.707 = RMS voltage

The RMS value of AC voltage or current is the amount of AC needed to provide the same heating effect as an equal amount of DC voltage or current. Thus the RMS value of AC voltage is comparable with DC voltage in considering the amount of heat it generates as it passes through various electronic components. Often it is necessary to convert RMS voltage to its equivalent peak value. To do so the following mathematic expression is used:

RMS voltage × 1.414 = peak voltage

For example, if a voltage from a wall outlet is measured to be 110 volts AC (VAC) using a volt-ohm milliammeter (i.e., the RMS value), what is the peak value?

Peak value = RMS value × 1.414

Peak value = 110 V × 1.41 = 155.1 VAC

The relationship of RMS voltage to peak voltage is an important concept when selecting electronic components to be used in an instrument. The rating of power lines is given in RMS values of AC voltage, whereas the voltage rating of most electronic components is given in DC voltage. Therefore if a selected component has a voltage rating less than the peak voltage of a given circuit, it will break down or burn out. The following example will be used to illustrate this point.

Example: If an electronic component has a voltage rating of 120 VDC, can it be connected into a circuit that receives 115 VAC?

Solution: RMS voltage = 115, therefore the peak voltage is equal to 1.414 × 115 or 162.6 V. Because the electronic component has a rating of 115 V, it will break down or burn out once the AC voltage exceeds 115 V. This will occur as the AC voltage approaches its peak value (either + or −). Thus it cannot be connected into the circuit.

Frequency. One complete waveform is one cycle; the number of cycles occurring each second is the known as the **frequency (F)** of the waveform. The alternating current that is commercially supplied in the United States has a frequency of 60 cycles/second (c/s). In the field of electronics, the unit of frequency (cycles/second) is called the **hertz (Hz).** Therefore 60 cycles/second is equal to 60 hertz or 60 Hz. In other countries, alternating current is generated at a frequency of 50 Hz.

The time required for one cycle is referred to as the **period (T).** The relationship of the period and the frequency of a signal is inversely proportional:

Period = 1/frequency or T = 1/F

Frequency = 1/period or F = 1/T

Referring to Fig. 1-16, if one cycle occurs every 0.25 seconds, then the period is 0.25 second. The frequency is 4 Hz because four cycles occur every second. These values are calculated below.

F = 1/T = 1/0.25 sec = 4 Hz

T = 1/f = 1/4 Hz = 0.25 sec

Phase. Using one signal as a reference, a time relationship or a phase difference can be determined between that signal and another signal or signals. Fig. 1-17, *A*, shows the periodic plotting of a waveform. Fig. 1-17, *B*, shows two waveforms, or signals, **in phase.** When signal 1 is at its maximum positive swing, so is signal 2; when signal 1 is at its maximum negative swing, so is signal 2. If these two signals were added together, the resultant signal would have an amplitude equal to the sum of the amplitudes of signals 1 and 2. That is:

Amplitude of signal 1 + Amplitude of signal 2 =
Amplitude of signal 3

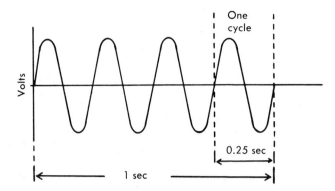

Fig. 1-16   Frequency and period of waveform; frequency (F) = 4 cycles/second (c/s) or hertz (Hz); period (T) = time required for 1 cycle = 0.25 second; equations: F = 1/T and T = 1/F.

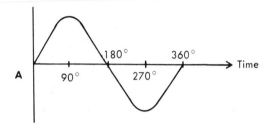

Relative degrees in ac sine wave

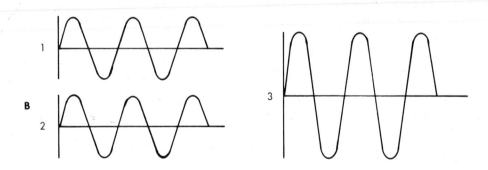

Signals 1 and 2 180° out of phase added to give signal 3

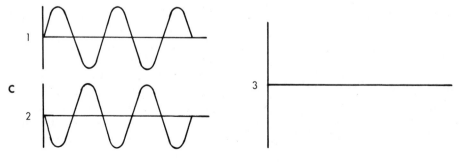

Signals 1 and 2 added to give signal 3

Fig. 1-17   Periodic plotting of sine wave.

Fig. 1-17, *C*, represents two signals that are **out of phase.** If two such voltages are 180 degrees out of phase (as is the case in Fig. 1-15, *C*), both voltages would be of equal magnitude but opposite in sign (Signal 1 = (+) VAC when Signal 2 = (−) VAC). If they were introduced into a circuit, the net effect of these two voltages would be 0 V because one signal cancels the other.

Review Questions

1. Electron flow in a conductor is due to the movement of its outer (valence).
   A. True
   B. False
2. The rate at which a charge moves through a conductor (flow of electrons) is called _____.
   A. Resistance
   B. EMF
   C. Current
   D. Voltage
3. The units of measure for EMF, current, resistance, and power are _____, respectively.
   A. Watts, volts, ohms, amperes
   B. Volts, amperes, ohms, watts
   C. Amperes, ohms, volts, watts
   D. Volts, watts, ohms, coulombs
4. Ohm's law states that the current in an electrical conductor is *inversely* proportional to the voltage between the ends of the conductor and *directly* proportional to the resistance.
   A. True
   B. False
5. A circuit with a power source of 20 V and a resistance of 100 Ω will carry a current of _____ A.
   A. 0.2
   B. 2
   C. 5
   D. 2000
6. An electrical circuit contains two resistors, R_A = 1.5 kΩ and R_B = 500 Ω. If the circuit carries a current of 0.05 A, what electrical potential (volts) is being used in the power source?
   A. 25
   B. 30
   C. 37.5
   D. 100
7. Given the following information, what is the voltage drop (in volts) over resistor No. 1?
   Power source: 5V   Resistor No. 1: 20 Ω
   Resistor No. 2: 80 Ω
   A. 1
   B. 4
   C. 16
   D. 20
8. The function of a fuse is to protect the AC power lines supplying a given circuit.
   A. True
   B. False
9. What is the power rating of a 120 V line carrying 10 amperes of current?
   A. 12 Watts
   B. 83.3 Watts
   C. 1200 Watts
   D. 12000 Watts
10. Direct current is characterized by:
    A. Voltage level constantly changing.
    B. Polarity remains unchanged.
    C. Voltage level remains unchanged.
    D. Polarity switches at a constant rate.
       1. Response A and C
       2. Response B and C
       3. Response B, C, and D
       4. All of the above
11. If the peak-to-peak voltage carried in an AC line is 340 volts, what is the equivalent DC voltage?
    A. 120 volts
    B. 168 volts
    C. 238 volts
    D. 240 volts
    E. 476 volts

Answers

1. A   2. C   3. B   4. B   5. A   6. D   7. A   8. B   9. C
10. 2   11. C

CHAPTER 2

Electronic Components

ROBERT H. WILLIAMS

Circuit Configurations
Wires as Resistors and Conductors
Resistors
Capacitors
Inductors
Transformers
Switches and Electromagnetic Relays
Diodes

The electronic circuitry of a laboratory instrument is composed of specific devices called electronic components. Each component is selected and configured in a circuit in such a way as to perform a particular function during an instrument's operation. These circuits and their respective components can vary from being quite simple to very complex. The components covered in this chapter are resistors, capacitors, inductors, transformers, and diodes. Their effect on direct and alternating current and their function in an electronic circuit is also described.

Circuit Configurations

Most modern circuitry is designed using a process called printed circuitry. Electronic components are prearranged on a chemically treated board and then connected by using a special soldering technique. This arrangement is called a printed circuit board, that when plugged into the electronic chassis of an instrument, performs a specific operation. The arrangement of electronic components on a printed circuit board refers to its configuration. Components may be connected in series, parallel, or in a combination of series and parallel.

A simplified approach is used to describe the basic types of arrangements that are common to many circuits and how they affect resistance, voltage, and current. These arrangements are illustrated by using a frequently used component, the resistor. Two accepted methods of representing connections in an electrical circuit are shown in Fig. 2-1, A and B. Circuits may be drawn so that a node or dot at the point of intersection of lines represents an electrical connection as shown in Fig. 2-1, A. In this circuit, the intersections at points a and b are not making electrical contact. In Fig. 2-1, B, intersecting straight lines represent electrical contact points, whereas the arched lines at points a and b indicate that these lines are not electrically connected. This latter type of circuit representation will be used throughout this text.

Series Circuits. The arrangement using the three resistors in Fig. 2-2 is called a **series circuit.** Components are connected in series if current flow has only one possible pathway. For example, in Fig. 2-2, the current passing through R_1 is the same as the current passing through R_2 and through R_3. In a series circuit, the current is always the same throughout the circuit, thus:

$$I_{total} = I_1 = I_2 = I_3 = \ldots I_n$$

The total resistance exerted by resistors in series is always equal to the sum of the individual resistances or:

$$R_{total} = R_1 + R_2 + R_3 + R_4 + \ldots R_n$$

In Fig. 2-2, the total resistance would be equal to the sum of R_1, R_2, and R_3 (50 ohms [Ω], 100 Ω, and 100 Ω) or 250 Ω. Using Ohm's law, the total current is then calculated by dividing the total voltage by the total resistance. Again, referring to Fig. 2-2, dividing 25 volts (V) by 250 Ω gives a total current of 0.1 amperes (A) (100 milliamperes [mA]). In this circuit 0.1 A will pass through each resistor regardless of the value of each resistor.

The concept of voltage drop and voltage division was discussed in Chapter 1. Using the principles described in that section, what are the voltage drops over each resistor (E_1, E_2, and E_3) in Fig. 2-2?

$$E_1 = I_1R_1 = (0.1 \text{ A}) \times (50 \text{ }\Omega) = 5 \text{ V}$$
$$E_2 = I_2R_2 = (0.1 \text{ A}) \times (100 \text{ }\Omega) = 10 \text{ V}$$
$$E_3 = I_3R_3 = (0.1 \text{ A}) \times (100 \text{ }\Omega) = 10 \text{ V}$$

The sum of the voltage drops occurring in a series circuit should always equal the total voltage. In the example above, the sum of 5, 10, and 10 V equals the total voltage of the circuit or 25 V. In general, the following rules are used when applying Ohm's law to components connected in series:

Resistance: The total resistance in a series circuit is equal to the sum of the individual resistances or, $R_t = R_1 + R_2 + R_3 \ldots$ etc.

Voltage: In a series circuit the sum of the individual voltage drops is equal to the applied voltage or, $E_t = E_1 + E_2 + E_3 \ldots$ etc.

Current: In a series circuit, the current is the same at all points in the circuit or, $I_t = I_1 = I_2 = I_3 \ldots$ etc.

Parallel Circuits. The arrangement using the two resistors in Fig. 2-3 is called a **parallel circuit.** The same voltage is dropped across each resistor. However, the current flow has two alternate paths to follow. When a circuit contains two or more paths for current to flow, the conducted pathways are connected in parallel. The total current in a circuit is equal to the sum of the current in all parallel pathways in the circuit. The total current in the circuit shown in Fig. 2-3 is equal to the sum of the current passing through R_1 and R_2:

$$I_{total} = I_1 + I_2$$

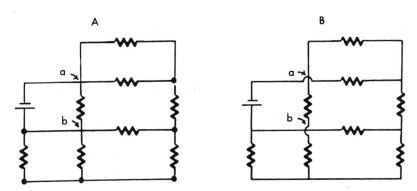

Fig. 2-1 Schematic representations of electrical connections.

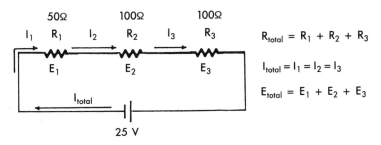

Fig. 2-2 Resistors connected in series circuit.

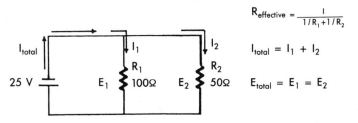

Fig. 2-3 Resistors connected in parallel circuit.

What are the values for I_1 and I_2?

$$I_1 = E/R_1 = 25 \text{ V}/100 = 0.25 \text{ A}$$
$$I_2 = E/R_2 = 25 \text{ V}/50 = 0.50 \text{ A}$$

What is the total current in this circuit?

$$I_{total} = I_1 + I_2 = 0.25 \text{ A} + 0.50 \text{ A} = 0.75 \text{ A}$$

The resistance to current flow in this circuit is less than if these resistors were connected in series.

When resistors are connected in series, the voltage from the voltage source is dropped proportionately across each resistor depending on its resistance (i.e., the voltage source "sees" an effective resistance equal to the sum of the resistors in series). However, when the resistors are in parallel, the full voltage is dropped across each resistor separately. In the parallel circuit a current flows in each resistor independently of the current in the other resistors. The total effective resistance (R_E) in a parallel circuit is always less than the smallest resistor composing the parallel branch. The formula for calculating the total effective resistance in a parallel circuit is:

$$R_E = \frac{1}{1/R_1 + 1/R_2 + 1/R_3 + \ldots 1/R_n}$$

Using the example in Fig. 2-3, what is the total effective resistance in this circuit?

$$R_E = \frac{1}{1/R_1 + 1/R_2}$$
$$R_E = \frac{1}{1/100 \ \Omega + 1/50 \ \Omega}$$
$$R_E = \frac{1}{1/100 \ \Omega + 2/100 \ \Omega} = \frac{1}{3/100 \ \Omega}$$
$$R_E = 100/3 = 33.33 \ \Omega$$

If the 100 Ω and 50 Ω resistors were replaced with a 33.33 Ω resistor, what current would flow in this circuit?

$$I = E/R = 25 \text{ V}/33.33 \ \Omega = 0.75 \text{ A}$$

Note that adding the current flowing through each resistor of this circuit results in the same value, 0.75 A.

In general, the following rules are used when applying Ohm's law to components connected in parallel:

1. Resistance: The "effective" resistance of parallel resistances is equal to the reciprocal of the sum of the reciprocals of the individual resistances:

$$R_E = \frac{1}{1/R_1 + 1/R_2 + 1/R_3 \ldots \text{etc.}}$$

The total effective resistance is less than the resistance contained in each branch. The effective resistance in each branch is always less than the smallest resistor composing a branch.

The effective resistance of parallel resistances in a given branch that have the same value ($R_1 = R_2 = R_3 = \ldots$ etc.) is equal to the total resistance in the branch divided by the number of resistors in the branch.

2. Voltage: In a parallel circuit the voltage across each leg or branch is the same.

3. Current: The total current in a parallel circuit is equal to the sum of the currents in the individual branches or, $I_t = I_1 + I_2 + I_3 \ldots$ etc.

Combination Series-Parallel Circuits. Although examples of individual series and parallel circuits have been discussed, such simple circuitry is rarely used in clinical laboratory instrumentation. Electrical circuits in most instruments are rather complex and often are composed of a combination of series and parallel circuits. This third possible variation of circuit design is shown in Fig. 2-4, *A*. If the effective resistance of R_2 and R_3 is calculated, the two parallel limbs are essentially changed to a resistor that is in series with R_1. In combination circuits the effective resistance of the parallel branches is

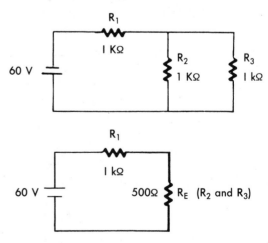

Fig. 2-4   Resistors connected in a combination series-parallel circuit.

always calculated first. The concept of circuit simplification involving parallel branches is illustrated in Fig. 2-4, *B*. The effective resistance (R_E) of the parallel branch (reciprocal of $1/R_2 + 1/R_3$) is:

$$R_E = \frac{1}{1/R_2 + 1/R_3}$$

$$R_E = \frac{1}{1/1000 \ \Omega + 1/1000 \ \Omega} \quad \text{NOTE: 1 k}\Omega = 1000 \ \Omega$$

$$R_E = \frac{1}{2/1000 \ \Omega}$$

$$= \frac{1}{1/500 \ \Omega}$$

$$R_E = 500 \ \Omega$$

The total effective resistance for the entire circuit (R_t) then becomes:

$$R_t = R_1 + R_E \text{ (effective resistance of } R_2 \text{ and } R_3)$$

$$R_t = 1000 \ \Omega + 500 \ \Omega$$

$$R_t = 1500 \ \Omega$$

Current division and voltage division are more complicated in combination circuits because of an increase in the number of legs or branch points. As shown in Fig. 2-4, *A*, current flow is more complex than in either a simple series or parallel circuit. The entire current of the circuit must first flow through R_1. This same current will then divide when it reaches the two paths, R_2 and R_3. The voltage drop occurring over each resistor will depend on the voltage division at R_1 and the parallel branch, R_2 and R_3, which is in series with R_1. Using the previously stated rules for series and parallel circuits, total current and voltage can be calculated for the entire system and individual current flow and voltage drops can be determined for each branch point and resistor.

Current flow in the entire system is calculated by using the total resistance of 1500 Ω.

$$I = E/R_t = 60 \text{ V}/1500 \ \Omega$$

$$= 0.040 \text{ A}$$

$$= 40 \text{ mA}$$

After calculating the total current, the amount of current passing through each branch point can be determined. Because R_1 is in series with the parallel branch, R_2 and R_3, the current passing through R_1 does not divide and thus receives the total current (I_{total}) of 40 mA. The parallel branch also receives the total current (I_p) of 40 mA. However, at the branch point, the current will divide between R_2 and R_3. Before current flow through

each parallel resistor (I_2 and I_3) is calculated, the voltage drop over each branch (E_p) is determined. The voltage drop is the same for each resistor in the parallel branch.

Resistor No. 1 (series)

$$I_1 = I_{total} = 0.04 \text{ A}$$

$$E_1 = I_1 R_1$$

$$= 0.04 \text{ A} \times 1000 \ \Omega$$

$$= 40 \text{ V (voltage drop over } R_1)$$

Resistors No. 2 and No. 3 (parallel) —

$$\text{use effective resistance} = R_E$$

$$I_2 + I_3 = I_{total} = I_p = 0.04 \text{ A}$$

$$E_2 = E_3 = E_p$$

$$E_p = I_p R_E$$

$$= 0.04 \text{ A} \times 500 \ \Omega$$

$$= 20 \text{ V (Voltage drop over } R_2 \text{ or } R_3)$$

$$I_2 = E_2/R_2 = 20 \text{ V}/1000 \ \Omega = 0.02 \text{ A}$$

$$I_3 = E_3/R_3 = 20 \text{ V}/1000 \ \Omega = 0.02 \text{ A}$$

$$I_p = I_2 + I_3 = 0.02 \text{ A} + 0.02 \text{ A} = 0.04 \text{ A}$$

Notice that the sum of the current in the parallel limbs is the same as that flowing through the series portion of the circuit, which must carry the total current. Using the above approach, a complex series-parallel combination of resistors can be analyzed and the effective resistance of the circuit calculated.

Voltage drop, voltage division, and current division are important electronic concepts. Understanding these concepts also provides a strong foundation on which other fundamental principles of electricity and electronics can be built. The following section presents a simplified analogy to electron flow to explain and clarify these concepts.

Current Division and Voltage Division. Because series and parallel circuits have been described, the concept of current division and voltage division can be discussed in greater detail. Figs. 2-5, *A* and *B* represent current division in a simple series circuit and in a parallel circuit. As previously mentioned, a series circuit has only one pathway for current flow. In Fig. 2-5, *A*, R_1 and R_2 are two resistors in series whereby the resistance of R_2 is two times ($2\times$) greater than R_1. No division of current occurs; therefore the same amount of current will pass through both resistors regardless of their size. In Fig. 2-5, *B*, the same two resistors are connected in parallel, and now, the total current has two different pathways that it can take. The amount of current that will enter each pathway (leg) of the parallel circuit will

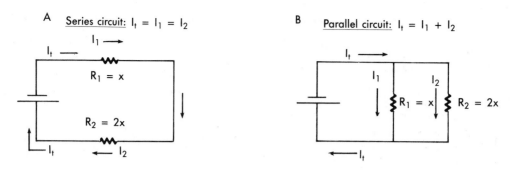

Fig. 2-5 Current division in a simple series circuit, **A**, and parallel circuit, **B**.

be dictated by the size of the resistor. Therefore in Fig. 2-5, *B*, R_2 will receive twice the amount of current as R_1. After the current has divided over the parallel branches, the individual currents will converge before they return to the battery and their sum will be equal to the total current of the power source.

Fig. 2-6, *A* and *B* represent voltage division in a simple series and in a parallel circuit. Recall that voltage is a force that is required to push electrons through a path of resistance. This force is due to a potential between the positive and the negative terminals of a voltage source (such as a battery). The voltage source gives the electrons at the negative terminal sufficient energy to do work if a complete circuit is connected across its terminals. When the electrons move around the circuit, they give up this energy so that when they finally return to the positive terminal, they have lost all of the energy that was supplied by the voltage source (i.e., they are at zero potential). The energy they have lost is converted to heat in the resistors of the circuit. This loss of energy is called a **voltage drop or IR drop.** The larger the resistor, the greater the loss of energy (as heat) of the elec-

trons entering that resistive pathway, and thus the greater the voltage drop.

Now referring to the series circuit in Fig. 2-6, *A*, the total voltage (E_t) on entering the first resistor (R_1) is reduced because a portion of the voltage is lost as heat. The amount of lost voltage is equal to E_1, the voltage drop over R_1. Only the remaining voltage ($E_t - E_1 = E_2$) is available to push electrons through R_2. This voltage is then lost as heat as electrons are pushed through R_2, causing another voltage drop (E_2). Having lost all their energy in a stepwise fashion, the electrons then enter the positive terminal of the voltage source. Thus in a series circuit, the total voltage has been divided proportionately among the resistive paths. Therefore in Fig. 2-6, *A*, the sum of the voltage drops ($E_1 + E_2$) is equal to the total voltage (E_t) of the power source serving that part of the circuit.

In a parallel circuit (Fig. 2-6, *B*), each resistor, R_1 and R_2, will receive the total voltage (E_t) coming from the power source, regardless of the resistor size (i.e., the force pushing the electrons through each resistor is the same even though R_2 is two times [2×] larger than R_1 and receives

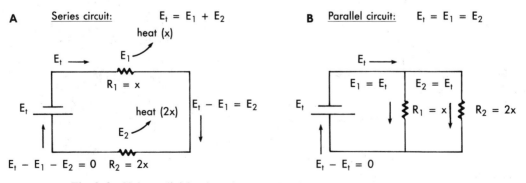

Fig. 2-6 Voltage division in a simple series circuit, **A**, and parallel circuit, **B**.

twice the number of electrons [current]. Because both resistors receive the same voltage, each resistor will dissipate the same amount of energy as heat. Therefore the voltage drop over each resistor will also be the same. After this voltage drops over both resistors, the electrons converge and enter the positive terminals at zero potential. Thus, in a parallel circuit, the voltage drop over each branch is always equal to the voltage entering the parallel circuit. In Fig. 2-6, *B*, the voltage drop for each resistor (E_1 or E_2) would be equal to the total voltage (E_t).

In summary, in a series circuit, the current is the same, but the voltage divides; in a parallel circuit, the current divides, but the voltage remains the same. Understanding the concept of current division and voltage division is important in the field of laboratory electronics because constructing the correct circuitry for a particular instrument's application or its electrical connection is based on these principles. For example, if several electronic devices or components need the same amount of current to operate properly, they have to be connected in series. However, if they require the same amount of voltage, they must be connected in parallel.

Wires as Resistors and Conductors

Wire Resistance. Wire offers a certain amount of resistance to the flow of current. It has been experimentally determined that the resistance of a wire is directly proportional to its length and inversely proportional to its cross-sectional area (i.e., its thickness). The resistance of a wire also depends on its inherent resistivity, ρ (pronounced rho). Resistivity is defined as the resistance of a wire of unit length and unit cross-sectional area. Thus resistance (R) in ohms can be calculated if a few dimensions and properties of the wire are known, including radius (r) or cross-sectional area ($A = \pi r^2$), length (l), and resistivity (ρ). The resistance of a given length of wire of a specific metal composition can be calculated with the equation:

$$R = \rho l/A$$

Conductance. It is sometimes convenient to speak of the conductance of a wire rather than its resistance. **Conductance (G)** is the reciprocal of resistance (R) and is expressed by the following formula:

$$G = 1/R$$

The unit of conductance is the **mho** (ohm spelled backward). A thousandth of a mho is millimho;

a millionth of a mho a micromho. Using this equation, any value expressed in ohms can be converted to mhos. For example, if a wire conductor has a resistance of 0.1 Ω, its conductance would be equal to 10 mhos. Copper is used as the standard for conductance and has arbitrarily been assigned a relative conductance of 1.00. All the other materials are compared with copper. For example, silver has a value of 1.08, and thus is a better conductor than copper.

Resistors

A **resistor** is an electronic component that impedes current flow. Thus the amount of current entering an instrument's circuit can be limited by the use of resistors. Resistors come in various types of construction and in many shapes and sizes. Resistors may be classified as fixed or variable. A fixed resistor has only one specified value that is unchanged during normal operation. A variable resistor allows for selection of resistance within a specified range of the resistor.

Fixed Resistors. Several different types and sizes of the more common fixed resistors are shown in Fig. 2-7. The symbol for a fixed value resistor is —⋀⋀— . They are generally made from carbon or nickel-chromium wire.

Carbon (Composition) Resistors. The resistive element is composed of a mixture of carbon (conducting material) and resin (nonconducting material), two wire leads, an insulator or ceramic casing, and an outer coating of a moisture-proofing material. The composition, not the size, of

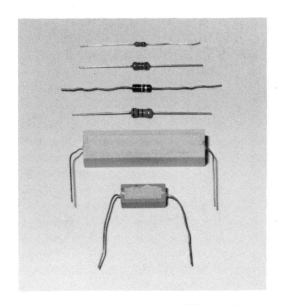

Fig. 2-7 Common assortment of fixed resistors.

the resistor determines the value of resistance; the greater the carbon content, the less the resistance, and vice versa.

The amount of insulator material and the surface area of the resistor dictate its ability to dissipate heat. Thus the wattage rating of a carbon resistor is not related to its resistance but rather to its physical size. The larger the diameter of a resistor, the higher its wattage rating. For example, a ⅛ inch resistor has a rating of ½ W, a ¼ inch resistor a rating of 1W, and a ⁵⁄₁₆ inch resistor a rating of 2 W. Fixed-value carbon resistors are generally used in instrument circuits where power dissipation is low and where precise resistance values are not needed. Values range from approximately 5 Ω to 22 MΩ, with tolerance values of ±5%, ±10%, or ±20%.

An internationally accepted series of colored bands is printed on most carbon resistors to indicate the value of the resistance and the degree of tolerance (Fig. 2-8, *A* and *B*). The color coding begins near one end of the cartridge. The first two bands indicate numerical values of resistance. The third band is called the multipler. The fourth band, which is gold (±5%) or silver (±10%), is the tolerance band; it indicates the end of the code. The tolerance of a color-coded resistor gives the maximum percent of deviation from the given value of the resistor. If the fourth band is not present, then a tolerance of ±20% is assumed. For example, refer to the resistor color code in Fig. 2-8 and note the following example. If a carbon resistor has the following colored bands printed on the casing, what is the value of the resistance?

> Band: (No. 1) Brown (No. 2) Black (No. 3) Red (No. 4) Silver
> Band No. 1 = brown = first digit = 1
> Band No. 2 = black = second digit = 0
> Band No. 3. = red = multiplier value of 10^2 = 00
> Band No. 4 = silver = tolerance value of ±10%

The rating of the resistor is: 1 + 0 + 00 = 1000 = 1.0×10^3 Ω or 1 kΩ. The fourth band indicates that the degree of tolerance is ±10%. Therefore the actual resistance is in the range of 1000 ± 100 Ω or 900 to 1100 Ω.

Wire-Wound Resistors. Because the resistance of a wire is a function of its length, a wire can be used to construct a resistor of a specified value by varying its length. A wire-wound resistor consists of a nickel-chromium wire tightly wrapped around a central insulating core, leads attached to each end of the nickel-chromium wire, and a casing of insulating and moisture-proofing material. This type of resistor is used where precise

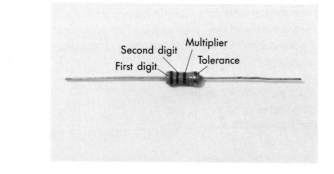

A

Second digit / Multiplier
First digit / Tolerance

	Color	Value		Tolerance	
	Black	0		Gold = 5%	
	Brown	1		Silver = 10%	
	Red	2		No band = 20%	
	Orange	3			
B	Yellow	4			
	Green	5			
	Blue	6			
	Violet	7		Multipler is the number of zeros	
	Gray	8		added to the first two digits	
	White	9			

Fig. 2-8 Common carbon resistor, **A**, and its color code, **B**.

values of resistance and/or high power dissipation is required. Wire-wound resistors have excellent stability, can be made with power ratings greater than 200 W, and are available in values up to about 100 kΩ. The resistors ratings are stamped on the resistor casing.

Variable Resistors. Some resistors are designed so that the total resistance can be varied. Some of the more common ones are pictured in Fig. 2-9. The circuits of laboratory instruments often require the resistance to be varied to change the voltage and/or current. All variable resistors operate by sliding a metal contact down the length of a resistive material. A variable resistor can be made of carbon or nickel-chromium wire wound on a bakelite circular form. With this type, a contact wiper arm follows the resistive element as the rotating shaft of the resistor is turned (Fig. 2-10, *A* and *B*). Carbon variable re-

sistors are used for small current requirements; wire-wound variable resistors are used for large ones.

Variable resistors can have two or three terminals. Those with two terminals are called **rhe-**

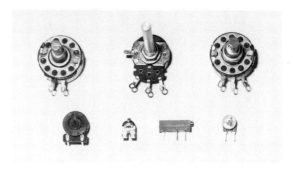

Fig. 2-9   Common assortment of variable resistors.

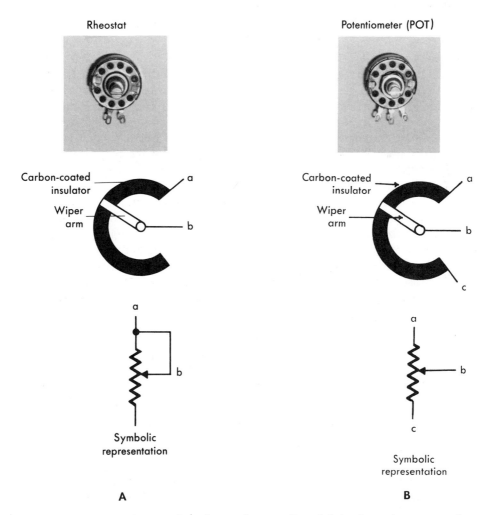

Rheostat	Potentiometer (POT)

Carbon-coated insulator

Wiper arm

a

b

Symbolic representation

A

Carbon-coated insulator

Wiper arm

a

b

c

Symbolic representation

B

Fig. 2-10   Common rheostat, **A**, and potentiometer, **B**, and their schematic representations.

ostats and those with three terminals are referred to as **potentiometers** (or **"POTS"**). The rheostat is used to vary the total resistance between the two terminals *a* and *b* (Fig. 2-10, *A*), and thus can be used to vary the current within a circuit. A rheostat is often used as a speed control device on various clinical laboratory instruments such as serofuges and centrifuges. The electrical symbol used to designate a rheostat is $\overbrace{\text{—}}$. Unlike the rheostat, the potentiometer does not simply vary the total resistance between the end terminals *a* and *b*, but rather the resistance between each end, *a* and *c* and the center contact *b* by using its three terminals (Fig. 2-10, *B*). Potentiometers are used to select voltage/current for application to another circuit. Therefore they are often used as voltage/current dividers. In the clinical laboratory, calibration of an instrument usually involves changing the voltage or current of a particular circuit. This is accomplished by selecting a specific amount of voltage/current by varying the resistance of a potentiometer. The electrical symbol of a potentiometer is $\overbrace{\text{—}}$

Carbon Rheostats and Potentiometers. A carbon rheostat or potentiometer is constructed by depositing a layer of carbon on a circular strip of insulation (Fig. 2-10, *A* and *B*). A metal wiper arm that slides on the carbon surface provides the means of selecting the desired resistance.

In Fig. 2-11, *A*, a rheostat has been arranged in a circuit for selection of current. As the wiper arm of the rheostat is moved downward, the resistance increases. However, the voltage at points *a* and *b* remains constant, regardless of the position of the wiper arm. Because the voltage remains constant while the resistance is increased, the current must decrease. When the wiper arm is moved upward, the resistance will decrease, the voltage across the resistor will still remain unchanged, and thus the current will increase.

In Fig. 2-11, *B*, a potentiometer has been configured in a circuit to vary the current and voltage. When the wiper arm is moved, the total resistance of the potentiometer does not change, but the total effective resistance in the circuit (between points *a* and *c*) varies. For example, if it is moved downward, the resistance between points *a* and *b* is increased, which causes a decrease in voltage at point *b*. Because the total effective resistance is increased, the current in the circuit will be decreased.

Carbon variable resistors are usually marked with a specified voltage or current. Carbon variable resistors are limited to applications that require low power dissipation and are used to regulate large resistances. They tend to become electrically "noisy" after considerable use because the carbon surfaces get worn during usage and the wiper arms become coated with loose carbon. However, they are commonly used on laboratory equipment because they are relatively inexpensive and easy to install.

Wire-Wound Rheostats and Potentiometers. When close regulation of resistance is essential in a circuit, a wire-wound rheostat or potentiometer is used. Wire-wound variable resistors are made by closely winding a coil of nickel-chromium wire around a strip of insulating material and then bending it into a circular form similar to that of the carbon variable resistors just described. An oxide coating on the wire insulates each turn of the wire, but bare metal is exposed to the wiper arm for good contact.

Wire-wound variable resistors are made in a vast array of physical sizes and shapes. They are available in values ranging from a few ohms to about 100 kΩ. Power ratings usually vary up to about 3 W. Tolerances range from $\pm 20\%$ to $\pm 1\%$. The increased stability and accuracy of wire-wound potentiometers make their use desir-

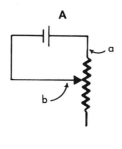

A

"Absolute" variable
resistor

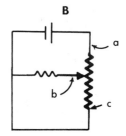

B

Variable resistor to obtain
wanted voltage and/or current

Fig. 2-11   Variable resistors in a circuit using a rheostat, **A**, and a potentiometer, **B**.

able in equipment where precise regulation/calibration of current or voltage is required.

Resistors in DC and AC Circuits. The resistance exerted by a resistor is independent of the frequency of the electrical signal. Therefore the opposition to current flow exerted by a resistor in either an alternating current (AC) or direct current (DC) circuit is the same. With a resistor, there is no phase difference observed between the generation of voltage and current (i.e., when a voltage is produced so is the current [they are in-phase]). However, in AC circuits, another type of opposition to current flow exists, which is called **reactance (X)**. Reactance is caused by the presence of components such as capacitors and inductors that are influenced by the frequency of the AC signal. They also affect the phase relationships between voltage and current (i.e., voltage and current are not generated at the same time [they are out-of-phase]). The combined current-opposing effects of reactance and resistance in an AC circuit are called **impedance (Z)**. Because resistors are not affected by the AC freqency, the impedance in an AC circuit containing only resistors is equivalent to the resistance. The effect of AC frequency on capacitor and inductor impedance is described later in this chapter. The unit of measure for both reactance and impedance is also the ohm.

Capacitors

A **capacitor** is a device used to store a quantity of electrical charge. It basically consists of two thin sheets of conducting material (plates) separated by a layer of insulating material called a **dielectric.** Dielectrics can be composed of air, plastic, mica, ceramic, or wax-saturated paper. One of the major functions of a capacitor in an electronic circuit is to separate AC from DC.

How a Capacitor Stores a Charge in DC and AC Circuits. When a capacitor is placed in a circuit without a source of potential, current does not flow (Fig. 2-12, *A*) (i.e., when the switch (S) is open). Normally, the two metal conducting plates will have an equal amount of positive and negative charges (electrically neutral). When the

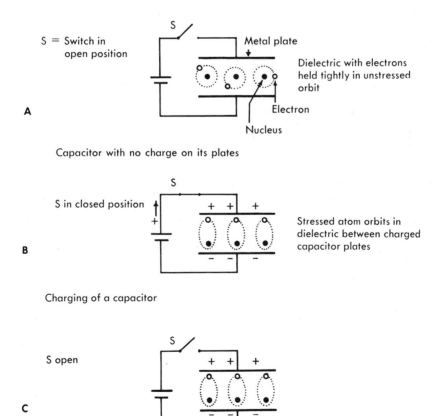

Fig. 2-12   Storage of a charge on a capacitor.

switch is closed (Fig. 2-12, *B*), a potential difference from the battery is applied to the two capacitor plates. The battery charges the plate connected to its negative terminal with electrons while it drives electrons away from the plate connected to its positive terminal. This occurs because the electrons on the second plate feel the electrical field of the electrons that have accumulated on the first plate. Because the dielectric is an insulator, it does not allow passage of current from one capacitor plate to the other. Current flows only as long as the potential between the capacitor plates does not equal that of the battery. Once the two potentials become equal, current no longer flows and the capacitor is considered to be charged. The force exerted between the charged plates and the atoms in the dielectric is called an **electrostatic field.** This force holds the charge on the capacitor plates even after the switch is opened (Fig. 2-12, *C*). A charged capacitor functions essentially as a DC voltage source and thus can discharge a current (i.e., the energy stored in the dielectric is released in the form of electron flow or current). The charge on the capacitor will remain for several days (even if it is removed from the circuit) unless a path is provided that will allow it to discharge its stored electrical energy.

When a pathway (shunt) is created between the negative and positive side of the capacitor, it can be discharged (Fig. 2-13). The potential difference across the capacitor causes a current to flow through the wire shunt from the negative to the positive side of the capacitor. The current will continue to flow until there is no longer a potential across the capacitor. A capacitor can also be discharged if its leads are "shorted" together. When the leads are shorted, a pathway has been provided that allows electrons from the negatively charged plate to flow through the leads and neutralize the positive charge on the other plate. The charging/discharging rate of a capacitor can be regulated by inserting a resistor in place of the wire shunt as shown in Fig. 2-13.

In a DC circuit a capacitor causes a break in the circuit once steady-state conditions have been reached. Under these conditions, DC current cannot pass through a capacitor. However, when an AC source is provided, it alternately charges one plate of the capacitor and then the other (Fig. 2-14, *A-D*). The plate that receives the electrons induces the movement of electrons away from the second plate. Current flow is at its maximum as the plate is just starting to charge with electrons. The instant the capacitor becomes fully charged, the current drops to zero. However, the AC voltage source changes directions and thus

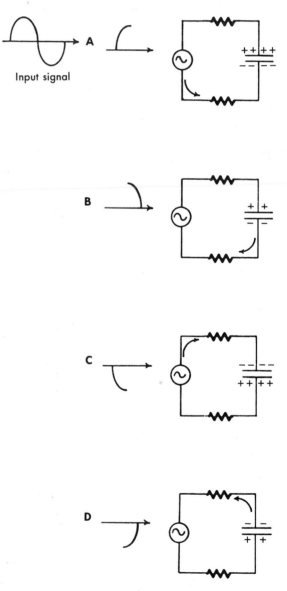

Fig. 2-14   Capacitor in an AC circuit, and the effect each quarter sine wave has on a capacitor.

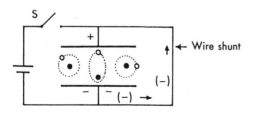

Fig. 2-13   Discharging a capacitor.

begins charging the opposite plate. This causes the charge on the first plate to decrease. Thus, when a capacitor is connected to an AC voltage source, it appears as though the current is passing through its dielectric. A charge of opposite sign is always induced on the opposite plate, although electrons do not actually move across the dielectric. For this reason a capacitor is considered an AC component.

Phase Relationship in a Capacitor. When a DC potential is applied to a capacitor, charge begins to collect on its plates. As the amount of charge increases, a voltage begins to develop on the capacitor. This voltage causes the current that flows toward the capacitor to decrease and thus is called a **counter-EMF**. Once the counter-EMF is equal to the potential of the DC voltage source, current flow ceases. When an AC voltage is applied across a capacitor, the capacitor alternately charges and discharges. The capacitor is charged by the peak voltage ($\pm$) of the AC signal (Fig. 2-14, *A* and *D*). When the amplitude of the AC signal's amplitude decreases (Fig. 2-14, *B*) and changes polarity (Fig. 2-14, *C*), the capacitor releases its charge in a direction opposite to the direction of the charging current. Current flow does not cease but rather changes direction. When AC is applied across a capacitor, the current always leads the voltage by 90 degrees. In other words current flows to the capacitor first, and then voltage collects on the capacitor.

Factors Affecting Capacitance. The ability of a capacitor to store electrical energy depends on the electrostatic field established between the plates. This electrostatic field is a function of the surface area of the plates, the distance between the plates, and the type of dielectric material used in the construction of the capacitor. The greater the electrostatic field, the greater the capacitance. Increasing the area of the plates or decreasing the distance between the plates, by using a thin dielectric layer, intensifies the electrostatic field and thus increases the capacitance. If the electrons of the dielectric tend to become easily distorted, then a higher electrostatic field is produced, which enhances the capacitance. Dielectrics that have atoms that become readily distorted have high dielectric constants. Those that have low dielectric constants have atoms that do not become readily distorted; they produce less capacitance. Air is used as the reference material to measure dielectric materials; it is assigned a dielectric constant of 1.

Units of Capacitance. The ability of a capacitor to store an electrical charge is called **capacitance (C)**. The unit of capacitance is the **farad (F)**. One farad is the capacitance that stores 1 coulomb of electrical energy when 1 V is applied. Recall that a coulomb is a unit of measure of electric charge that is equal to that of 6.24×10^{18} electrons. In more practical terms, a coulomb is equal to 1 A of current flowing past a point in 1 second. The equation used to calculate capacitance is:

$$C \text{ (farads)} = Q \text{ (coulombs)}/V \text{ (volts)}$$

The farad is too large for most applications. Units commonly used are either the microfarad, designated μF (a millionth of a farad or 10^{-6} farad), or the picofarad, designated a pF (a millionth of a microfarad or 10^{-12} farad).

Common Types of Capacitors. Capacitors are not only composed of different materials but also come in different shapes and sizes (Fig. 2-15). Capacitors can be classified as fixed or variable. A fixed capacitor has only one specified value; a variable capacitor allows for selection of different capacitance values within a specified range. The schematic symbols used to represent capacitors follow. When the symbols on the right are used, the curved side represents the plate connected either to ground or to the low voltage side of the circuit.

Fixed value capacitors: ⊣⊢ or ⊣⊢
Variable capacitors: ⇥ or ⇥

Fixed Capacitors. The tubular paper capacitor is the most common fixed capacitor. The dielectric consists of a strip of paper saturated with any one of a variety of materials, such as petroleum jelly or parafilm wax, sandwiched between strips of metal foil. Generally, aluminum is used to make the metal foils. A black band is usually painted on the end where the lead is connected to the outside layer of foil. Values, tolerance, and voltage rating are stamped on the surface. This type of capacitor is available in sizes from a few

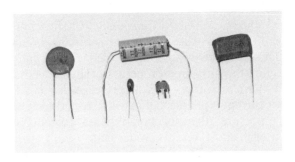

Fig. 2-15 Common fixed and variable capacitors.

picofarads to 100 μF. Tolerances generally range from $\pm 10\%$ to $\pm 25\%$. The mica capacitor, as the name implies, uses mica as the dielectric sandwiched between plates of silver metal. These capacitors are very efficient and reliable but are expensive. The capacitor is usually encased in molded Bakelite. Mica capacitors are usually available in values from a few picofarads to about 10,000 pF and can be made to a tolerance of $\pm 2\%$. The two types of capacitors mentioned previously are also known as "dry" capacitors.

When larger capacitances are required, "wet," or electrolytic capacitors are used. An aluminum electrolytic capacitor consists of a loosely rolled or folded sheet of aluminum that is immersed in a borax solution (electrolyte). The borax solution causes an extremely thin layer of aluminum oxide to form on the aluminum surface. The aluminum sheet becomes one plate of the capacitor, the borax solution becomes the other plate, and the layer of aluminum oxide becomes the dielectric. The dielectric layer, being so thin, greatly enhances the capacitance. The tantalum electrolytic capacitor substitutes tantalum foil for aluminum. It has greater stability, less "noise," and less "leakage current." It also can be completely sealed and is generally physically smaller than aluminum electrolytic capacitors of similar value.

Electrolytic capacitors are more expensive than the dry capacitors. They are available in a value range of 1 to 5000 μF and generally have tolerances of -20% to $+50\%$. Polarity must be observed when electrolytic capacitors are used. If an electrolytic capacitor has been incorrectly connected (polarity reversed), it should be discarded.

Variable Capacitors. Some circuit functions require capacitors that can adjust the value of capacitance. There are two general types: those that can change the effective area of the plates, and those that vary the distance between plates. Both types use aluminum plates and air as the dielectric.

Voltage Rating of Capacitors. All capacitors are given a voltage rating that is the maximum DC voltage that can be safely used without damaging the insulating properties of the dielectric. When a certain level of voltage is exceeded, an arc of current is produced that will "break down" or "puncture" the capacitor. When a capacitor is used in an AC line, AC voltages are usually given as root mean square (rms) values. Therefore the maximum voltage that will be generated by the

line must be accounted for. For example, a capacitor that is rated at 400 volts direct current (VDC) cannot be placed across a 400 volt alternating current (VAC) source. The VAC source has a peak voltage of 565.5 V (400 V $\times$ 1.414) that far exceeds the rating of the capacitor. A capacitor rating should always exceed the peak value of the AC voltage source.

Capacitors in Series and Parallel. To obtain a desired value of capacitance, capacitors are often connected in series and parallel combinations. Fig. 2-16, *A* shows three capacitors connected in series across a battery. When capacitors are connected in series, the positive conducting plate of one capacitor influences the negative plate of an adjacent capacitor (Fig. 2-16, *A*). The three inner plates of these capacitors are connected such that they effectively act as one plate (Fig. 2-16, *B*). In essence, the three capacitors behave as though they were a single capacitor whose plates are separated in distance equivalent to all three plate separations. Because the greater the distance between conducting plates the lower the capacitance, the total capacitance of any series combination of capacitors is less than that of any individual capacitor in the circuit. The rule for adding capacitors in series (Fig. 2-16, *B*) is the same as the rule for adding resistors in parallel and is described below.

Series: For any number of capacitors connected in series, the total capacitance is equal to the reciprocal of the sum of the reciprocals of the individual capacitances or,

$$C_{total} = \frac{1}{1/C_1 + 1/C_2 + 1/C_3 \ldots \text{etc.}}$$

For example, what is the total capacitance in a circuit that contains the following capacitors connected in series?

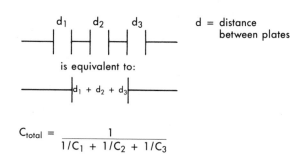

$$C_{total} = \frac{1}{1/C_1 + 1/C_2 + 1/C_3}$$

Fig. 2-16   Three capacitors in series.

$$C_1 = 45 \ \mu F \qquad C_2 = 90 \ \mu F \qquad C_3 = 15 \ \mu F$$

$$C_{total} = \cfrac{1}{1/45 \ \mu F + 1/90 \ \mu F + 1/15 \ \mu F}$$

$$= \cfrac{1}{2/90 \ \mu F + 1/90 \ \mu F + 6/90 \ \mu F}$$

$$= \cfrac{1}{9/90 \ \mu F} = \cfrac{1}{1/10 \ \mu F}$$

$$= 10 \ \mu F$$

Fig. 2-17, *A*, shows three capacitors connected in parallel. When capacitors are connected in parallel the positive and negative plate of each capacitor is affected by the entire voltage source. Each capacitor is charging independently of the others. When the conducting plates are wired together in tandem, a parallel connection of capacitors acts like a single capacitor having a total plate area equivalent to the sum of the plate areas of the individual capacitors (Fig. 2-17, *B*). Because capacitance varies directly with the plate area, the total capacitance of several capacitors connected in parallel is found by adding all the individual capacitances (Fig. 2-17, *B*), using the same rule as with series resistors. The rule for calculating capacitors in parallel is given below.

Parallel: For any number of capacitors connected in parallel, the total capacitance is equal to the sum of the individual capacitances or,

$$C_{total} = C_1 + C_2 + C_3 \ldots \text{etc.}$$

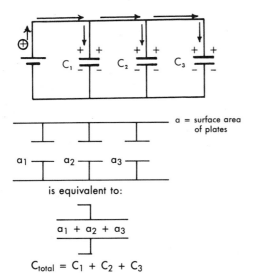

$$C_{total} = C_1 + C_2 + C_3$$

Fig. 2-17 Three capacitors in parallel.

For example, if the three capacitors given in the problem above were connected in series instead of parallel, what would be the total capacitance of the circuit?

$$C_{total} = 45 \ \mu F + 90 \ \mu F + 15 \ \mu F$$
$$= 150 \ \mu F$$

Capacitive Reactance. A capacitor offers resistance to the flow of current through its dielectric. This resistance is called **capacitance reactance** (X_c) and is measured in ohms. The capacitive reactance can be determined by the following equation:

$$X_c = 1/\left(2\pi fC\right)$$

where:

X_c = Capacitive reactance in ohms

π = A constant of 3.14

f = Frequency of applied voltage in cycles/second

C = Capacitance in farads

Note there is an inverse relationship between capacitive reactance and frequency. As the frequency of polarity switching increases, there is less time available for the capacitor to reach a full charge. As the electrostatic charge on the capacitor decreases, so does the counter-EMF that opposes the AC voltage source. In effect, there is less hindrance to current flow as the frequency increases. The following problem illustrates this concept.

Given the following frequencies of a 120 VAC signal, what is the capacitive reactance of a 200 μF capacitor?

1. 50 Hz
2. 100 Hz
3. 200 Hz

Solutions:

$$X_c = 1/\left(2\pi fC\right)$$

1. $X_c = (1/2)(3.14)(50 \text{ Hz})(0.0002) = 15.92 \ \Omega$
2. $X_c = (1/2)(3.14)(100 \text{ Hz})(0.0002) = 7.96 \ \Omega$
3. $X_c = (1/2)(3.14)(200 \text{ Hz})(0.0002) = 3.98 \ \Omega$

In a purely capacitive circuit, capacitive reactance (X_c) can be substituted for the term impedance in Z = E/I, so that Ohm's law for AC circuits becomes:

$$X_c = E/I$$

In a circuit that contains both capacitors and resistors in series, the total impedance is:

$$Z = \sqrt{R^2 + X_c^2}$$

Resistance and capacitive reactance in parallel are added by using the equation:

$$Z = 1 / \sqrt{(1/R)^2 + (1/X_c)^2}$$

Inductors

When a potential is applied to a wire, its inherent resistance tends to impede current flow. However, an additional opposition to current flow can occur when this wire is coiled into an electrical device called an **inductor**. An inductor is also called a **choke** or **coil**. The name of the device is dictated by the way it is used in a circuit. Several types of inductors are shown in Fig. 2-18. The usefulness of an inductor in an electrical circuit is related to its additional opposition to current flow as a coiled conductor that creates and interacts with its magnetic field.

Inductors, like capacitors, are referred to as **reactors** because they store energy and then deliver it back to the circuit. Whereas a capacitor stores electrical energy as electrostatic charge, an inductor stores it as electromagnetic energy. Time is required to accumulate, store, and then release this energy. This explains why reactors produce changes in phase relationships between current and voltage, and components like resistors do not. Also, unlike resistors, they do not dissipate electrical energy in the form of heat.

Electricity, Magnetism, and Induction of Current. When an electrical current flows through a conductor, a magnetic field is formed that surrounds the conductor. The strength of this magnetic field is directly proportional to the quantity of current passing through the conductor. When the wire stops conducting, the magnetic field collapses. It is also possible to produce current using a magnetic field. When a magnetic field cuts across a conductor, a current is generated (i.e., a current has been induced). There are two basic mechanisms that can be used to induce current using a magnetic field and a conductor: (1) a wire can be kept stationary and the magnet moved so that lines of force cut across the conductor to induce current; or (2) a magnet can be kept stationary and the conductor moved so as to cross perpendicularly the lines of magnetic force, cutting them in a downward (*A*), or upward (*B*), motion (Fig. 2-19).

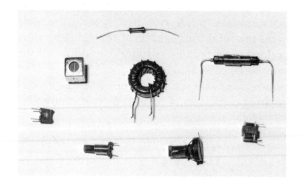

Fig. 2-18   Common assortment of inductors.

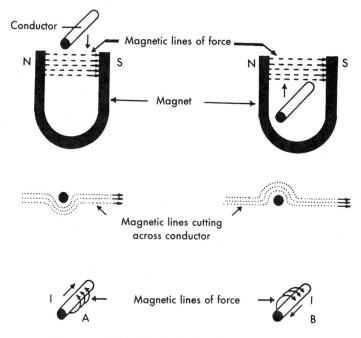

Fig. 2-19   Induction of current.

Inductors in DC and AC Circuits. When a DC voltage source generates current flow through an inductor, a magnetic field is generated. As a magnetic field develops around the coiled wire, a counter-EMF is induced that produces a current that opposes the direction of current flow from the voltage source (Fig. 2-20). The only other time a counter-EMF is generated with a DC source is when the current stops and the magnetic field collapses. When the field collapses, a counter-EMF is momentarily established that produces a brief opposing current. A continuous counter-EMF can be produced only when the induced magnetic field is constantly changing. This condition does not exist in a DC circuit, and thus for all practical purposes an inductor exhibits an effect comparable to a straight wire. For this reason, an inductor in a DC circuit acts as a resistor of low resistance.

With an AC voltage source, the production and strength of the magnetic field will vary at the same rate (frequency) and in proportion to the magnitude of the current. The result is a constantly moving magnetic field that causes a continuous counter-EMF (potential difference) to develop in the inductor. The greater the frequency of AC passing through the inductor, the greater the counter-EMF, and thus the greater the hindrance to current flow. An inductor exerts an impedance to AC that is directly proportional to the frequency of the AC passing through the inductor. At any given instance the induced potential difference is in direct opposition to the applied potential difference. It is for this reason that inductors are referred to as chokes. An inductor in an AC circuit, unlike a DC circuit, behaves like a resistor of high resistance. In a laboratory instrument they essentially serve as an AC-DC separator (filter) (i.e., isolate AC that is superimposed on DC). They are also used as part of an instrument's power supply where AC must be converted to DC. For these reasons, inductors are considered AC components.

Phase Relationship in an Inductor. When voltage is applied to an inductor, the current causes the formation of a magnetic field. As the magnetic field develops, a counter-EMF is induced that opposes an increase in current flow. The production of the counter-EMF occurs before it gives rise to a current that opposes the current coming from the voltage source. When AC is applied across an inductor, a continuous supply of counter-EMF is produced in which the voltage leads the current by 90 degrees. The effects of an inductor on AC current are opposite to those seen with a capacitor where the current leads the voltage by 90 degrees.

Units of Inductance. The ability of a coil to store electromagnetic energy and then oppose a change in AC current flow by releasing this energy as a counter-EMF is called **inductance (L)**. The unit of measure for inductance is called the **henry (H)**. One henry is equal to the induction of 1 V from a current variation of 1 A/second. Other units of inductance are the millihenry (mH) and the microhenry (μH).

The inductance of a coil is determined primarily by the number of coils, their diameter, and the core material. The construction of a coil depends on its particular application for a given circuit. The core material may be air or a magnetic material such as iron. Air-core inductors are made by winding wire on a nonmagnetic material to serve as a support, or by using wire sufficiently heavy to be self-supporting A magnetic core increases the inductance by concentrating the magnetic field within the coil. An inductor having a movable iron core is a variable inductor, the inductance of which can be varied by adjusting the length of the iron core inside the coil.

An inductor that uses air as its central core is called an air-core inductor. The electrical symbol

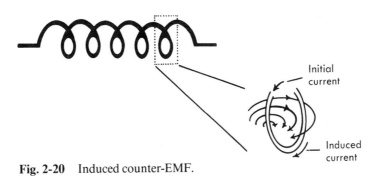

Fig. 2-20   Induced counter-EMF.

An inductor that uses air as its central core is called an air-core inductor. The electrical symbol for such an inductor is ⎍⎍⎍ . An inductor that uses an iron core is called a magnetic-core inductor. The symbol for an inductor with a central core of iron is ⎍⎍⎍ . Variable inductors are shown by one of the following two symbols: or ⎍⎍ ⎍⎍ .

Inductive Reactance. The specific opposition, impedance, or effective resistance offered by an inductor (coil) to AC is called **inductive reactance (X_L)**. Its unit of measure is the ohm. The formula used to calculate inductive reactance is:

$$X_L = 2\pi fL$$

where:

X_L = Inductive reactance in ohms

π = A constant of (3.14)

f = Frequency of applied voltage in hertz

L = Inductance in henrys

Note that once a fixed inductor is constructed, the frequency of the applied voltage is the only variable capable of changing the inductive reactance. To fully appreciate the meaning of this equation, note the effect of changing AC voltage frequency on inductive reactance in the problem given below.

Given the following frequencies of a 120 VAC signal, what is the inductive reactance of a 200 mH inductor?

1. 50 Hz
2. 100 Hz
3. 200 Hz

Solutions:

$$X_L = 2\pi fL$$

1. $X_1 = (2)(3.14)(50 \text{ Hz})(0.2 \text{ H}) = 62.8$
2. $X_1 = (2)(3.14)(100 \text{ Hz})(0.2 \text{H}) = 125.6$
3. $X_1 = (2)(3.14)(200 \text{ Hz})(0.2 \text{ H}) = 251.2$

Note that a direct relationship exists between frequency and inductance reactance; as the frequency increases, the inductive reactance increases and vice versa. In a purely inductive circuit, inductive reactance (X_L) can be substituted for impedance (Z) so that for AC circuits, Ohm's law is changed from $Z = E/I$ to $X_L = E/I$.

Inductors in Series, Parallel, and Series-Parallel. The rules for adding an inductor in series and in parallel are the same as those for adding resistances. However, these rules are applicable only if the magnetic fields of inductors do not interact with each other.

Series: The total effective inductance of inductors connected in series is equal to the sum of the individual inductances or,

$$L_{total} = L_1 + L_2 + L_3 \ldots \text{etc.}$$

Parallel: The total effective inductance of inductors connected in parallel is equal to the reciprocal of the sum of the reciprocals of the individual inductances or,

$$L_{total} = \frac{1}{1/L_1 + 1/L_2 + 1/L_3 \ldots \text{etc.}}$$

The following problems will demonstrate the use of these rules:

1. If three inductors are connected in series ($L_1 = 3.0$ H, $L_2 = 2.0$ H, $L_3 = 6.0$ H), what would be the value of an equivalent single inductor?
Solution:

$$L_{total} = 3.0 \text{ H} + 2.0 \text{ H} + 6.0 \text{ H}$$
$$= \cancel{10.0} \text{ H}$$

2. For example, if the three inductors given in the problem No. 1 are connected in parallel instead of series, what would be the total inductance of the circuit?
Solution:

$$L_{total} = \frac{1}{1/3 \text{ H} + 1/2 \text{ H} + 1/6 \text{ H}}$$
$$= \frac{1}{2/6 \text{ H} + 3/6 \text{ H} + 1/6 \text{ H}}$$
$$= \frac{1}{6/6 \text{ H}} = \frac{1}{1/1 \text{ H}}$$
$$= 1.0 \text{ H}$$

Resistance and Impedance. The total effective impedance exerted by an inductor and a resistor connected in series is determined by using the following equation:

$$Z = \sqrt{R^2 + X_L^2}$$

The total effective impedance exerted by an inductor and a resistor connected in parallel is determined by using the following equation:

$$Z = (R)(X_L) / \sqrt{R^2 + X_L^2}$$

Transformers

Transformers are used extensively in laboratory equipment (Fig. 2-21). Their primary function is to meet the voltage level requirements of various circuits in an instrument by changing the level of input voltage. The input AC voltage ap-

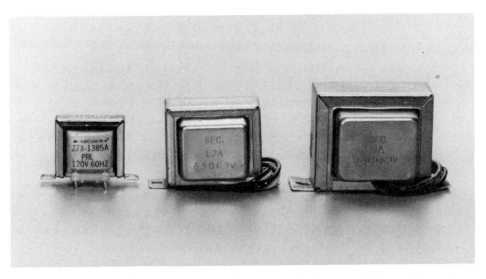

Fig. 2-21 Common transformer in various sizes. (Courtesy Radio Shack, a division of Tandy Corporation.)

plied across a transformer may be decreased or increased or may remain unchanged. Transformers may also serve to block unwanted DC from passing from one circuit to another or provide protection from electrical shock.

Induction of Current. When AC passes through a coil, it produces a magnetic field that is constantly changing. The expanding and collapsing of this magnetic field around a coiled wire that is carrying AC induces a counter-EMF. Production of a counter-EMF within a coil is called **self-inductance.** However, it is also possible for one coil to induce a counter-EMF in an adjacent coil. This process is called **mutual inductance.** To induce a current by mutual induction, an adjacent coil must be arranged in a parallel orientation and in close proximity to another coil. The coil connected to the AC power source is called the primary coil; the adjacent coil that is not attached to the AC voltage source but has had a current induced in it by the first coil is called the secondary coil (Fig. 2-22).

Transformer Construction. The design of a transformer allows for maximum power transfer from one coil to the other. Two factors that influence the voltage output of a transformer are the proximity of the coils and the strength of the magnetic field. The closer the coils, the greater the effectiveness of current induction. Therefore the coils of a transformer are made by winding insulated wires over each other and around a central core. A central and peripheral iron core is used to concentrate the magnetic field about the coils (Fig. 2-23). The schematic symbols that are used to represent transformers are:

Air-core: Iron core:

Transformer Action. Induction of current is accompanied by induction of voltage and dissipation of power. Although these three parameters are interrelated, the preferred electrical parameter that is used to describe induced energy is voltage. The input voltage in the primary coil in-

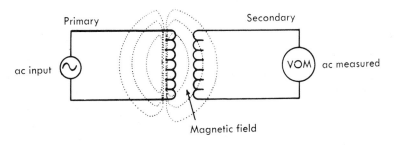

Fig. 2-22 Current induction in a transformer.

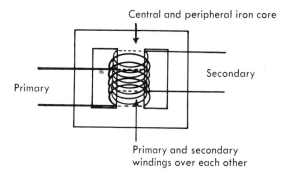

Central and peripheral iron core

Secondary

Primary

Primary and secondary
windings over each other

Fig. 2-23 An iron-core transformer depicting primary and secondary windings.

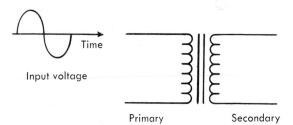

Time

Input voltage

Primary   Secondary

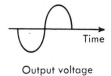

Time

Output voltage

Fig. 2-24 Transformer action.

duces current and thus voltage in the secondary coil. The positive half of an AC voltage source generates a magnetic field that cuts across the secondary coil in a direction that is opposite to that generated from the primary coil. Therefore when the input voltage of the primary coil is positive, the voltage across the secondary coil is negative, and vice versa (Fig. 2-24). Thus the AC voltage induced in the secondary coil is 180 degrees out of phase with the AC voltage across the primary coil.

To calculate the voltage induced in the secondary coil by the primary coil, use the following equation:

$$E_s/E_p = N_s/N_p$$

where:

E_s = Voltage in secondary coil
E_p = Voltage in primary coil
N_s = Number of turns in secondary coil
N_p = Number of turns in primary coil

As shown in the equation, the induced voltage is directly related to the number of turns in both coils. If there are more turns in the secondary coil than in the primary coil, the magnetic field of the primary coil will cut across more conducting wires in the secondary coil. Therefore it will induce a larger voltage. This type of transformer is called a **"step-up" transformer** (Fig. 2-25). On the other hand, if there are fewer turns in the secondary coil than in the primary coil, the transformer

Primary   Secondary

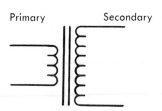

Fig. 2-25 Step-up transformer.

Primary   Secondary

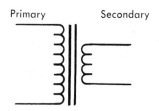

Fig. 2-26 Step-down transformer.

Primary   Secondary

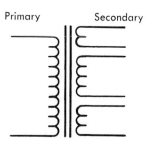

Fig. 2-27 Transformer with multiple secondary windings.

is a **"step-down" transformer** (Fig. 2-26). A transformer can have more than one secondary coil. Such multiple secondary windings can provide several levels of induced voltage to various parts of an instrument's circuit (Fig. 2-27). The following examples will help to illustrate the use of a transformer:

1. What voltage is induced in a secondary coil of 150 turns if 120 VAC is applied across a primary coil of 100 turns? (Step-up transformer)
   Solution:

   $$E_s/E_p = N_s/N_p$$
   $$E_s/120 \text{ VAC} = 150/100$$
   $$E_s = 18000/100 = 180 \text{ VAC}$$

2. What voltage is induced in a secondary coil of 75 turns if 120 VAC is applied across a primary coil of 100 turns? (Step-down transformer)
   Solution:

   $$E_s/E_p = N_s/N_p$$
   $$E_s/120 \text{ VAC} = 75/100$$
   $$E_s = 9000/100 = 90 \text{ VAC}$$

In both step-up and step-down transformers it appears that the voltage has been magnified or diminished without regard to the law of conservation of energy. However, the energy transferred between the primary and secondary coils is power. The power in the primary coil (P_p) equals the power in the secondary coil (P_s) if the transformer is 100% efficient. Consider the ideal situation where:

$$P_p = P_s$$

Because power is the product of current and voltage, the following relationship exists:

$$I_p \times E_p = I_s \times E_s$$

Thus, if voltage is stepped up, the current is proportionately stepped down, and if the voltage is stepped down, the current is stepped up. To demonstrate this concept, consider the following problem:

1. In each of the previous problems, if the power in the primary coil was 60 W, what would be the current in the primary coil and in the secondary coil?
   Current in the primary coil (Problem No. 1)

Solution:

$$I_p = P_p/E_p$$
$$I_p = 60 \text{ W}/120 \text{ V} = 0.5 \text{ A}$$

Current in the secondary coil (Problem No. 1)
Solution:

$$I_p \times E_p = I_s \times E_s$$
$$I_s = I_p \times E_p/E_s$$
$$I_s = P_p/E_p$$
$$I_s = 60 \text{ W}/180 \text{ V} = 0.333 \text{ A}$$

Note that in the secondary coil the voltage increased and the current decreased.

Current in the primary coil (Problem No. 2)
Solution:

$$I_p = P_p/E_p$$
$$I_p = 60 \text{ W}/120 \text{ V} = 0.5 \text{ A}$$

Current in the secondary coil (Problem No. 2)
Solution:

$$I_s = P_s/E_s \text{ and } P_s = P_p$$
$$I_s = P_p/E_s$$
$$I_s = 60 \text{ W}/90 \text{ V} = 0.667 \text{ A}$$

Note that in the secondary coil the current increased and the voltage decreased.

As previously mentioned, a DC voltage source cannot sustain a constantly changing magnetic field, which is prerequisite for the production of a continuous counter-EMF. Consequently, DC is unable to induce a current. For this reason a transformer is considered an AC component. Although AC will be transmitted through a transformer, DC will be blocked. Thus another useful application of transformers is the isolation of certain AC circuits and/or components from unwanted direct current.

Switches and Electromagnetic Relays

Switches. Electronic circuits can be controlled by several different types of mechanical or electronic switches. A **switch** is a device that turns current "on or off" or redirects current flow. The switch controls the circuit operations. When closed, a switch allows current to flow. When it is opened, current stops. Switches are rated according to their voltage and current capabilities. There are four types of manual switches. They are classified according to their mode of operation. A single-pole-single-throw (SPST) switch is a single control device that regulates current flow at one point in the circuit. For example, the "on/off" power switch of most laboratory instruments is a SPST switch. A single-pole-double-throw (SPDT) switch is used to control the operation of two separate circuits. When the switch is in one position, power is provided to one of the circuits but not the other. In the other position, power is directed to the other circuit, but is removed from the previous one. A SPDT switch cannot be used to power both circuits. To direct power to more than one circuit, a three-way device called a double-pole-single-throw (DPST) switch or a four-way device called a double-pole-double-throw (DPDT) switch is used. The DPST switch is used to control current flow at two different locations. The DPDT switch is used to control the operation of up to four different circuits.

Electromagnetic Relays. With many clinical laboratory instruments it is not always practical to operate a switch manually to control a circuit's operation. Often a remote-controlled switch called a **relay** is used (Fig. 2-28). Relays come in many shapes and sizes and have numerous applications (e.g., in many clinical laboratory instruments, electronic switches must be opened and closed in a synchronized manner to direct current to specific locations within the instrument). Often it is necessary for a smaller current in one circuit to control a larger current in another circuit. The device that is used for these types of operations is the relay.

The operation of all relays is based on the principle of induction. A basic relay circuit is shown in Fig. 2-29. It consists of a coil, an iron core, movable magnetic contacts, an armature, and a tension spring. When the switch in the primary circuit is closed, current flow in the coil creates a magnetic field that pulls the contacts together. Closing the contacts allows current to flow through the secondary circuit causing the lamp to glow (Fig. 2-29). To turn off the lamp, the switch in the primary circuit must be opened. This stops the flow of current in the coil, which in turn

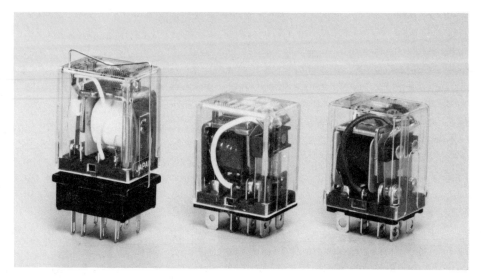

Fig. 2-28 Common relay in various sizes. (Courtesy Radio Shack, a division of Tandy Corporation.)

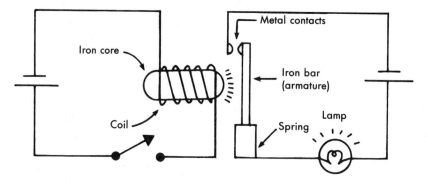

Fig. 2-29 Basic circuitry of a relay (electromagnetic switch).

causes the magnetic field to decay. As soon as the field is weak enough, the spring takes over and "breaks" (opens) the circuit, thus turning off the lamp.

Diodes

Diodes are electronic components that play a major role in rectification (conversion) of AC to DC. The derivation of diode comes from "di" meaning two and "ode" from electrode, which indicates that the component is a two-electrode unit (negative electrode or cathode and a positive electrode or anode). Diodes provide for unidirectional current flow. Although there are two basic types of diodes, vacuum tube and **semiconductor,** vacuum tube diodes are no longer used in the electronic circuits of newer laboratory instruments. Therefore the discussion of this electronic component will be limited to the process of semiconduction and semiconductor diodes.

Semiconductor Diodes. A semiconductor electronic component is also called a solid-state device, and thus the names **semiconductor diode** and "solid state diode" are interchangeable. Semiconductor diodes serve two basic functions in the circuits of laboratory equipment: (1) rectifying AC to DC and (2) regulating voltage. The latter function requires a special type of diode that will be described later in this section. Some examples of the more common semiconductor diodes are shown in Fig. 2-30.

The operation of a semiconductor diode is based on its crystalline structure and composition. Semiconductors are generally made of pure silicon or germanium. The conductivity of a semiconductor is between that of an insulator and that of a conductor. The conductivity of the pure crystal can be enhanced by adding a specific impurity via a process called "doping." The impurity, often a pentavalent or trivalent element, must have a structure compatible with the crystalline structure of the pure crystal. The addition of an impurity to a pure crystal does not change the electrical neutrality of the crystal because the impurities have an equal number of electrons and protons. A pure crystal doped with a pentavalent or trivalent impurity is referred to as an extrinsic or impurity semiconductor (Fig. 2-31, *A* and *B*).

A doping element that provides one free electron/crystalline atom is called a donor impurity. The excess electrons are not covalently bonded and thus are available to freely move within the crystal as negatively charged carriers. The number of electron carriers depends on the amount of impurity introduced into the crystal. Donor impurities are generally pentavalent elements such as arsenic, antimony, or phosphorus, and are used to manufacture N-type semiconductors (see Fig. 2-31, *A*).

A doping element that provides a deficit of one electron/crystalline atom is called an acceptor impurity. This electron deficit is often referred to as a "hole" because the acceptor impurity contains an unpaired electron. Because this electron is unpaired, it will attract other electrons from the crystal, causing holes or electron deficiencies to occur throughout the crystal. The number of holes generated in the crystal will depend on the amount of impurity introduced into the crystal. This electronic hole can be thought of as a positive charge because there is a relative lack of mobile electrons. Acceptor impurities are usually tri-

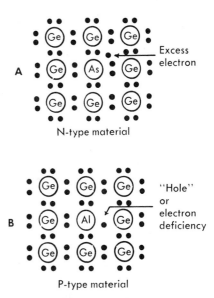

N-type material

P-type material

Fig. 2-31 Impurity (doping) semiconductor crystals.

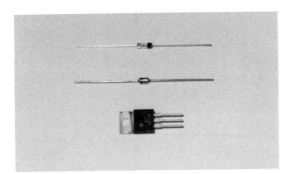

Fig. 2-30 Common semiconductor diodes. (From top to bottom: germanium P-N junction diode, Zener diode, adjustable voltage regulator.)

valent elements such as aluminum, gallium, or boron, and are used to produce P-type semiconductors (see Fig. 2-31, *B*).

When a potential is placed across an N-type or P-type semiconductor, both conduct a current; however, the method of current conduction differs. Current flow through a N-type semiconductor is caused by the movement of negative carriers (Fig. 2-32, *A*); in a P-type semiconductor, it is due to the apparent movement of positive carriers (holes) (Fig. 2-32, *B*).

P-type and N-type crystals chemically fused to construct a semiconductor diode are called a P-N junction diode (Fig. 2-33). After the two materials have been joined, a few carriers of each type of crystal diffuse across the interface of the junction forming a voltage or potential barrier. This barrier prevents further movement of the electrons from the N material to the P material and

vice versa. The schematic symbol for a P-N junction diode is ——▶|—— . Note that in Fig. 2-33, the P-material is often called the plate and the N-material the cathode.

The potential across the semiconductor diode is referred to as the bias, which can occur in a forward or reverse direction. When sufficient voltage is applied in the forward direction, the diode's barrier is overcome and electrons flow from the N-type to the P-type crystal. Fig. 2-34, *A*, represents a circuit that is conducting a current through a forward-biased semiconductor diode. The positive terminal of the battery is connected to the P-type semiconductor (plate), and the negative terminal is connected to the N-type semiconductor (cathode). The positive and negative charges from the battery repel the positive and negative carriers of the diode. The positive holes and the negative electrons cross the barrier poten-

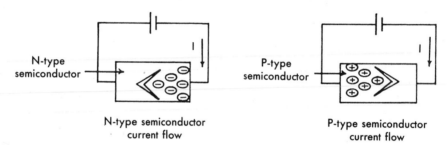

Fig. 2-32   Current flow through N-type and P-type semiconductors.

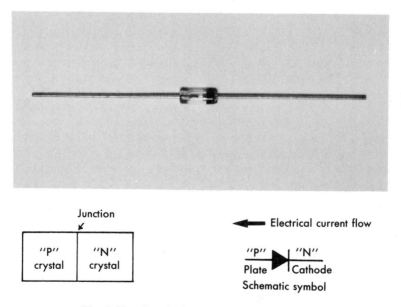

Fig. 2-33   Germanium P-N junction diode.

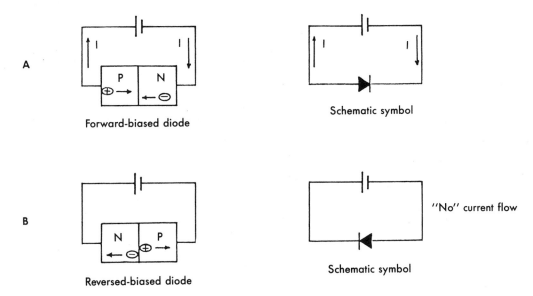

Fig. 2-34   P-N junction diodes in a circuit.

tial where they combine and become neutralized. The electrons that have been lost by combining with the holes at the diode junction are continuously replaced with electrons from the negative terminal of the battery. These electrons move toward the junction, where they again combine with new holes arriving there. As a consequence, current flows through the junction. The net result is current flow from the negative terminal to the positive terminal of the battery. This overall process is called semiconduction.

A semiconductor diode is reverse-biased when the positive terminal of the battery is connected to the N-type semiconductor, and the negative terminal is connected to the P-type semiconductor (Fig. 2-34, *B*). The positive carriers are attracted to the negative terminal of the battery, whereas the negative carriers are attracted to the positive terminal. Because both types of carrier charges move away from the P-N junction, no current is conducted through the diode.

If a potential in excess (breakdown voltage) is placed across a reverse-biased semiconductor diode, the covalent bonds near the junction are broken, causing an abrupt increase in current. This avalanche current will destroy the integrity of a conventional P-N junction diode. There is a special type of semiconductor diode, however, called a **Zener diode,** which is designed to conduct only avalanche current. The Zener diode consists of a reverse-biased silicon P-N junction diode that operates at the breakdown voltage. It

is strategically placed in a circuit where a specific voltage level must not be exceeded. When that level is exceeded, an avalanche current or Zener current occurs, which causes the voltage to drop through the Zener diode. This process maintains a constant voltage in the main circuit. Zener diodes are used in laboratory instruments to regulate voltage. The schematic symbol for a Zener diode is

Diode Applications. Although specially designed diodes can be used for voltage regulation, the primary function of diodes in an instrument's circuit is to rectify AC to DC. Because semiconductor diodes are unidirectional current devices (i.e., they allow current to flow in only one direction), they can convert AC voltage to DC voltage via the process called **rectification** (Fig. 2-35). For this reason, diodes are also known as rectifiers.

Before describing the process of rectification in detail, it is important to remember that a diode will conduct a current in a circuit only if it is in a forward-biased orientation relative to the polarity of the voltage source (i.e., the cathode [⊢] must be connected to the negative side of the circuit [negative pole of the voltage source] and the plate [→] must be connected to the positive side [positive pole of the voltage source]). When it is connected to an AC voltage source, the polarity (poles) will periodically switch. Therefore the orientation of the diode will change from forward-biased to reverse-biased and vice versa, thus affecting its ability to conduct a current.

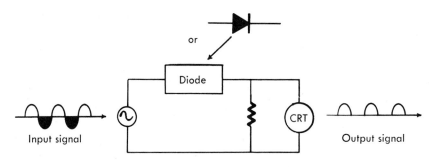

Fig. 2-35 Rectification.

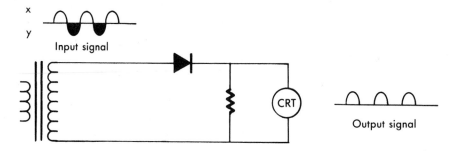

Fig. 2-36 Half-wave rectifier.

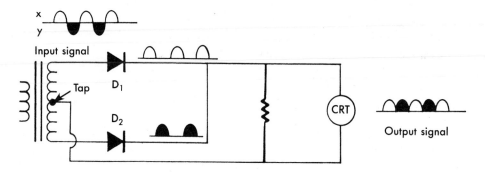

Fig. 2-37 Full-wave rectifier.

The use of a diode as a **half-wave rectifier** is shown in Fig. 2-36. The input of an AC signal to the circuit occurs by inducing a current from the primary winding to the secondary winding of the transformer. When the half cycle of the input signal is positive (*X*), the diode is forward-biased. Therefore it can conduct a current and produce an output voltage. When the half cycle of the input signal becomes negative (*Y*), the diode will be in a reverse-biased orientation because the polarity of the AC voltage source has switched. The cathode of the diode will now be connected to the positive side of the circuit and the plate will be connected to the negative side. Therefore no current will be conducted and no output voltage generated. In this example, during the full AC cycle,

only the positive half will conduct through the diode. This process, called half-wave rectification, is illustrated in Fig. 2-36; one half of the AC cycle is represented by a white semicircle, the other by a black semicircle.

In Fig. 2-37 two diodes have been connected in a circuit to function as a **full-wave rectifier**. During the first half of the cycle (*X*), diode No. 1 (*D₁*) is forward-biased, and therefore it can conduct a current, whereas diode No. 2 (*D₂*) is in a reverse-biased orientation, and thus cannot conduct a current. The opposite is true during the second half of the cycle (*Y*). D₂ now is forward-biased, and thus can conduct a current, whereas D₁ becomes reverse-biased and therefore cannot.

The output voltage of a full-wave rectifier contains the voltage of both half cycles of the input AC voltage. Because the output voltage has not changed polarity, it is considered DC voltage. Note that the DC voltage produced by rectification does not maintain a constant level of potential, but instead occurs as a series of unidirectional pulses. DC voltage that is produced through the process of rectification is known as **pulsating DC voltage** or **ripple.** Pulsating DC voltage can be converted to constant DC voltage by the action of reactors such as capacitors and inductors.

Note that with a full-wave rectifier (see Fig. 2-37) the plates of both P-N junction diodes are connected together, and the common junction is connected to one side of the load resistor (R_L). The other end of R_L is connected to the center tap of the secondary winding of the transformer. Because each diode is connected to one end of the transformer winding and the center tap, only one half of the secondary voltage of the transformer appears over each diode. This means that the secondary winding of the transformer must supply a total voltage that is twice the value of the voltage required for the load. Thus to produce sufficient voltage for the circuit, the transformer would have to have two times the step-up ratio between the primary and the secondary winding.

To resolve this problem, another electrical component called a **full-wave bridge rectifier** is used instead (Fig. 2-38). The main difference is that four diodes are configured in the circuit instead of two, and there is no need to center tap the power transformer (Fig. 2-39). The bridge circuitry is pictured in Fig. 2-39, *A* and *B*, to describe its operation during the positive and negative half of the AC cycle. AC voltage is applied to opposite corners of the bridge circuit (points *a* and *b*), while the output to the resistor load R_L is taken from the remaining two corners (points *c* and *d*). With a full-wave bridge rectifier, full-wave rectification can be obtained with the switching action of the diodes in the circuit (see Fig. 2-39, *A* and *B*).

During the positive half cycle (see Fig. 2-39, *A*), current leaves the lower (negative) terminal of the AC voltage source and enters point *b* of the 4-diode network (called a bridge). The bridge is positive to negative from top to bottom because of the polarity of the AC source. Remember, current will flow through the diode only if it is forward-biased (i.e., when the cathode is negative and the plate is positive). Diode D_2 has a negative cathode and a positive plate, but the polarity of diode D_4 is reversed. Thus current can flow through only diode D_2 to reach point *c*. This current then flows through the resistor load (R_L), to point *d*. After point *d*, it must flow through diode D_3 because diodes D_4 and D_1 are of the wrong polarity. Eventually the current enters the positive terminal of the AC source.

During the negative half cycle (see Fig. 2-39, *B*), the polarities of the voltages on the four diodes are reversed. Current leaves the upper negative terminal of the AC voltage source and ar-

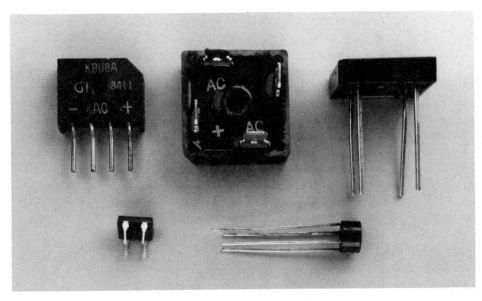

Fig. 2-38 Full-bridge rectifier. (Courtesy Radio Shack, a division of Tandy Corporation.)

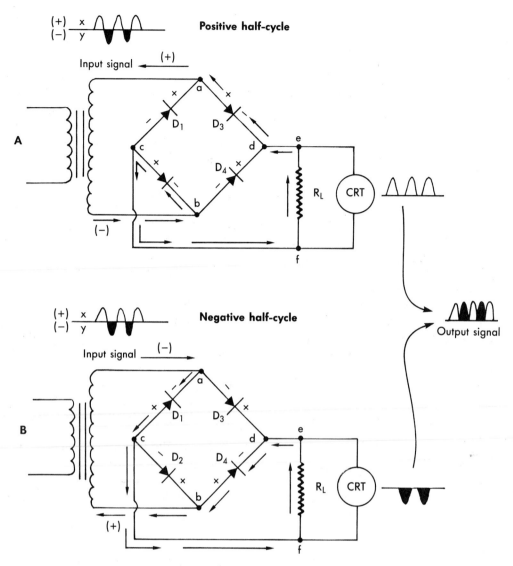

Fig. 2-39 Circuitry of a full-wave bridge rectifier showing positive half-cycle **A** and negative half-cycle **B**.

rives at point *a*. The voltage on diode D_3 is of the wrong polarity; however, diode D_1 is forward-biased, and thus will conduct a current. After passing through point *c*, the current follows the same path as the positive half cycle current, flowing through R_L toward point *d* (because D_2 is reverse-biased). At point *d*, the diode that has the correct voltage polarity to conduct a current is D_4. After the current flows through diode D_4 it proceeds to point *c*, and eventually to the positive terminal of the AC source.

One of the advantages of using a bridge rectifier rather than a conventional full-wave rectifier is that it produces twice the voltage output. This is because the entire voltage of the transformer secondary winding is applied across two con-

ducting diodes during each half cycle. The other advantage is that it is a very small component that allows for miniaturization of the complex circuitry required for sophisticated laboratory instruments.

Review Questions

1. Which of the following statements concerning the application of Ohm's law in either a series or parallel circuit is (are) true?
   A. The current in a series circuit is the same throughout the entire circuit.
   B. The voltage drop over each resistor in a parallel branch is the same.
   C. The total effective resistance in a parallel circuit is equal to the sum of the individual resistances.

D. The total voltage in a series circuit is equal to the sum of the individual voltage drops over each resistor.
   1. A, B, and C
   2. A, B, and D
   3. C and D
   4. Only C
2. Given the following circuit, calculate the voltage drop over resistor No. 3.

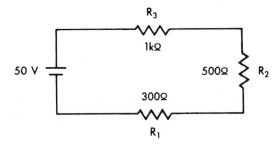

A. 125 volts
B. 25 volts
C. 50 volts
D. 250 volts

Use the following circuit to answer questions 3 through 5.

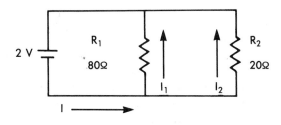

3. What is the voltage drop over resistor No. 2?
   A. 0.025 V
   B. 0.4 V
   C. 1.0 V
   D. 2.0 V
4. What is the total current in milliamperes?
   A. 0.02
   B. 0.125
   C. 20
   D. 125
5. The current passing through resistor No. 2 is _____ A?
   A. 0.025
   B. 0.100
   C. 25
   D. 100
6. The function of a capacitor is to _____.
   A. Block the flow of AC
   B. Store electrical energy
   C. Convert AC voltage to DC voltage
   D. Store electromagnetic energy

7. Which of the following electronic components uses electromagnetic energy to produce a counter EMF when supplied with AC voltage?
   A. Capacitor
   B. Resistor
   C. Diode
   D. Inductor
8. Which of the following electronic devices is used to rectify AC voltage to DC voltage?
   A. Resistor
   B. Diode
   C. Inductor
   D. Transformer
9. What voltage is induced in a secondary coil of 250 turns if 120 VAC is applied across the primary coil of a transformer that has 100 turns?
   A. 96
   B. 120
   C. 300
   D. 600
10. Which of the following electronic components functions as an electromagnetic switch?
   A. Transformer
   B. Coil
   C. Choke
   D. Relay
11. Which of the following electronic components can function as a voltage/current divider?
   A. Inductor
   B. Capacitor
   C. Rheostat
   D. Potentiometer
12. Conversion of alternating current to direct current is called:
   A. Rectification
   B. Induction
   C. Electromagnetism
   D. Mutual induction
12. Components that store energy and then deliver it back to the circuit are called:
   A. Resistors
   B. Reactors
   C. Diodes
   D. Rectifiers

Answers

1. 2 2. B 3. D 4. D 5. B 6. B 7. D 8. B 9. C
10. D 11. D 12. A 13. B

CHAPTER 3

Electronic Functional Units

ROBERT H. WILLIAMS

Power Supplies
Detectors
Signal Processing Units
Readout Devices

Individual electronic components have been discussed in previous chapters. However, to perform a particular function they must interact in a specific circuit configuration called an electronic unit. In this chapter the electronic principles and design of these components are applied to the operation of electronic units such as power supplies, detectors, amplifiers, and readout devices.

Power Supplies

Because an instrument performs a variety of functions, it requires a power source that can produce an assortment of AC and DC voltage levels, a source of direct current, and a means of regulating voltage levels at specific circuit locations. Thus most instruments are designed to contain an electronic **power supply**. Electronic power supplies characteristically consist of five stages: transformer, rectifier, filter, voltage regulator, and voltage divider (Fig. 3-1). These five stages are summarized below.

Transformer. The primary function of the transformer is to increase or decrease the input AC voltage supplied from commercial power generators. Thus specific voltage levels can be directed to different parts of an instrument circuitry. This component has already been discussed in detail in Chapter 2.

Rectifier. The rectifier converts alternating current into unidirectional, or direct current. The design and operation of the component that is responsible for the rectification process, the diode, has also been discussed in Chapter 2. Both half-wave and full-wave rectifiers produce pulsating direct current that requires additional processing in order for the DC voltage to become uniformly constant. This requires the use of electronic filters.

Filter Network. The **filter network** converts pulsating direct current to smooth direct current. As previously discussed, the variation in DC voltage that is produced after the rectification process is called ripple. To provide the constant direct current that is essential for the operation of most instruments, the ripple must be removed. The filtering process removes unwanted ripple by using electronic components such as reactors (capacitors, inductors) that can store current during the conduction part of the diode's cycle and then release it back to the circuit during the nonconduction part of the diode's cycle. Fig. 3-2, *A-D* represents several different circuits that contain different combinations of electronic components used during the process of rectification and filtering.

Fig. 3-2, *A*, represents a circuit that is composed of a half-wave rectifier and no filtering components. A cathode ray tube (CRT) is connected across the resistor (R) to monitor the voltage output of the circuit as a waveform. When the diode is forward-biased relative to the AC signal, it conducts a current and a voltage is generated.

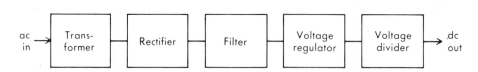

Fig. 3-1 Five stages of an electronic power supply.

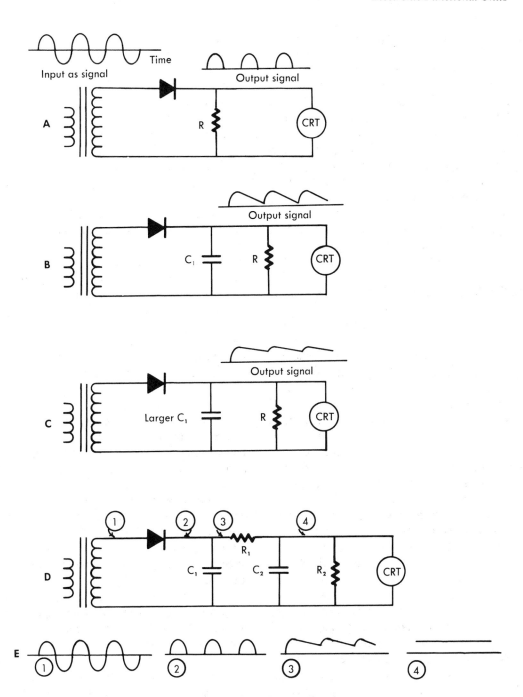

Fig. 3-2 Rectification and filtering.

When the diode is reverse-biased, it does not conduct a current and thus no output voltage is produced. The CRT registers the voltage output of the rectified circuit as a half-waveform that contains only the positive portion of the original AC signal. Note that the voltage level is discontinuous and not constant.

In Fig. 3-2, *B*, a capacitor (C_1) in parallel to R has been added to the circuit. When the diode

conducts a current, the capacitor becomes charged. When the conduction of the diode declines, the capacitor discharges its stored charge through R. The discharging of the capacitor has, in effect, "filled the voltage gap" that occurs when the diode is reverse-biased and thus not conducting a current. In Fig. 3-2, *C*, the capacitor in Fig. 3-2, *B*, has been replaced by a larger capacitor. The larger capacitor is capable of storing a larger charge. The current discharged from this capacitor fills the voltage gap better than the current discharged from the first (smaller) capacitor.

In Fig. 3-2, *D*, the filtering network is composed of two parallel capacitors, C_1 and C_2. The parallel configuration increases the overall capacitance. Also, having two capacitors in the circuit influences the amount of DC voltage variation received by each. For example, as C_1 charges and then discharges through R_1, C_2 receives a pulsating current of less variation than that of C_1. The function of C_2 is to discharge at a rate that will further reduce the amount of ripple. Frequently, electrolytic capacitors are used because of their ability to store a greater amount of electrostatic charge.

In Fig. 3-3, the resistor (R_1) from Fig. 3-2, *D*, has been replaced by an inductor. An inductor can also be used in the filtering process because it can also store electrical energy (as electromagnetic energy). The inductor, like the capacitor, stores energy when the diode conducts a current, and releases its stored energy when the diode does not conduct a current. Thus, as the magnetic field around the coil expands and contracts, current is either impeded or supplied to the circuit depending on the AC cycle. The release of the electrical energy stored in the inductor during the nonconducting phase of the diode helps to further reduce the amount ripple.

Different combinations of electronic filters can be used to obtain nearly pure direct current (i.e., direct current with an extremely low amount of ripple). However, the need to store very large quantities of energy over longer periods of time would require the use of large capacitors and inductors if half-wave rectification were used. In other words, large voltage gaps would have to be filled over time during the nonconducting phase of the diode(s). However, if a full-wave rectifier is substituted in the circuits described above, several other benefits can be achieved. Because both halves of the AC input sine wave would be used, the efficiency of the

power supply would double. The diodes would also conduct more frequently, and thus the total current provided by each would decrease substantially. This would increase the life expectancy of these electronic components because of less wear. Finally, a shorter period of time would be required to filter the power supply, therefore inductors and capacitors could be used that are smaller and less expensive.

Voltage Regulator. Constant DC current output would be obtained from power supplies if the AC input were always constant. Unfortunately, line voltage fluctuations can occur that ultimately cause a fluctuation of the output voltage from the power. Because most instruments require some form of constant DC voltage within a narrow range, the output voltage from the power supply must be regulated. This can be obtained by using electronic components called **voltage regulators**. Examples of these devices are the Zener diode and transistors. The use of transistors as electronic voltage regulators plays an important role in the regulation of current flow and thus can be used to maintain a constant voltage level. For the sake of simplicity, this discussion will be limited to the use of the Zener diode as a voltage regulating device. However, the basic underlying principle is similar.

A voltage regulator is an electronic device composed of a resistive element that responds to current change in an inverse manner. Its principle of operation is based on Ohm's law and the interrelationship of current, voltage, and resistance. When current flow through a voltage regulator increases, its resistance will decrease proportionately. Thus the voltage drop across the regulator remains constant. If strategically placed in a circuit, it will maintain a constant voltage at that point. In essence, all voltage regulators operate in this manner.

In Fig. 3-4, the resistor R in Fig. 3-3 has been replaced with a Zener diode. Current will flow through a reverse-biased Zener diode when its specific breakdown voltage (Zener voltage) is ex-

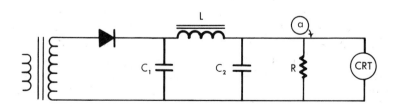

Fig. 3-3 Rectifier and filter.

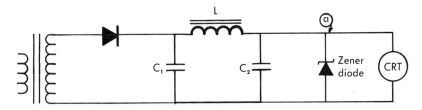

Fig. 3-4 Rectifier and filter with Zener diode voltage regulator.

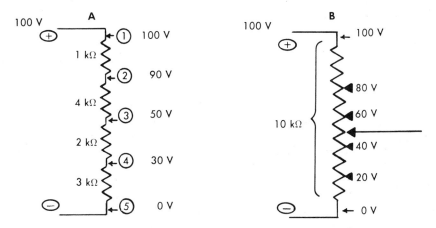

Fig. 3-5 Voltage divider.

ceeded. When this occurs, a large (avalanche) current will begin to flow through the Zener diode. However, its resistance will also decrease. Thus in Fig. 3-4 a constant voltage at point *a* is maintained.

Voltage Divider. The application of voltage division enables a power supply to meet specific DC voltage requirements of each circuit within an instrument. As shown in Fig. 3-5, different voltages may be obtained by dropping voltage across a series of resistors. Voltage may also be varied by using a potentiometer. The use of resistive components as **voltage dividers** has already been addressed in Chapter 2 and thus will not be reiterated here.

Detectors

Analysis of biologic fluids in the clinical laboratory is based on the detection of physicochemical properties that are characteristic of the analyte of interest. The primary mode of detection in most clinical laboratory instruments is the detection of light or radiant energy (photodetection). Detectors of temperature, gas composition, and radiation are also commonly used. Each mode of analysis requires a specific type of detector. Al-

though detectors differ in design, construction, and operational principle, the one characteristic they all have in common is their ability to detect one form of energy and convert it to another form. Such an electronic device is called a **transducer.** The detectors used in clinical laboratory instruments usually detect a physical or chemical property (i.e., light, heat, gas molecules, or radiation), which then is usually converted into electrical energy. An exception is the transducer that detects radiation: radiant energy is first converted to light or electromagnetic radiation by one type of transducer (i.e., the fluor of a scintillation counter), and is then converted to electrical energy by another transducer (i.e., photodetector). The electrical signal produced by the transducer is usually processed by a signal handling device (i.e., the signal is usually amplified before being directed to a readout device).

Photosensitive Detectors. Spectrophotometers, fluorometers, emission flame photometers, atomic absorption spectrophotometers, and optical cell counters are examples of instruments that use photodetectors. The photodetectors that will be covered in this section include the barrier-layer cell, phototube, photomultiplier tube, and a

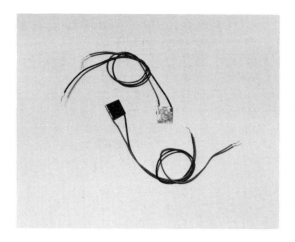

Fig. 3-6 Common selenium barrier-layer (photovoltaic) cell.

variety of semiconductor photodetectors (i.e., photoresistors, photodiodes, and phototransistors). All of these devices use photosensitive or photoemissive materials that release electrons when they are exposed to light energy. When a closed circuit is provided, the free electrons produce a photocurrent.

Photovoltaic Cell. The **photovoltaic cell,** also called the **barrier-layer cell,** generates its electrical output directly from light energy (Fig. 3-6), and thus does not require an external power source. Construction of the barrier-layer cell is shown in Fig. 3-7. A thin layer of semiconductor, usually selenium, is deposited on a metal base, usually iron. The selenium is coated with a very thin transparent layer of silver lacquer. A glass protective window is placed over the lacquered surface, and the cell is encased in plastic. The iron

acts as the positive electrode and the selenium as the negative electrode or collector. A wire lead extends through the plastic case from each of the two electrodes. When light passes through the glass and the lacquer and impinges upon the selenium surface, enough energy is provided to the selenium to cause liberation of some electrons. The emitted electrons are collected by the silver lacquer. When the photovoltaic cell is connected in a circuit, electrons flow from the collector, through the circuit, to the iron electrode, and finally back to the selenium. The current that is produced is directly proportional to the intensity of radiant energy striking the cell's photosensitive surface.

The spectral response of a selenium photovoltaic cell is from 380 to 700 nm. Its optimum response occurs at wavelengths between 500 to 600 nm (i.e., the colors green and yellow, which is similar to the human eye). The selenium barrier-layer cell is used mainly by older colorimeters or spectrophotometers that measure relatively high levels of illumination. Sophisticated instruments, such as spectrophotometers with narrow band passes, cannot use a barrier-layer cell as a photodetector because of the low level of radiant energy directed to the detector. It also exhibits a phenomenon known as "fatigue," which refers to the gradual decrease in a photocell's output voltage because of its continued exposure to radiant energy. High levels of illumination accentuate this fatigue effect. The voltage output of a photovoltaic cell is also highly sensitive to temperature changes.

Phototube. A **phototube** consists of a curved sheet of photosensitive material that serves as an emitter or cathode and a positively charged thin

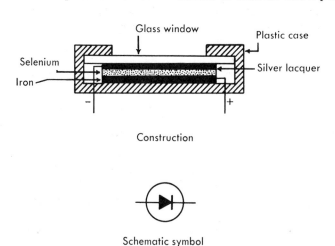

Construction

Schematic symbol

Fig. 3-7 Construction of barrier-layer (photovoltaic) cell.

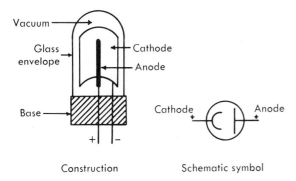

Fig. 3-8 Phototube construction and schematic symbol.

tube that serves as a collector or anode. The construction and schematic symbol of a phototube are shown in Fig. 3-8. The cathode of the phototube is coated with a photosensitive material (i.e., cesium-antimony and multi-alkali [Sb/K/Na/Cs]), that emits electrons when illuminated. The number of electrons emitted is directly proportional to the intensity of the radiant energy striking the cathode. The anode attracts or collects the electrons emitted from the cathode. Both cathode and anode are encased in an evacuated glass envelope. Both electrodes receive a DC potential that is provided by the instrument's power supply. One of the major drawbacks of a conventional phototube is the amount of photocurrent generated; it is very small and therefore must undergo considerable amplification before a suitable signal is obtained.

Photomultiplier Tube (PMT). Because of the inherent problems associated with the conventional phototube, most of these devices have been replaced with a photodetector called a **photomultiplier tube (PMT)**. The design and schematic symbols for the linear and circular PMT tubes are shown in Figs. 3-9 and 3-10. The photomultiplier tube consists of a cathode and anode and 9 to 16 photosensitive electrodes, called **dynodes,** which are all encased in an evacuated glass envelope. When radiant energy strikes the cathode, emitted electrons are attracted to the first dynode. Upon striking the dynode, each "primary" electron causes the emission of three to six "secondary" electrons. The electrons emitted from the first dynode are then focused and attracted to the second dynode, where the process is repeated. The chain reaction continues through the entire series of dynodes until the anode is reached. The result is an internal amplification of the initial signal (see Figs. 3-9 and 3-10). The internal amplification achieved by a photomultiplier tube can be as great as 10^6.

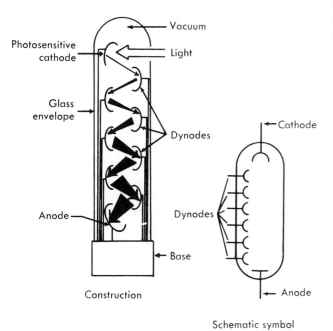

Fig. 3-9 Photomultiplier tube, linear design, and amplification process.

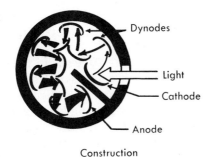

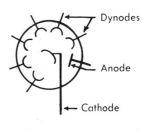

Fig. 3-10 Photomultiplier tube, circular cage design, and amplification process.

Electrons are directed to successive dynodes in two ways. First, the dynodes are orientated and designed so that electrons tend to be focused toward the next one. Second, each successive dynode has a higher positive potential than the previous one, thus attracting the electrons to the next dynode. Normally, the number of dynodes in a photomultiplier tube is limited to a maximum of 16. Like the conventional phototube, the number of emitted electrons/unit of time is directly proportional to the light intensity impinging on the photoemissive surface. However, the PMT is 200 times more sensitive than the conventional phototube-amplifier system. Also, the photomultiplier tube can respond to light interruptions of 10^9 per second. Conventional photomultiplier tubes are still used in many laboratory instruments that use photodetection as a means of specimen analysis.

Semiconductor Detectors. A semiconductor primarily is used in a circuit to regulate current flow by changing its internal resistance. This is accomplished by changing the potential bias across its P-N junction. The internal resistance of a transistor is also controlled in a similar manner. Unlike conventional semiconductors that respond to direct changes in voltage, semiconductor photodetectors such as photoresistors, photodiodes, and phototransistors respond to bias changes resulting from absorption of radiant energy. Semiconductor photodetectors have virtually replaced conventional phototubes and in many cases photomultiplier tubes in modern laboratory instruments. Some of the more common types of these photodetectors that regulate current are depicted in Fig. 3-11.

Photoresistor. The simplest semiconductor photodetector is the **photoresistor.** A photoresistor is an evacuated cell containing two leads attached to a thin layer of photoconductive material (i.e., selenides of cadmium or lead), deposited on a transparent material such as quartz or glass. The device is connected in the circuit so that it receives a constant potential. When photons impinge on the exposed photoconductive material, an increase or decrease in its resistance occurs. With a change in resistance there is a change in current that corresponds to the intensity of impinging light. The photoresistor's photoconductive material characteristically responds to ultraviolet, visible, and infrared radiant energy.

Photodiode. A conventional P-N junction diode is converted to a photodiode by adding a collimating lens that focuses incident light on the

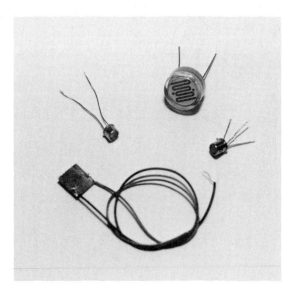

Fig. 3-11   Common types of semiconductor photodetectors.

junction. The photodiode is placed in a reverse-biased orientation in the detection circuit. When light impinges on the photodiode, electrons are freed from covalent bonds of the semiconducting materials composing its junction. The liberated electrons cause current to flow through the circuit. As the radiant energy of the incident light increases, the current increases and vice versa.

Phototransistors. Phototransistors (PT) and photo-field effect transistors (PFET) use their collimating lenses to focus incident light onto a photosensitive material in an area called the base or gate. To function properly, they must be appropriately "biased" in the circuit (biasing will be discussed later in this chapter). When radiant energy strikes the photosensitive material in the base or gate, electrons are excited and move into the collector-to-emitter (in the PT) or drain-to-source (in the PFET) conduction area. The result is a current that is proportional to the incident radiant energy. Unlike photodiodes, phototransistors can also amplify the signal. Typically the signal is increased 50 to 500 times that of most photodiodes.

Temperature Detector. In the clinical laboratory, it is often necessary to determine the osmolality of various biologic fluids. Osmolality is influenced by the number of particles of the solution, which in turn is inversely related to its freezing point. The osmolality of a fluid can be indirectly determined by using a detector called a **thermistor,** which is found in an instrument called a freezing point osmometer. A thermistor is a transducer that converts changes in temperature (heat) to resistance (Fig. 3-12). Therefore a change in temperature can be used to quantify the number of particles in a solution and thus its osmolality.

The thermistor consists of a small button constructed of a fused mixture of metal oxides, attached to two leads, and encapsulated in glass

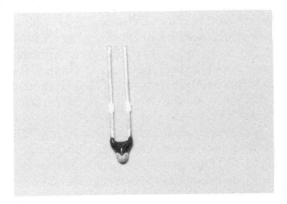

Fig. 3-12 Thermistor.

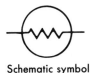

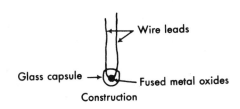

Fig. 3-13 Construction of thermistor and electrical symbol.

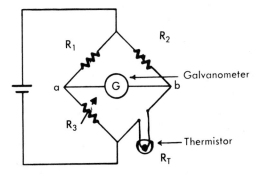

Fig. 3-14 Thermistor in a Wheatstone bridge circuit.

(Fig. 3-13). The metal oxide mixture has a large negative temperature coefficient of resistance, meaning that a small decrease in temperature causes a relatively large increase in the resistance of the thermistor. This characteristic and its small size make this device a useful thermodetector, especially when small quantities of material are measured.

Because a change in temperature can be determined indirectly by measuring the thermistor's resistance, a special circuit called a **Wheatstone bridge** can be used to measure this resistance (Fig. 3-14). R_1 and R_2 are fixed resistors of known value; R_3 is a variable resistor that is used as a rheostat, and R_T is the resistance of the thermistor (see Fig. 3-14). If R_1 equals R_2, and R_3 equals R_T, the circuit is then balanced; there is no voltage difference between points a and b, and thus no current flows through the galvanometer. As the temperature changes, the thermistor's resistance changes and a current flows through the galvanometer. After the circuit is rebalanced using the variable resistor R_3, the resistance of the thermistor R_T is once again equal to R_3. The current can then be related to resistance change (as measured by the variable resistor) and is then converted to a change in temperature. If the value of R_3 is read on a scale that is calibrated in units of osmolality, the temperature change of a solution can then be related to its osmolality.

Gas Detectors. A gas chromatograph is an instrument used in the clinical laboratory to separate, identify, and quantify volatile compounds in biologic fluids. The fluid is first vaporized and then carried through a column by the constant flow of an inert gas. Identification of the compound is based on the time required for it to reach the detector. Quantitation of the compound is based on the detector's response and subsequent conversion of this signal into an electrical parameter. The detector must be very sensitive because a small sample size is often used. Detectors that are commonly used in gas chromatography are one of the following types: thermal conductivity, flame ionization, nitrogen-phosphorous, or electron capture.

Thermal Conductivity Detector (TCD). Analysis by thermal conductivity is based on the difference in the rate of heat conduction (thermal conductivity) between pure carrier gas and the carrier with a sample mixture. The thermal conductivity of the pure carrier gas is greater than that of the gas containing sample (effluent from the column). If each of these gases were to flow at a constant rate over a heated filament, the carrier gas would cool the filament faster than the gas containing the sample. The resistance of most metals increases with an increase in temperature. Therefore the difference in the rates at which gases cool a metal filament can be measured as a difference in resistance. The difference in resistances between that generated by pure carrier and carrier containing vaporized sample can in turn be related to the molecular concentration of the sample.

Fig. 3-15 illustrates a **thermal conductivity detector.** Usually four heat-sensing filaments with closely matched resistances are connected to form the arms of a Wheatstone bridge circuit. The bridge arrangement is enclosed in a temperature regulated chamber. The pure carrier gas and the gas containing sample from the column (effluent) flow at a constant rate over filaments 3 and 4 and filaments 1 and 2. When a gas containing sample passes over filaments 1 and 2, the mixture has a lower thermal conductivity compared with the pure gas passing over filaments 3 and 4. The mixture does not cool the filament as well as pure carrier gas. The increase in filament temperature causes an increase in the filament resistance. The Wheatstone bridge becomes unbalanced, a current is amplified, and then is directed to the readout device. This variation in current is directly proportional to the sample concentration in the carrier gas.

Flame Ionization Detector (FID). The operation of the **flame ionization detector** (Fig. 3-16) is based on the principle that combustion of organic compounds produces ionic fragmentation and free electrons. Ions and electrons between two oppositely charged electrodes will conduct a current between those electrodes. The flame ion-

ization detector consists of a hydrogen flame positioned between two electrodes that are charged with a high polarizing voltage. The eluted components in the carrier gas are ionized by burning them in a mixture of hydrogen and air. The ionic fragments and free electrons conduct current between the two electrodes, which then decreases the effective resistance between them. The more ions and electrons that are generated, the greater the decrease in resistance, and thus the greater the increase in current through the circuit. The increased current causes an increase in the voltage drop across resistor R in Fig. 3-16. The increased output voltage is amplified before being directed to a readout device. The response of the FID is directly proportional to the number of carbons in a molecule bound to hydrogen or other carbon atoms.

Nitrogen Phosphorous Detector (NPD). The **nitrogen-phosphorous detector** is illustrated in Fig. 3-17. This type of detector is similar to a flame ionization detector except that ions of an alkali metal (rubidium) are introduced into a hydrogen flame. When a compound containing nitrogen or phosphorous is burned in the flame, alkali metal vapor is released at an increased rate and then becomes ionized. The increase in ionization causes an increase in current flow. This overall process results in an enhanced sensitivity for detecting nitrogen and phosphorous containing compounds.

Electron-Capture Detector (ECD). The **electron-capture detector** is used to quantify large organic molecules, particularly halogens, by capturing electrons and thus forming negatively

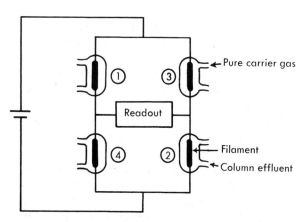

Fig. 3-15   Thermal conductivity detector (TCD).

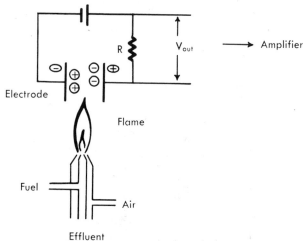

Fig. 3-16   Flame ionization detector (FID).

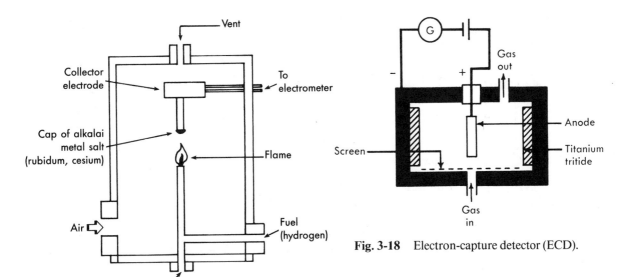

Fig. 3-17 Nitrogen-phosphorous detector (NPD).

Fig. 3-18 Electron-capture detector (ECD).

charged ions. The construction of the electron-capture detector is represented in Fig. 3-18. Within the chamber are a cathode, an anode, and a source of beta particles (β), which are high speed electrons emitted from the nucleus of a radioactive material such as titanium tritide. As the carrier gas (nitrogen or argon) flows through the detector, the beta particles cause ionization of the gas molecules, thereby producing electrons and positive ions. The electrons are attracted to the anode. The large positive ions are usually swept out of the chamber before reaching the cathode and thus contribute very little to the current in the circuit. While the carrier gas flows through the chamber, a constant current flows through the circuit. When a column effluent containing organic molecules enters the chamber, the organic molecules capture the free electrons to form large negative ions that are removed from the chamber before reaching the anode. This results in fewer negative charges reaching the anode and therefore a decrease in the current in the circuit. Thus there is an inverse relationship between current flow and the quantity of organic molecules in the column effluent.

Radiation Detectors. Some clinical laboratory tests require instruments that detect gamma or beta radiation. All instruments for the detection and measurement of radiation require a sensing element that converts radiation energy to electrical energy. First, a special type of transducer is needed to detect the radiation. A **fluor** is a substance that emits light when exposed to radiation.

Therefore it behaves as a transducer because it converts radiation to light energy. The light energy can then be converted to electrical energy by using a photosensitive device (i.e., photomultiplier tube).

A fluor can be a solid or a liquid depending on the type of radiation (i.e., gamma or beta emission) to be detected. The most common means of detecting radiation is via the production of flashes of light or **scintillations.** Detection of gamma radiation (solid scintillation counting) requires the use of a solid fluor that is usually composed of a single large crystal of sodium iodide containing thallium. The thallium-activated sodium iodide crystal characteristically emits photons at a visible wavelength suitable for detection by photomultiplier tubes. Detection of beta radiation involves the use of a liquid fluor that is added to a solvent (often toluene). These fluors, when excited, emit photons in the near ultraviolet and visible regions. They generally compose less than 1% of the solvent-fluor mixture.

Signal Processing Units

After conversion of physical or chemical energy to electrical energy by the detector, the electrical signal is changed in various ways by devices called signal processing units. Signal processing units perform specific functions such as amplification, counting and mathematical manipulations, including addition, subtraction, multiplication, division, integration, and differentiation. This section reviews the principles of amplification with solid state devices; it also briefly describes integrated circuits, printed circuit boards, operational amplifiers, and several types of signal

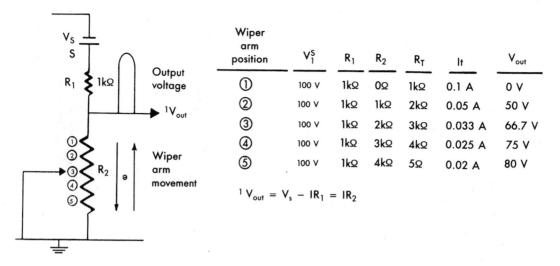

Wiper arm position	V_1^S	R_1	R_2	R_T	It	V_{out}
①	100 V	1kΩ	0Ω	1kΩ	0.1 A	0 V
②	100 V	1kΩ	1kΩ	2kΩ	0.05 A	50 V
③	100 V	1kΩ	2kΩ	3kΩ	0.033 A	66.7 V
④	100 V	1kΩ	3kΩ	4kΩ	0.025 A	75 V
⑤	100 V	1kΩ	4kΩ	5Ω	0.02 A	80 V

$$^1 V_{out} = V_s - IR_1 = IR_2$$

Fig. 3-19   Conceptual amplification.

processing circuits used in mathematical operations.

Amplification. Often the signal of an electronic circuit of an instrument needs to be amplified. As previously mentioned, output signals from detectors may be amplified before being directed to readout devices. **Amplification** is simply changing a small input signal into an output signal of larger magnitude. The concept of amplification uses the application of voltage division. Fig. 3-19 illustrates the concept of amplification. The voltage source (V_s) is a constant DC source of 100 V, R_1 is a fixed resistor, and R_2 is a variable resistor that can change from 0 Ω to 4 KΩ. R_T and I_T represent the total resistance and current of the circuit. Note that the output voltage (V_{out}) is equal to the voltage drop over the variable resistor R_2. When the wiper arm of R_2 is moved completely upward, its resistance is zero. Thus the entire voltage from the DC source is dropped over R_1. Because zero volts are dropped over R_2, the output voltage (V_{out}) is also zero. As the wiper arm on R_2 is moved downward, its resistance increases. This increase in the resistance of R_2 causes a greater portion of the DC voltage to be dropped over that resistor, thus increasing V_{out}. In essence it is the change in the "effective" resistance of the variable resistor that is affecting the amplification of the output signal. If R_2 is very sensitive to changes in resistance, a small change in the wiper arm position produces a large change in its resistance. Therefore a small movement of the R_2 wiper arm would result in a large voltage change at the output. This is essentially how a small input voltage affects a semiconductor transistor amplifier, which will be discussed in a later section of this chapter.

The degree to which a signal can be increased by an amplifier is referred to as its **gain**. The amplifier gain is the ratio of output voltage to input voltage or:

$$\text{Gain} = V_{out}/V_{in}$$

For example, if an input voltage of 0.1 V results in an output voltage of 10 V, the gain of the amplifier is:

$$\text{Gain} = V_{out}/V_{in} = 10 \text{ V}/0.1 \text{ V} = 100$$

Several types of amplifiers have been developed, including semiconductor transistor and operational amplifiers. Construction, schematic representation, and operational principles of each type are briefly discussed in the following sections.

Semiconductor Transistors. The name **transistor** is derived from its functional application. When this semiconductor device was first developed in 1948, it was recognized that its resistance could be changed to regulate current flow in a circuit. The device was initially called a transfer resistor. This functional description later changed to transistor.

Bipolar Transistors. The first semiconductor transistors to be developed were called NPN and PNP junction transistors. They are called junction transistors because charge movement is regulated internally at the junction where the semiconductor materials are fused. An NPN transistor consists of two N-type semiconductor wafers sandwiched between a P-type semicon-

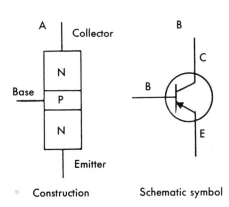 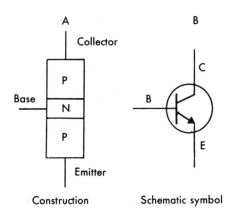

Fig. 3-20 NPN transistor; arrow in schematic symbol represents direction of electron flow.

Fig. 3-21 PNP transistor; arrow in schematic symbol represents direction of electron flow.

ductor (Fig. 3-20, *A*). A **PNP transistor** is composed of N-type semiconductor material sandwiched between two P-type semiconductor wafers (Fig. 3-21, *A*). In both types of transistors, the middle semiconductor material layer, called the base *B*, is very thin (approximately 0.001 inch thick). The other two semiconductor elements in the transistor are called the collector *C*, and the emitter *E*. Schematic symbols for NPN and PNP transistors are shown in Fig. 3-20, *B*, and Fig. 3-21, *B*.

The emitter of the transistor is functionally equivalent to the cathode, and the collector is equivalent to the plate. The direction of electron current flow through a transistor is indicated by the emitter arrows in the schematic symbol. The emitter is the source of free electrons and "holes" in NPN and PNP transistors. Current flow through a transistor is from emitter to base and then to the collector. In the NPN transistor, it is the flow of electrons (negative charges), whereas in the PNP transistor, it is the holes (positive

charges). Movement of charges in the direction indicated above is achieved by biasing the electrodes of the transistors (i.e., applying fixed DC potentials of different levels on each of the three electrodes). The base controls the current flow through the transistor by biasing the base-emitter potential. Transistors must be correctly biased to allow current flow. If a positive potential is applied to the P-type semiconductor and a negative potential is applied to the N-type semiconductor, the P-N junction will be forward-biased. If a positive potential is applied to the N-type semiconductor and a negative potential is applied to the P-type semiconductor, the P-N junction will be reverse-biased.

If an NPN transistor is properly biased, the emitter will be at a negative potential (Fig. 3-22, *A*). This will repel electrons toward the base, which is positively charged. The electrons from the emitter thus pass through the very thin base region to the collector, which has a potential that is more positive than the base. Current flow

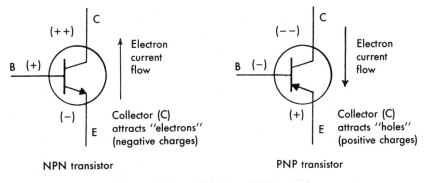

Fig. 3-22 Biasing of PNP and NPN transistors.

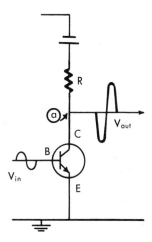

Fig. 3-23 NPN transistor amplifier.

tive half-cycle), the base becomes more positive with respect to the emitter. It therefore attracts more electrons from the emitter, causing an increase in current flow within the circuit. With an increase in current, the voltage drop over R is greater and thus the voltage at point *a* decreases. When the input signal swings negative, the emitter-base bias decreases, which causes fewer electrons to be attracted to the base and thus to the collector. The net effect is to reduce current flow, and therefore less voltage is dropped across R. In this case the voltage at point *a* increases. Note that a small input signal produces an output signal not only of greater amplitude, but also one that is 180 degrees out of phase with the input signal. A similar process occurs with a PNP transistor. The difference is that "hole" movement rather than electron movement is regulated at the base.

Field Effect Transistor (FET). The junction transistors discussed previously have limited usefulness if a signal must be amplified without significantly draining the current from the signal source. To limit the current drain from the voltage source, an amplifier with high input impedance must be used. A semiconductor amplifier that provides a high input impedance is the **field effect transistor** (Fig. 3-24). Frequently, an FET is used as the first stage (at the input) of a multistage amplifier. A multistage amplifier consists of many individual amplifying transistors connected collector-to-base in series, with each transistor amplifying the output signal of the previous one.

Field effect transistors are of two types, N-channel and P-channel. The construction and the schematic symbol of an N-channel semicon-

through a PNP transistor is somewhat different (Fig. 3-22, *B*). In the PNP transistor the charges that move through the transistor are holes (positive charges) rather than electrons. The positive potential on the emitter of the PNP transistor repels the holes into the base region. The holes are attracted first by the negative potential on the base, and then by the more negative potential on the collector.

When an AC input source is connected to the base, the potential difference between the base and the emitter will change depending on the half-cycle (positive vs negative) and the amplitude of the AC signal. In an NPN transistor (Fig. 3-23) a change in the emitter-base bias changes the current flow through the transistor and thus the output voltage at point *a*. With an AC input signal having been introduced at the base (posi-

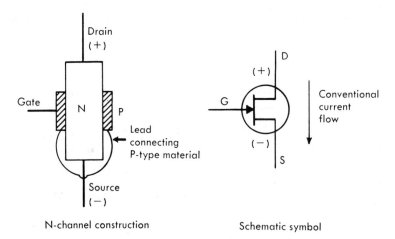

N-channel construction   Schematic symbol

Fig. 3-24 Field effect transistor (FET).

ductor FET are shown in Fig. 3-24. The FET consists of a bar of semiconductor material called the channel, which is N-type (for N-channel) or P-type (for P-channel). An electrode is connected to each end of the channel. These electrodes are called the source (S) and the drain (D). The N-channel is fused between two layers of P-type semiconductor called the gate (G). Some FETs are designed with a gate consisting of a sleeve of P-type material around the N-channel.

The effective resistance of the FET is controlled by the potential applied to the gate. In the N-channel FET, the electrons flow from the negatively charged source to the positively charged drain. When a negative voltage is applied to the gate, electron flow through the N-channel is hindered. The greater the negative potential on the gate, the greater the impedance to electron flow. Thus current flow decreases. The gate therefore controls the flow of current through the channel.

Another FET that has an extremely high impedance is an insulated-gate FET called a **metal oxide semiconductor field effect transistor (MOSFET).** This modified FET consists of a gate insulated from the channel by a thin film of metal oxide. Like an FET, the gate's electrostatic field controls charge flow through the channel. The MOSFET has the highest input impedance (as high as 10^{10} Ω) of any transistor. Examples of different types of transistors are shown in Fig. 3-25.

Integrated Circuits. The evolution of electronic devices that led to the development of specifically designed semiconductors, discrete transistors, and associated circuitry has given rise to the **integrated circuit** (IC). An integrated circuit (Fig. 3-26) is a tiny electronic circuit fabricated on a piece of a semiconductor made of silicon or gallium, referred to as a **chip.** Today, diodes, transistors, FETs, resistors, capacitors, and asso-

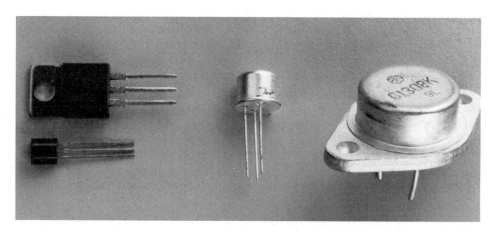

Fig. 3-25 Different types of transistors. (Courtesy Radio Shack, a division of Tandy Corporation.)

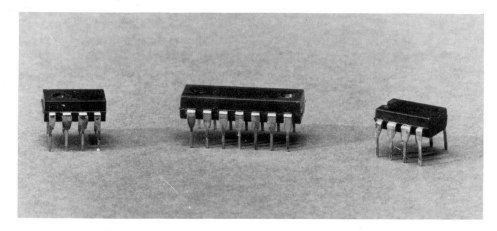

Fig. 3-26 Integrated circuits. (Courtesy Radio Shack, a division of Tandy Corporation.)

ciated connections can be built into such small devices. Repair of ICs is virtually impossible; therefore they are usually replaced. Such disposable electronic circuits are feasible because they are relatively inexpensive. Integrated circuits are used in all modern instruments of the clinical laboratory. With the development of integrated circuits, miniaturization in electronics has become a reality. Another example of a more sophisticated IC is the large-scale integrated circuit (LSI), which is an IC chip containing an entire instrument circuit or a major portion of it. LSI circuitry permits microminiaturization of instruments. Digital computers and small calculators were the first instruments to contain the LSI circuit. Now, most laboratory instruments contain such circuitry.

Printed Circuit Boards. By combining these miniaturized, simplified devices on **printed circuit boards,** instruments can be repaired in the field by simply replacing the entire board (Fig. 3-27). This enables the field service engineer or even in some cases a competent medical technologist to reduce the time involved diagnosing the cause of instrument failure. Replacing an instrument board is not always a complicated procedure and can reduce extensive instrument downtime, especially if service personnel are not readily available. However, it is important to receive some kind of guidance by the manufacturer for board replacement and to use electrical safety precautions.

Operational Amplifiers (QA or Op Amp). The **operational amplifier** is a multistage amplifier system contained within one small unit or package (Fig. 3-28). Like the solid-state devices dis-

cussed earlier, the Op Amp is replaced rather than repaired. The name "operational amplifier" was derived from its ability to perform mathematical "operations" on a signal or signals. The flexibility and versatility of the Op Amp provide for a multitude of applications, all of which are used in the signal processing units of clinical laboratory instruments. A few of the many mathematical operations performed by the Op Amp include addition, subtraction, integration, differentiation, logarithm derivation, antilogarithm derivation, multiplication, and division.

The Op Amp unit is available in different shapes and sizes, each having several (8 to 16) terminals (Fig. 3-28). These terminals are connected to biasing voltages and associated circuitry. The terminals discussed in this brief section are the two input terminals and one output terminal. As shown in Fig. 3-29, the output terminals are conventionally marked $-$ and $+$ for inverting input and noninverting input. A signal applied to the inverting input terminal produces a signal of the opposite sign at the output terminal (i.e., the output signal compared with the input signal is inverted). If a signal is applied to the noninverting input terminal, the output signals have the same sign.

The function performed by an Op Amp is determined by the external circuitry. Fig. 3-30 shows an amplifier circuit that is commonly used to increase an input signal. The Op Amp has a large input impedance of at least 10^5 and a high gain of at least 10^4 Ω. The gain of an operational amplifier circuit is calculated using the following expression:

$$Gain_{Op\ Amp} = R_2/R_1$$

where:

R_1 = Resistance of input resistor

R_2 = Feedback resistance

Examples of mathematical operations performed by Op Amp circuits are described using Fig. 3-31 as a reference guide. A detailed understanding of the operation of each sample Op

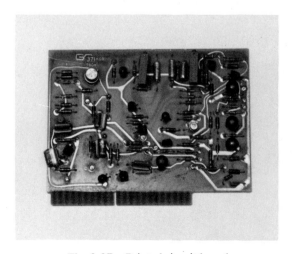

Fig. 3-27 Printed circuit board.

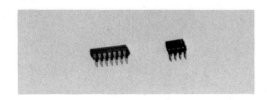

Fig. 3-28 Common operational amplifiers.

Amp circuit is not necessary. The examples are provided only to demonstrate the versatility of the Op Amp in performing different functions by changing and/or rearranging associated circuit components.

Addition of signals is achieved by establishing a circuit with a resistor in the feedback loop at *b* and parallel resistors at *a*, with each resistor conducting one of the input signals to be added. The output of the Op Amp will be the negative sum of the input signals. Two signals can be subtracted in an Op Amp circuit by placing a resistor at *b* and two parallel resistors at *a*, with one input signal having a positive sign and the other a negative sign. Integration is achieved in an Op Amp circuit by having a resistor at *a* and a capacitor at *b*. Measurement of area is obtained through the operation of integration. Differentiation is obtained by exchanging the components in the integration circuit. Thus an Op Amp circuit that contains a differentiator has a capacitor at *a* and a resistor at

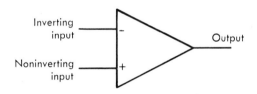

Fig. 3-29 Operational amplifier schematic symbol.

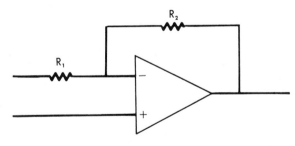

Fig. 3-30 Common operational amplifier circuit.

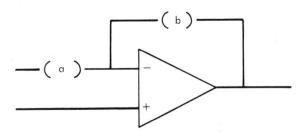

Fig. 3-31 Operational amplifier; optional associated circuitry for mathematical operations.

b. Measurement of slope or rate change is achieved through the operation of differentiation. Logarithmic function is obtained from a log Op Amp circuit, which has a resistor at *a* and a P-N junction diode in a forward-biased orientation at *b*. This operation makes possible the direct conversion of transmittance to absorbance in spectrophotometry. Antilogarithms can be obtained from an Op Amp circuit with a forward-biased P-N junction diode at *a* and a resistor at *b*. Multiplication and division are more complex operations and require the application of three Op Amp circuits. To multiply or divide, first the logarithms of the variables are obtained. Then, these logs are added for multiplication or subtracted for division, and finally, the antilogarithms are extracted.

Basic Circuits Used in Signal Manipulation. The modular design of modern instrumentation has developed through the use of operational amplifiers and integrated circuitry. Because operational amplifiers have a multiplicity of applications, they are found in most instruments in which signal handling, simple or complex, is required. In clinical laboratory instruments, the signal generated or affected during sample analysis is processed through a number of signal manipulations before being presented to the readout device. Some of the basic types of circuits that are involved in signal manipulation are described below.

Amplifier Circuits. When the term amplifier is referred to in a broader sense, all the components in a complex circuit that are necessary to amplify the signal are considered including devices such as conventional transistors, power transistors, FETs, and MOSFETs. The amplifier circuit may have more than one amplifying electronic component. If so, it is said to have more than one stage of amplification.

Log-to-Linear Converters. With a photodetector, the proportion of the light that reaches the detector is known as the percent transmittance (%T). Unlike absorbance, the relationship between %T and concentration is not linear, but rather logarithmic. It is possible to pass the photosignal from a light detector through a log-to-linear converter and produce an electric signal that is linear with concentration. This allows the technologist to read the concentration of a solution directly on a digital meter.

Analog-to-Digital Converters. Whenever the current from a photocell, pH electrode, or other type of transducer is measured, a signal is received that is analogous to the parameter being measured. To know what that electric signal means, a comparison must be made to a similar one from a standard. The electric signal that is comparable with, or analogous to, the parameter being measured is called an analog signal. If it is necessary to tell a computer, for example, what this signal means, the signal must be converted into numbers or digits (signal becomes digitized). An analog-to-digital (A-to-D) converter is a circuit that performs this task.

Integrators. An integrator is an electronic device that continuously sums the product of time vs rate to give a cumulative total of some variable (i.e., determining the area under the curve of the graph). Because many of the measured phenomena are variables, this is an important device. Integration is accomplished electronically by a battery of capacitors that digitize a variable electric signal into units that can be counted.

Discriminator Circuit. Whenever a cell counter senses a blood cell or a gamma detector senses a radioactive emission, the detection process may be thought of as an electronic event that produces a signal or pulse. The amplitude of the pulse can be measured, and if the technologist is looking for a specific size of cell or one isotope, all impulses that do not meet the set criteria can be screened out. For example, the pulse from a white blood cell will be considerably larger than that of a red blood cell. Thus the two cell types can be distinguished by measuring their electrical pulses using a **discriminator circuit.** A capacitor can be set up in the circuit in such a way that only impulses exceeding a predetermined level pass onto a detector. All smaller pulses are shorted out to ground. This arrangement would be called a lower, or threshold, discriminator. Another capacitor arrangement can be used whereby all signals that exceed a given level are shorted out to ground. This arrangement would be called an upper discriminator. Both lower and upper discriminators can be used in a circuit that allows only signals that exceed a predetermined minimum level but are less than a predetermined maximum level to pass onto a detector. This would leave an electrical window through which only the pulses of interest would pass.

If a large number of signals are being processed in a brief period of time, sometimes two signals will occur at exactly the same instant and appear to be one signal that is twice as large. This coincidence can be anticipated if the duration of the impulse and the approximate number of im-

pulses that occur each second are known. If the number/second is large, so will be the number of coincidences. It is mathematically possible to calculate the probability of coincidence and electronically correct for the error involved. Hence, the use of an anticoincidence circuit may be added to a discriminator to correct for coincidence.

Counting Circuits. After the pulses have been discriminated in the manner just described, it may be necessary to count them (i.e., the blood cells or gamma emissions that the pulses represent). This function requires some sort of counting circuit. The selected pulses can occur so rapidly that it is difficult to count them accurately. For this reason, a scaler, which selects only a representative number of pulses for counting, may be added. Two types are common. The binary scaler can be set to select every second pulse so that a count of two, four, eight, sixteen, thirty-two, etc. can be taken. The decade scaler will count every tenth impulse; the progression is 1, 10, 100, 1000, 10,000, etc.

Current-Summing Devices. These circuits generally make use of capacitors to store all of the current involved in an operation, such as the counting of impulses of a given size during a selected interval. This electrical total can then be used for further operations such as averaging or integration.

Feedback Circuits. When part of the output of an amplifier is returned to the input side to achieve some desirable effect, it is termed a **feedback circuit.** Negative feedback is often used in amplifiers to stabilize the gain of the amplifier. Feedback information can also be used to inform the instrument of changes in conditions that can cause it to modify its performance. These types of circuits are incorporated into instruments that use robotics and sensing devices during their operation. When connected to a readout device (i.e., a computer), it can provide invaluable information pertaining to instrument status and potential problems.

Readout Devices

Readout systems that are currently used in clinical laboratory instrumentation have become very sophisticated and increasingly complex. However, all **readout devices** serve the same purpose: to measure an electrical signal such as a change in current, voltage, or resistance, that has been generated by the instrument's detector and then convert it into a presentable format. Note that a proportionality exists between the concentration of the analyte of interest and the generated electrical signal that eventually reaches the readout. Thus an electrical signal can be related to the concentration of the analyte by calibrating an instrument in the proper units (i.e., concentration, transmittance, absorbance, etc.).

Analog vs Digital Devices. An **analog device** produces an electrical signal that has continuous values. The continuous signal can then be used to rotate a mechanical device such as a meter pointer. A **digital device** produces an electrical signal that is converted to a binary system (i.e., using a binary code, digits 0 and 1). Many solid-state readout devices require conversion of an analog signal to a digital signal before they can be activated (i.e., a set of light-emitting diodes [LEDs]). Although some analog devices are discussed in this section, the readouts of most modern instruments and many measuring devices now contain sophisticated digitalized components. Some of the instrument readout or display devices that will be covered in this section include analog meters and recorders, digital displays, and oscilloscopes.

Meters. The meter face and the meter movement are housed within a case that is usually made of an insulating material such as plastic. A calibrated scale using the appropriate units is displayed on the meter face. The meter movement is an internal device that deflects from a preset position when current is applied. The degree of deflection is related to the current flow through the meter movement. The operation of most meter movements used in clinical laboratory instruments is based on electromagnetic theory.

Meters that measure current flow are based on the interaction of the poles of a permanent magnetic field with those of an induced electromag-

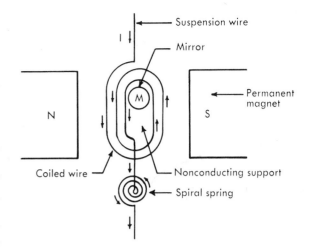

Fig. 3-32 d'Arsonval galvanometer.

netic field. It consists of a coiled wire positioned between the two poles of a permanent magnet. The induced electromagnetic poles of the coil are in close proximity to the corresponding poles of the permanent magnet. Thus, when a current flows through the coiled wire, the like poles will repel and the coil will deflect, or rotate. A coiled spring is attached to the coiled wire assembly to control its degree of deflection and return it to its original position once current no longer flows through the coiled wire. This is the principle of the **d'Arsonval,** or **moving coil meter movement,** which is used in galvanometers, electronic measuring devices, and clinical laboratory instruments with meter readouts.

Galvanometer. A **galvanometer** is a device capable of detecting very small amounts of current. The galvanometer moving element assembly and its optical arrangement are illustrated in Figs. 3-32 and 3-33. The assembly consists of a perma-

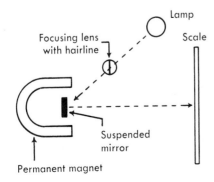

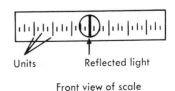

Fig. 3-33 Galvanometer optical arrangement.

nent magnet and a delicately suspended moving element. Its degree of rotation is controlled by a very flexible spiral spring that carries a current. The moving element consists of a fine wire wound around a lightweight nonconducting material on which is mounted a small mirror. The principle of operation is identical to that of the moving coil movement described above. As current flows through the suspension wire, the coil, and the spring of the galvanometer, a magnetic field is generated around the coil that causes the mirror attached to the moving coil assembly to rotate (see Fig. 3-32). A light beam is reflected from the mirror and is then directed to a translucent readout scale. A hairline on the focusing lens is used to indicate the readout point on the scale. As the moving assembly rotates, the reflected light from the mirror moves across the readout scale. When the current through the coil stops, the electromagnetic field around the coil collapses and the moving assembly is returned to its initial or zero position by the spiral spring. The "zero adjust" on the galvanometer is used to adjust the spiral spring tension when no current is flowing through the coil. Because of its delicate nature, the galvanometer is susceptible to damage from small mechanical shocks. Therefore instruments that contain galvanometers (some spectrophotometers and osmometers) should be handled carefully.

d'Arsonval Meter. The *d'Arsonval meter* is a modified galvanometer, and thus its operation is based on the same principle as the moving coil movement (Fig. 3-34). The meter movement assembly is positioned between the curved magnetic poles of a permanent magnet. The meter movement assembly consists of a coil of fine wire wound on an iron mandrel support fitted with hardened-steel pivots and mounted on jeweled bearings. The jeweled bearings allow the moving element to rotate with minimum friction. A pointer attached to the moving assembly deflects across the meter face as the moving element rotates. Matched coiled hair springs are attached above and below the coiled assembly to control its degree of rotation and return to a fixed reference point where no current flow exists.

The d'Arsonval meter is not as sensitive as the galvanometer, therefore it is used in instruments if the amount of measured current does not require a high degree of sensitivity. This meter can also be damaged by mechanical shock or excess current being applied to its circuitry. The principle of the d'Arsonval meter movement is used in a device called the "analog" volt-ohm-milliammeter (VOM), which is used to measure current, voltage, and resistance in electrical circuits (discussed in Chapter 4). Some laboratory instrument meters also use this principle. However, their meter faces are usually calibrated in units of absorbance, transmittance, and concentration.

Recorders. Recorders are readout devices that are still used in some clinical laboratory instruments (i.e., gas chromatographs, high performance liquid chromatographs [HPLCs], and spectrophotometers). However, in newer instru-

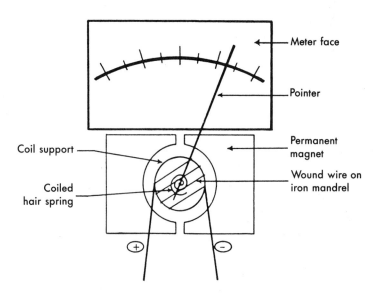

Fig. 3-34 d'Arsonval meter.

ments, many recorders have been replaced by dot matrix, laser, or thermal printers. Functionally, meters and recorders are the same (i.e., a signal is produced by the detector and then processed by the signal processing unit to display the data in a clear and descriptive manner). Unlike meters, recorders present data in the form of a permanent record. The two major classifications of recorders are the galvanometer recorders and the potentiometric recorders, the latter being used more often in the clinical laboratory.

Galvanometric (Moving Coil) Recorders. The moving coil or galvanometer recorder is based on the same electromagnetic principle as the operation of the moving coil meter. A transcribing device records the rotation of the moving coil assembly. These devices are of two types, indirect writing and direct writing. The type of galvanometric recorder is dictated by the type of indicator attached to the moving coil. The indicator element on an "indirect" writing recorder is usually an ink jet expelled from a capillary onto the moving chart paper. The recorder is classified as a high frequency recorder, which means that its signal recording occurs at a rate of up to 1 kHz or 1000 signals/second.

The "direct" writing recorders are classified as medium frequency recorders. They respond to frequencies up to a maximum of 105 Hz. Direct writing recorders are available with an ink pen or a heated stylus attached to the moving coil assembly. The ink pen type uses untreated chart paper on which the ink flows by capillary action to produce a permanent chart tracing. The heat stylus indicator requires the use of "heat sensitive" paper. Both types of recorders use chart paper as the permanent record. A chart drive moves the chart paper at a constant rate. The indicator element traces the output data onto the chart paper. Thus the recorded data are presented on a time axis.

Potentiometric Recorders. The potentiometric recorder is classified as a low-frequency recorder, responding to signals from 0 to approximately 5 Hz. The potentiometric recorder uses a null-balancing measuring system, which is illustrated in Fig. 3-35 as a simple block diagram. The input voltage is from an analytical instrument (e.g., a spectrophotometer). The reference voltage is a constant voltage source supplied by a mercury cell or generated by the power supply within the circuit. The difference between the input voltage (V_{in}) and the reference voltage (V_{ref}) is called the error voltage (V_{error}):

$$V_{in} - V_{ref} = V_{error}$$

The input voltage and reference voltage are compared, and the error voltage is converted by a chopper (i.e., a device that permits intermittent passage of two signals that are being compared with each other), to a pulsating DC signal. This signal is then amplified, usually by an operational amplifier. The amplified error voltage drives a servomotor. The greater the error voltage, the faster the servomotor rotates, and vice versa. An error voltage of zero provides no force to the servomotor, and the servomotor stops. The servomotor is mechanically connected to both the slidewire contact and the recorder pen, as indicated by the dotted line in Fig. 3-35. The servomotor drives the pen and the slidewire contact simultaneously. As the servomotor drives the slidewire contact, the resistance of the slidewire changes, thus altering the reference voltage to the circuit. The continuous change in reference voltage is compared with the input voltage. Once the slidewire contact reaches the null position (where the reference voltage equals the input voltage), the error voltage is zero, and the servomotor, recorder pen, and slidewire contact no longer move. The servomotor does not operate again until a different input voltage is applied. This re-

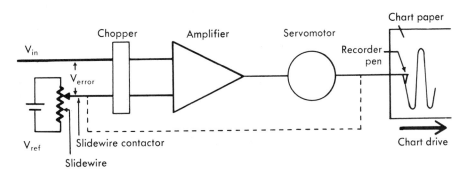

Fig. 3-35 Simplified block diagram of a null-balancing potentiometric recorder.

balancing is continuous and begins immediately with any change in input voltage.

Three adjustments on a potentiometric recorder, the **range,** the **zero,** and the **gain,** are indicated in Fig. 3-36. The range of a recorder is defined as the full scale deflection (FSD) of the pen across the graph paper, which is equal to the input voltage. For example, a range setting of 1 mV represents a FSD caused by an input voltage of 1 mV. As indicated in Fig. 3-36, the range is determined by introducing resistances over which the input voltage will be dropped to a maximum value of 1 mV at point *a*. All recorders have a maximum operating voltage. In this example, the maximum voltage is equal to 1 mV. The range selector provides a mechanism by which a large input voltage is reduced to the operating voltage of the recorder. For example, if the input voltage is 10 mV, the resistance of R_1 must be able to drop 9 mV so that the output voltage at point *a* is equal to 1 mV. In this example, setting the range selector to the 10 mV position connects the circuit to R_1, a resistor with a value that will drop 9 mV. The same is true for the 100 mV range. When 100 mV is the input voltage, the voltage drop over R_2 must be 99 mV.

If the range needs to be selected from a continuous scale (i.e., in this case 0 to 100 V) then a variable resistor would be used in place of the fixed resistors shown in Fig. 3-36. This type of range se-

lector is required if full deflection of the pen must be set on the chart paper. For example, when using a recording spectrophotometer, the operator often sets the pen at full deflection (100% T) when using a reagent blank for a colorimetric reaction. This setting dictates the maximum voltage to be recorded throughout the procedure.

The zero adjust is used to set the recorder pen at a baseline. This setting dictates the minimum voltage to be applied during a procedure. All the light should be blocked from the photodetector of the spectrophotometer before this adjustment is made. The gain control adjusts the amplification of the signal and thus the response of the servomotor to the error voltage. If it is increased, so is the amplification of the signal, and vice versa. When the gain control is too high, the pen via the servomotor will respond to the signal change by vibrating, or oscillating, even though no apparent input signal has been received. This phenomenon is called electronic "noise." The gain must be reduced until the pen stops oscillating. On the other hand, if the gain is too low, the pen will respond sluggishly or not at all to input signals.

In addition to frequency response described earlier, there are three other recorder characteristics that should be considered: chart speed, pen response, and sensitivity. The chart speed of a recorder is the rate at which the chart paper moves, usually expressed in inches or centimeters/min-

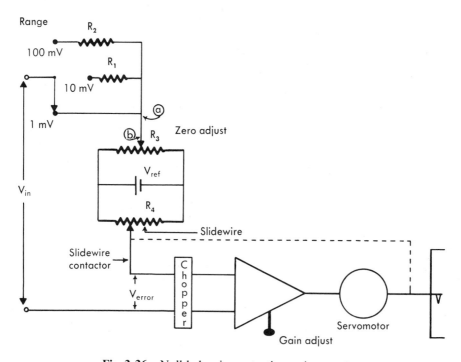

Fig. 3-36   Null-balancing potentiometric recorder.

ute. Pen response is the time (in seconds or milliseconds) required for the pen to move from one edge of the paper to the other when full-scale voltage is applied. Recorder sensitivity is a measurement of the degree of deflection caused by a unit of current and is expressed in centimeters/microampere or milliampere.

In most potentiometric recorders a motor drive moves the chart at a constant rate. This produces a linear time axis with time (T) being on one axis, and a variable (Y) on the other. Thus these recorders are called TY recorders or, more often, "stripchart" recorders. This recorder has been modified to produce two other types, the X-Y recorder and the linear-logarithmic recorder. The modification is the addition of another set of slidewires and servomotor. Although these types of recorders can be found in the clinical laboratory, an explanation of their operation is beyond the scope of this text.

Integrators. Sometimes a recorder or other readout device (i.e., a computer monitor) converts the detector signal as a graphic display in the form of a peak. The concentration of an analyte can be determined by relating its concentration to peak height (as absorbance) or peak area. Relating peak height to concentration presents no particular problems because it can be accomplished simply by using the absorbance change that is relayed to a conventional recorder via a detector. However, to relate the area under the peak to concentration, an electronic device called an **integrator** must be used in conjunction with the readout system. The function of an integrator is to determine the area under a curve (i.e., a peak) by measuring a change in some parameter in intervals (such as absorbance) over time or distance, and then summing them to produce a total area. There are several types of electronic integrators that are currently available. One type consists of extremely accurate capacitors that store a representative portion of the output signal and then discharges it into circuits. These circuits record this current fraction as an event such as open stroke. The discharge of the capacitor can be recorded as blips on the edge of the recorder paper, as digits on a dial, or as some other form of record. Electronic integrators possess the advantages of having very few moving parts and being trouble free. Integrators are used in densitometers to quantify protein fractions separated by protein electrophoresis, in gas chromatographs and HPLC systems, and in cell sorters.

Most state of the art instruments use inte-

grated circuits to process electronic signals and integrate the area under a curve. Microprocessors are then used to manipulate the information as it is collected. If an actual graphic display is not needed, the recorder may be eliminated entirely and the data processed, integrated, and reported as a digital display. These sophisticated electronic devices can sense the valley denoting the end of a peak, measure peak height, and measure changes in slope with a great degree of accuracy and reliability.

Digital Displays. Clinical laboratory instruments that are designed today use digital readouts. Thus conventional meters containing meter movements have virtually been replaced. Digital readouts are capable of displaying information in alphabetic or numeric form. An analog-to-digital convertor, which is part of digital circuitry, changes electric signals to digital binary form. The digital circuitry then converts the binary information to arithmetic numbers. Digital displays contain an electronic circuit, called the drive circuitry, that they require for accepting input information and applying required voltages to the appropriate readout elements.

Digital readouts have several advantages over conventional meters. Unlike meter movement assemblies, they are not susceptible to mechanical shock. They are also more accurate than meters, and unlike analog meters, they are not affected by **parallax,** which is an optical illusion that makes an object appear displaced when viewed from an angle. The pointer position of a meter on a readout scale depends on the angle from which it is read. To eliminate such errors, the eye should be aligned directly above the meter pointer. Data presented in digital form eliminates possible reading errors caused by parallax. In this section a brief description of common types of digital displays is presented. Digital readout systems are generally classified as electromechanical or electronic. Because electromechanical digital readouts have almost become obsolete, they will not be discussed. However, this type of readout was quite popular in the older versions of such instruments as the flame emission photometer where a coupled-wheel or drum type mechanical register(s) displayed the information.

Neon Filamentous Digital Displays. Electronic digital readouts are displays that are found in almost all modern instrumentation. The first to be developed was the NIXIE tube, which consisted of a glass tube containing neon gas and a maximum of 12 stacked filaments in the form of numbers or letters. A specific letter or number could be illuminated by applying a potential of 100 to 180 V to that alphabetic or numeric filament. The filament segment tube was developed later. Its operating voltage was only to 15 to 25 V, although its driving circuitry was more complex. This display, shown in Fig. 3-37, consisted of seven filaments that could be selectively illuminated for an alphanumeric or numeric display.

Semiconductor Digital Displays. Today, however, there are two types of solid-state displays that are used routinely in the design of clinical laboratory instruments, the **light-emitting diode** (LED) and the planar glow panel. The solid-state light-emitting diode is available as a seven-segmented display (Fig. 3-38) or as a 36-diode X-Y

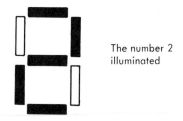

Fig. 3-37 Seven-segment light emitting diode displaying the number 2.

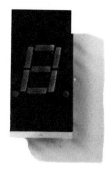

Fig. 3-38 Common solid-state LED as a seven-segmented digital display.

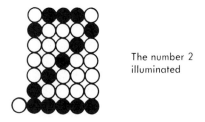

Fig. 3-39 X-Y array of light-emitting diodes displaying the number 2.

array readout (Fig. 3-39). Alphanumeric characters are displayed with the selective illumination of the diodes in the array. The diodes used in these readout devices are made of gallium arsenide. When the voltage applied across a LED exceeds a certain threshold level, a current can cross the semiconductor junction. For gallium arsenide, which emits in the near-infrared region, the threshold is 1.3 V. At this level the voltage excites the semiconductor electrons. When the electrons cross the junction and combine with the positive holes, they emit photons. Because the LED converts an electrical current directly into light, it is more efficient than many other light sources that are used as digital displays. It also has very low power consumption. The usual operating voltage is around 1.75 V at 50 mA for the seven-segment display; only 5 to 10 mA current is required to illuminate one character in the X-Y display.

Planar glow panel or planar panel solid-state displays consist of double-anode, single-cathode gas discharge diodes arranged in an 111-dot X-Y array. The anodes are oriented with one toward the front of the panel and the other toward the back. The dot in the array becomes visible when its front anode is illuminated; a dot is not visible when the back anode is illuminated.

Oscilloscope or Cathode Ray Tube. The **oscilloscope** is a readout device used for viewing electrical waveforms, measuring voltage, current, or frequency, and determining phase relationships between signals. Another name for the oscilloscope is **cathode ray tube** (CRT). CRTs are included in clinical laboratory instruments when the visualization of electrical signals is required during sample analyses. For example, most electronic particle counters have a CRT on which are displayed the electrical impulses produced by individual particles.

The cathode ray tube consists of three major parts enclosed in an evacuated tube: an electron gun, two sets of deflection plates, and a screen (Fig. 3-40). The electron gun generates a well-focused electron beam. The gun consists of a heated cathode and an accelerating anode. Free electrons are emitted from the hot cathode and then enter an aperture in the control grid. This aperture controls the stream of electrons that eventually pass onto the anode. The potential of the control grid is negative with respect to the cathode, and therefore is used to control the number of electrons passing to the anode. The electron beam intensity is controlled by adjusting the potential on the control grid.

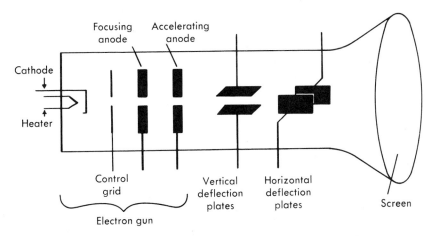

Fig. 3-40 Construction of the cathode ray tube (CRT) or oscilloscope.

The focusing anode is the first anode beyond the grid. The potential of the focusing anode is very positive with respect to the cathode. Thus the electrons are accelerated and the beam is concentrated as it passes through the anode's aperture. Adjustment of the potential on this anode controls the sharpness of the electron beam. The next anode, called the accelerating anode, has an even greater positive potential, and thus increases the acceleration electron flow. The electron beam produced by the electron gun is directed to the center of the screen.

Before reaching the screen, the electron beam passes through the horizontal and vertical deflection plates: two pairs of parallel plates oriented at right angles to each other. One horizontal and vertical plate is set at a fixed potential. The other horizontal or vertical plate can be made positive or negative. When either plate is made positive, the electron beam is attracted toward that plate, thus causing the electron beam to be deflected horizontally or vertically; deflection in the opposite direction occurs when applying a negative potential (repels the electron beam). By applying voltages to both the vertical and horizontal deflection plates simultaneously, the electron beam can be deflected in any direction, the extent of which depends on the relative magnitudes of the two voltages. The interior surface of the screen is coated with a fluorescent or phosphorescent material that emits visible light when its molecules are bombarded by electrons. Thus the electron beam appears as an intense spot on the CRT screen. An associated circuit of the oscilloscope, called a **time base generator,** applies a sawtooth voltage signal to the horizontal deflection plate. This signal causes the electron beam to move at a constant rate across the screen, and then returns it rapidly to the starting position where it begins another sweep across the screen. This way, the signal displayed on a CRT is a measure of the change in voltage with respect to time.

Review Questions

1. Which of the following devices is not considered a major component of a power supply:
   A. Transformer
   B. Voltage regulator
   C. Rectifier
   D. Wheatstone bridge
2. An electronic device that converts one form of energy to another is called a:
   A. Diode
   B. Transducer
   C. Transformer
   D. Voltage regulator
3. Which of the following electronic components serves as a voltage regulator?
   A. Capacitor
   B. Zener diode
   C. Inductor
   D. Operational amplifier
4. An electronic device that is used to measure unknown resistances by nulling (balancing) the circuit is called a:
   A. Wheatstone bridge
   B. Thermistor
   C. Photoconductive cell
   D. Transistor
5. In an NPN semiconductor transistor, electron current flow is from the _____, to the _____, and finally to the _____

   A. Base, emitter, collector
   B. Collector, emitter, base
   C. Emitter, base, collector
   D. Collector, base, emitter

6. An electronic device that is used to sort out electronic signals is called a(n):
   A. Discriminator
   B. Counting circuit
   C. Feedback circuit
   D. Integrator

7. Which of the following electronic devices is not considered a digital display?
   A. NIXIE tube
   B. LED
   C. Oscilloscope
   D. Planar glow panel

8. Which of the following is not a component of the cathode ray tube (CRT)?
   A. Electron gun
   B. Control grid
   C. Horizontal deflection plate
   D. Vertical deflection plate
   E. Accelerating dynode

9. The function of the filter network in a power supply is to:
   A. Step-up or step-down the voltage.
   B. Convert alternating current to direct current.
   C. Convert pulsating direct current to smooth direct current.
   D. Direct current to various parts of the circuit.

10. The function of the dynode in a phototube is to _____the signal.
    A. Filter
    B. Convert
    C. Amlify
    D. Rectify

11. If an input voltage of 0.15 volts results in an output voltage of 30 volts, the "gain" of the amplifier is:
    A. 0.005
    B. 4.5
    C. 20
    D. 200

12. One of the primary functions of a transistor is to _____ an electronic signal.
    A. Block
    B. Amplify
    C. Integrate
    D. Smooth

13. The electronic component that converts a change in temperature to a change in resistance is called a(n):
    A. Integrator
    B. Transistor
    C. Fluor
    D. Thermistor

14. The purpose of a readout device is to convert an electronic signal to a presentable format.
    A. True
    B. False

Answers

1. D   2. B   3. B   4. A   5. C   6. A   7. C   8. E   9. C
10. C   11. D   12. B   13. D   14. A

CHAPTER 4

Measurement of Electricity

ROBERT H. WILLIAMS

The Volt-Ohmmeter (VOM) or Multimeter
The Oscilloscope

Sometimes it is necessary to make electrical measurements of a circuit to determine if it is functioning correctly. The test equipment that is used to make such measurements can be influenced by the polarity of the power source. Unlike resistance, measurement of voltage and current is affected by polarity. For this reason, a brief review of the concept of polarity and how it is related to measuring devices is given below. The sections that follow will then introduce to the reader the most common electrical measuring devices, the volt-ohm-milliammeter (VOM) or multimeter and the oscilloscope.

Concept of Polarity. The term **polarity** can refer to the direction of current flow or describe a voltage as being negative or positive with respect to some reference point such as a power source. It also is used to denote points in a circuit as being relatively positive or negative with respect to each other. For example, to observe polarity with a VOM means that the negative or common lead (usually black) is connected to the negative side of the circuit or the negative terminal of the voltage source, whereas the positive lead (usually red) is connected to a positive side of the circuit or the positive terminal. This allows current to flow in the proper direction through the VOM. This concept is best understood by noting the basic types of current flow and how they are related to polarity. The distinguishing feature between a direct current and an alternating current is not the change in the magnitude of voltage in relation to time but rather the change in polarity. If the polarity does not change, then current flow is considered direct whether it be fixed or pulsating.

The Volt-Ohm-Milliammeter (VOM) or Multimeter

Definition. Modern instrumentation is composed of electronic units such as power supplies, amplifiers, and microcomputers. These units are

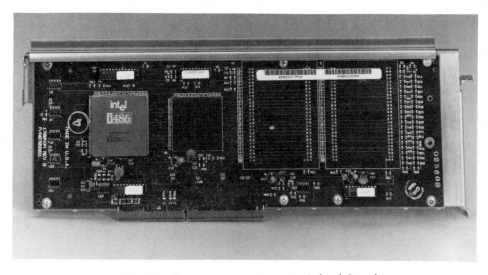

Fig. 4-1   Common computer control circuit board.

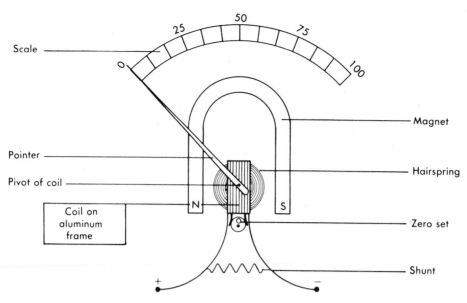

Fig. 4-2 Basic d'Arsonval movement. Range extension using resistor shunt.

often constructed on printed circuit boards that plug into an instrument's electronic chassis. A computer control board is shown in Fig. 4-1. Today, service work primarily involves determining the cause of the malfunction and then replacing the appropriate circuit board. Although many instruments have self-diagnostic capabilities via their dedicated computer, others require that voltage and/or resistance measurements be taken between two test points on a circuit board. These electrical measurements are then compared with the manufacturer's specifications to determine those boards that must be replaced. The device that is frequently used to make these measurements is the **volt-ohm-milliammeter (VOM)** or multimeter.

Theory of Operation. The common VOM is basically a d'Arsonval meter that has been configured to measure current, voltage, or resistance. Its ability to measure electrical current and thus serve as an **ammeter** has already been described in Chapter 3. In general, the meter consists of a coil of wire that is wound on an iron mandrel surrounded by a permanent magnet (Fig. 4-2). The iron mandrel and its coil are supported on a low-friction pivot system. Attached to the mandrel is a pointer that is associated with the scale of the meter face. A suspension spring is attached to the mandrel and permanent magnet in such a way that in the absence of current, the mandrel and pointer return to zero. When current passes through the meter coil, a concentrated magnetic

field is induced that turns the mandrel and thus the pointer until the spring force counteracts the magnetic force. Current is read from the meter face scale using the pointer.

When the d'Arsonval meter is used as an ammeter to measure current in a circuit, it must be connected in series, as shown in Fig. 4-3. This arrangement allows the total current in the circuit to flow through the meter and thus become registered on the meter scale. An ammeter has a very small inherent resistance. This characteristic prevents the meter from imparting additional resistance to the circuit that would significantly alter the current flow in the test circuit.

Although the d'Arsonval meter is considered a current measuring device, it can be used to measure voltage and thus serves as a **voltmeter.** When the meter resistance is held constant, the current that is measured, multiplied by the meter's internal resistance, is equal to the voltage. To be used as a voltage measuring device, the meter must have a very high inherent resistance. The high inherent resistance of the meter prevents an appreciable drain of current from the circuit, which would ultimately alter the measured voltage. For this to occur, the voltmeter must be connected in parallel across the two points where the potential difference is to be measured. Fig. 4-4 shows a voltmeter connected in parallel to R_1 to measure the potential difference (voltage) between points *a* and *b*. This parallel arrangement allows for measurement of voltage with minimal effect on the current flow. (Remember the effect of a larger resistor on total resistance and voltage when it is connected in parallel to another resistor that is considerably smaller: it contributes very little to the overall effective resistance and yet it drops the same amount of voltage.)

All meters have an internal resistance that is a result of the resistance of the current-carrying elements. The internal resistance that is based on the length, the cross-sectional diameter, and the resistivity of the wire used in the construction of the coil is indicated on the meter face or in the meter specifications provided by the manufacturer. Because each meter has a fixed internal resistance and can detect current, Ohm's law ($E = IR$) can be used to measure the voltage indirectly. Because this calculation is an inconvenience, meters that measure voltage have a voltage scale placed under the pointer. This scale accounts for the meter's internal resistance. Multirange meters can be made as well.

The amount of current required to deflect a meter movement full-scale is referred to as the meter's **sensitivity**: the lower the current required for full-scale deflection the greater its sensitivity. Meter sensitivity is expressed in amperes, milliamperes, or microamperes. Meter sensitivity can also be related to meter voltage drop and meter internal resistance. Meter voltage drop, usually given in millivolts, is the amount of voltage dropped across the internal resistance when current flows at full-scale deflection. The meter internal resistance, often expressed as ohms/volt, is determined by dividing the meter internal resistance by its full-scale voltage. The higher the ohms/volt ratio, the less current is required for full-scale deflection and thus the more sensitive the meter. The ohms/volt value is frequently indicated on the meter face.

The design and construction of a meter determine its sensitivity and therefore its range of operation. Meters with only one range are of limited application. For example, a meter with an internal resistance (R_m) of 100 Ω and a sensitivity of 5 mA can be used to measure currents of no more than 5 mA and voltages of no more than 500 mV.

$$E = IR = (5 \text{ mA})(100 \text{ Ω}) = 500 \text{ mV}$$

To expand its range, the meter must contain a number of series and parallel resistors. The configuration of these resistors depends on how the meter will be used. If the meter is used as an ammeter, the resistors are connected in parallel to the meter movement; if it is used as a voltmeter

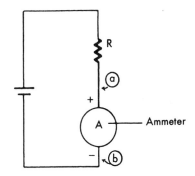

Fig. 4-3   Series connection of an ammeter in a circuit.

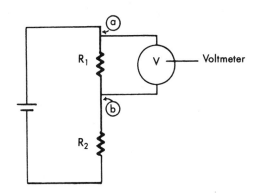

Fig. 4-4   Parallel connection of a voltmeter in a circuit.

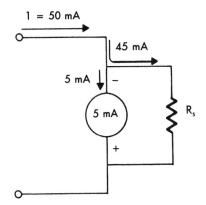

Fig. 4-5   Range extension of an ammeter.

the resistors are connected in series. Moving the selector switch on a VOM in essence sets the range by selecting the appropriate resistor(s) and its (their) configuration.

Fig. 4-5 illustrates how to extend the range of an ammeter by adding a resistor. In this example the range of the ammeter needs to be extended to 50 mA. Note that the resistor is connected in parallel to divert or shunt from the meter any current

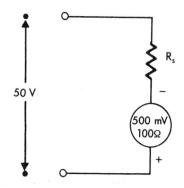

Fig. 4-6 Range extension of a voltmeter.

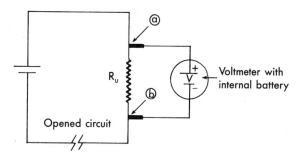

Fig. 4-7 Connection of an ohmmeter in a circuit.

that exceeds 5 mA, which in this case amounts to 45 mA. Thus a shunt resistor (R_s) must be incorporated into the meter circuit that diverts this amount of current. Because the voltage drop across the meter of 500 mV is the same as that across the parallel shunt, the value of the shunt resistor can be determined using the following form of Ohm's law:

$$R_s = E_{fs}/I_s$$

where:

R_s = Value of shunt resistor
E_{fs} = Full-scale deflection voltage
I_s = Current through shunt
R_s = 500 mV/45 mA = 11.11 Ω

Fig. 4-6 illustrates how to extend the range of a voltmeter. In this example, the full-scale voltage is only 500 mV. To extend the range, a resistor, R_s (known as the "multiplier"), must be connected in series with the meter's circuit. Because the range needs to be extended to 50 V, R_s must drop 49.5 V. To determine the value of R_s, the total resistance is calculated using a voltage of 50 V and a current of 5 mA. The meter's resistance (R_m) is then subtracted from the total resistance (R_t) as shown below.

R_t = E/I = 50 V/5 mA = 10,000 Ω
R_s = R_t − R_m
R_s = 10,000 Ω − 100 Ω = 9,900 Ω

The d'Arsonval meter can also be configured to measure resistance and thus be used as an **ohmmeter** (Fig. 4-7). The meter contains an internal battery that is connected to the meter movement and to the resistor of unknown value (R_u). Because the battery provides a constant source of voltage and the current can be directly measured by the meter, the resistance can be calculated using Ohm's law (R = E/I). The meter's circuit also contains a variable resistor for adjusting the meter to read zero ohms. To set this circuit up for

measurement of resistor (R_u), probes *a* and *b* are connected together. This connection provides a completed pathway for current to flow from the meter's internal battery. The variable resistor is then adjusted to make the meter scale read maximum current, which corresponds to zero ohms. When the probes are disconnected, the meter reads zero amperage; this corresponds to a resistance of infinity. After this initial calibration, probes *a* and *b* can be connected to the unknown resistance (R_u). Because the battery voltage is constant, the current that flows through R_u can be measured and then correlated to its resistance. However, this relationship is nonlinear. Consequently, the scale of the meter face found on an ohmmeter reflects this nonlinearity with resistance values (in ohms) being more crowded at the high resistance end of the scale.

General Operation of the VOM. The VOM or multimeter is probably the most useful piece of test equipment available for troubleshooting electronic malfunctions. The design of this device makes it suitable for measuring several electrical parameters. A conventional multimeter (VOM) can be used as a DC ammeter for measuring direct current, as a DC voltmeter for assessing DC voltage, as an AC voltmeter for analyzing AC voltage, as an ohmmeter for resistance and continuity measurements, and as a decibel meter for measuring electric power in an apparatus that produces sound.

A conventional multimeter is shown in Fig. 4-8 with a meter scale for volts, amps, and ohms; plus (+) and minus (−) jacks; a zero ohms adjust; a switch labeled +DC, −DC, AC; and a switch used to select different ranges for measurement. Other conventional meters may not have the same knobs or switches; however, they are still capable of analyzing the same parameters (Fig. 4-9). Referring to either Fig. 4-8 or Fig. 4-9, the topmost scale on the meter's face is used to

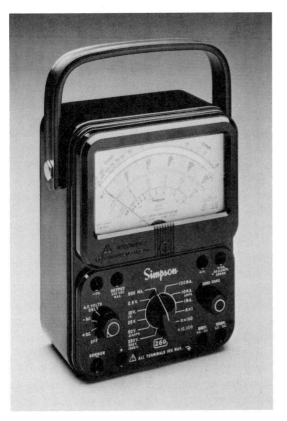

Fig. 4-8 Conventional analog multimeter with polarity selector switch. (Courtesy Simpson Electric Company.)

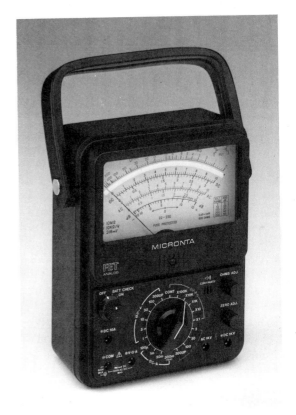

Fig. 4-9 Analog multimeter with optional battery check. (Courtesy Radio Shack, a division of Tandy Corporation.)

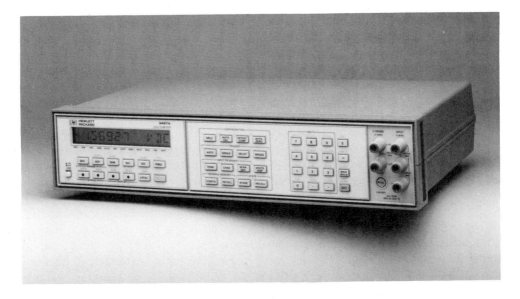

Fig. 4-10 Digital volt-ohm-milliammeter. (Courtesy Hewlett-Packard Company.)

make all measurements of resistance (ohms) and is the only scale that is nonlinear. The scale below the ohms scale is used for all DC voltage and current measurements and contains two to three different scaler ranges depending on the range that is required during measurement. The scale below the DC scale is used for all AC voltage measurements. The bottom scale is for measuring decibels. Many of the newer electronic and digital multimeters (Fig. 4-10) also have an AC ammeter function and a low-power ohms function. The use of the VOM as an ammeter, voltmeter, and ohmmeter, and the precautions that should be taken during its use will be described in some detail.

The VOM as an Ammeter. Ammeters are devices used to measure electron flow (current flow) in a circuit. It can be envisioned as a flow meter because it samples the current flowing through the circuit. An ammeter (or milliammeter) has an extremely small internal resistance and must be connected in series with the circuit that is being measured. Before any attachments are made, power to the circuit must be turned off. Power is restored after the meter is connected into the circuit. When direct current flow is measured, polarity must be observed. This does not apply to measurements of alternating current. Fig. 4-11 shows the correct way to hook up an ammeter for measuring direct current. Most VOMs only measure direct current. Using a DC ammeter to measure alternating current or an AC ammeter to measure direct current can damage the instrument. Therefore care should be taken to note the type of current that needs to be measured. Always remember that the ammeter has a very low resistance and can be damaged by small currents. The ammeter must have low resistance because it is connected in series in the circuit. High resistance would interfere with the normal operation of the circuit.

When measuring unknown currents, the range selector switch should be on the highest possible position. With the VOM pictured in Fig. 4-8 this is 500 mA. The range for each amperage is selected by positioning the range switch to a DC amperage position: 1 mA, 10 mA, 100 mA, or 500 mA. Readings are taken from indications along the DC scale. Note that the scale is linear. The quantities marked at the right end of the scale are the **full-scale deflection (FSD)** values. They are a series of numbers used to make readings when the meter is set to that range. The po-

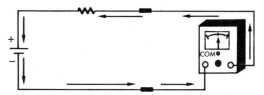

Ammeter

Series connection allows all
circuit current to flow through meter

Fig. 4-11   Proper method of connecting the VOM as an ammeter to measure current in a circuit.

sition of the range selector switch dictates the actual FSD value. It serves as an electronic multiplier and divider that prevents excess current (or voltage) from affecting the meter movement. For example, using the multimeter in Fig. 4-8, readings on the 10 mA range are taken directly from the series of numbers starting at zero and leading up to the number 10 (last series of numbers at the bottom of the second scale). For 100 mA, the same group of numbers is used, but this time the reading is multiplied by 10. For the 1 mA range, the same scale is used, but all readings must be divided by 10. If the 500 mA range is required, the middle DC scale (0 to 50) is chosen. The value is then multiplied by 10.

With the VOM shown in Fig. 4-9, a similar approach is used. Note that there are two scales; the first digit corresponds to one of the FSD values and the second correlates with one of the range settings. The range selector switch serves as a divider or multiplier of the FSD value depending on the range needed for measurement. For example, using this multimeter, readings taken on the 1 mA range are taken directly from the series of numbers starting with zero and leading up to the number 10. However, the reading is then divided by 10 to get the appropriate value. Dividing by 10 is equivalent to an FSD of 1. For the 100 μA setting the same group of numbers is used, but this time the reading is multiplied by 10; multiplying by 10 is equivalent to a full-scale deflection of 100. For the 30 mA and 300 mA range the zero to three scale is used; the only difference is that all readings must be multiplied by 10 and 100, respectively. Because each meter has its own specific operating instructions for measuring current, they will not be described. However, regardless of the type of meter used, the following precautions must be observed when using the VOM as an ammeter:

Ammeters must be connected in series with the circuit under test.

When measuring unknown currents, always begin with the highest possible range setting (lowest sensitivity) and decrease the range setting until an accurate reading can be made.

When direct current flow is measured, polarity must be observed.

Always turn the power "off" before inserting an ammeter in a circuit unless there is no way to avoid it.

Failure to adhere to these rules will damage the VOM and cause erratic readings.

The VOM as a Voltmeter. The voltmeter in most modern multimeters (Fig. 4-8) is actually three voltmeters in one. Located on some instruments (upper left-hand corner in Fig. 4-8) is a switch labeled DC+, DC−, AC. By positioning this switch properly, it is possible to measure any one of these voltages. Some units provide separate "jacks" for reversing the VOM leads and thus the polarity. Others do not have the capability of switching polarities for DC. In such cases it is necessary to know if the point of measurement is positive or negative relative to the power source of the circuit. Before making voltage checks in a circuit, be aware of the types of voltage, the point to be checked, and the normal voltage at that point.

Referring to the VOM in Fig. 4-8, the range for each voltage is selected by positioning the range switch to a DC position: 2.5 V, 10 V, 25 V, 50 V, and 250 V. Readings are taken from indications along the DC scale. Note that this scale, like the one for amperage, is linear. Reading the scale is similar to the protocol that is used for the VOM as an ammeter: the divisions along the scale are marked in scaler quantities. Quantities marked at the right end of the scale are the FSD quantities, and ranges selected by the switch selector correlate with these FSD values. For example, readings on the 250 V range are taken directly from the series of numbers leading up to the number 250. For 25 V, the same group of numbers is used, but this time when the 250 V scale is used, all readings must be divided by 10. The approach to the problem using the multimeter shown in Fig. 4-9 is very similar.

A voltmeter can be imagined as being a pressure sampler because it measures the electrical pressure between two points in a circuit. A voltmeter has a very high internal resistance and thus

must be connected in parallel with the voltage to be measured. When measuring DC voltage, polarity must be observed (red lead to positive and black lead to negative if +DC setting is used). If the polarity of the circuit is unknown, the pointer may deflect to the left when connected to the circuit. It can be made to deflect to the right by (1) reversing the position of the +DC, −DC, AC switch, or (2) reversing the position of the test leads: putting the red lead where the black lead is connected and the black lead where the red lead is connected in the circuit. When measuring an AC voltage, readings are taken from the AC scale and polarity need not be observed (it is compensated for within the meter). Fig. 4-12 shows the correct way to connect a voltmeter.

Regardless of the type of VOM used, the following precautions must be observed when it is used as a voltmeter:

Voltmeters must be connected in parallel with the circuit.

Polarity must be observed when measuring DC voltage.

Polarity need not be observed when measuring AC voltage.

When measuring unknown voltages, always begin with the highest possible range (lowest sensitivity) and decrease the range setting until an accurate reading can be attained.

As with the ammeter, using a voltmeter inappropriately will result in permanent damage and erratic readings.

The VOM as an Ohmmeter. An ohmmeter is used to measure resistance and to check for continuity ("shorted" or "open") circuits. It contains its own power source and does not require cur-

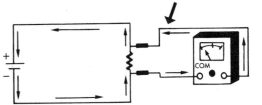

Voltmeter

Parallel connection allows a portion
of the circuit to flow through meter

NOTE: A portion of the circuit current flows through the meter

Fig. 4-12 Proper method of connecting the VOM as a voltmeter to measure voltage in a circuit.

rent from the test circuit as part of its use. A combination of batteries and circuits is part of the design of the ohmmeter that provides the correct range of current for operating the meter in each range of resistance (ohms). Thus it is used only when power to the circuit under test has been removed (because it supplies its own power source). When resistance is to be measured, one end of the component under test must be disconnected from the circuit.

The ohms scale, usually at the top of the meter, is called an inverse scale. An inverse scale is one in which the zero is located at the right end of the scale; all other scales such as amperage and voltage have a left-side zero (Figs. 4-8 and 4-9). Note that the scale is highly nonlinear. The most accurate readings are taken from the right one third of the scale. On many meters the scale is "green" to distinguish it from the others.

For ohms readings to be accurate, the meter should be calibrated (zeroed) before each measurement. To perform this calibration, the test leads are first connected (shorted) together. This allows current from the internal battery to flow through a completed circuit. The pointer will deflect to the right (near zero ohms). A zero (ohms) adjust knob, located on the meter, is then used to adjust the pointer to the zero position while the test leads are still connected. When the test leads are disconnected (i.e., when the current path is open), the pointer will deflect back to the left, or the infinity side of the scale. Once these steps have been performed, the meter is calibrated for use. It is not necessary to observe polarity when connecting the test leads to an ohmmeter. The current source is internal. Consequently, the direction of current flow is established by the ohmmeter. Fig. 4-13 shows the correct method for measuring resistance.

Ohmmeter

Circuit must be broken (power removed) or component must be disconnected from the circuit. Meter supplies current!

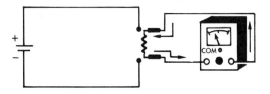

Fig. 4-13 Correct method for measuring resistance with a VOM as an ohmmeter.

Using the VOM as an ohmmeter and interpreting the resistance scale is similar to that of an ammeter or voltmeter. For example, using the multimeter in Fig. 4-8 or Fig. 4-9, if the R × 1 is selected, then the reading is multiplied by 1 (i.e., no multiplier is used and the reading is taken directly from the scale). If R × 100 is chosen, then the reading is multiplied by 100, etc.

There are many types of ohmmeters, and their directions for their use may vary slightly. However, the following precautions should always be observed when using a VOM as an ohmmeter to prevent damage to the meter movement:

Because ohmmeters have their own power source, the power to the circuit must be removed before making any resistance measurement.

A component in a complex circuit must be isolated from other components before a resistance measurement.

When measuring unknown voltages, always begin with the highest possible range setting (lowest sensitivity setting) and decrease the range setting until an accurate reading can be made.

Anytime the resistance range is changed, the ohmmeter must be rezeroed.

The most accurate readings are taken from the right one third of the scale.

These steps are also applicable to the VOM when it is used to check continuity within a circuit. The purpose of doing a continuity check is to determine if there is a completed path for current flow. Therefore in contrast to checking an individual component, a continuity check determines the circuit's ability to conduct current. Three possibilities exist when the VOM is used to check continuity. A reading of infinity indicates that an **opened circuit** exists (i.e., the path for current flow is broken). This reading should be considered reliable only when the measurement is made on the highest ohms range available. A zero reading indicates that a **short** or zero resistance exists between the test leads (only possible in the case of a solid piece of wire). Other components lying in the path are an indication of a defective circuit. This reading is only reliable when measurements are made using the smallest possible ohms range. If some resistance value is determined, then there is continuity within that part of the circuit. It is the most common indication observed when performing a continuity check.

The Oscilloscope

The operation of the oscilloscope or cathode ray tube (CRT) has been described in Chapter 3. The purpose of this section is to cover the basic applications of the oscilloscope as a measuring and troubleshooting device for electrical circuits. It is not intended to suggest that laboratory personnel will use such a device. However, having a basic working knowledge of the oscilloscope will help the technologist understand how a service representative uses such equipment as part of the troubleshooting process.

With alternating current it is often necessary to view the waveshape, determine its amplitude, and measure its operating frequency to determine the cause of a malfunctioning instrument, especially one that is computerized. This can be accomplished with an oscilloscope such as those

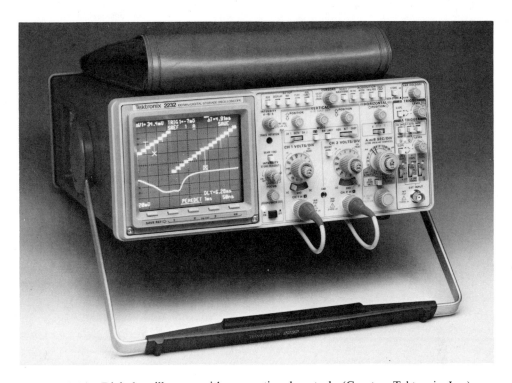

Fig. 4-14 Digital oscilloscope with conventional controls. (Courtesy Tektronix, Inc.)

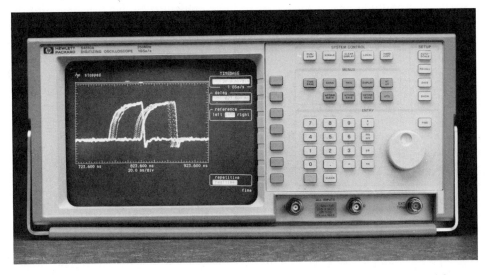

Fig. 4-15 Digitizing oscilloscope with push-button functions. (Courtesy Hewlett-Packard Company.)

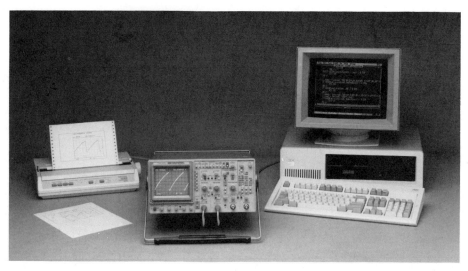

Fig. 4-16   Oscilloscope interfaced with a computer. (Courtesy Tektronix, Inc.)

shown in Figs. 4-14 and 4-15. For complex troubleshooting a more sophisticated setup may be required that involves interfacing the oscilloscope with a computer (Fig. 4-16). This type of test equipment allows for faster and more reliable comparison of signals between the malfunctioning instrument and the manufacturer's specifications, which are usually part of the computer's database.

Oscilloscopes can be used to measure several electrical signal parameters generated by AC or DC voltage (fixed or pulsating) sources. To measure voltage, an operator first calibrates the oscilloscope by observing the amplitude of a known voltage on the screen. Because there is a direct relationship between amplitude and voltage, the unknown voltage can determined by comparing its amplitude with that of the known voltage and then multiplying the known voltage by this ratio. Current in a circuit is calculated by measuring the voltage drop across a known resistance in the circuit. To determine the frequency of a signal, the operator first calibrates the oscilloscope screen with a signal of known frequency. The unknown frequency of the signal can then be measured on the calibrated screen of the oscilloscope.

Characteristics of a Basic Oscilloscope. There are many different types of oscilloscopes. Some oscilloscopes are basic, whereas others are highly automated and complex. However, all have certain common characteristics. As previously mentioned, all oscilloscopes have a CRT that presents

a waveshape for observation. The CRT functions in a similar manner to the picture tube of a television set. There are some additional features that relate to controlling the signal that is projected on its screen. All oscilloscopes and any equipment using CRTs for display purposes usually have seven basic controls: horizontal position, vertical position, intensity, focus, astigmatism, volt/cm, and time/cm.

Operations Performed with the Oscilloscope. The oscilloscope can perform several different types of measurements and calculations. For example, it can be used to measure peak-to-peak voltage, determine the operating frequency of circuits, or view waveforms by plotting the voltage characteristics of a signal against time (Fig. 4-17). Many oscilloscopes can display more than one waveform simultaneously. This allows comparison of the waves or signals to ensure that they are identical. The proper use of an oscilloscope serves as an important diagnostic tool for anyone involved in electronic troubleshooting.

Review Questions

1. The term "polarity" refers to:
   A. The magnitude of current flow
   B. The positive/negative direction of current flow
   C. The positivity/negativity of points in a circuit with respect to each other
   D. B and C
2. When the VOM is used as a voltmeter it must always be:
   A. Connected in parallel with the test circuit

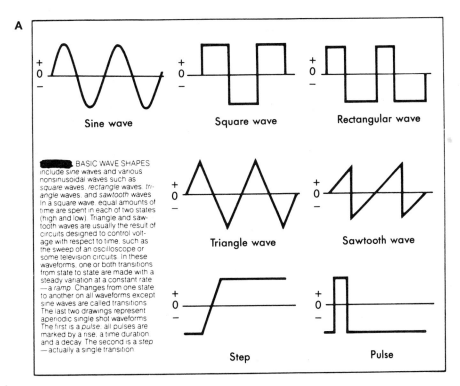

A

Sine wave

Square wave

Rectangular wave

Triangle wave

Sawtooth wave

Step

Pulse

██████ BASIC WAVE SHAPES include *sine* waves and various nonsinusoidal waves such as *square* waves. *rectangle* waves. *triangle* waves. and *sawtooth* waves In a square wave. equal amounts of time are spent in each of two states (high and low). Triangle and sawtooth waves are usually the result of circuits designed to control voltage with respect to time. such as the sweep of an oscilloscope or some television circuits. In these waveforms. one or both transitions from state to state are made with a steady variation at a constant rate —a *ramp.* Changes from one state to another on all waveforms except sine waves are called transitions The last two drawings represent aperiodic single shot waveforms The first is a *pulse.* all pulses are marked by a rise. a time duration. and a decay. The second is a *step* —actually a single transition

B

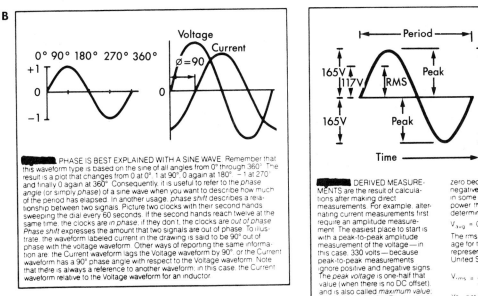

0° 90° 180° 270° 360°

+1
0
−1

Voltage
Current
∅ = 90

██████ PHASE IS BEST EXPLAINED WITH A SINE WAVE. Remember that this waveform type is based on the sine of all angles from 0° through 360°. The result is a plot that changes from 0 at 0°. 1 at 90°. 0 again at 180°. −1 at 270° and finally 0 again at 360° Consequently. it is useful to refer to the *phase angle* (or simply *phase*) of a sine wave when you want to describe how much of the period has elapsed. In another usage. *phase shift* describes a relationship between two signals. Picture two clocks with their second hands sweeping the dial every 60 seconds. If the second hands reach twelve at the same time. the clocks are *in phase.* if they don t. the clocks are *out of phase Phase shift* expresses the amount that two signals are out of phase. To illustrate. the waveform labeled current in the drawing is said to be 90° out of phase with the voltage waveform. Other ways of reporting the same information are: the Current waveform lags the Voltage waveform by 90°. or the Current waveform has a 90° phase angle with respect to the Voltage waveform. Note that there is always a reference to another waveform; in this case. the Current waveform relative to the Voltage waveform for an inductor.

C

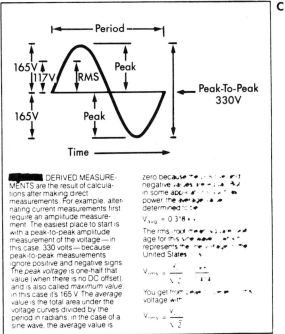

Period

165V
117V RMS
Peak

165V
Peak

Peak-To-Peak
330V

Time

██████ DERIVED MEASUREMENTS are the result of calculations after making direct measurements. For example. alternating current measurements first require an amplitude measurement. The easiest place to start is with a peak-to-peak amplitude measurement of the voltage—in this case. 330 volts—because peak-to-peak measurements ignore positive and negative signs The *peak voltage* is one-half that value (when there is no DC offset). and is also called *maximum value;* in this case it's 165 V. The *average value* is the total area under the voltage curves divided by the period in radians; in the case of a sine wave, the average value is

zero because the ███ ███ ███ negative ██████ ███ ██ in some ████ ██ ███ ██ power the average ██ ██ determined ██ ██

$V_{avg} = 0.318 \cdot \cdot$

The rms ███ ███ ███ ███ age for this sine ████ ██ ███ represents ███ ██ ███ ██ United States ███

$V_{rms} = \dfrac{V_{\cdot}}{\sqrt{2}} \quad \text{███}$

You get ███ ███ ██ ███ voltage ███

$V_{rms} = \dfrac{V_{\cdot}}{\sqrt{2}}$

Fig. 4-17 Common parameters viewed and measured with an oscilloscope. **A,** Basic wave shapes, **B,** phase relationships, and **C,** derived measurements. (Courtesy Tektronix, Inc.)

B. Connected in series with the test circuit
C. Used with a test circuit that has had its power source turned "off"
D. Rezeroed each time a different range is selected

3. Which of the following VOM scales is "nonlinear"?
   A. DC voltage
   B. AC voltage
   C. DC current
   D. Resistance

4. Which of the following statements concerning the use of the VOM as an ohmmeter is false?
   A. The meter must be rezeroed each time the range selector is changed
   B. The meter should be connected in parallel with the component that is being measured
   C. The power source must be removed from the circuit/component that is being tested
   D. The meter should be connected in series with the component/circuit being analyzed

   1. A, B, C
   2. B, C, D
   3. A and C
   4. B and D

5. Which portion of the ohms scale of a VOM is considered the most accurate?
   A. Upper (left) ½
   B. Lower (right) ⅓
   C. Upper (left) ⅓
   D. The entire scale is considered satisfactory

6. Another name for an oscilloscope is a:
   A. Volt-ohm-milliammeter
   B. Diode
   C. d'Arsonval meter
   D. Cathode ray tube

7. A "short" circuit is one in which there is no path of resistance.
   A. True
   B. False

8. Which of the following parameters can be measured/determined by using an oscilloscope?
   A. Frequency
   B. Amplitude
   C. Phase differences
   D. All of the above

9. Which of the following statements is false concerning the use of the VOM as an ammeter?
   A. The meter should always be connected in parallel at the point the current is to be measured.
   B. The range selector should always be set on the highest setting (less sensitive) and then moved to the lowest setting (most sensitive) until an accurate reading can be made.
   C. When the meter is connected in a circuit polarity must be observed.
   D. It is not neccessary to remove the power before conneting an ammeter.

   1. A, B, C
   2. B, C, D
   3. A and D
   4. B and C
   5. None of the above

Answers

1. D   2. A   3. D   4. 4   5. B   6. D   7. A   8. E   9. 3

5

Electrical Safety and Troubleshooting Rules

ROBERT H. WILLIAMS

Electric Shock
Electrical Safety Precautions
Basic Troubleshooting Principles

With the widespread use of sophisticated electronic instruments in the clinical laboratory, it becomes paramount that the technologist recognizes the hazards associated with their operation. Laboratory personnel should be aware of the danger of electric shock and informed of the precautionary measures that should be taken when working with electrical instruments. Safety precautions should always be observed and taken very seriously. Although equipment manufacturers include safety devices designed to stop current flow in case of a circuit overload, these devices do not always protect the operator. Therefore, along with the causes of electrical shock, some of the preventative measures associated with electrical safety are also discussed in this chapter and include recognition of training limitations, adequate grounding, insulation of conductors, self-protection and hazardous components, circuit modifications, exceeding power line voltages, and extinguishing electrical fires. A brief discussion covering basic troubleshooting principles follows the safety section.

Electric Shock

Although electric shock is not always fatal, it is responsible for hundreds of fatalities each year. Body fluids contain electrolytes and therefore can act as electrical conductors. When the body makes contact with two points that differ in potential, it serves as a conducting pathway for current flow. The conduction of electrical current through human tissue results in the unpleasant sensation called **electric shock.** It is important to remember that current, not voltage, kills. Every precaution should be taken to prevent current from passing through the body when working with electrical devices. Therefore the body should never be put into a position where it can serve to complete a circuit and thus function as a conductor.

Although body fluids are considered good conductors of electricity, the body is also provided with an effective defense mechanism against shock. Dry, unbroken skin is a good insulator and thus provides a large resistance to current flow. However, when the skin becomes wet, the resistance of the body decreases dramatically from the megohm range to as low as 300 ohms (Ω). Such a change in body resistance will affect the amount of current produced by a given potential if it is applied across the body. For example, if an AC potential of 120 V at 60 Hz is applied across the body when the skin is wet, a current as high as 400 mA could be produced.

Electrical shock causes two types of injuries: burns and paralysis. The severity of the injury in either case can range from minor, temporary harm to death. People in excellent health can die from small currents; however, those in poor health are often at greater risk. It is difficult to state a definite level of current that is capable of killing a person. The ability to withstand a shock also varies widely over short periods of time. In general, the magnitude, the pathway, and the duration of current passing through the body dictate the type and severity of the injury.

The heat that is generated during current flow causes the burns often observed with electric shock victims. High currents (100 to 200 mA) can burn entry and exit holes through the skin and, if high enough, will destroy all cellular structures. Action potentials generated by nerve and muscle tissues are electrochemical in nature and thus can be disrupted by electrical current that has been introduced by an external voltage source. The disruption of action potentials exerts a direct effect at the neuromuscular junction, causing paralysis or inducing muscular contraction. Stimulation of the neuromuscular system with as little as 1 mA of current is felt as a tingling sensation. Currents above 10 mA will cause muscle contractions sufficiently severe to cause temporary paralysis. This electrically induced paralysis prevents the victim from releasing the electrical source, which produces a more severe shock. The most serious types of electrical shocks are those that involve the chest cavity and brain. An amount of current in the range of 100 to 150 mA passing through the body arm-to-arm or arm-to-opposite leg will alter the muscle-contracting electrical impulses of the heart, producing severe ventricular fibrillation and often death. Disruption of the electrical activity of the brain generally produces a similar outcome.

Electrical Safety Precautions

There are several safety precautions that should be recognized by laboratory personnel when they work with or troubleshoot any piece of electrical equipment. Being aware of electrical safety is not sufficient grounds to allow just anyone to operate or probe into an electrical instrument. Electrical safety precautions should not only be practiced by instrument operators but also should become an integral part of the routine operation of any clinical laboratory. Some of these safety precautions are briefly discussed below.

Recognition of Training Limitations. One of the most important safety measures that can be observed by instrument operators is to perform only those functions within their capabilities. It is also essential that they recognize their limited training in troubleshooting any electrical instrument that appears to be malfunctioning. Knowledge of the basic principles of electricity and electronics and use of the VOM does not automatically qualify an individual to probe irresponsibly into the circuits of an instrument. The repair of any electrical piece of equipment should be performed only by those individuals who are adequately trained. Some minor repairs such as replacing a blown fuse or a burned out light bulb or lamp in a spectrophotometer may be within the capabilities of medical technologists. However, replacing electronic components and circuit boards, adjusting voltages, or fixing a

power supply would most likely require a qualified electronics technician or field service engineer.

Most instruments that are manufactured today are menu-driven by computers. It now has become virtually impossible for any laboratorian to fix any type of electronic malfunction regardless of how simple the problem may seem to be. Consequently, most clinical laboratory instruments are fixed under a service contract that not only covers the service but also the parts necessary for the repair. The basic troubleshooting section that is covered later in this chapter primarily pertains to approaches that are used by a qualified electronics technician.

Adequate Grounding. It is important that the laboratorian understand the concept of **"ground"** and how it is related to electrical safety. Because the earth (or ground) contains a tremendous amount of electrical charge, it can gain or lose these charges and yet maintain its electrical neutrality. The earth is thus regarded as being a "charge neutralizer." Because of its infinite capacity to neutralize charge, **earth ground** is considered to be at zero potential. An **electrical ground** is a conducting material connected to the earth. If a charged conductor is connected to the earth, it will lose its charge to the ground. On losing its charge, it will have a neutral or zero potential relative to the earth or to ground. Schematically a ground is represented as $\perp$. To make voltage measurements within a circuit, a reference point must be established. Because of its zero potential this reference point is usually earth ground (or simply ground) or the negative side of the power source.

The primary purpose of grounding an instrument is to afford protection against electric shock. The chassis of an instrument may accumulate electrical charge if there is a short in the circuit or the metal chassis is being used as part of a circuit. The accumulation of charge on the chassis of an instrument is referred to as **leaking voltage**. The potential danger of leaking voltage is that an instrument operator may receive an electric shock by touching the chassis and a ground (i.e., a water pipe) simultaneously, especially if the instrument is not adequately grounded. To prevent this from happening, a connection (ground) is made between the metal chassis and the earth ground that provides a pathway for the potentially dangerous charge to flow from instrument to ground. This type of connection is referred to as **chassis ground** and its schematic symbol is   /π . Proper grounding is essential to prevent leaking voltage from inducing an electrical shock to an instrument operator.

An electric shock can also result from touching the metal chassis of two different instruments that carry different potentials even though they appear to be properly grounded. The difference in potential is caused by varying degrees of "grounding effectiveness." If both instruments are touched at the same time, current will flow hand-to-hand from the instrument with the higher potential to the one with the lower potential. In general, to avoid the possibility of an electrical shock, the instrument operator should never touch an instrument and a potential ground, or two instruments, simultaneously.

To prevent electric shock, a continuous ground connection must exist between the instrument and its outlet and between the outlet and its ground conductor, which is attached to the earth. These connections and the adequacy of grounding should be checked periodically by a competent electrician. In most modern buildings a three-pronged outlet is provided for electrical devices to prevent electrical shock. One of the flat prong spaces in the receptacle is connected to earth ground and thus has zero potential; the other is connected to the AC voltage source and thus has a potential of about 115 to 120 V. When contact is made between the two via the plug of the power cord, the circuit is completed and electricity will flow. The third prong space is slightly rounded and is used as a chassis ground. This socket space makes contact with a wire that is connected to a water pipe or other conductor that has good contact with the earth under the building. Any electrical charge that accumulates onto the chassis is subsequently released to the earth.

For this reason power cords on most instruments have three-prong plugs. The third (round) prong serves as the connector between the ground lead attachment to the instrument chassis and the ground conductor into the earth. It is important that a continuous conducting pathway from the instrument to the grounded outlet exists. Removing the ground pin on the three-prong plug to use it with a two-prong outlet prevents adequate grounding and thus defeats its purpose. The use of the so-called cheater plugs or two-to-three-prong adapters (Fig. 5-1) causes the same problem if not used properly. The grounding lead on the cheater plug must be connected to ground, usually by attaching it to a screw on the outlet receptacle plate. However, such ground attach-

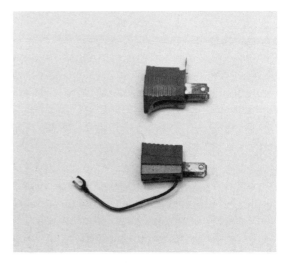

Fig. 5-1 Two-to-three prong adapter ("cheater") plugs.

ments are not always reliable. If the screw is coated with paint (an insulating material) or does not make sufficient contact with the receptacle, the ground lead is of little or no value. Therefore the use of the cheater plug should be avoided if at all possible.

The grounding of a power cord or an extension cord can be ruined by pulling on the cord to expedite the removal of a plug from an outlet receptacle. Often this technique leads to a broken or loosened ground wire. Use of extension cords may also jeopardize grounding protection, in addition to presenting a tripping hazard. Never use an extension cord that has a two-prong socket with an electrical device that has a three-prong plug. If extension cords need to be used they should be heavy-duty and have a three-prong plug.

The ground lead of the power cord that is connected to the instrument should be securely attached to the instrument chassis via a metal-to-metal connector or a three-prong socket. If this lead becomes loose or disconnected or the cord becomes frayed, it should be fixed or replaced immediately. An instrument that is not adequately grounded can collect charge and transfer this charge if it comes in contact with another conductor. For this reason an instrument should never be operated on any metal surface such as a metal cart, a bench, or a table.

Insulation of Conductors. All conducting leads in an instrument should be insulated. If they become exposed, a short can occur (i.e., an exposed conducting wire making contact with the instrument chassis). This is because a **shorted circuit** provides for a path of zero resistance for current to flow that circumvents the normal resistive paths of the circuit. The result is that an excessive amount of current is drawn and a large amount of heat is generated. It is this excess heat that damages or ruins electronic components or the entire circuit. Also, if an exposed conducting wire is touched by a person in contact with a ground, an electric shock will most likely occur. To avoid an electric shock and/or circuit damage caused by exposed conductors, circuit wiring should be inspected periodically for frayed wires and cracked or melted insulation coatings on electrical leads. Wires with damaged insulation should be replaced immediately by a competent electronics engineer or service representative.

A conscious effort should be made to keep not only the circuit wiring but also the electrical cables in good condition. Electrical cables should not be stepped on or run over with carts. Electrical sockets that appear to be damaged should be reported to the proper authorities immediately. Organic solvents should not be used to clean electrical equipment because they can damage most types of insulation and are potentially explosive in the presence of any electrical sparking.

Self-Protection and Hazardous Components. Observing electrical safety rules can be lifesaving and therefore should be practiced consistently by all instrument operators. Any time the laboratory receives a new instrument, the operator should read the instruction manual thoroughly before operating the instrument. Special instructions pertaining not only to its operation but also to its maintenance should also be noted. Any electrical shock felt by the instrument operator should be reported immediately. When working on circuits, the operator should keep one hand away from conducting surfaces to avoid hand-to-hand electric shock (i.e., use the lab coat pocket as a place to put the other hand). Use only insulated tools. Keep the work area and hands and clothes dry. If standing on a damp surface, such as a concrete basement floor, wear rubber-soled shoes. Do not wear metal jewelry such as rings, wristwatches, or loose necklaces and bracelets because a short circuit can result by touching metallic objects to conducting parts of the circuit. Turn off and unplug instruments before performing repairs.

Never assume that the circuit of an unplugged and/or turned off instrument is safe to probe into indiscriminately. Capacitors in electronic equipment can remain charged for a long time even after the equipment is turned off. This will occur if there are no resistive paths in parallel with the capacitors to release the stored electricity to ground. Thus in high voltage circuits charge capacitors can present a lethal source of electricity even though the main power to the equipment is turned "off." Another reason for discharging capacitors is to prevent damage to measuring instruments such as a VOM when it is used as an ohmmeter. As previously discussed, an ohmmeter should never be connected to a source of current. If an ohmmeter is inadvertently connected across a charged capacitor, the capacitor will discharge its stored current through the meter, causing considerable damage.

To prevent possible human injury and/or damage to measuring equipment, a qualified electronics technician should discharge all high voltage capacitors (electrolytic) before attempting to work on any electrical equipment. Discharging a capacitor can be accomplished by short circuiting its terminals with the blade of an insulated screwdriver or an insulated clip lead. Often circuits will be designed to include so-called **bleeder resistors,** which are connected in parallel to capacitors and discharge the capacitor to ground when the circuit is turned off. However, if the circuit design is not well understood, it is best to assume that charged capacitors exist within the circuit and to approach any troubleshooting with extreme caution.

Another electronic component that is considered to be a potential hazard is the cathode ray tube (CRT). Extreme care should be taken when troubleshooting instruments that contain these electronic devices. To accelerate the electrons that are generated by the cathode to the anode to form the electron beam, a very high voltage is required. This high voltage can be lethal. Also, the CRT is surrounded by a glass envelope that is under a high vacuum. Any mechanical shock to the large glass envelope that surrounds the inner working components can result in "implosion" of the tube causing serious injury to anyone in the nearby area. Only experienced electronics technicians should be permitted to work on any instrument that contains cathode ray tubes.

Regardless of the instrument, only qualified personnel should work on high voltage circuits. They should never work alone, and medical assistance should always be immediately available if required. They should also know the whereabouts of all circuit breakers and fuse boxes that provide power to the instrument that is being serviced. Failure to use common sense more often than not will result in lethal electric shock.

Circuit Modifications. Circuit modifications should be left to the field service engineer. Replacement of any instrument components should be in compliance with the manufacturer's specifications. However, the one electronic component that usually can be replaced by laboratory personnel is a fuse. Most electronic instruments have a fuse in series with the 115 to 120 VAC power supply to the instrument. Other fuses may be located throughout the circuitry as protection for separate electronic circuits and/or components. Although fuses are made in different shapes and sizes (Fig. 5-2), they all contain a wire that melts if the current through the fuse exceeds a certain level. The fuse contains a resistive element that melts ("blows") at a certain temperature, causing a gap or break in the circuit, which stops the flow of current. Therefore the purpose of the fuse is to prevent excessive current from being drawn should the instrument malfunction.

Fuses are marked with their current and voltage ratings. The current rating is the level of current above which the fuse filament will melt. The voltage rating is the maximum voltage that can be present in the circuit (i.e., 32 V, 125 V, 250 V) and is related to the size of the break or gap produced when the fuse filament melts. The larger the voltage rating, the wider the gap that is produced. The gap ensures against "electrical arcing" (i.e., electrons jumping from one end of the break to the other). If the gap is not sufficient, the circuit would continue to operate under excessive voltage, thus damaging the instrument. Fuses

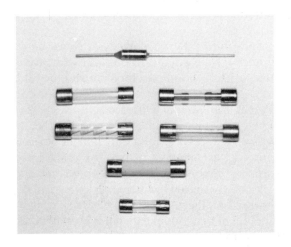

Fig. 5-2 Fuses commonly used in clinical laboratory equipment.

should be replaced with those of the same ratings. Never replace a fuse with one that has a higher current rating or a lower voltage rating. If the current rating is too high, a larger amount of current will be allowed to enter the circuit, causing serious damage to the circuitry. If the fuse has a voltage rating that is too low, the current can bypass its protective function by "electrical arcing." Jumper connectors or other conducting substitutes should never be used to bypass a fuse.

The fuse that is most commonly used in laboratory instruments is called a **slow-blowing fuse.** This fuse does not blow immediately with a surge of current because it has a high lag time. It will, however, blow immediately if the circuit is drawing abnormally high current. A slow-blowing fuse is used to prevent unnecessary instrument downtime because of increased current demands when an instrument is first turned on or from the normal surges that occur in a commercial power supply. A **fast-blowing fuse** or standard fuse has a short lag time. It will blow very quickly with any increase in current. This type of fuse is used to protect sensitive electronic equipment and delicate meters or components within a circuit.

The fuse is the first electronic component that should be checked if an instrument goes completely "dead." However, it is important to realize that a blown fuse indicates that a more serious electronic problem exists, which must be identified and corrected before the fuse is replaced. It is important to realize that replacement of a fuse should be performed in a judicious manner.

Exceeding Power Line Voltages. It is important that the total power expended by all instruments on a given circuit does not exceed the power rating of that circuit line to prevent a circuit overload. The overload is caused by the instruments drawing an excessive amount of current from the power line. When the amount of current exceeds a predetermined value, an electromagnetic switch called a circuit breaker is opened ("tripped"). The function of the circuit breaker is similar to that of a fuse except it protects the power line rather than an instrument or other device. Also, unlike a fuse, the circuit breaker can be reset after the overload is corrected.

Everyone knows that equipment will cease to operate if a fuse blows or circuit breaker is tripped. However, low power line voltage can also cause equipment to operate erratically or not at all. Low line voltage is often caused by too much equipment being operated from the same power line. The power consumed by each piece of electrical equipment is usually marked on its surface. The total current drawn by a number of pieces of equipment can be found by adding up the power consumed by each piece of equipment and dividing the total by the line voltage. This current should then be compared with the current capability of the power line to determine if it is within specified ratings.

For example, if the following equipment is plugged into a 120 V line carrying 12 A, how much current is drawn by the equipment and is the line operating within its capacity?

Instrument power rating:

Osmometer 250 W
Flame photometer 400 W
Blood gas analyzer 300 W
Random access analyzer 550 W
Solution:
Total power consumed: 250 W + 400 W +
    300 W + 550 W = 1500 W
Current (I) = P/E: 1550 W/120 V = 12.5 A

Because the total amperage required by the four instruments is 12.5 A and the line is carrying 12.0 A, the line is being operated beyond its rating. Thus the circuit breaker protecting this line would be tripped.

There is another approach to the problem. If the total power of the line is calculated (P = IE = 12.0 A × 120 V = 1440 W) and then compared with the total power being consumed by the instruments (250 W + 400 W + 300 W + 550 W = 1500 W), a similar conclusion can be drawn. The power rating of the line has been exceeded, and thus there is a circuit overload.

Extinguishing Electrical Fires. The generation of excess heat by high current may cause an electrical fire. If smoke and/or odor indicate burning within a circuit, the instrument should be turned off and unplugged immediately. A carbon dioxide-type fire extinguisher should be used on all electrical fires; water and foams are electrical conductors and therefore should never be used.

Poisonous selenium dioxide fumes having a characteristic pungent odor are liberated from a selenium rectifier when it burns out. The fumes should not be inhaled. Therefore adequate ventilation is of immediate importance. Replacement of the burned out rectifier should not be attempted until after it has cooled.

A common cause of electrical fires with laboratory instruments is a lack of adequate ventilation. If sufficient space is not provided for instruments that generate large amounts of heat, they will tend to overheat. The generation of an excessive amount of heat can melt the insulation of wires and other electronic components. Most instruments that produce large amounts of heat are equipped with fans that help circulate the air and thus maintain the instrument at an appropriate operating temperature. However, for them to function properly, the instrument must be located in an area that allows for adequate airflow.

Basic Troubleshooting Principles

The purpose of troubleshooting an instrument is to determine which module, circuit, or component is defective. It requires common sense and a basic understanding of troubleshooting principles. The first rule of troubleshooting any piece of equipment is to check the simplest and most obvious things first: Is the power cord plugged in, is the instrument plugged into the correct line voltage (i.e., 120 V vs 220 V), are the cables and connectors properly connected to the instrument, is a bulb or lamp burned out, or has the fuse blown. These types of problems can usually be resolved by a competent technologist. If these possibilities have been ruled out and the instrument is still not operating properly, a more sophisticated approach must be taken.

Several approaches have been devised to isolate the cause of the malfunction and determine which component or circuit is defective. The following section deals with some of those basic techniques. However, these techniques should be performed only by an individual well-versed in electrical and electronic procedures and are not recommended to be practiced by most medical technologists.

Substituting Parts or Modules Based on the Problem. Often a malfunctioning instrument can be repaired by noting the problem and then substituting a spare part or plug-in module. Some instruments are manufactured with identical parts or modules that are interchangeable. Other instruments, especially if they are bought or leased with a service contract, come with replacement parts or components. If the problem in one module can be corrected by interchanging with that of another, or if the problem is directly related to the function of that module, then it is most likely defective. Many instruments such as the Technicon SMAC System or Beckman Astra have modules that are accessible and easily replaced.

Voltage Measurements at Test Points. Often it is necessary to compare measured voltages at various test points with those specified in the electrical schematics of the manufacturer's maintenance manual. The proper type of meter must be used in this method to ensure that voltage measurements are accurate. The modern analog VOM is usually adequate for most measurements. However, digital meters are preferred when measuring small voltages.

Today's sophisticated instruments are constructed on printed circuit boards that plug into the chassis as modules. Often it is extremely difficult to measure voltages on these boards when they are plugged into the instrument because they are placed in electrical sockets that are in parallel and in close proximity to each other. One solution is to place the printed circuit modules on racks that can slide out from the instrument, thereby making the components more accessible for electrical measurements. Another approach is to use an **extender board.** To use an extender board, the power is first turned off. Then the printed circuit board is removed and attached to the extender board. Finally, the extender board is plugged into the instrument and the power is turned on. By using the extender board, the printed circuit board is placed outside the instrument's enclosure where voltages may be conveniently measured. Extender boards usually are encoded with a system of letters, numbers, or colors to ensure they are not plugged into the instrument or the printed circuit board in the reverse direction. If either the extender board or the circuit board is reversed, electrical damage to the instrument will most likely occur.

Resistance Measurements and Continuity Checks. This approach is similar to the one previously mentioned except resistance measurements are compared with the specified values provided by the manufacturer. Because an ohmmeter is used for these purposes, the equipment must be turned off and capacitors that do not contain bleeder resistors have to be discharged before taking any measurements. Because modern instruments contain semiconductor circuits that are composed of diodes and transistors, the polarity of the circuit and the ohmmeter must be known. This is because an internal battery is used as the voltage source, and diodes and transistor biasing are affected by the direction of current flow. The polarity of the circuit is usually given in the electrical schematics provided by the manufacturer. The polarity of the ohmmeter can be determined by measuring the ohmmeter voltage output with a DC voltmeter and then observing the polarity of the voltage. If the needle on an analog meter deflects in a negative direction or a negative sign appears on the readout of a digital meter, then the polarity needs to be reversed. On most modern VOMs the polarity can be reversed by changing the position of a selector switch.

Sometimes it is necessary to perform a continuity check using the ohmmeter. Continuity checks are important in determining if there is a completed path to conduct current flow. A reading of infinity indicates that an open circuit exists (the path for current flow is broken), and a zero reading means that a short exists (there is zero resistance between the test leads). Performing a continuity check may help to determine which component is malfunctioning.

Comparing Signal Tracings and Waveforms. This method of troubleshooting requires the use of an oscilloscope that can monitor the various waveforms that are often encountered in complex AC and DC circuits. It requires the services of a skilled electronics technician.

Most clinical laboratory instruments are menu-driven by computers and therefore are too complex to be repaired by most clinical laboratory personnel. Furthermore, many of these computerized instruments have self-diagnostic checks that help to pinpoint the location of the problem. Even with these self-diagnostic capabilities, most service personnel from the manufacturer will inevitably elect to replace an entire board or module rather than attempt to repair or replace an individual component. In general, troubleshooting and repairing a malfunctioning instrument is best performed by a service engineer unless it involves the simple replacement of a fuse, a lamp, or an entire analytic module.

Review Questions

1. Which of the following factors can affect the severity of an electric shock?
   A. Magnitude of current
   B. Duration of current
   C. Pathway of current
   D. All of the above
2. Which of the following statements concerning electrical safety is false?
   A. A "cheater" plug can be used with the three-prong power cord of an instrument provided that its grounding lead is connected to a ground.
   B. When working on circuits, keep one hand away from conducting surfaces.

C. Only qualified electronic personnel should work on instruments that contain cathode ray tubes.

D. A foam extinguisher can be used on an electrical fire.

3. Capacitors do not have to be discharged before working on an instrument that has malfunctioned provided that the instrument is turned off.
   A. True
   B. False

4. What is the rating of a 120 VAC power line carrying 20 A of current?
   A. 48 kW
   B. 120 W
   C. 720 W
   D. 2400 W

5. The function of a "bleeder" resistor is to discharge a _____ to ground when the circuit is turned off.
   A. Diode
   B. Capacitor
   C. Inductor
   D. Cathode ray tube

6. What is the minimum current rating required of a 115 VAC power line if it is to supply power to the following instruments?
   Cell sorter 500 W
   Flame photometer 350 W
   Oven 560 W
   A. 1.61 A

B. 11.5 A
C. 14.0 A
D. 16.1 A

7. A "blown" fuse can be replaced with one that has a higher amperage rating or lower voltage rating.
   A. True
   B. False

8. Solvents containing alcohol can be used to clean electrical equipment.
   A. True
   B. False

9. The resistance of components in a circuit containing capacitors can be measured only if the _____.
   A. Instrument has been turned off.
   B. Circuit contains "bleeder" resistors.
   C. Instrument has adequate grounding.
   D. Capacitors have been discharged.
   E. A, B, and D

10. Which of the following devices is used to protect power lines from experiencing an overload?
    A. Diode
    B. Transformer
    C. Rectifier
    D. Circuit breaker

Answers

1. D   2. D   3. B   4. D   5. B   6. C   7. B   8. B   9. E
10. D

Bibliography for Chapters 1 to 5

Accreditation manual for hospitals, 1982, Joint Commission on Accreditation of Hospitals, Chicago, Ill.

Ackerman PG: Electronic instrumentation in the clinical laboratory, Waltham, Mass, 1972, Little, Brown.

Bibbero RJ: Microprocessors in instruments and control, New York, 1977, John Wiley & Sons.

Bender GT: Principles of chemical instrumentation, Philadelphia. 1987, WB Saunders.

Boyce JC: Microprocessor and microcomputer basics, Englewood Cliffs, NJ, 1979, Prentice Hall.

Cromwell L, Weibell FJ, Pfeiffer EA, et al: Biomedical instrumentation and measurements, Englewood Cliffs, NJ, 1973, Prentice Hall.

Eggert AA: Electronics and instrumentation for the clinical laboratory, New York, 1983, John Wiley & Sons.

Ferris CD: Guide to medical laboratory instruments, Waltham, Mass, 1980, Little, Brown.

Fullton SR, Rawlins, JC: AC circuits, vol I, Basic circuit concepts, Fort Worth, Tex, 1981, Radio Shack, Division of Tandy Corporation.

Fullton SR, Rawlins JC: AC circuits, vol II, Circuit analysis methods, Fort Worth, Tex, 1981, Radio Shack, Division of Tandy Corporation.

Hicks MR, Schenken JR, and Steinrauf MA: Laboratory instrumentation, New York, 1980, Harper & Row.

Hodges DA: Microelectronic memories, Sci Am, Sept. 1977, 130.

Holton WC: The large-scale integration of microelectronic circuits. Sci Am, Sept. 1977, p. 82.

Jacobowitz H: Electricity made simple, Garden City, NY, 1959, Doubleday & Company.

Jacobowitz H: Electronics made simple, Garden City, NY, 1965, Doubleday & Company.

Jacobson B, Webster JG: Medicine and clinical engineering, Englewood Cliffs, NJ, 1977, Prentice Hall.

Jeffers DM, Lowe FB: Basic electronics for medical technologists, Houston, Tex, 1975, The American Society of Medical Technology and the ASMT Education & Research Fund.

Jeffers DM, Lowe FB: Clinical laboratory electronics, Houston, Tex, 1972, The American Society of Medical Technology and the ASMT Education & Research Fund.

Johnson DE, Hillburn JL, and Julich PM: Digital circuits and microcomputers, Englewood Cliffs, NJ, 1979, Prentice Hall.

Lackey JE, Hehn MD, and Massey JL: Fundamentals of electricity and electronics, New York, 1983, Holt, Rinehart & Winston.

Malmstadt HY, Enke CG: Electronics for scientists, New York, 1962, WA Benjamin.

Manville RR: Basic electricity/electronics, vol I, Basic principles, ed 2, Indianapolis, 1981, Howard W. Sams.

Meloan CE: Instrumental analysis using physical properties, Philadelphia, 1968, Lea & Febiger.

Meloan CE: Instrumental analysis using spectroscopy, Philadelphia, 1968, Lea & Febiger.

Mims FM: Getting started in electronics, Fort Worth, Tex, 1988, Radio Shack, Division of Tandy Corporation.

Oliva RA, Dale CW: DC circuits, vol I, Basic electricity and circuit concepts, Fort Worth, Tex, 1979, Radio Shack, Division of Tandy Corporation.

Oliva RA, Dale CW: DC circuits, vol II, Circuit analysis methods, Fort Worth, Tex, 1979, Radio Shack, Division of Tandy Corporation.

Tammes AR: Electronics for medical and biology laboratory personnel, Baltimore, 1971, Williams & Wilkins.

TEK Multipurpose Oscilloscopes—Oscilloscope Primer: The XYZ's of using a scope, Beaverton, OR, 1986, Tektronix.

Yanof HM: Biomedical electronics, Philadelphia, 1965, FA Davis.

PRINCIPLES OF INSTRUMENTATION

CHAPTER 6

Light and Its Measurement

LARRY E. SCHOEFF

Properties of Light
Dispersion of Light
Measurement of Light

Properties of Light

The majority of the instruments discussed in this book are devices that measure light in some way. Before the actual instrumentation is approached, think about light as a form of energy. An understanding of its nature, origin, and behavior is helpful later, as its emission, absorption, and quantitation in laboratory instruments are considered.

Energy. Light is a form of energy known as **electromagnetic radiation (EMR).** This radiant energy exhibits both wavelike properties and particle-like behavior. These particles, or packets of light energy, are known as **photons,** and their energies are directly related to their frequencies. The photons of radiant energy are produced by vibrating electrical charges that may be inner, middle, or valence electrons in atoms, or the vibrations of molecular atoms (Fig. 6-1).

The electrons of an atom possess most of the energy of the atom. When these electrons move from one orbital position to another, some energy is always absorbed or given up. If an element is heated in a flame, certain valence electrons will move from their normal position, which is usually referred to as **ground state,** to a new characteristic orbital position, or **excited state.** This means that the atom has absorbed a certain, definable amount of heat energy. When the atom cools, this energy is released as light. This very specific amount of energy corresponds to an exact color of light.

Each electron of each element requires a characteristic amount of energy to perform this transition. The electrons of some molecules may have more than one discrete and definable new orbital position they can occupy. Some electrons of the molecule are in bonding orbitals where they are controlled by two atoms. The transition from each of these orbital positions to ground state is characterized by emission of a very specific amount of light energy that corresponds to a characteristic color (Fig. 6-2). Emitted radiation from atoms is pure monochromatic radiation (i.e., one color light of a single wavelength), which produces line spectra; whereas molecules that contain many kinds of atoms produce band spectra as a result of overlapping lines or wavelengths of emission energy (Fig. 6-3).

Wavelength. Light is generally described in terms of color. However, when the color must be described with precision or when the radiant energy is beyond our visible range, we designate the radiant energy in terms of wavelength. Light or EMR waves are often described as being similar to the waves produced by dropping a pebble into water. The distance between two successive tops (crests) of the waves is defined as the **wavelength.** The height of each wave is called the **amplitude.** The other essential characteristic of a wave is the **frequency,** which is the number of waves, or crest-trough cycles, that will pass an observation point in 1 second (Fig. 6-4).

Frequency. The very high gamma rays of radioactivity are quite dangerous, and considerable caution should be exercised in exposure to x-rays. Even the lower frequencies of ultraviolet light can cause severe damage to the eye if a person looks directly into the source for more than a few seconds. The low-frequency rays of the infrared and the even longer radio waves may warm or pass through a person with no damage at all unless they are very intense.

It has been noted that visible light is produced when a valence electron is involved in a transition. Other energy levels in the electromagnetic spectrum derive from other atomic and molecular energy sources, shown in Fig. 6-5. Gamma ra-

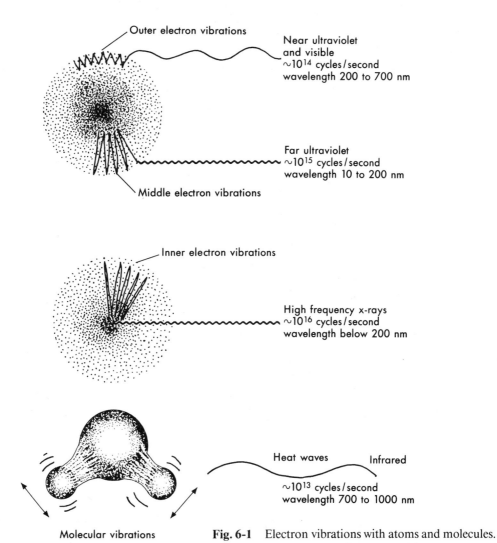

Fig. 6-1 Electron vibrations with atoms and molecules.

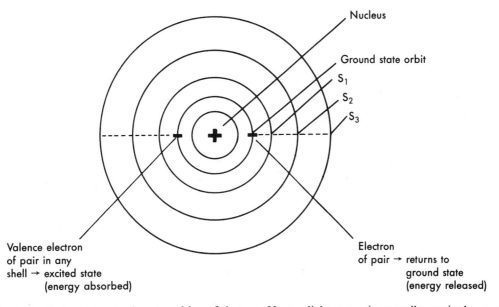

Fig. 6-2 Hypothetical atom to show transition of electron. Heat or light energy is generally required to move an electron from ground state to a new orbital position of S_1, S_2, or higher. As the electron returns to ground state, light is emitted; its wavelength will be determined by the energy given up. Violet is of higher energy than red.

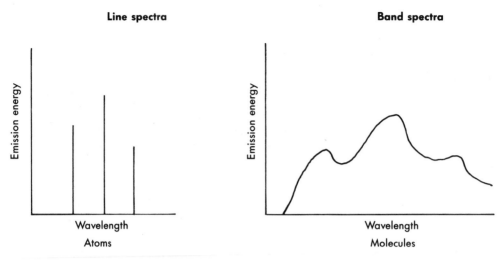

Fig. 6-3   Line spectra vs band spectra.

diation, which is the most potent form of electromagnetic energy, derives from the transition of a proton from the nucleus of the atom, which is a very fundamental change.

The frequency of light remains constant regardless of the medium through which it travels. The speed, however, may vary slightly and, as a consequence, the wavelength will also change. Also, the frequency may be expressed as cycles/second (c/s), but wavelength is expressed in number of units: centimeters, nanometers, and angstrom units. It is for these reasons that physicists like to refer to the frequency of the electromagnetic energy. In biology and medicine the wavelength is commonly used as the term of reference. In practice, the change in wavelength in different media mentioned before is not significant for most purposes. Furthermore, the visible and near-ultraviolet light, which is usually used, can be described in all cases in terms of nanometers. Hence the wavelength designation is adequate and is easier to visualize. The Greek letter lambda

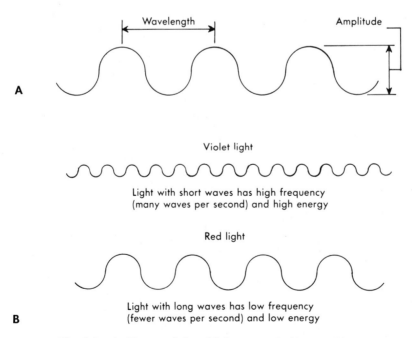

Fig. 6-4   **A,** Characteristics of light waves. **B,** Short and long waves.

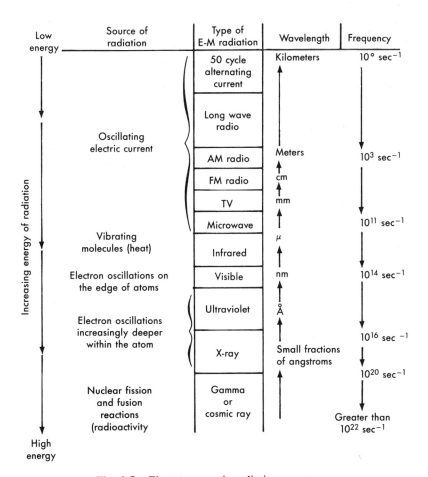

Fig. 6-5   Electromagnetic radiation spectrum.

(λ) is used as a symbol for wavelength. The symbol Å is used for angstrom unit, which is equal to one tenth of a nanometer.

Energy/Wavelength/Frequency Relationships. The wavelength is inversely related to frequency and energy (i.e., the shorter the wavelength, the higher the frequency and energy generated by this wavelength and vice versa), as seen in Fig. 6-4. For example, radiant energy occurring in the ultraviolet region will have a shorter wavelength, a higher frequency, and will contain more energy than radiant energy occurring in the infrared region. As stated earlier, the wavelike properties of light are interrelated with the photonlike or energetic properties of light. A German physicist, Max Planck, expressed the relationship between energy and frequency of light by saying that the energy of a photon (E) was directly proportional to the frequency (V).

$$E \propto V$$

The proportionality constant that resulted is known as **Planck's constant (h).** Consequently,

several equations were derived that quantitatively expressed the interrelationships among energy, frequency, and wavelength. These equations are given below:

A. *Energy and Frequency*

$$E = h\nu$$

where:

E = energy (photons)
h = Planck's constant
ν = frequency

B. *Energy and wavelength*

$$E = \frac{hc}{\lambda}$$

where:

E = energy (photons)
h = Planck's constant
c = speed of light
λ = wavelength

C. *Frequency and wavelength*

$$V = \frac{c}{\lambda}$$

where:

$$V = \text{frequency}$$
$$c = \text{speed of light}$$
$$\lambda = \text{wavelength}$$

In a vacuum all light travels at a constant speed, which is about 3×10^{10} cm, or 186,000 miles/second. If the distance light travels in 1 second is divided by the length of one wave, the number of waves/second or frequency is determined. The energy of light depends on its frequency and wavelength. To reiterate this, the higher the frequency (shorter wavelength), the higher its energy. Thus, light has been defined in terms of its wavelength, its frequency, or its energy. Physicists and engineers often express electromagnetic energy in terms of its frequency, or cycles/second.

When discussing very short wavelength (e.g., radiation such as gamma rays and x-rays), it is more convenient to refer to their energy, which is measured in thousands of electron volts (keV) or millions of electron volts (meV). One electron volt equals the amount of energy gained by one electron in passing through a potential difference field of one volt. When light is transmitted through matter, whether a liquid, a gas, or a solid, its speed is somewhat slower than in a vacuum, but its frequency is always constant. The ratio of the speed of light in a vacuum to its speed in a substance is referred to as the **refractive index** of the substance. This varies slightly with the wavelength under consideration and with the composition of the substance.

Intensity. Early students of light used the intensity of a candle made in a specific way as a term of reference. The term "standard candle" is still used, although it has since been more scientifically defined. Illumination is measured in footcandles. A footcandle is the illumination provided by one standard candle at a distance of 1 foot. Illumination varies inversely with the square of the distance from the source.

The total amount of light hitting a surface at a given distance is called the "luminous flux." A lumen is the luminous flux on 1 square foot of surface, all points of which are 1 foot from a light source of one candle.

$$\text{Total luminous flux} = \text{Candles} \times \frac{4R^2}{R^2}$$
$$= \text{Candles} \times 4$$

The surface of a sphere is equal to $4R^2$, and the flux decreases as the square of the distance (R = radius) increases.

As the number of candles (or candlepower) of a light is increased, the intensity of the light obviously increases. If a photocell is placed 1 foot from a light source and the light intensity is steadily increased, the output of electricity from the cell increases; this increase in electricity is directly proportional to the light intensity. Note that this output depends on the intensity of the light source, not on the wavelength or the energy level. If the light intensity is kept constant and the cell is first located 1 inch from the light, then 2 inches, and later 3 inches, it can be seen that the output of the photocell varies inversely with the square of the distance from the light. This becomes a critical factor in the design of photometric instruments.

Dispersion of Light

EMR Spectrum. When light hits a surface that causes it to diffract, or bend, there is a tendency for the different wavelengths to bend at slightly different angles and form a spectrum. This happens because of the difference in the refractive index of a substance for various wavelengths of light, mentioned previously. The colors in the spectrum normally listed are violet, blue, green, yellow, orange, red. The blue, green, and red are, of course, the primary colors that stand out. The human eye can see green at a wavelength of around 555 nm better than any other color. The sensitivity of the eye falls off rather symmetrically in both directions, and the human eye cannot see much below 400 or above 700 nm.

In the clinical laboratory, the wavelength regions that mainly concern the technologist in regard to the spectrophotometric measurements are the ultraviolet, the visible, and the near infrared regions. The visible region is further subdivided into various regions of "color." The visual sensation known as the color red is caused by light with a wavelength of 650 nm. Light with a wavelength of 400 nm causes the sensation of violet; other wavelengths in the visible region cause the other colors. The wavelength from 150 nm to 2500 nm is the clinical application range. This range of wavelengths includes those not visible to the human eye. As previously illustrated (see Fig. 6-5), the ultraviolet end of the range has wavelengths shorter than the visible, and the infrared and heat energy range has wavelengths longer than the visible. The visible range lies approximately between 350 nm and 750 nm (Fig. 6-6).

When light entering the eye consists of more than one wavelength, the sensation produced is

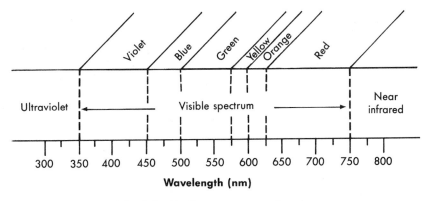

Fig. 6-6 Radiant energy wavelengths.

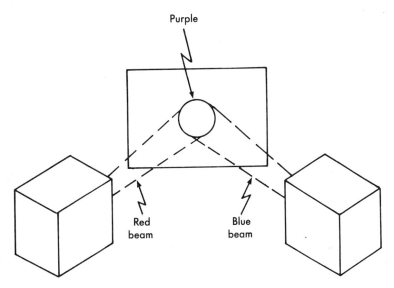

Fig. 6-7 Combining colored light.

caused by the combination. As an example, when red and blue wavelengths of visible light are contained in a light beam, the sensation is known as the color purple (Fig. 6-7). When all of the wavelengths of visible light are contained in a light beam, the sensation of white light is created.

Transmission vs Absorption. What has been described so far is how light is perceived as color. The question arises as to why a particular substance or object appears a certain color to the eye; for example, why does an apple appear red to the eye and not blue, or why do some objects appear black (lacking in color)? This question can be answered in terms of the wave nature of light and the phenomena caused by its wave nature as it passes through a substance. The ability of a substance to permit light to travel through it is referred to as transmission (Fig. 6-8). The light that

does not travel through the substance is said to be absorbed by the substance. Thus the effect of the substance on light is measured in two ways, transmission and absorption. This is illustrated in Fig. 6-9. The light that is transmitted is the color of the substance seen; the light that is absorbed is the complementary color of the transmitted light (Table 6-1). For example, an apple appears red to the eye because it transmits colors in the red region and it absorbs colors (wavelengths) in the blue-green region. An object appears black to the eye because it has transmitted no colors. Instead, it has absorbed all the colors of the visible spectrum. The opposite condition occurs with "white" objects. In spectrophotometry, it is often necessary to exclude (by absorption) some wavelengths while transmitting other desirable wavelengths. The device used to "screen out" undesir-

Fig. 6-8 Light transmitted through a substance.

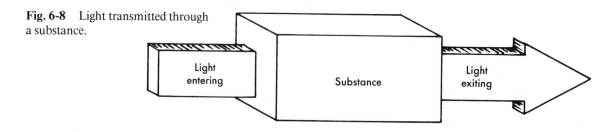

Fig. 6-9 Transmission and absorption of light.

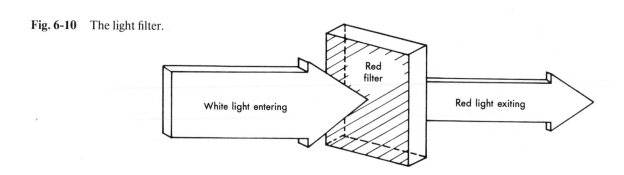

Fig. 6-10 The light filter.

Table 6-1 UV-visible spectrum characteristics

Wavelength (nm)	Region name	Color absorbed	Complementary color
180-220	Short UV	Not visible	—
220-380	UV	Not visible	—
380-430	Visible	Violet	Yellow-green
430-475	Visible	Blue	Yellow
475-495	Visible	Green-blue	Orange
495-505	Visible	Blue-green	Red
505-555	Visible	Green	Purple
555-575	Visible	Yellow-green	Violet
575-600	Visible	Yellow	Blue
600-620	Visible	Orange	Green-blue
620-700	Visible	Red	Blue-green

From Lee LW, Schmidt LM: *Elementary principles of laboratory instruments,* ed 5, 1983, CV Mosby.

able wavelengths is called a **filter.** Colored glasses and liquids are good examples of filters. In essence, the "red filter" appears red because only red light is transmitted by the glass; the other wavelengths, predominantly from the blue-green region are absorbed (Fig. 6-10). It is important to recognize that light is transmitted or absorbed by various forms of matter (i.e., gases, liquids, and solids); however, in a vacuum, only transmission occurs.

Reflection/Refraction. Sometimes light is neither transmitted nor absorbed but instead is deflected by the surface of a substance. This phenomenon is referred to as **reflection** (Fig. 6-11). For example, a mirror surface reflects light. When light travels from one medium or substance into another, it undergoes **refraction** (i.e., the light beam is deviated, being transmitted through the medium or substance in a direction different from the original [Fig. 6-12]). The refraction capability of a **prism** is used to spread a white beam of light into a spectrum (rainbow)

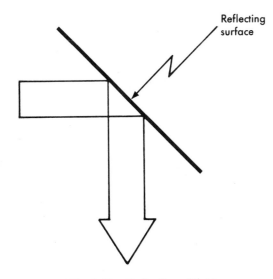

Fig. 6-11 Reflection of light.

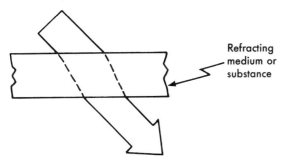

Fig. 6-12 Refraction of light.

(Fig. 6-13). This is known as **dispersion** and is achieved by the prism because the prism refracts each color of the spectrum to a different degree. Violet light is refracted (bent) farther than red. The actual separation between two wavelengths depends on the dispersive power of the prism and the apical angle of the prism. A nonlinear wavelength scale results. The longer wavelengths are not refracted as much and thus are crowded. Dispersion by glass is about 3 times that of quartz. Quartz or fused silica is mandatory for inclusion of the spectra below 350 nm.

Diffraction. Another phenomenon of radiant light energy results when it passes through very small openings called **slits.** As a light beam passes through any very narrow slit, the light is diffracted. **Diffraction** is a deviation, or change, in direction of the light beam as it passes by the edge of an opaque body. In addition a slit can deviate the beam in such a manner that the exiting beam is made up of light and dark areas. This has the effect of splitting the original beam into several beams (Fig. 6-14). The ability of a slit to disperse radiant energy is dependent on the size of the slit in comparison with the wavelength of the radiant energy going through the slit.

The ability to produce multiple beams of radiant energy depends on the wavelike properties of the radiant energy. When two waves are in phase, they are traveling so that their crests and

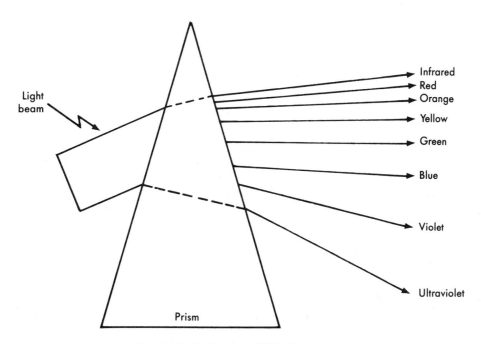

Fig. 6-13 Refraction of light by a prism.

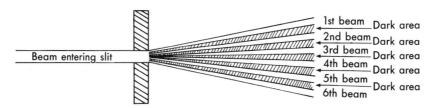

Fig. 6-14 Slit dispersing a light beam.

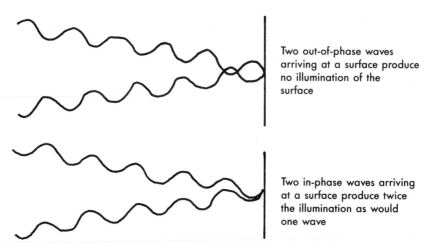

Fig. 6-15 Reinforcing and canceling waves.

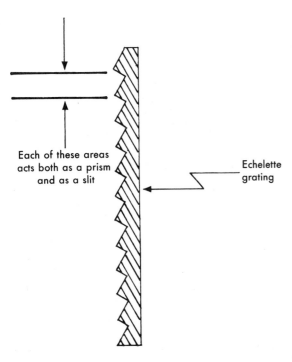

Fig. 6-16 Echelette transmission grating.

valleys are in coincidence. When two in phase waves of the same wavelength strike a surface, the energy at the surface is the sum of the energies of the two waves. If two waves are completely out of phase, the crest of one wave is opposite the valley of the other wave. When two waves of the same wavelength are completely out of phase on striking a surface, they cancel each other and no energy can be detected at the surface (Fig. 6-15). This accounts for the dark bands between the beams of visible energy produced by a narrow slit. This can be demonstrated visually with radiant energy in the visible range. When two in phase light rays arrive at a surface, the surface illumination is twice as great as it would be for a single light ray.

A device that incorporates the light principles of dispersion and diffraction is called a **grating.** A grating is generally used to produce the spectrum within a spectrophotometer of good quality. It disperses light by prism action and creates several spectra by using the characteristics of the narrow slit (Fig. 6-16). A linear dispersion of light results from a grating. When a beam of energy, containing many wavelengths, strikes a grating, many tiny spectra are produced, one for each line of the grating. Each ascending-order spectrum is more distorted and more diffuse than the preceding one. As a result, some interference can be produced by second and third order spectrum wavelengths overlapping at various primary wavelengths. In general, within the visible range, with a good quality grating, this problem is not as apparent because most of the secondary and tertiary wavelengths generated are not found within the visible range. As the wavelengths move past the corners, wavefronts are formed. Where these cross, those that are in phase reinforce one another and those that are not cancel out and disappear, thus leaving a complete spectrum to display on the exit slit, much the same as with a prism. Only the strongest spectrum produced by the grating is used in the spectrophotometer.

Measurement of Light

Devices. Photosensitive devices are subject to the same sort of limitations as the eye, and most have an optimum range at which they are most sensitive. In a photometer, the 100% transmittance (T) reading must be reset each time the wavelength is changed. This is because of the difference in sensitivity of the photocell at different wavelengths. To compensate for this difference in sensitivity, scanning spectrophotometers may have a cam-driven slit or other device to regulate total light falling on the phototube.

Devices that are capable of breaking up white light to form a spectrum are called **monochromators.** Two that are commonly used in spectrophotometers are the prism and the diffraction grating. The prism is a piece of glass or quartz cut in such a way as to have interfaces at very precise angles. These can produce the fine quality of spectrum seen in some of the better instruments.

The diffraction grating is a highly polished surface into which a large number of parallel grooves have been cut. Such a surface is able to scatter light and produce a spectrum. The grating may either reflect light or transmit it.

Photometric instruments used in the clinical laboratory measure light in a variety of ways. In addition to spectrophotometers, there are flame photometers, fluorometers, atomic absorption photometers, isotope-counting analyzers, cell counters, coagulation-measuring devices, and many other instruments that are either light sensing or light measuring. All of these are discussed in detail in later chapters.

A **photometer** is literally an instrument for measuring light intensity, and in the medical laboratory the term is often used in its generic sense as any instrument that measures light. In the clinical laboratory a **colorimeter** refers to an instrument that measures the absorption of a colored light by a solution, in which the colored light is produced by simple or compound glass filters. A **spectrophotometer** is an instrument that measures the absorption of monochromatic light, which has been defined by selecting a band from a spectrum produced by a monochromator. General usage of these terms has given them legitimacy in the laboratory, but think clearly about what is meant by each one.

Flame photometers measure the emission of single atomic elements burned in a flame. Atomic absorption photometers measure the light absorbed by certain atoms when excited by heat. Fluorometers measure light of a specific wavelength that is emitted by a molecular compound when it is excited by light of a given energy or wavelength. Thus spectroscopy can be classified into four categories: absorption or emission by atoms, and absorption or emission by molecules.

Overview of Components. Any device for measuring the absorption of light by a solution will have certain basic components (Fig. 6-17). A source of power of some sort is required for the **exciter lamp.** An exciter lamp, *A*, provides light containing many colors or wavelengths (represented by many arrows at *B*). This light passes through a filter or other device, *C*, that allows one color of light (represented by the single arrow at *D*) to impinge on the sample, *E*. This light is called the **incident light.** Some of the incident light is transmitted through the sample and is called **transmitted light.** The remainder of the light energy is absorbed by the molecules in the sample. This energy absorption represents energy used up in the displacement of valence electrons in the sample molecules. It is obvious that more energy would be used up if more molecules were in the path of the light. It would make little difference whether this increase in molecules were due to a longer light path through the solution or to the higher concentration of molecules in the solution.

The transmitted light, represented by the intermittent line, *F*, strikes the photosensitive surface of the photocell, *G*, where it produces an electric current that is proportional to the amount of light. This current, called the **photo-**

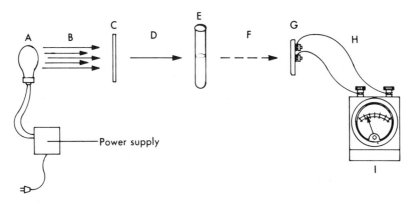

Fig. 6-17 Process of absorption measurement.

current, *H*, flows through the meter circuit and causes the needle to move up scale on the meter, *I*.

Molecular Absorption. Specific molecules or molecular compounds in a solution absorb specific light energy. The same kind of molecules will absorb the same wavelength of light. Light of a specific wavelength must be used because each substance absorbs light optimally at its characteristic wavelength(s). Producing monochromatic light is necessary to measure absorption of substances accurately.

It is necessary to identify an intensity of light as a norm (100% T) and then measure how much of the light is absorbed. Ideally, the incident light that falls on the sample is pure monochromatic light, but in practice it will contain some **stray light** of various wavelengths that has somehow reached the sample. Usually the internal surfaces of a monochromator are painted black in an effort to make them ideal black-body radiators, or surfaces able to absorb all wavelengths of light, but this is an ideal that is never completely effected. The transmittance of a sample, designated as T, is the percent of incident light that is transmitted through it. The **percent transmittance,** or **%T,** of a sample is its transmittance over the transmittance of its solvent alone.

Absorbance is a measure of the monochromatic light that has been absorbed by the sample. It can be thought of as the reciprocal of transmittance, but it is expressed as the log to the base 10 of the reciprocal of transmittance. Mathematically, A = 2 − log 1/T, or 2 − log %T. Absorbance is designated by the capital letter A. In earlier years the terms optical density (OD), absorbency, and extinction were used to denote absorbance. All of these terms are ambiguous and obsolete and should not be used.

Laws of Absorbance. Two laws of absorbance govern the measurement of light relative to a sample's concentration. The first law is known as **Beer's law,** which simply stated, means that absorbance varies directly with the concentration of the solution in question. For example, if a 0.5% solution of a substance has an absorbance of 0.20, then a 1.0% solution of the same substance would have an absorbance reading of 0.40. Beer's law implies linearity with respect to concentration and absorbance. If a test solution obeys Beer's law, then a plot of various concentrations (abscissa) vs absorbance values (ordinate) will give a straight line on cartesian graph paper. However, if transmittance is used instead of absorbance, this linear relationship does not hold. A straight line can be achieved by plotting transmittance vs concentration on semilogarithmic graph paper, which implies a logarithmic relationship and not a linear relationship (Fig. 6-18).

The second law is known as the **Bouguer-Lambert law** or simply the Lambert law. This law, basically stated, means that absorbance increases exponentially with increases in the light path (i.e., the absorbance of a given solution in a 2 cm light path will be twice that given by the same solution in a 1 cm light path). Because the number of individual molecules of the substance absorbing light determines absorbance, it stands to reason that either increasing the concentration twofold of a given substance or doubling the light path through that substance would in fact have the same effect on the absorption of the substance. Consequently, reference is often made to the Beer-Lambert law, which implies that similarity between the two laws exists. The overall equation, which incorporates both laws, is given by the following expression:

$$A = abc$$

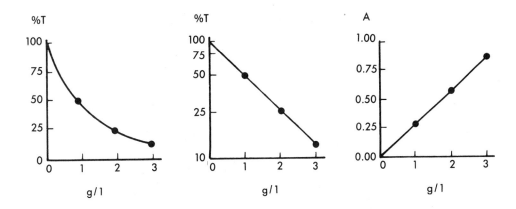

Fig. 6-18 Transmittance and absorbance as a function of concentration. **A**, % T, linear scale. **B**, % T, logarithmic scale. **C**, Absorbance, linear scale.

where:

A = Absorbance
a = Absorptivity of a substance under standard conditions
b = Light path in cm
c = Concentration of the substance

Typically, $b = 1$ cm and c is expressed in mmole/L. The value for a is a constant for a given compound at a given wavelength under prescribed conditions of solvent, temperature, pH, etc., and is called the **molar absorptivity.** By definition, molar absorptivity is the absorbance of 1 g/L of a substance (1 molar), measured in a 1 cm light path at a specific wavelength. Often the molar absorptivity may be a number (such as 4.6) that can not be read on most spectrophotometers. In practice a dilution of the one molar solution is made, and the absorbance value is multiplied by the dilution factor. Molar absorptivity is a convenient expression, but not usually practical for direct measurement. In the English literature absorptivity is often called extinction coefficient.

The Beer-Lambert law gives rise to a series of expressions routinely used in spectrophotometry. If conditions are kept constant such that the molar absorptivity of a given measured substance does not change and if the length of the light path remains constant, then the only remaining variables in the expression are the absorbance, A, and the concentration, c. If the absorbance of a standard and an unknown containing the same substance are measured, the two can be equated by the following expression:

$$\frac{A_u}{C_u} = \frac{A_s}{C_s}$$

where:

A_u = Absorbance (unknown)
C_u = Concentration (unknown)
A_s = Absorbance (standard)
C_s = Concentration (standard)

The expression A_s/C_s represents what is known as the constant K, which represents the slope of a standard calibrative curve (concentration vs absorbance). If A_u is divided by K, the result is C_u. This equation is illustrated as:

$$\frac{A_u}{A_s/C_s} = C_u \qquad \text{or} \qquad \frac{A_u}{K} = C_u$$

A more convenient expression to use involves multiplying the absorbance of the unknown by the reciprocal of K or (C_s/A_s). This factor is sometimes referred to as the F constant and is commonly used in spectrophotometers of good quality, which are capable of giving direct concentration readout. This equation is given below.

$$A_u \times \frac{C_s}{A_s} = C_u \qquad \text{or} \qquad A_u \times F \text{ (or } 1/K) = C_u$$

Fig. 6-19 will help illustrate the use of these equations. This graph represents the calibration (standard) curve for various standard concentrations of Evans blue dye. To calculate K or the slope of the line, simply do the following:

1. Pick out two standards and their respective absorbances.
2. Calculate the delta between the two concentrations.
3. Calculate the delta between the two respective absorbances.

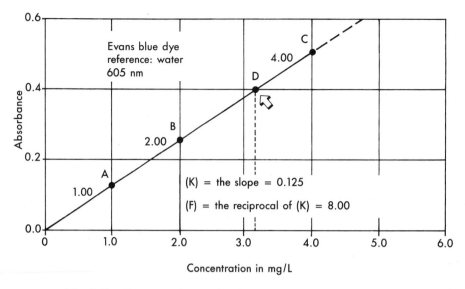

Fig. 6-19 Concentration vs absorbance graph. K = Slope of line.

4. The ratio between the delta of the absorbances of these standards and the delta of their respective concentrations is the slope of the line K.

In the example given in Fig. 6-19, the slope K and F constant would be calculated as follows:

	Std. (A)	Std. (C)	(Delta)
Absorbance:	0.125	0.500	0.375
Standard			
concentration:	1.00	4.00	3.00

For this particular substance (Evans blue dye):

$$K = \frac{A_s}{C_s} = 0.125$$

$$F = \frac{C_s}{A_s} = 8.00$$

To obtain the concentration at point D where absorbance = 0.4:

$$C_u = \frac{A_u}{K} = \frac{0.4}{0.125} = 3.20$$

or

$$C_u = A_u \times F = 0.4 \times 8.00 = 3.20$$

These relationships only hold true for substances that obey Beer's law. Some substances and mixtures do not follow Beer's law because of their nature. These are the materials that are susceptible to changes in temperature, pressure, pH level, dissociation, etc. Stray light within the instrument will also cause results to wander from the ideal situation expressed by Beer's law. It should be noted that point C in Fig. 6-19 represents the highest standard used in computing the linearity of the calibration curve. Therefore any unknown sample that has an absorbance reading beyond this point cannot be read and its corresponding concentration cannot be calculated using this standard line. It is inappropriate to extrapolate beyond the last standard point because doing so would only assume linearity beyond the highest standard. Most reactions have an upper limit of linearity. Therefore, to properly use this calibration curve, the high unknown sample should be diluted before reacting it with reagent(s). There may also be limitations/restrictions concerning sample dilution and the method of interest. Always refer to the appropriate reference before diluting the sample.

In this chapter the basic properties of light and how various types of media and devices affect the dispersion, transmission, and absorption of light have been examined. The last section included discussion of how light is measured in photometers and the laws of absorbance that govern its measurement. In the next chapter a detailed description of spectrophotometers is presented, along with various conditions and problems that are encountered in operating these instruments.

Review Questions

1. What role do electrons that surround atoms play in the light measurement process?
2. What regions of the electromagnetic spectrum are of clinical interest for measurement devices?

3. What type of emission spectra are produced by atoms? Molecules? Solids?

4. Differentiate absorbance from % transmittance and diagram a graph of each vs concentration.

5. Describe the relationship between energy, frequency, and wavelength of light.

6. Diagram, in sequence, the basic components of a photometer.

7. List three types of monochromators in increasing order of resolution.

CHAPTER 7

Molecular Absorption Spectroscopy

LARRY E. SCHOEFF

Components of Spectrophotometers
**Single Beam versus Double Beam Spectropho-
tometers**
Parameters of Operation
Common Instruments in Use

Most determinations made in the clinical laboratory are based on the measurements of radiant energy transmitted or absorbed under controlled conditions. The device that is used to detect transmitted or absorbed radiant light energy is called a spectrophotometer. Because this instrument is so widely used in the clinical laboratory, it is essential that the technologist has a good understanding as to how it functions. The prerequisites that are needed to have a good working knowledge of this system, its application, and its instrumental maintenance are a good understanding of the basic principles of spectrophotometry, and a good working knowledge of each component part and its respective function as a part of the system as a whole. In this chapter the major components of a spectrophotometer and their respective functions are described in detail. In addition, problems with a single beam spectrophotometer are discussed, along with solutions (i.e., the use of a dual-beam system). Finally, calibration and operation of spectrophotometers are covered, followed by a description of common spectrophotometers in use.

Components of Spectrophotometers

Power Supply and Exciter Lamp. Some supply of electricity to operate the exciter lamp is necessary. Details of power supplies are discussed in Chapter 3. The exciter lamp must furnish an intense, reasonably cool, constant beam of light that can be easily collimated. The filament must be small and provide an intense light; it must be of such a design that it can be exactly aligned

when replaced, and it must be highly reproducible in all respects.

As any object changes temperature, it emits a somewhat different spectrum. This is apparent when house lights dim during a power failure. Lamps take on a yellow color, and if the power surges back past its normal value, the light becomes whiter. If the spectra produced by the lamp in such cases could be compared, it would be immediately obvious that the same area of the spectrum does not give the same distribution of wavelengths. Hence the temperature of the lamp is important. The quality and uniformity of construction of the exciter lamp are significant factors in the uniform performance of the spectrophotometric instrument. For work in the visible and near infrared ranges, tungsten and halogen quartz lamps are good sources of radiant energy. The quartz lamp is preferred because it provides a more intense beam of light and a better source of white light in the near ultraviolet region. Both lamps may be used down to about 340 nm.

Several other sources are available for ultraviolet (UV) work. The hydrogen lamp is probably one of the best choices. The mercury lamp has a much more uneven emission spectrum and is less desirable. A xenon lamp gives a brilliant light that is ideal for narrow slit work but is almost too brilliant for routine application because there is a large stray light problem with such an intense beam. The xenon lamp requires a high voltage to ignite or fire. Ozone is produced by ionization of oxygen around the lamp in dangerous quantities and must be dissipated in some way. Hydrogen, mercury, and xenon lamps are all vapor lamps. In lamps of this sort a high voltage is applied through the envelope that contains the vapor of the element named. The molecules of gas are ionized and emit a characteristic light, which will contain the same wavelengths that would be seen if the element were burned in a hot flame. There is no filament in a vapor lamp. The high firing or ionization voltage is required only initially, after which a low voltage is adequate to maintain ionization and cause the lamp to glow.

For IR spectrophotometers a silicone carbide rod heated to about 1200° C works well. When the exciter lamp is changed in a photometer, the calibration of the instrument should be rechecked. Calibration is included in the discussion of spectrophotometers.

Most colorimetric instruments now use a prefocused lamp. This is a lamp with the characteristics just discussed with its base configured to fit only one way in the socket for alignment. Because the lamp may be locked in only one position, any lamp of the same design will be positioned and centered in the identical way. The filament in each lamp is positioned in the same place in relation to the base. Even with the prefocused lamp there may be some slight but important error of alignment. The angle at which light strikes a diffraction grating determines the position of the spectrum and hence the color of light striking the sample. Recalibration is therefore necessary each time a lamp is changed.

A few newer instruments make use of light emitted by lasers. Others may use light-emitting diodes as a source of light. The use of these unusual energy sources is discussed as it applies to specific instruments.

Between the exciter lamp and the monochromator, **collimating lenses** are often inserted. These lenses collect the light rays and focus them in such a way that the light passing into the monochromator will be an organized beam of parallel light (Fig. 7-1). A heat filter may also be placed in the light beam close to the exciter lamp to protect the monochromator from radiant heat. A heat filter is clear glass designed to absorb or reject heat-producing infrared rays while allowing visible light to pass.

Monochromator. A monochromator is a device for producing light of a single color from an impure source. The word monochromatic means "of one color." As mentioned earlier, it is difficult to identify the point at which one color begins and another ends. Monochromatic light is identified specifically when its wavelength is specified. It is unlikely, however, that a light of one uniform wavelength will be isolated. It must be explained what range of wavelengths is being discussed. This range is the **bandpass.** A monochromatic light that appears to be grass green in color would have a wavelength of about 550 nm, but wavelengths of 525 to 575 nm in length might also be present. The bandpass would be from 525 to 575 nm, or 50 nm wide.

The term bandpass needs to be defined still more specifically. Consider the green light passing through a glass filter. All the light of 550 nm wavelength passes but the somewhat less blue-green light also passes. Blue light may pass in small amounts, and a trace of violet (400 nm) may pass. In the same way yellow-green, yellow, and orange (600 nm) may be present in decreasing amounts. If transmitted light were plotted against wavelength, there would be a curve similar to that in Fig. 7-2. Because the outer edges of the curve extend more or less to infinity, the previous explanation of bandpass is vague. By defi-

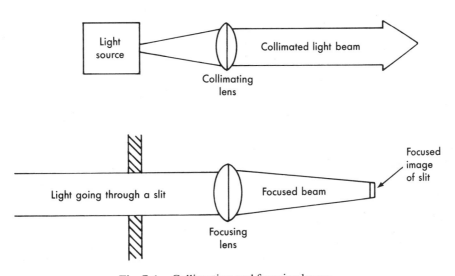

Fig. 7-1 Collimating and focusing lenses.

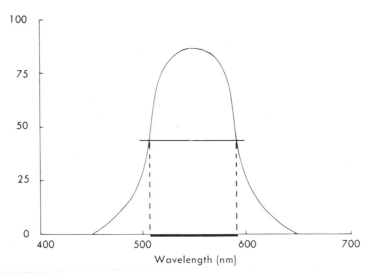

Fig. 7-2   Light transmitted through green filter. Heavy line at base indicates bandpass.

nition the bandpass is the range of wavelengths between the points at which transmittance is one half the peak transmittance (Fig. 7-2).

The simplest monochromator is a single glass filter, although it may not appear to be a monochromator because the bandpass of a filter is wide and the light that passes will include more than one color. Glass filters are made by suspending a coloring agent in molten glass. The thickness of the filter, molded from the mixture, determines how much light will be absorbed. The filter is identified by (1) peak transmittance, (2) bandpass, and (3) thickness and/or opacity.

A narrower bandpass may be obtained by cementing two glass filters of different colors together. Only the wavelengths that are passed in common by both filters will constitute the bandpass for this compound filter.

Glass filters are used only for transmitting visible and near-visible light. Both UV-absorbing and IR-absorbing, visible light-transmitting filters are available, and near UV-transmitting, visible light-absorbing filters also exist. For some purposes filter colorimeters are quite adequate. A good filter colorimeter is sufficiently accurate and economical for doing routine tests such as hemoglobin concentration.

Interference filters, made by placing semitransparent silver films on both sides of a thin transparent layer of magnesium fluoride, will give a narrow bandpass. Side bands (harmonics) occur at other wavelengths, however, and may be the thickness and refractive index of the magnesium fluoride and the angle at which the incident light strikes the filter. This type of filter may have an extremely narrow bandpass. The most widely used true monochromator is composed of an **entrance slit,** a **prism** or **diffraction grating** to disperse the light, and an **exit slit** to select the bandpass (Fig. 7-3).

The entrance slit is generally fixed and is designed to limit the collimated light allowed to strike the prism or grating. Reflected light is thus reduced to a minimum. One measure of the quality of a monochromator is the amount of stray light it allows to pass. Usually this is expressed in terms of percent of total light. Less than 1% is acceptable for most routine purposes.

When it strikes a prism, white light is dispersed to form a spectrum. This occurs because the angle of refraction of light at an interface (such as that between air and a glass prism) varies with the wavelength. Thus violet is refracted more than red, and the spectrum is formed. The index of refraction determines the spread of the spectrum and the relative width of the color bands. Glass is the material of choice for visible light; ultraviolet light is absorbed by glass. Quartz and fused silica are preferable for ultraviolet light; but when they are used in the near-IR and IR regions, the color bands produced are too narrow for practical use. The reason for this is apparent in Fig. 7-3. The spectrum is distorted as it is projected at an angle onto the back wall of the monochromator. The red end of the spectrum shows the least distortion; the blue end shows the most. A slit of consistent width placed at the red end and the blue end would produce a significantly different band-

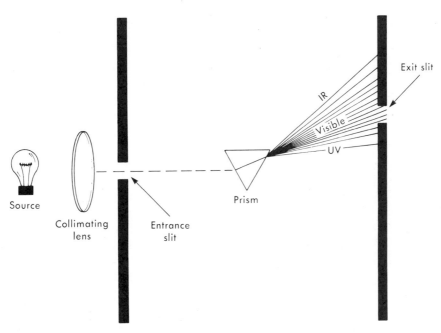

Fig. 7-3 Principal elements of a monochromator. Changing the position of the prism causes the spectrum to move up or down on the back wall of the monochromator so that another color passes through the exit slit.

pass of light. In past years most high-quality spectrophotometers have used glass or quartz prisms in their monochromators. A very clean spectrum can be produced. The mechanics must be very precise. Because high-quality diffraction gratings can now be produced economically, most spectrophotometers of good quality incorporate diffraction gratings.

Glass diffraction gratings are made by cutting tiny furrows into the aluminized face of a perfect, flat piece of crown glass. These furrows are cut at a precise angle and at an accurate distance from each other. Cutting is done with a diamond point, and there are usually 1000 to 50,000 furrows to the inch. These original glass gratings may be used as master gratings in the production of a molded product called a replica grating.

As white light strikes the grating, it is diffracted to form several spectra (Fig. 7-4). Each of these is at a different angle from the grating. The brightest of these is called the first-order spectrum. It is generally used rather than the more diffuse, higher-order spectra. The angle at which the first order spectrum is diffracted depends on the angle at which the white light hits the grating and on the blaze angle of the grating. The **blaze angle** is the angle at which the furrows are cut in the grating (Fig. 7-5). If the grating surface is coated with a layer of silver or aluminum, the spectrum will be

reflected instead of passed through the grating.

The spectrum, whether transmitted or reflected, falls onto the wall of the monochromator. A tiny exit slit in this wall allows a small portion of the spectrum to pass through and into the sam-

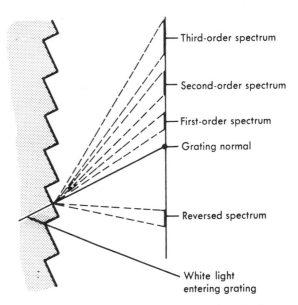

Fig. 7-4 Diffraction of light by a grating. Each ascending-order spectrum is more distorted and more diffuse than the preceding.

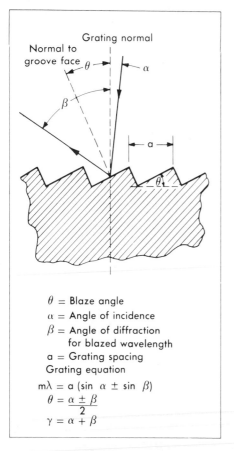

θ = Blaze angle
α = Angle of incidence
β = Angle of diffraction
    for blazed wavelength
a = Grating spacing
Grating equation
$$m\lambda = a \,(\sin \alpha \pm \sin \beta)$$
$$\theta = \frac{\alpha \pm \beta}{2}$$
$$\gamma = \alpha + \beta$$

Fig. 7-5 Greatly magnified cross section of a diffraction grating. (Courtesy Bausch & Lomb.)

ple to be measured. The particular portion of the spectrum (wavelength) that passes the slit is determined by the position of the spectrum; this in turn is determined by the relative positions of the light, the grating, and the slit. Some spectrophotometers move the light, whereas others move the grating to select the light that passes through the exit slit.

The bandpass of the monochromator depends on the width of the slit in relation to the length of the spectrum. A narrow bandpass is generally desirable. (The discussion on spectral scanning explains this.) Hence a narrow slit is used. There is a practical limit to the size of the slit, however. For example one fleck of dust in a very narrow slit may occlude it. Also the amount of light energy passing a very narrow slit may not be adequate to measure accurately. If the monochromator wall and slit are moved farther from the prism, the spectrum becomes larger and a wider slit may be used. This may not help much because light in-

tensity decreases as the square of the distance traveled (as mentioned earlier) and the light energy of a narrow bandpass are still not adequate. The best solution to this dilemma is the production of better detectors and amplifiers.

Many of the better monochromators have adjustable slits that allow the operator to determine the bandpass. Some slits are adjustable in two directions, allowing adjustment of both the bandpass and the total amount of light the wavelengths can pass.

In general grating monochromators are capable of better **resolution** than those that use prisms. Resolution is best in gratings with the most lines or furrows to the inch. Some stray light in grating monochromators is because of the first- and second-order spectra overlapping and reflecting light of other wavelengths through the slit. Sometimes a double monochromator or a glass filter is used to reduce the stray light. Gratings have the additional advantage of being practical for all wavelengths of light, in contrast to the glass or quartz prisms, which cannot be used in the UV region.

Transmittance gratings lose some light efficiency because a certain amount of energy is lost in passage through the grating. Narrow bandpass instruments generally use reflectance gratings for this reason, but transmittance gratings allow a simpler instrument design.

Sample Holder. A few observations concerning cells or **cuvettes** used for samples is pertinent. A square cuvette, which presents a flat surface to the incident light, has less light loss from reflection than does the round cell. This loss is more noticeable in an empty cuvette because the difference in the index of refraction between air and glass is greater than between glass and a solvent. In routine work this loss is probably not significant, being fairly constant at about 4% for most round cuvettes. It should be obvious that the cuvette must be thoroughly clean and free of fingerprints, etching, and clouding and that the sample and reference cells must be matched for transmittance. It should also be apparent that a longer light path through the sample will allow more accurate readings in dilute samples. Various types of horizontal cells and spacers are manufactured to provide long light paths for small samples. For routine work a light path of 1 cm has become standard. Most definitions and values are expressed in this term of reference. Ultraviolet light, as noted earlier, is absorbed strongly by lime glass. For this reason quartz or special-type glass cells must be used to hold the sample in this range.

An obvious but often ignored error is room light entering from the top of the cuvette or elsewhere. A light shield over the cuvette well should be provided and used whenever a reading is being made, otherwise a change in lighting may cause odd and mysterious errors, loss of accuracy, and confusion.

Many types of flow-through and flush-out cuvettes are available. These provide a constant light path and constant absorbance characteristics in addition to the obvious advantages of speed and facility of sample handling. In routine use care must be exercised not to allow them to become cloudy. Cells of this sort should be flushed thoroughly between types of samples and should not be left dry unless they have been rinsed several times with distilled water. Blanks should be run regularly.

Aside from the optical problems of the automatic sample-handling systems, there are often mechanical problems. These devices may suffer from various annoying handicaps that render them awkward for routine use. Totally automated chemistry systems are rapidly taking the place of these semiautomated sample handlers.

Photodetector. Photo cells, phototubes, photodiodes, photomultiplier tubes, and other types of detectors are discussed in Chapter 3.

Readout Device. In the past nearly all spectrophotometers used ammeters or galvanometers. Newer digital devices and printers have now replaced these, and many instruments relay their electrical output directly to computer circuits where calculations are performed, allowing direct reporting of sample concentrations. Readout devices are discussed in Chapter 3.

Single Beam vs Double Beam Spectrophotometer

Single beam spectrophotometers (Fig. 7-6) can be modified and improved to solve various problems that arise during operation and moreover provide additional capabilities of the instrument. These problems are identified below, along with instrument design modifications to solve these problems.

Problems and Solutions in Design. When a heavy load is placed on an electric power system, lights dim and later brighten. If readings are being made on a photometer at this moment, results will be completely unreliable, or if an aging exciter lamp flickers momentarily, readings on the photometer will be unstable and erroneous. Thus voltage fluctuation and changes in the light source, as well as instrument drift, can cause significant problems in measurements. If two photocells are positioned at equal distances from the exciter lamp and are attached to the same meter so that they oppose each other, this instability can be canceled. Photocell No. 1 will drive the meter upscale, and photocell No. 2 will drive it downscale. By using variable resistors the needle can be

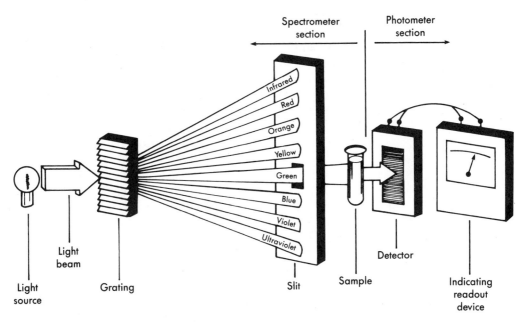

Fig. 7-6 A simplified single-beam spectrophotometer.

located at 100% T with the blank in the cuvette well. If the two cells are balanced, a change in light intensity will not cause the needle to move because both photocells will be affected equally. This is a very simple dual-beam photometer.

It is not quite true that the two photocells in a simple dual-beam photometer will balance each other. One beam is passing through a monochromator, and the photodetectors will not respond equally to the white light at the reference cell and the monochromatic light at the sample cell. Two monochromators could be used to solve this problem. If filters were being used, this might be a workable idea and the cells would balance better.

Using two grating monochromators to solve the problem mentioned previously would be quite expensive, and the two monochromators might not be exactly correlated. It is easy to insert a **beam splitter** into the light path between the monochromator and the sample so that the light will go to both the sample and the reference detectors. Beam splitters may be made in any of several ways. One of the simplest beam splitters is a half-silvered mirror, called a **dichroid mirror,** that allows half the light to pass through to the sample and the rest to be reflected to the reference cell.

Having two detectors can also be expensive, and if phototubes or photomultipliers are used, the wiring detail and power supply become complicated. Also, the two detectors are difficult to balance. One phototube can be used to read both the reference and the sample photocurrent. The net current is being read when the two currents are presented to the meter biased against each other. If one detector output is 40 μA and the other is 50 μA, there will be a net current of 10 μA when they oppose each other.

This signal comparison through one detector is accomplished by means of a **photochopper,**

which may work in several ways. One common light chopper is a mirror that rotates very rapidly. At one moment it directs the light beam past the sample, into a mirror, and then into the phototube. At the next moment it directs the beam through the sample and into the phototube (Fig. 7-7). When the beam is going directly to the phototube through the reference (position *1*), 50 μA of current flows. When the light passes through the sample (position *2*), only 40 μA of current flows. The output of the phototube is a square-wave current alternating between 40 and 50 μA. The difference between the two signals is the true absorbance signal from the sample's concentration of analyte.

In a single beam photometer the operator had to insert the blank solution in the sample beam, adjust it to 100% T, and substitute the sample to be read. With the sophisticated arrangement described previously this process is no longer necessary. All that is needed now is to provide a sample well for the reference, and the reference beam with the blank in it can be compared with the sample beam with the sample in it. The two can be compared without changing tubes, and a ratio can be established between them. If the output of the detector is fed to a recorder, the system can be called a **ratio-recording photometer.** This system is ideal for following a kinetic reaction in which the sample is changing absorbance as a function of time in response to enzyme activity, heat, or some other force.

To automatically produce a spectral absorbance curve, a drive motor is geared to the diffraction grating to turn it very slowly in the light path so that each color of the spectrum passes through the slit in succession. With the ratio-recording system, the instrument is continuously recording the relationship between the sample and the blank as different wavelengths pass through the sample. This geared motor attachment is called a **wavelength drive.** The recording that is produced is called a **spectral scan** of the sample. The spectral scan usually identifies a pure substance positively, and hence is a valuable tool. Concentration of the substance can also be calculated from known data.

There is some difficulty in reading peak heights at 400 and 700 nm on the chart. As noted earlier, detectors have a spectral response similar to the human eye. At the center of the spectrum the response will be high, but at the ends the response will be considerably lower. This inconvenience can be eliminated by installing a variable

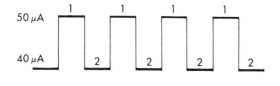

Fig. 7-7 Square-wave signal from a phototube receiving "chopped" light first from a reference cell and then from sample cell.

slit in the light beam before it reaches the detector. This variable slit is operated by a cam or eccentric wheel whose shape is a function of the shape of the spectral response curve. The cam is turned by and coordinated with the wavelength drive motor so that the slit is widest at the ends of the spectrum and narrowest in the middle. Now the spectral scan will be true, and the absorbance peaks in all wavelengths will be relative. This variable slit controls the intensity of the light but

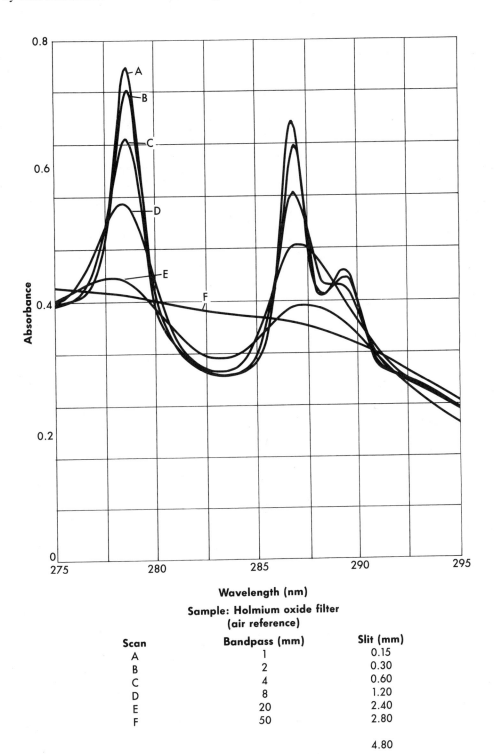

Sample: Holmium oxide filter (air reference)

Scan	Bandpass (mm)	Slit (mm)
A	1	0.15
B	2	0.30
C	4	0.60
D	8	1.20
E	20	2.40
F	50	2.80
		4.80

Fig. 7-8 Resolution as a function of bandpass or width (courtesy Beckman Instruments, Inc.).

does not change the bandpass because it is regulating the amount of white light before it reaches the monochromator.

Spectral scans have value only when there is good resolution (i.e., the absorbance at a specific wavelength must be specified), compared with another wavelength 20 nm shorter or longer. To resolve absorbance peaks, the bandpass must be short (Fig. 7-8). The relation of bandpass to resolution might be illustrated by comparing rides in two cars with long and short wheel bases. A car with a long wheel base evens out bumps and holes in the road, but a car with a short wheel base seems to climb every bump and go to the bottom of every hole. By the same token, the wide bandpass levels out all the peaks and valleys of the spectral scan. However, every peak and valley should be seen. Often a very sharp, narrow peak may be characteristic of a compound that positively identifies it. This would be completely missed if a wide bandpasss were used. The peaks of an absorbance curve that show high absorbance are called **absorbance maxima,** and the points of lowest absorbance are the **absorbance minima.** Compounds may be identified in the literature by the exact wavelength of their principal absorbance maxima.

Mechanics of Double Beam. In a double beam system monochromatic light from either a single or double monochromator is focused through both a reference and a sample compartment. The intensity of these two beams of light is then measured by either one or two detectors, and the sample beam is compared with the reference side as a ratio. This ratio may be fed into a meter or directly into a ratio-recording instrument. Double beam designs of instruments may use either a double beam in space or a double beam in time.

In a **double beam in space** spectrophotometer (Fig. 7-9), the light is split with a half mirror that allows half the beam to pass through the sample and the other half is deflected to another detector that is balanced against the sample detector. The detectors are balanced with the blank solution in the sample cell by adjusting the light intensity of the reference beam with the reference detector current. Two separate light paths are created by a beam splitter; two separate detectors measure the radiant power of each beam. The light may be split after it has passed through the monochromator as pictured, or it may split after the light source and each beam have a separate monochromator. Any voltage fluctuation to the lamp will affect both detectors equally. However, as discussed before, the detectors may age differently resulting in different responses, and this design does not compensate for fluctuation in detector power. Also, if two monochromators are used, it is very unlikely that they would match perfectly.

A **double beam in time** design (Fig. 7-10) attempts to solve these problems by splitting the beam with a rotating photochopper that alternately presents a mirror and an opening. The split beams through the sample and through the reference are recombined to strike a single detector. The output of the detector is an alternating signal or pulse that has amplitude proportional to the differences in intensity of the two beams (i.e., the ratio between the sample and reference beams is a direct measurement of the absorbed light). The advantage of this system is that power

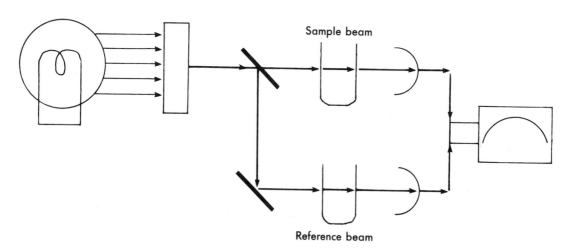

Sample beam

Reference beam

Fig. 7-9 Double beam in space.

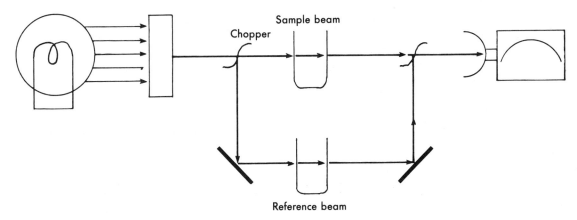

Fig. 7-10 Double beam in time.

fluctuation to either the lamp or detector will affect both beams equally, thus not affecting the ratio of reference to the sample beam. Another advantage is ease of operation. The reference cell for blank solvent makes it unnecessary to replace the blank to check the balance.

Most double beam spectrophotometers use a single photodetector and a beam splitting and reuniting system of choppers (spinning mirrors) (i.e., a double beam in time), to overcome the problem of balancing two phototubes to an exactly equal spectral response. Figure 7-11 shows the optical system of a popular double beam in time spectrophotometer. Instead of a rotating chopper to split the light beam, this design uses a set of mirrors mounted on a motorized fork that vibrate rapidly and continuously in and out of the sample and reference paths.

Parameters of Operation

Absorbance Spectra. In preparing a graph with absorbance on the vertical axis and wavelengths from 400 to 750 nm on the horizontal axis, the absorbance readings of a solution plotted at each

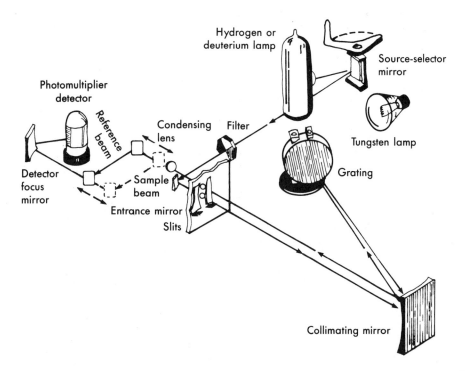

Fig. 7-11 Optical system of a dual beam spectrophotometer (courtesy Beckman Instruments, Inc.).

wavelength would form the solution's unique spectral absorbance curve. Some absorbance maxima, or peaks where the solution absorbed strongly, would be found. These absorbance maxima are characteristic; the whole spectral absorbance curve is exactly characteristic of the substance being measured (Fig. 7-12). In toxicology a substance is often identified by absorbance maxima and their relative heights when compared with each other. The absolute peak height (i.e., the absorbance at a given wavelength), depends on the concentration of the substance in the solution. When a concentration curve is set up (e.g., blood glucose) the absorbance peak height at an optimum wavelength is being measured, which means at an absorbance maximum or peak.

When a plot of the spectral absorbance curve is set up, it is necessary to take a number of individual absorbance readings to more resolutely define the curve. If readings were taken at 50 nm intervals only, there would be a very poor curve that might completely miss some of the absorbance peaks. If readings were taken every 25 nm, there would be a better defined curve. If 10 nm intervals were used, it would be even better.

As these readings are taken, set the spectrophotometer's monochromator at given points. When the reading is taken at 500 nm, light that is nominally 500 nm is being used but actually the bandpass may have been from 490 to 510 nm. If the bandpass had been very wide (e.g., 50 nm), the **resolution** would have been very poor and few peaks would be seen. If a 2 nm bandpass had been used, the resolution would have been excellent. Thus resolution depends on bandpass (see Fig. 7-8).

Calibration. Unfortunately no one has ever developed a monochromator that is always true in all circumstances. If small changes are made in the light, the diffraction grating, and the slit, the geometry is changed and the band of color pass-

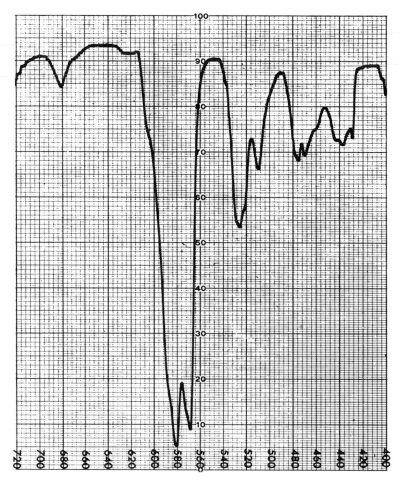

Fig. 7-12   Spectral absorbance curve of didymium, using the Beckman DB and the automatic adjustment option.

ing through the exit slit may be altered. Hence, when the wavelength dial signals that light at 520 nm is passing through the slit, there may actually be light at 500 nm instead. It is necessary to have a means of telling whether the monochromator is true and properly calibrated.

It has been pointed out that absorbance maxima or peaks are highly characteristic. The result is that each solution of nickel sulfate, for example, will have a peak at exactly the same wavelength. This information can be used to calibrate monochromators. If absorbance values are checked around this typical absorbance peak, the highest value should be found at the characteristic, defined wavelength. If this does not prove to be the case, the position of the lamp or grating can be adjusted to correct the wavelength setting to correspond to true values.

It is possible to use, as a calibrating standard, almost any substance for which there is a spectral absorbance curve. If a solution is used, there is a risk that there are impurities or that a change in pH has changed the absorbance curve. If a pure crystalline substance is used, this is not a problem; in most cases the crystal will remain unchanged with time and conditions. The rare earth crystal called didymium has a stable crystalline form and also has some sharp characteristic peaks. It is therefore a good standard of reference. Holmium oxide is another crystalline compound with similar good characteristics. Fig. 7-12 is a spectral absorbance curve of didymium.

There are also neutral-density filters manufactured specifically for calibrating spectrophotometers. These filters allow a very narrow band of light to pass; this transmittance peak can be used in the same manner as the absorbance peaks of didymium. Also, the U.S. Bureau of Standards sells glass filters that may be used for calibrating.

How an instrument is checked for wavelength calibration depends on the instrument itself and the type of scan it can produce. The first and most obvious means of checking is to identify a very characteristic, sharp absorption peak of a substance and see whether the spectrophotometer actually does show maximum absorption at this point. If methyl orange, for example, has an absorption maximum at 460 nm, put a sample of methyl orange in a cuvette, turn the wavelength selector knob slowly through the wavelengths from 440 to 480 nm, and observe whether the meter shows maximum absorbance at 460 nm.

This check presupposes, however, that (1) there is only one significant absorption peak in this general area; (2) the instrument has sufficient resolution to discern it as a sharp peak; (3) the absorbance value is on the scale (i.e., readable at the concentration used); and (4) if one point of the spectral scan is correct, all others will be. These assumptions are not necessarily true or attainable in all cases and are examined below.

Many compounds have a great many peaks at close intervals, and it is hard to be sure whether the area of maximum absorbance is actually the wavelength sought. Various precautions may be taken. First, the scan of the substance should be examined to ascertain that the peak to be used is well separated from any other. Second, the color of the light should be noted to verify that it is the approximate wavelength under consideration. If the wavelength dial reads 650 nm and the color of light passing through the cuvette is green, the instrument is badly out of calibration, and the meter response is irrelevant. Third, the whole spectral scan should be followed to be certain that peaks are in proper relation to each other, in terms of both peak location and peak height.

The second problem—whether the spectrophotometer is capable of discerning the peak—can be better visualized looking at Fig. 7-10. Notice that the very broad absorbance bands in some areas of the spectrum are not truly peaks; it would be difficult to identify a point of maximum absorbance. This is true of all scans done at a wide bandpass. With wide bandpass instruments it is probably less important that calibration be absolutely correct, but every effort should be made to achieve the maximum that the system will allow.

Calibration of these instruments is done on a different basis. For example, if the spectral scan of didymium (see Fig. 7-12) is examined carefully, it can be seen that there is an abrupt change in absorbance between 580 and 620 nm. This characteristic can be used to calibrate roughly; if enough information is available, even a fairly close calibration can be attained. By turning the wavelength dial with didymium in the light path, it is fairly easy to locate the general area where absorbance drops off precipitously. Exactly when the absorbance reading will be at any one point, of course, depends on such variables as the bandpass and grating characteristics. If a didymium scan made on an instrument with the same bandpass, grating, and other construction details is available for reference, it is reasonable to assume that the trace can be duplicated and that the absorbance of the instrument being calibrated will be the same at a test wavelength as that of the sample curve.

The next problem that may occur in looking for the test absorbance peak would be that it is off scale or that the peak is so small it is of little value for reference. When using a calibrating material in a strange instrument this is often the case, and if the material is a glass filter no dilution or concentration of the sample can be done to solve the problem. If absorbance is too high or too low, change the absorbance by (1) using a brighter light (if the slit can be opened farther), (2) changing the attenuation of the detector by turning the control pots, or (3) using neutral-density filters. Neutral-density filters decrease the total light without selectively decreasing intensity at any given wavelength. Filters of this sort can be purchased in varying thicknesses. With experimentation using neutral-density filters and the standard controls of the instrument, it is possible to get a usable scan on the commercially available calibration filters.

The last problem is that the instrument may not be in calibration at all points throughout the spectrum if only one point has been calibrated. This is a major concern with some spectrophotometers but only an occasional problem with others because of the construction of the instrument. It is sound practice to occasionally check more than one calibration point on any instrument. If either the light source or the grating is moved slightly, the spectrum will move, allowing a different band of color to pass. If properly done, the same proportion of the entire spectrum can still pass through the slit but it will be a different color band. If, during movement of the light source, grating, or slit width, the slit wall is no longer parallel to the surface of the grating, the spectrum is distorted with the blue portion very short, narrow, and bright and the red portion wider, longer, and more diffuse. If the movement of the light or the grating is repeated, the bandpass is no longer in the same proportion of the spectrum at the two ends of the scale. The geometry of the monochromator is complicated, and the movement of any of these components must be made carefully if the spectrum is not to be distorted. In some instruments all these relationships are so rigidly positioned that only one element can be moved in one plane. In this case, barring major damage, a one-point calibration is probably adequate in all cases. In other instruments more than one element may be movable, and calibration at several points is advisable.

Several techniques for checking multiple points are available, and different filter materials can be purchased or prepared. Didymium is probably the most common of the commercially available filter materials. The principal absorption peak is around 500 nm, and there are four maxima that are usable as calibration points.

Holmium oxide glass is another specially prepared filter with about 10 sharp major maxima that can be used. Some of these are in the near UV, giving it some value for calibration in this area.

Maintenance. In the normal operation of photometric instruments several checks should be made from time to time to ensure accurate, reliable operation. Essentially there are four photometric characteristics that should be monitored.

Several methods of wavelength calibration have been discussed. Once the instrument is in routine, daily use, some type of wavelength check should be performed each day. Use of a didymium filter or some such standard to check absorbance wavelengths is probably sufficient for routine calibration. These values should be recorded. If there is any significant change, it should be investigated. Most quality instruments will go for long periods of time without need of recalibration, but the routine checking must be done. Whenever lamps are changed or instruments repaired or moved about, the wavelength calibration must be rechecked.

Each time a standard curve is prepared, the linearity of the instrument is being checked. If the material being used follows Beer's law, the absorbance plotted against concentration should be a straight line. When the plot is not quite linear, there is the inclination to assume a slight error in measurement and to dismiss it if it does not seem significant. It is wise to watch these deviations carefully to see if there is a tendency for repeated plots to show the same deviation from linearity, which might indicate a lack of linearity of the instrument. Remember that readings below 20% T and over 60% T are inherently somewhat in error, the error being more pronounced at the ends of the scale. Very accurate prepared standards may be purchased; these should be used occasionally as a careful linearity check. These results should be made a matter of permanent record.

To check bandwidth, a standard source lamp, which may be purchased for use, or a sharp cutoff filter should be available. If a mercury lamp is used, a good isolated peak should be found at 546 nm. Turn the 100% T adjustment knob to set the meter on 100. Then move the wavelength setting toward 700 nm until the meter reads 50% T. Record the wavelength. Now move the wavelength setting toward 400 nm until the meter again reads 50% T. Record this wavelength. The difference between the two recorded wavelengths is the bandwidth. It should correspond closely to the bandwidth claimed by the manufacturer. Remember, however, that in most instruments the spectrum is significantly distorted, so the bandwidth at the red end of the spectrum may be noticeably narrower than at the violet end. There is probably little point in checking this characteristic on fixed-slit spectrophotometers. Instruments with variable slits should be checked occasionally.

Stray light may be caused by reflection within the instrument, light from the next higher-order spectrum, or room light reaching the detector. Filters can be obtained that almost completely absorb light at a given wavelength. These are called blocking filters. Set the wavelength knob at the value of the blocking filter. Zero the instrument in the usual manner and, with nothing in the cuvette well, set the meter at 100% T. Now insert the blocking filter. Any stray light will cause the meter to move away from zero. Over 2% is generally considered unacceptable. This measurement should be made periodically to ensure proper function of the instrument.

Many simple, common sense observations can be made that can reveal potentially serious problems.

Warm-up Time. Turn the instrument on and set the readout at 100% T. Check for several minutes to see how long it requires to stabilize. Do not use until the readout stays at zero.

Fatigue. If the instrument is left on for some time with the readout on 100% T, does it have a tendency to fade below the initial setting? If the fading is very slow the instrument may be usable, but 100% T should be reset often during use.

Readout Repeatibility. Insert a sample in the cuvette well and set the readout at 50% T. Remove the sample and reinsert it. Check the readout. If the needle does not return to 50% T, the instrument should be serviced by an instrument repair person. Be sure the cuvette is oriented in the well the same way each time.

Wavelength Repeatability. With a sample in the well set the readout at 50% T and note the wavelength. Turn the wavelength knob and then bring it back to its exact original wavelength.

Does the readout return to 50% T? If not, the instrument should be serviced.

Grating Deterioriation. Insert a slip of white paper into the cuvette well so the color of light entering the well can be observed. Rotate the wavelength knob slowly from 400 to 750 nm. Learn to recognize the approximate colors of various wavelengths. At 555 nm the color should be grass green. At 610 nm it should be yellow-orange. Colors should be sharp and clear. If they are streaky or if more than one color appears at the same time, the grating may be deteriorating or dusty. The instrument should be checked by a competent repair person.

Low Energy. Place an empty cuvette in the well and set the wavelength at 400 nm. Turn the 100% T knob fully clockwise. The readout should go past 100% T with ease well before the knob is fully clockwise. Repeat at 700 nm. If the readout reaches 100% T only when the knob is fully rotated clockwise, there is insufficient energy. The exciter lamp may be dirty or going bad, the slit may be dusty, the amplifier (if any) may be weak, or the detector may be defective. Steps should be taken to locate the trouble.

Scratched or Defective Cuvettes. Place a water blank in the well and set the meter at 50% T. Rotate the cuvette slowly and watch the needle. If it moves more than 1% T, it should be discarded. Some cuvettes have an index line, and they should be oriented in the well the same way each time. If this is carefully done each time, some latitude might be allowed, but the technologist should nonetheless be alert to this source of error.

Common Instruments in Use

In recent years automated, computer-assisted chemistry analyzers have reduced the number of spectrophotometers in medical laboratories. However, for those tests that have not been automated, spectrophotometers are still essential in a laboratory.

With the introduction of integrated circuits and microprocessors, spectrophotometers have undergone radical changes. It has become fairly easy to design instruments that monitor their own performances, cycle through entire sequences, and perform a variety of calculations. There is a trend back to single-beam instruments because computer circuits can store reference data and compensate at all times. These newer instruments are more compact, faster, and more accurate, and they can provide many timesaving conveniences.

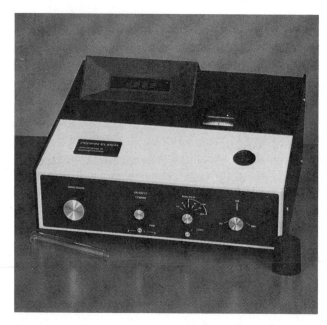

Fig. 7-13   Coleman Model 35 Digital Spectrophotometer (courtesy Perkin-Elmer Corp.).

Coleman Spectrophotometers (Perkin-Elmer Corp). The Coleman, Perkin-Elmer, Hitachi group has produced more spectrophotometers for the medical laboratory than any other manufacturer. In past years the Coleman Junior Models 6 and 35 had been the most common spectrophotometers in the clinical laboratory. There are still some of these instruments in use today.

The newer Coleman Model 35 (Fig. 7-13) has a digital readout that presents % T, absorbance, and concentration. It has a wavelength range of 335 to 825 nm and much improved resolution and accuracy in its 8 nm spectral bandpass. A more sensitive phototube detector provides an improved signal-to-noise ratio, and stray light is less than 0.1% T at 340 nm. The quartz halogen lamp does not darken with age and requires no wavelength calibration on replacement. All electronics are on two circuit boards, which are easily replaceable and result in less downtime and easy servicing. A continuously variable concentration knob allows scale expansion of 0.1 to 5 times.

Gilford Micro-Sample Spectrophotometer. The Gilford Micro-Sample Spectrophotometer has gained acceptance in most laboratories (Fig. 7-14). It is one of the first popular sepectrophotometers designed primarily for microsamples. A 500 microliter (μl) sample allows a 1 cm light path. The spectral range is from 340 to 700 nm,

with a bandpass of 8 nm. A linear, digital voltmeter is used for the readout, allowing absorbance values from 0 to 2 to be read to 0.001 A. Concentration can also be read directly. Adjustment of the zero A end of the scale is made by varying the intensity of the lamp. Lamp temperature is kept low so that failure is unusual. Samples are drawn through a measuring cell by a vacuum pump outside the instrument. This instrument has been coupled with samplers, microprocessor, and printers to produce small automated chemistry analyzer systems. This model and its newer versions have functioned well and have been very popular.

Beckman Model 35 UH/His Spectrophotometers. The Beckman Model 35 UH/His Spectrophotometer is a dual-beam, scanning, and recording spectrophotometer. It is adaptable for scanning gels by suppressing the reference beam. It has an operating range of 190 to 700 nm. The monochromator uses a single filter grating with 1200 lines/mm blazed at 250 nm. The Model 35 (Fig. 7-15) has variable slits with a normal and a wide program, which allows a 0.125 to 5 nm bandwidth. The photometric range is from 0.0 to 3 A with an accuracy of 0.5%. Scanning speeds can be set in six steps, from 1 to 250 nm/minute. If the absorptivity of a compound is known, the K-factor (1/absorptivity) can be entered into the digital display and concentrations will be directly calculated, saving the time of preparing and reading calibrating standards. Model 35 can also be used for kinetic measurements, spectral scanning, chromatography gel scanning, or rapid endpoint analyses. The light path schematic diagram for the Beckman double-beam Model 35 spectrophotometer is shown in Fig. 7-11.

Beckman DU-70 Scanning Spectrophotometer. This is an example of a highly sophisticated, computer-directed spectrophotometer (Fig. 7-16). This single-beam instrument with automatic zeroing and blank subtraction, has a UV-visible range of 200 to 900 nm and a fixed 2 nm bandpass (Fig. 7-17). The computer includes a high-

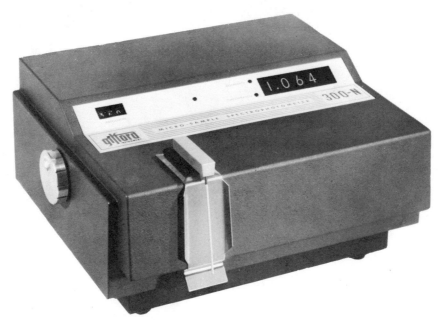

Fig. 7-14 Gilford Micro-Sample Spectrophotometer (courtesy Ciba-Corning, Inc.).

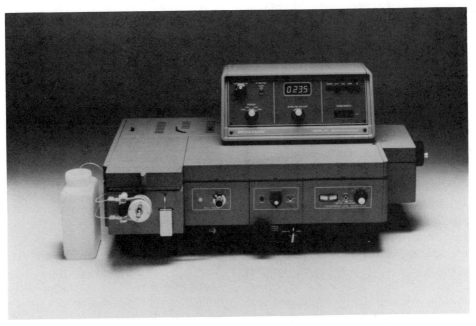

Fig. 7-15 Beckman Model 35 UH/His spectrophotometer (courtesy Beckman Instruments, Inc.).

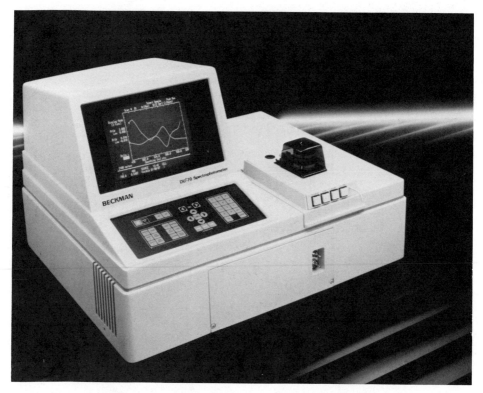

Fig. 7-16 Beckman DU-70 spectrophotometer (courtesy Beckman Instruments, Inc.).

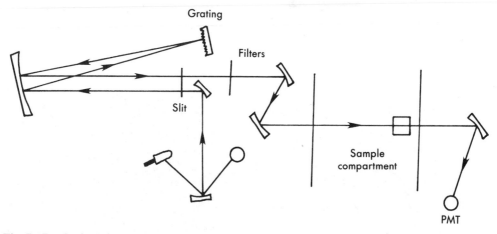

Fig. 7-17 Optical diagram of the Beckman Model DU-70 (courtesy Beckman Instruments, Inc.).

resolution graphic video display for presentation and manipulation of the spectral data in % T and absorbance. Scan speeds from 60 to 240 nm/ minute are standard with a response time of 0.05 seconds. The operator has a choice of 10 calculation options including peak pick, derivatives, and smoothing without delays associated with changing screens. Overlay of up to six spectra at a time, plus overlay of multiple functions, is pos-

sible. Spectral storage of 40 full-range scans is possible or up to 99 short-range scans within the standard memory.

Repetitive scans for six samples at chosen time intervals and selected spectral interpolation are standard for the DU-70. Net absorbance calculations and ratios or subtractions of wavelength readings are also provided. Multiwavelength readings at up to eight selected wavelengths and read-averaging of up to 99 readings ensures the best possible precision in extreme cases of signal noise. Concentration calculations at single wavelengths, using a factor or a standard, is standard along with the time drive of kinetic rate determinations. Standard within the software library of the DU-70 is complete control and final answer computational capabilities for kinetics: quantitative single-component and multicomponent analysis and gel scanning.

This instrument lends itself to research activity as well as routine analysis, making it ideal in medical laboratories where developmental activities are conducted. Perkin-Elmer Corporation also makes an equally sophisticated spectrophotometer with similar capabilities.

The photometers discussed in this chapter range from very basic, inexpensive instruments to advanced, computer-driven models. Each of the companies mentioned offers several other models with variable features and accessories to accommodate the full spectrum needs of clients. Many other companies such as Milton-Roy with its spectronic series, Sequoia-Turner, Hewlett-Packard, and Varian-Techtron, all make excellent spectrophotometers with each company offering many models with basic to advanced features.

Review Questions

1. Compare and contrast the various exciter lamps used in UV to infrared spectrophotometers.
2. What is "bandpass," and why is it so important to the accuracy of the sample measurement?
3. Why does a diffraction grating disperse light in a linear fashion and a prism disperse it nonlinearly?
4. What are second and third order spectra? Are they desirable? Why or why not?
5. What are the advantages of a double beam spectrophotometer over a single beam spectrophotometer?
6. Describe the double beam in time design of a spectrophotometer. Why is it more desirable than a double beam in space?
7. How is wavelength calibration performed on spectrophotometers?
8. List at least eight "common sense" checks to monitor the accurate performance of spectrophotometers.

Bibliography

Bender J: Principles of chemical instrumentation, Philadelphia, 1987, WB Saunders.

Hicks R et al: Laboratory instrumentation, Philadelphia, 1987, JB Lippincott.

Kaplan L, Pesce A: Clinical chemistry—theory, analysis and correlation, St. Louis, 1989, CV Mosby.

Narayanan S: Principles and applications of laboratory instrumentation, Chicago, 1989, ASCP Press.

Tietz N: Textbook of clinical chemistry, Philadelphia, 1986, WB Saunders.

CHAPTER 8

Atomic Emission and Absorption Spectroscopy

LARRY E. SCHOEFF

Emission Flame Photometry
Atomic Absorption Photometry

Emission Flame Photometry

Emission flame photometry is still used in the clinical laboratory to determine sodium, potassium, and lithium concentrations in biologic fluids, although ion specific electrode (ISE) analysis is rapidly replacing this technology.

In previous years calcium was also analyzed by flame photometry; however, chemical methods and ISE instruments have long ago replaced this technique for calcium because of multiple emission spectra and interferences that were very difficult to correct.

Principle. When a metallic salt is burned in a flame, colors are produced. These colors are at very specific wavelengths and are characteristic of the atom being burned. The heat energy that the atom absorbs drives one or more electrons out of their usual orbital positions. As the atom cools, the absorbed energy is released in the form of light and the electrons return to their normal positions (ground state). Any particular atom may have more than one excited electron. The heat energy absorbed and the light emitted on cooling are characteristic of the particular electron orbit involved, as well as the atomic species. For this reason each metal, when heated, has its own **emission spectrum** showing emission at various characteristic wavelengths. The number of emission bands may increase as the temperature of the flame is increased and more stable electrons in the atom are excited. If the temperature becomes high enough, the electrons may be thrown out of their orbits, whereby the atom becomes **ionized** and the electrons do not return to their proper positions with the characteristic emission of light. Electrons thrown out of position assume charac-

teristic new orbits until they return to ground state. They may return to normal by dropping to one or more intermediate new orbital positions before finally returning to ground state. These partial energy releases cause the emission of light at other characteristic wavelengths.

Instrumentation. The flame photometer is a device that analyzes burning solutions and measures the wavelength and intensity of their emissions. The design of the instrument is not complicated, but the details of construction must be precise. There are two major parts: the **atomizer-burner assembly** must introduce a constant amount of solution into the flame that must burn at a constant temperature, and the **colorimeter** portion of the instrument must measure the color and intensity of the light emitted by the flame (Fig. 8-1). Because only one element/light path is analyzed, an interference filter for the wavelength of the brightest emission peak of the selected element is placed between the flame and the detector so that only this characteristic wavelength passes.

In the atomizer-burner a fuel gas, propane, is brought together with an oxidizing agent, compressed air, and burned to produce a flame of predictable heat. The choice of gases and the mixture of fuel and oxidant determine the temperature. The solution to be burned is pulled into the flame by **Venturi action** as the gases rush by the tip of a capillary tube whose other end is immersed in the test solution.

A **premix burner** is used in which the gases rushing past the tip of the capillary **nebulize** the sample and spray it in a fine mist into a closed chamber beneath the flame (Fig. 8-2). The larger droplets fall to the floor of the chamber, and only the very fine droplets are carried upward into the flame by the flow of gas.

124

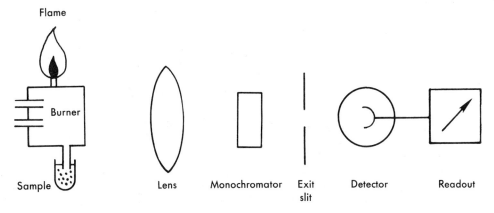

Fig. 8-1 Components of a flame photometer.

The fuel content of the gas and the pressure and composition of the gas mixture are critical. Both gases should be accurately and consistently metered, and all gas lines and the burner should be clear and unobstructed. Moisture in compressed air can be a serious problem, and a moisture trap and filter should be used. Where piped gas is used, care should be taken that the gas be relatively clean and consistent as to fuel content.

The total pressure of the gas mixture will determine the flame height, and it is important that the right portion of the flame be in front of the detector. In the base of the flame, where it is hottest, the element absorbs heat energy. As the element rises, it moves into the cooler part where it gives off its light energy; it is in this area that the emission should be monitored. The flame is the light source and the sample holder of the photometer; it breaks the chemical bonds of the element being analyzed and brings the element to its excited state.

In most instruments fewer than 5% of the ions passing through the flames are energized. If the temperature falls slightly because of changes in gas pressure, fuel content, or water in the flame, the accuracy of the instrument may be seriously

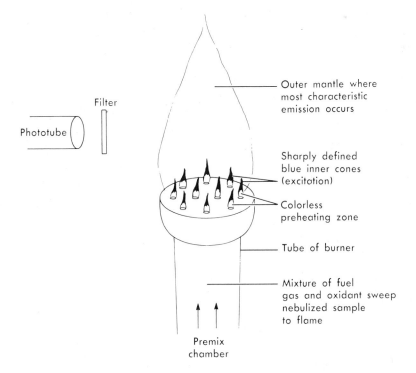

Fig. 8-2 Cross-section of premix burner and flame, showing where detector should be relative to flame.

impaired. If this happens, there will be insufficient energy to activate the photometer properly and, when a precalibrated scale panel is used, it becomes impossible to set the high and low ends of the scale using the high and low standards.

The photometer part of the instrument must be designed to detect and measure a very small light signal. The light intensity of a flame is much less than that of an exciter lamp. Also, an interference filter with a very narrow band pass is generally used to isolate the specific energy peak (wavelength) that is characteristic of the element being measured. Hence the light reaching the detector is very weak. For this reason a phototube or photomultiplier is generally used, and the output is amplified considerably before it is presented to the readout device.

Internal Standard Technique. Because the light source is represented by the sample itself, it is impossible in flame photometry to simultaneously compare sample with blank without duplicating some of the components (i.e., at least the light source or flame). Double-beam photometry is not very helpful in this case and would not compensate for variations in stability of the instrument (i.e., those caused by light source fluctuations).

An **internal standard** has been used to control some of these problems. It contains a known concentration of an element with an emission peak appreciably different from the unknown so that the two can be readily differentiated. A separate wavelength filter and photodetection system is provided. The internal standard is mixed with the test solution; when the test solution with the internal standard is burned, the two photosignals are compared electronically as a ratio signal. Because the internal standard and test are affected similarly, variations in sample-aspiration rate, atomization rate, and solution viscosity will virtually be canceled out and eliminated. Although the intensity of emitted light for both the internal standard and the analyte will vary, the ratio of the two will not. Therefore only the true signal of the test solution will be measured. The effect of variation in flame temperature and stability is also canceled. Because the optimum emission temperature for the internal standard and the element being tested may not be quite the same, a disproportionate percentage of the two atomic species may be excited. In the case of sodium and potassium compared with lithium as an internal standard, this variation is minimal. The internal standard technique, in effect, acts like a double-beam photometer to control fluctuations.

An internal standard can also be used to minimize the effect of **mutual excitation.** This phenomenon is the result of photons emitted by excited sodium atoms, in turn exciting potassium atoms. This can result in falsely elevated potassium values unless concentrations of sodium and potassium in the standards closely approximate the concentrations of these analytes in unknowns, which is a difficult achievement for urine specimens. The internal standard acts to absorb the radiation and buffer the potassium atoms from the effect of mutual excitation.

The conditions for a good internal standard are as follows: its concentration should be the same in the test samples and calibration standard; its excitation energy should be comparable with that of the element being measured; its emission lines should be distinct and separate from that of the measured element; and it should not be present in vivo in the patient sample to be analyzed.

For many years lithium was used as an internal standard with flame photometers. It worked well because its emission spectrum of 671 nm was equidistant between sodium (589 nm) and potassium (767 nm). In recent years lithium has become commonly used as a therapeutic drug in psychiatric medicine, which prevents its use as an internal standard in those patients receiving it therapeutically.

By modifying the preparation of diluted specimens for analyses and throwing a switch on the flame photometer to change the signal from K/Li to Li/K, potassium may be used as an internal standard whenever lithium needs to be measured for therapeutic drug monitoring reasons.

Newer flame photometers now use cesium

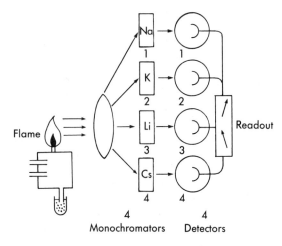

Fig. 8-3 Flame photometer with cesium internal standard.

(852 nm) as the internal standard, which eliminates the need for modifications to the technique and allows for direct measurement simultaneously of sodium, potassium, and lithium. The design of a flame photometer using cesium as the internal standard requires four separate monochromators and photodetectors (Fig. 8-3).

Emission Flame Photometers in Common Use. The IL Model 143 by Instrumentation Laboratory, Inc. was the first instrument in general use to employ an internal standard. For several years it was the most common flame photometer in hospital laboratories. Most of the flame photometers used today are of the same basic design. A few Model 143s and the later Model 443 (with LED readout) flame photometers are still in use. Instrumentation Laboratory, Inc. and other manufacturers have introduced newer models with automatic sampling capability, self-standardization, and electronic readout.

IL Model 643 Flame Photometer. The IL Model 643 Flame Photometer (Fig. 8-4) and its predecessor the IL 343 were designed to provide a direct method for the determination of sodium, potassium, and lithium in serum and urine by using cesium as the internal standard. By analyzing four elements rather than three, the same internal standard can be used for analyzing each of

the three most common flame emission elements: sodium, potassium, and lithium. This eliminates the variables normally introduced by alternating internal standard solutions during the analysis of sodium, potassium, or lithium. Employing cesium for each analytic mode also eliminates the lengthy aspirator bowl flush-out procedures required during the changeover procedures from one internal standard to another. The IL 643, by using a 1.5 mmol/l cesium solution rather than the traditional 15 mmol/l lithium solution, reduces the input concentration of salts by tenfold. This reduction in aspirated salts will greatly reduce salt buildup in the aspiration and burner section of the instrument thus reducing the frequency of cleaning procedures.

IL 943 Flame Photometer. The IL 943 Flame Photometer (Fig. 8-5) is the only model that Instrumentation Laboratory, Inc. currently markets. It is an updated instrument that has replaced the IL 643. Improved mechanics and electronics have resulted in less maintenance and greater precision and accuracy of measurements. More sophisticated software allows for automatic fault monitoring and self-diagnostics.

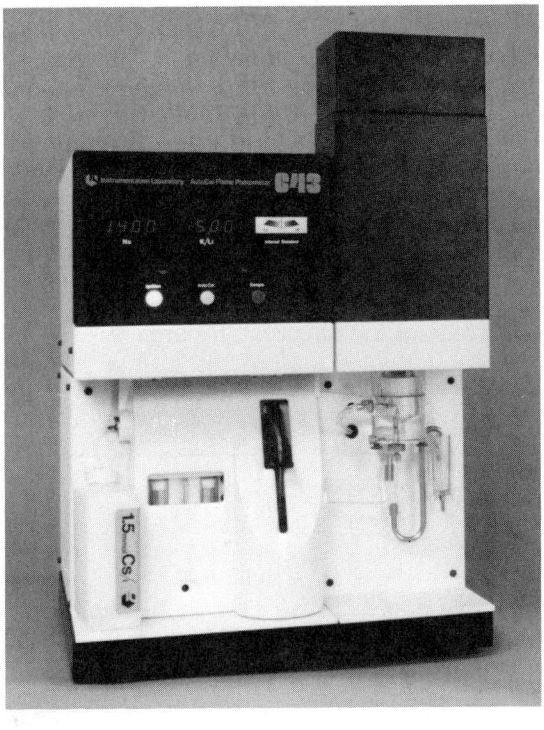

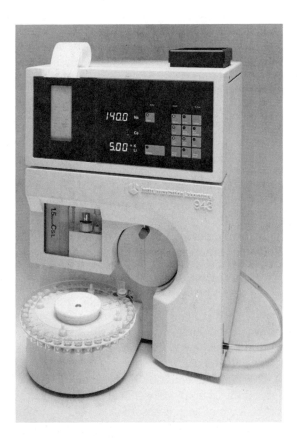

Fig. 8-4 IL 643 Flame Photometer. (Courtesy Instrumentation Laboratory, Inc.)

Fig. 8-5 IL 943 Flame Photometer. (Courtesy Instrumentation Laboratory, Inc.)

The plumbing assembly mechanics on the IL 943 have been improved to provide a more stable fuel and air system. The aspiration system has been redesigned and now employs an integral one-piston dilutor that automatically aspirates, mixes, feeds the sample to the flame, and then disposes of the waste. One button automatically activates the dilution cycle, the detection and computation of analyte concentration, the verification of internal standard preset concentration range, and the display of results.

Added computer software on the IL 943 controls autocalibration, stat interpretation, automatic fault monitoring, which includes checking for unstable data in any channel and improper operating sequence, and automatic shutdown if fuel or air is interrupted. The system also automatically monitors fuel and air and tests aspiration rate.

The low diluent requirements for cesium make the IL 943 and IL 643 flame photometers less expensive to run than lithium-internal standard flames that require 10 times as much diluent for 5 times as much sample. They are also less expensive to operate and easier to maintain than ion selective electrode (ISE) analyzers.

Many clinical laboratories purchase and use modern flame photometers for several reasons. The newer flame photometers provide more accurate and reliable lithium measurements than ISE instruments. They offer more precise sodium and potassium measurements in urines, especially at low concentrations because the flame photometer is not affected by interferences from the urine constituents, as seen with ISE methodologies. The flame photometer is useful for documenting the accuracy of ISE analyzers. Finally, the flame photometer remains the reference instrument for sodium and potassium measurements.

Instrumentation Laboratory, Inc. is now the only major manufacturer of flame photometers.

Atomic Absorption Photometry

Atomic absorption spectrophotometry is widely used in the clinical laboratory for determining concentrations of calcium, magnesium, lithium, copper, zinc, lead, mercury, and several other trace metals.

Principle. In **emission flame photometry** (see preceding section), a specific amount of energy, in the form of heat, is absorbed by an atom. This energy causes certain valence electrons to move to new orbital positions more distant from the nucleus. The atom is **excited,** or in a higher energy state. Because this is an unstable state, the extra energy is given up in a very short time as the atom moves to a cooler part of the flame. This energy is released as light, and the wavelength (energy level) is the precise energy involved in the electron transition.

In **atomic absorption photometry** the process is essentially reversed. If the atom in question can be dissociated from its chemical bonds, an unexcited ground state atom will absorb light of a specific wavelength (i.e., of a certain energy level). This is the exact energy required, in emission flame photometry, to excite the atom by moving certain valence electrons to new, defined orbital positions. In other words, the unexcited atom will absorb light of the wavelength that it would emit if emission flame photometry were used.

The best way found, until recently, to cause the atom to dissociate from its chemical bonds was to heat it in a flame. When heated, some of the atoms emit, but it is estimated that only about 1% to 2% do so, and all of them will absorb light energy. Thus the error is small, reasonably constant, and can be compensated for. The energy band that is absorbed is very narrow (i.e., 0.0001 nm) and at exactly the wavelength that would be emitted if the atom were excited. Because the disassociated atom will absorb exactly the wavelength (energy) that an excited atom of the same element emits, it is most convenient to produce the energy band by heating that element.

These very fine emission lines are produced in the atomic absorption photometer by a **hollow cathode lamp.** This is a neon or argon lamp with a cathode consisting of the metal in question (Fig. 8-6). The lamp will emit only the spectrum of the gas plus that of the heated metal. The emission process is illustrated in Fig. 8-7. When an electrical potential is applied between anode and cathode, some of the fill gas atoms are ionized. The

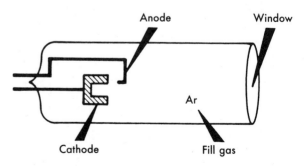

Fig. 8-6 Hollow cathode lamp. (Courtesy Perkin-Elmer Corp.)

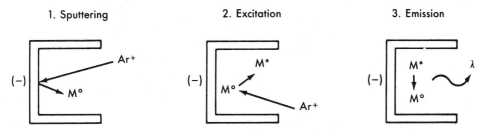

Fig. 8-7 Hollow cathode lamp process.

positively charged fill gas ions accelerate through the electrical field to collide with the negatively charged cathode and dislodge individual metal atoms in a process called **"sputtering."** Sputtered metal atoms are then excited to an emission state through a kinetic energy transfer by impact with fill gas ions. If this emitted light is directed into the flame containing the metal, the atoms of the metal in question will absorb the emission from the metal in the hollow cathode lamp. Absorption will follow Beer's law so that there is a linear relationship between absorption and concentration of the element in the light path, just as in spectrophotometry.

For this arrangement to work accurately, it is imperative that a very narrow emission peak of the hollow cathode lamp be measured and that all extraneous light be rejected. To accomplish this a high-quality monochromator with a very narrow band pass is necessary. Figure 8-8 compares emission flame photometry with atomic absorption photometry.

Instrumentation. The atomic absorption (AA) flame photometer in its simplest form consists of a hollow cathode lamp, a **chopper,** an atomizer-burner, a monochromator, a detector, and a readout (Fig. 8-8, *B*). It is similar to a spectrophotometer. The hollow cathode lamp acts as the exciter lamp, and the flame acts as the cuvette.

In actual practice most AA photometers include many additions, refinements, and details. Most of these are considered further in the following sections.

A hollow cathode lamp is made for virtually every metallic element. Until recently the life of one of these lamps was about 100 hours of burning time. Because there was a rather long warm-up time for lamps of many elements, the actual use time was shorter. Lamps are now produced with a much longer life, and in most cases the

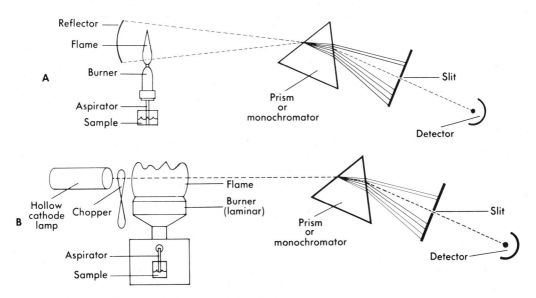

Fig. 8-8 Atomic absorption technique. **A,** Emission flame photometer measures light emitted by the flame. **B,** Atomic absorption photometer measures absorption of light from the hollow cathode by the flame.

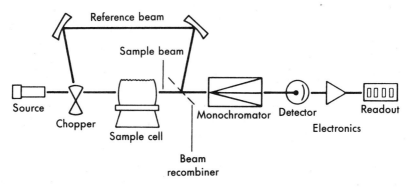

Fig. 8-9   Double-beam AA spectrophotometer. (Courtesy Perkin-Elmer Corp.)

warm-up time has been reduced. These lamps are rather expensive. More than one element has been inserted in one cathode in some cases so that one lamp can be used for two or more elements. This practice saves somewhat on initial cost; however, the lamp life is still the same. Also, the multielement lamps containing metal alloys may have interference between the elements.

The importance of lamp warm-up time has been somewhat controversial. The spectral emission of the lamps of certain elements fluctuates considerably during the first few minutes after the lamps are ignited. With some elements this instability has lasted for 30 minutes or more. In an effort to obviate the need for a long warm-up time, some companies have produced a double-beam instrument that works very much like a double-beam spectrophotometer (Fig. 8-9). The emission from the hollow cathode lamp is directed to a beam splitter, which routes half the light around the flame. Regardless of the variations of the cathode lamp output, the reference beam and the beam passing through the flame are now comparable. The electronic output appears as the ratio of the sample and reference beams. The effects of changes in lamp emission and detector sensitivity are thereby eliminated. Compared with the single-beam system, double-beam gives better precision and detection limits.

Although many previous difficulties with single-beam optical design have been largely overcome with modern engineering, there are still advantages that can be claimed for double-beam. Automated instruments can automatically change lamps, reset instrument parameters, and introduce samples for high throughput multielement analysis. Double-beam technology, which automatically compensates for lamp source and common electronics drift, allows these instru-

ments to change lamps and begin an analysis immediately with little or no lamp warm-up. This not only reduces analysis time but also prolongs lamp life because lamp warm-up time is eliminated.

As the flame burns the sample, a few atoms of the element to be tested are excited and give off light of the same wavelength as the hollow cathode lamp. Also, some stray light from the room and the burner may coincide with the cathode lamp emission. To eliminate these sources of error, the beam from the hollow cathode lamp is chopped, or modulated, either mechanically or electronically to differentiate it from unchopped light emission from the flame. Only the chopped light, which is a selectively amplified lamp emission signal, reaches the detector and is measured. As mentioned earlier, this is fairly easy to do. In the double-beam instruments, the chop may be the alternative viewing of the reference and sample beams.

The **modulation** is accomplished mechanically by using a rotating chopper or electronically by pulsing the current supplied to the hollow cathode lamp (Fig. 8-10).

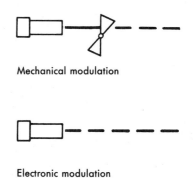

Mechanical modulation

Electronic modulation

Fig. 8-10   Modulation of hollow cathode lamp beam.

Burner design has been studied extensively over the years. Because absorbance varies directly with the optical path through the flame, it has seemed expedient to use a "curtain" or "fishtail" flame, with the hollow cathode beam passing through the length of the flame. Some instruments have the ability to turn the flame at an angle to shorten the path if this becomes desirable. The burner designed to give a curtain of flame is called a **laminar flow burner.** Some burners have three slots in the head, which give the curtain of flame more width. A higher-temperature, nitrous oxide burner is made for those refractory elements that will not atomize at lower flame temperature.

Within the burner's chamber the sample solution is nebulized, and once aspirated into the flame the sample is atomized. Under the influence of the heat the sample's molecular bonds are broken to yield ground state atoms for absorption of light. Acetylene is the commonly used fuel in the burner, whereas compressed air is the primary oxidant for combustion. Temperatures of 2300° C are usually achieved in flame atomic absorption. The most critical component in the flame atomic absorption spectrophotometer is the flame and its associated nebulizer. A steady flame is essential, and controlled gas flows are required for both oxidant and fuel. A clean burner head is essential for precise and accurate analysis.

The monochromator is tuned to select the resonance line of the element being determined. It is important that the monochromator of the AA spectrophotometer be of high quality because the emission bands that are being measured are very narrow. A band pass of about 0.2 nm or less may be required for good resolution.

The grating monochromator and photomultiplier tube detector can isolate a pure radiant energy signal and measure the intensity of that signal. Extraneous radiant energy, both from other wavelengths of the line spectrum and from light generated by the flame, is kept from reaching the photomultiplier tube by the monochromator. The photomultiplier tube converts the radiant energy that was not absorbed in the flame into a signal and amplifies this signal to drive a readout device. The chopped lamplight presents a separately recognizable alternating current flow to the photomultiplier detector for quantitation.

Flameless Atomic Absorption. Determinations of analyte concentrations in mmoles/L are routine for most elements. However, the need for trace metal analyses at μmoles/L or lower calls

for a more sensitive technique. The sensitivity of atomic absorption can be improved by improving the sampling efficiency and/or constraining analyte atoms to the light path for a longer time; therefore a greater absorption for the same analyte concentration can be achieved.

The purpose of the flame is to convert the sample into an atomic vapor. The flame, however, can be replaced by other atomization processes that result in greater sensitivity of measurement. One process applicable to mercury analysis uses chemical reactions to convert mercury into an atomic vapor. The sample is decomposed by digestion with acids, then a reducing agent is added to convert mercury to the elemental state, and finally a stream of gas is bubbled through the apparatus pushing mercury vapor into a sealed cell with quartz windows in the optical beam. Absorbance measurements are then made.

The most advanced and widely used high-sensitivity sampling technique for atomic absorption is the **graphite furnace.** In this technique a tube of graphite is located in the sample compartment of the AA spectrophotometer with the light path passing through it. A small volume of sample solution is placed in the tube where the sample is vaporized in an inert atmosphere when an electric current is passed through the support. This creates an instantaneous temperature sufficient to vaporize the analyte. These atomizers are in the space normally occupied by the flame. The temperatures achieved by flameless atomic absorption (up to 2700° C) are necessary to vaporize heavier metals.

The graphite furnace is made up of three major components: the atomizer, the power supply, and the programmer. The atomizer is located in the sampling compartment of the atomic absorption spectrophotometer where sample atomization and light absorption occur. The power supply controls the power, temperature, and gas flow to the atomizer under the direction of the programmer.

The atomizer's cylindrical tube is aligned horizontally in the optical path of the spectrophotometer and serves as the sampling cell (Fig. 8-11). The sample is dispensed through a hole in the center of the tube wall onto the inner tube wall or a graphite platform. The tube is held in place between two graphite contact cylinders, which provide electrical connection. An electrical potential applied to the contacts causes current to flow through the tube, which heats the tube and sample.

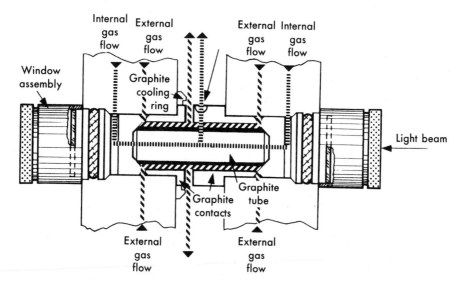

Fig. 8-11 Graphite furnace atomizer. (Courtesy Perkin-Elmer Corp.)

The entire assembly is mounted within an enclosed, water-cooled housing. Quartz windows at each end of the housing allow light to pass through the tube. The heated graphite is protected from air oxidation by the end windows and two streams of argon. An external gas flow surrounds the outside of the tube, and a separately controllable internal gas flow purges the inside of the tube so that the internal flow is interrupted during atomization.

Sources of Error. Chemical, ionization, matrix, and spectral interferences can occur in atomic absorption measurements. With some elements the presence of certain anions in the sample results in the formation of compounds that are not completely dissociated in the flame. The result is a decrease in the number of ground-state atoms present in the flame. The most common example of **chemical interference** in atomic absorbance is the formation of a tight complex of calcium with anions, especially phosphate ions. The effect of tightly complexing anions can be minimized or eliminated when lanthanum or strontium is added to the sample to displace calcium from the complex. Lanthanum forms a more stable complex with phosphate than calcium does.

When atoms in the flame become ionized (A^+), instead of remaining in the ground state (A°) they will not absorb the incident light. This is termed **ionization interference,** and this effect will result in an apparent decrease in analyte concentration. Ionization interference can be corrected when an excess of a substance that is more

easily ionized is added thus providing free electrons. Thus the excess free electrons shift the reaction

$$A^+ + e^- \rightarrow A^\circ$$

to the formation of ground-state atoms. Ionization interference is minimized by operation of the flame at the lower temperatures of acetylene-air combustion.

Differences in the matrix between the sample and the standard can result in errors. Factors that may cause variable behavior from sample to sample or between unknowns and standards include temperature, solvent composition, salt content, viscosity, and surface tension. Protein is sometimes included in the standards when the serum dilution factor is small. **Matrix interference** is minimized as composition differences between the standard and the sample become negligible. Calcium standards must contain physiologic concentrations of sodium because sodium will cause a negative interference. Organic solvents increase nebulization efficiency and therefore increase light absorption. High acid concentration increases viscosity, which decreases sample uptake rate, thereby decreasing light absorption.

Nonspecific, or background absorption, caused by solids and undissociated molecular complexes formed in the flame, is the most common type of **spectral interference.** Solids can also scatter light. Continuous emission from hydrogen in the fill gas of the lamp can cause background problems as well. The solution for this type of broad band spectral interference is to

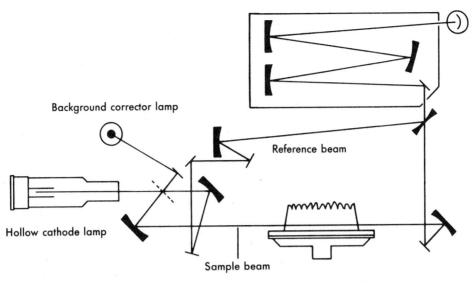

Fig. 8-12 Double-beam system with continuum source background corrector. (Courtesy Varian-Techtron Co.)

measure the background absorbance and subtract it from the total absorbance.

Continuum source background correction incorporates a continuum light source in a modified optical system (Fig. 8-12). The broad band continuum ("white" light) source differs from the primary (atomic line) source in that it emits light over a broad spectrum of wavelengths instead of at specific lines. Background absorption, which has very broad absorption spectra, will absorb the continuum emission and the line emission. True atomic absorption absorbs the primary source emission and negligibly absorbs the broad band continuum source emission. Instrument electronics then automatically remove the unwanted background contribution, providing a background corrected AA result. Continuum source background correction is widely applied and, except in some very unusual circumstances, is fully adequate for all flame AA applications. There are some limitations to continuum source background correction however that especially impact graphite furnace atomic absorption and require more sophisticated correction techniques.

Zeeman effect background correction can correct for higher and more spectrally complicated background absorption in complex matrices and provide more precise and accurate analytic results. Zeeman effect background correction uses the principle that the electronic energy levels of an atom placed in a strong magnetic field are changed, thereby changing the atomic spectra that are a measure of these energy levels. When an atom is placed in a magnetic field and its atomic absorption observed with polarized light, the normal single-line atomic absorption profile is split into two or more components symmetrically displayed about the normal position. The spectral nature of background absorption, on the other hand, is usually unaffected by a magnetic field. By placing the poles of an electromagnet around the atomizer and making alternating absorption measurements with the magnet off and then on, the uncorrected total absorbance (magnet off) and "background only" absorbance (magnet on) can be made. The automatic comparison is then made by the instrument to compensate for background correction.

Note that the uncorrected (AA + BG) and background (BG) measurements are not made at precisely the same time because the spectrophotometer alternates between measuring these two signals. For flame AA this has little impact because flame signals are steady state. However, with the graphite furnace, background and atomic absorption signals are changing rapidly as the atomization process proceeds. This means that the background in the uncorrected total signal measurement (AA + BG) and the background during background only measurement (BG) are not necessarily the same. Therefore the corrected signal (AA) may not be accurate if a correction for the timing offset is not made.

To compensate for this timing problem, an interpolation technique can be used to determine the background present at the time that the total uncorrected signal was measured. With an interpolation technique (BG) readings taken before and after the (AA + BF) reading are used to mathematically estimate the (BG) reading at the same time as the (AA + BG) reading. This technique improves the accuracy of correction when the background absorption varies significantly with time.

Other spectral interference occurs whenever the absorption wavelength of the element being analyzed overlaps the emission wavelengths of another element present in the sample. This is more frequent with multielement lamps. Interference is resolved by using a narrower slit width or another wavelength for measurement, if possible.

Atomic Absorption Spectrophotometers in Common Use. There are probably more Perkin-Elmer atomic absorption spectrophotometers used today in U.S. clinical laboratories than any other. This company has produced instruments for study of atomic absorption since 1960. Varian Techtron of Australia is the other major manufacturer of AA spectrophotometers. In the 1950s Techtron specialists worked with the Australian government and Dr. Alan Walsh in the original development of the atomic absorption technique. During 1960 the first complete atomic absorption instruments were manufactured by Techtron (now Varian Techtron) in Melbourne, Australia. Both companies offer flame and flame-less models with a vast array of add-on accessories and options. Basic and advanced models from both companies are described in the following sections.

PE Model 3100. As Perkin-Elmer's basic clinical instrument the Model 3100 (Fig. 8-13) offers exceptional analytic performance. The double-beam optics of the 3100 provide the stability and precision required for quality analyses. The system's high-light throughput monochromator with a dual-blazed grating delivers excellent signal-to-noise levels over the entire AA wavelength range. The 3100 accommodates all the popular sampling techniques including flame, mercury/hydride, graphite furnace, and flame emission capability. In the 3100 the sample beam travels through the sample compartment while the reference beams travel around it (Fig. 8-14). The beams are recombined before entering the monochromator. The double-beam system compensates for any changes that may occur in lamp intensity during an analysis.

The light beams in Model 3100 are transmitted through the system by front-surfaced quartz-coated mirrors. The advantages of using reflecting optics are that the efficiency in energy throughput is unaffected by the wavelength being considered and that no additional focusing optics are required. All mirrors used in the system are also specially coated with silicon oxide to protect the surface in a corrosive laboratory atmosphere.

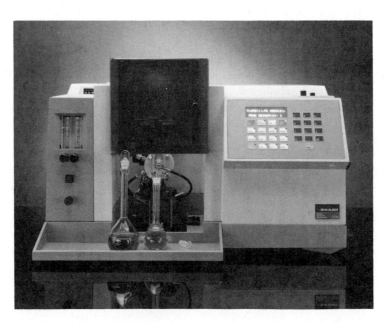

Fig. 8-13 PE 3100 AA Spectrophotometer. (Courtesy Perkin-Elmer Corp.)

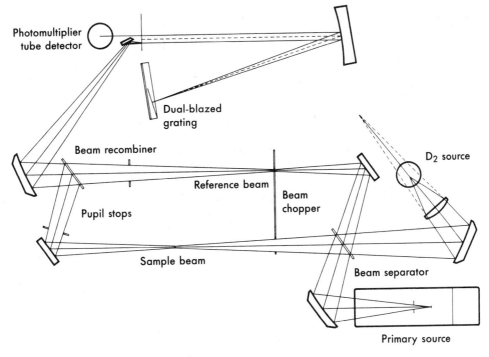

Fig. 8-14 The PE Model 3100 Optical Layout. (Courtesy Perkin-Elmer Corp.)

The photometer and monochromator optics are also enclosed with special covers for additional protection.

A large, finely ruled grating is the heart of the 3100's high-dispersion monochromator. Its wider mechanical slits capture more source energy. Analytic performance is enhanced without sacrificing resolution. A dual-blazed grating with two blaze angles—one in the ultraviolet at 236 nm and the other in the visible at 597 nm—enhances energy throughput over the entire useful wavelength range for better precision at low concentrations.

Two sets of slit heights, high and low, are standard with the Model 3100. High slits are selected when analyzing samples with the flame. Low slits are selected for graphite furnace analyses because the furnace requires a reduced beam geometry. A high-performance photomultiplier complements the optical system, providing detection capabilities over the complete wavelength range of the Model 3100.

The burner system accommodates an impact bead or a flow spoiler for maximum flexibility. Either system may be selected for analysis. An auxiliary oxidant flow can be used for improved flame stability and precision, as well as for a simple means of obtaining proper flame conditions when using combustible organic solvents. The solid titanium burner head comes with a 10 cm single-slot for use with air and acetylene. It is equipped with a standard adjustable nebulizer so that the uptake rate may be varied to optimize nebulization of any type of solution, aqueous or organic.

Automatic calibration with up to 8 standards is provided for both linear and nonlinear working curves.

Many optical accessories can extend the flexibility of the Model 3100 even further by enhancing analytic performance or adding automation capabilities. A stabilized temperature platform graphite furnace and continuum source background corrector result in more sensitive performance and freedom from interference. Autosamplers for flame or furnace sampling save operator time and add consistency to the results.

PE Model 5100 PC. The Model 5100 PC (Fig. 8-15) is Perkin-Elmer's most advanced and versatile atomic absorption spectrophotomer. It represents a new generation of AA instrumentation, with its powerful dual-grating double-beam optical system providing optimized conditions for both flame, furnace, and mercury/hydride sampling techniques. The high resolution monochromator also provides excellent flame emission per-

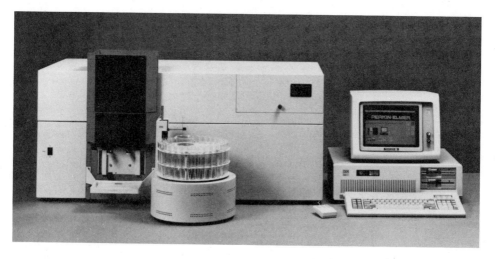

Fig. 8-15 PE 5100 AA Spectrophotometer with Flame Autosampler. (Courtesy Perkin-Elmer Corp.)

formance. The 5100 PC has full-wavelength range background correction capabilities by using continuum source or Zeeman effect techniques. Use of the dual-option burner system and optical stabilized temperature platform graphite furnace results in optimal precision and detection limits.

All instrument parameters are fully automated, allowing the instrument to determine a series of up to 12 elements with wavelength, slit, lamp and flame conditions, or graphite furnace program changes automatically set to provide optimum performance for each element. The integrated personal computer and built-in high resolution screen graphics allow the operator to monitor, compare, and manipulate fast transient signals.

Add-on options to the 5100 PC include the graphite furnace and mercury/hydride analysis units. The furnace autosampler automatically prepares calibration standards, adds matrix modifiers and diluent for up to 40 samples, and performs spike recoveries. With the flame autosampler up to 50 solutions can be introduced into the 5100 PC's flame system automatically with sequential or random access. The 5100 PC was designed to be capable of accommodating future expansion with new hardware and software as it is developed.

SpectrAA-20. The single-beam SpectrAA-10 and the double-beam SpectrAA-20 spectrophotometers made by Varian Techtron offer varying degrees of automation for flame, furnace, and hydride analysis for the budget-conscious laboratory.

The SpectrAA-20 (Fig. 8-16), with its integrated computer and keyboard, provides system control and data processing. The manually operated turret holds four hollow cathode lamps prealigned for automatic set-up and operation. In automated analysis, the next lamp in sequence is automatically warmed up. The optical system incorporates a holographic reflectance grating of 1200 lines/mm with a wavelength range of 190 to 900 nm.

The flame atomizer incorporates a high sensitivity pneumatic nebulizer with an externally adjustable impact bead. Mixing occurs as the fuel is injected tangentially into the turbulent aerosol, providing outstanding signal-to-noise performance. The nebulizer uses a platinum-iridium capillary and a ceramic venturi for long, reliable operation. The flame atomization system incorporates a comprehensive series of safety interlocks. A programmable sample changer is available for flame or hydride atomization.

Changing from flame operation to the graphite tube atomizer takes no more than a minute or two. The important differences are selecting the optimum heating program for the furnace and programming the sample dispenser.

During the analysis the system will display the temperature profile of the heating program with the analytic signal superimposed. Combining the SpectrAA-20 with the furnace saves operator time, reduces contamination problems, and eliminates dilution errors.

The vapor generation accessory is fully compatible with the SpectrAA-20. The peristaltic pumping system produces a continuous signal

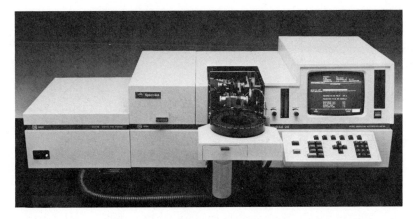

Fig. 8-16 SpectrAA 20 AA Spectrophotometer with graphite tube and atomizer and autosampler (Courtesy Varian-Techtron Co.)

that may be integrated over a selected time period.

To increase efficiency of time and sample use, Varian has developed a unique approach to signal integration called Precision Optimized Measurement Time (PROMPT). The operator specifies the precision required for the analysis, and SpectrAA measures each sample for only the length of time required to achieve that precision. High concentrations may require only a second or two, but low levels will require a longer period.

The operator is guided through the method selection sequence by a series of help messages on the display screen. The element to be analyzed is selected; the instrument parameters, including wavelength and spectral bandwidth are set; the autosampler (if used) parameters are set; up to five standards values are selected for autocalibration; all of the above is then stored on disk. To perform an analysis the operator simply recalls the method from the disk, selects the samples to be analyzed, sets the report format parameters, and presses the start button.

SpectrAA-400. Varian now markets the computerized SpectrAA-400 as their most advanced AA spectrophotometer for centralized instrument control and report management capability. The SpectrAA-400 offers multielement analysis (i.e., an automatic run sequence of up to 12 elements can be selected for samples). The high resolution color graphics on the video monitor can display flame and furnace signals in real time with background signals in a contrasting color. The computer's hard disk can store up to 90 methods for both flame and furnace work from which the parameters can be automatically recalled or modified as needed for analysis.

The IBM PS/2 Model 30 is the central com-

mand station for the operation of the SpectrAA-400 spectrophotometer, furnace and sampler, as well as the center for data processing and report generation.

The SpectrAA-400 has a fully automated eight-lamp turret that automatically recognizes the position of each lamp in the turret. During automated analysis, the next lamp to be used is warmed up. The double-beam optical system's synchronous beam-switching mirror provides twice the optical throughput of conventional beam splitters. The monochromator uses a holographic grating of 1800 lines/mm for very efficient isolation of spectral lines. Seven slits from 0.1 nm bandwidth provide optimum conditions for either flame or furnace operation.

The high speed deuterium background correction system can be selected at will to provide correction of background up to two absorbance units. Its 2 ms high speed response ensures accurate correction of rapidly changing background signals. In the double-beam system (see Fig. 8-12) radiation from the continuum source traverses the same sample and reference paths as radiation from the hollow cathode lamp. The intensities of both sources can thus be concurrently monitored. Any drift in the intensity of either source can be automatically corrected so as to maintain the accuracy of background correction.

The flame atomization system of the SpectrAA-400 is similar to that of the SpectrAA-20. Numerous interlocks monitor gas supplies, nebulizer bung, burner, flame shield, and the liquid trap to protect the operator. Accessories for the SpectrAA-400 include a flame autosampler, vapor hydride generator, graphite furnace, and furnace autosampler.

For difficult samples in the graphite furnace

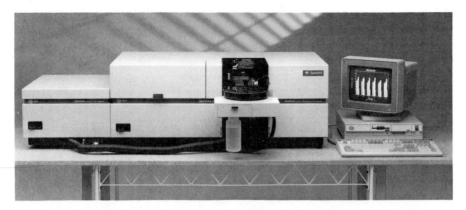

Fig. 8-17 SpectrAA-400-Zeeman AA Spectrophotometer with graphite tube atomizer and auto-sample. (Courtesy Varian-Techtron Co.)

air ashing may be selected in a program of up to 20 stages. Special gas mixtures may be introduced to the furnace to control the chemistry of chemical modifiers.

The unique furnace sampler features hot injection and a programmable injection rate, thereby reducing furnace program times and making the determination of analytes in organic solvents easier. For low-level determinations the analyst can dispense, dry, and ash the sample again and again using multiple inject and then atomize to obtain the ultimate in detection limits. A chemical modifier can be preinjected into the furnace to control the chemistry of the sample matrix.

In 1988, Varian, the pioneers in Zeeman technology, introduced the SpectrAA-400 Zeeman (Fig. 8-17), providing the benefits of fast Zeeman background correction. With Varian's patented Zeeman technology accurate correction is accomplished by polynomial interpolation of background signals coupled with a high measurement frequency and regulated magnetic field strength. Conventional Zeeman systems perform background correction at the main frequency of 50 or 60 Hz; SpectrAA-400 Zeeman instruments modulate the magnetic field at twice that frequency, so that 100 or 120 measurements/second are taken. The more measurements, the greater the accuracy of correction.

To ensure the accuracy of correction, the polynomial interpolation routine determines the actual background signal magnitude at the time of total absorbance measurement by measuring the background before and after a total absorbance measurement (analyte plus background). Thus rapid changes in background peaks are accurately monitored and corrected. Variations in the magnetic field strength because of main voltage variations would seriously influence background correction accuracy and hence the validity of the results. The SpectrAA-400 Zeeman incorporates a comprehensive monitoring and controlling circuitry to maintain a constant magnetic field strength.

Review Questions

1. What is the purpose of the flame in an atomic absorption photometer?
2. What is the purpose of an internal standard in a flame photometer?
3. What is the purpose of modulation of the light beam in an atomic absorption photometer?
4. How does a hollow cathode lamp differ from a ordinary tungsten lamp?
5. How does atomic emission photometry differ from atomic absorption photometry?
6. What is the main advantage of flameless atomic absorption over flame type atomic absorption?
7. What is the difference between continuum source and Zeeman effect background correction techniques?

Bibliography

Beaty RD: Concepts, instrumentation and techniques in atomic absorption spectrophotometry, Norwalk, Conn, 1988, Perkin-Elmer.

Bennett PA, Rothery E: Introducing atomic absorption analysis, Mulgrave, Australia, 1983, Varian Techtron.

Holmes T: PC applications for AA data management, Am Lab, 21(2):36–43, 90–97, 1989.

Kaplan LA and Pesce AJ: Clinical chemistry: theory, analysis, and correlation, St Louis, 1987, Mosby-Year Book.

Liddell PR: System integration for atomic absorption, Am Lab, 17(5):57–63, 1985.

CHAPTER 9

Molecular Emission Spectroscopy

LEMUEL J. BOWIE

Fluorometer Design
Variables Affecting Fluorescence
Applications

To understand the process of fluorescence, it is necessary to understand the properties of molecules in their ground (unexcited) and in their excited states. When molecules absorb electromagnetic radiation of suitable wavelengths, the electrons are excited to higher electronic states or energy levels. Within each of these electronic energy levels are closely spaced vibrational and rotational levels. Because these excited states are unstable, molecules dissipate this energy rapidly and return to the ground state. Many molecules can dissipate this energy by imparting it to the environment as heat. However, certain molecules, particularly those that have multiple aromatic rings, are able to release this energy in the form of photons of electromagnetic radiation. As a consequence, when these excited molecules dissipate this excess energy by reemission of radiation, the energy of the radiation is not of a single wavelength but is composed of several wavelengths representing the difference in energy between these multiple excited state levels and the multiple levels of the ground state (Fig. 9-1).

Because some energy is lost before emission from the excited state by collision with solvent or other molecules, the wavelength of the emitted light is longer (lower energy) than that of the light used to excite the molecules. This shift to longer wavelengths is called the **Stokes shift.** Because the collisional deactivation of higher vibrational and rotational states is so efficient (e.g., a lifetime of vibrational excited state is approximately 10^{-13} to 10^{-10} seconds), most emission occurs from the lowest lying vibrational level (see Fig. 9-1).

There are two types of emission processes based on the average length of time the molecule remains excited before reemission of light. This time is referred to as the lifetime of the excited state. Most uncharged molecules contain an even number of electrons in the ground state. The electrons fill molecular orbitals in pairs, and their spins are in opposite directions (paired) as dictated by the Pauli exclusion principle. When spins are paired in this manner, the electronic state is referred to as the singlet state because there is no difference in the energies of the electrons detectable by application of a magnetic field. Similarly, if an electron becomes excited by absorption and its spin remains paired with the ground state, the excited state is referred to as a singlet excited state. For singlet excited states, the lifetime of the excited state is in the order of 10^{-7} to 10^{-9} seconds. The reemission of light from singlet excited states is called **fluorescence.** The reemission is so rapid that to the naked eye the reemission appears to stop as soon as the exciting light is removed. Molecules that are capable of absorbing light and reemitting it as fluorescence are called **fluorophores.**

When the spins of the electrons occupying an excited electronic state are unpaired, the resulting excited state is called a triplet state because the energy levels would be split if a magnetic field were applied. If the excited state is originally an excited state singlet but the spins become unpaired during the lifetime of the excited state, the process is called **intersystem crossing.** In contrast to the singlet excited state, the lifetime of the excited state triplet ranges from 10^{-4} seconds to greater than 1 second. As a consequence, emission can be observed for some time after the removal of the exciting light and is called **phosphorescence.** Because of the extended lifetime of the excited state, there is a greater opportunity for collisions and other deactivation processes to occur so that phosphorescence is best observed at

139

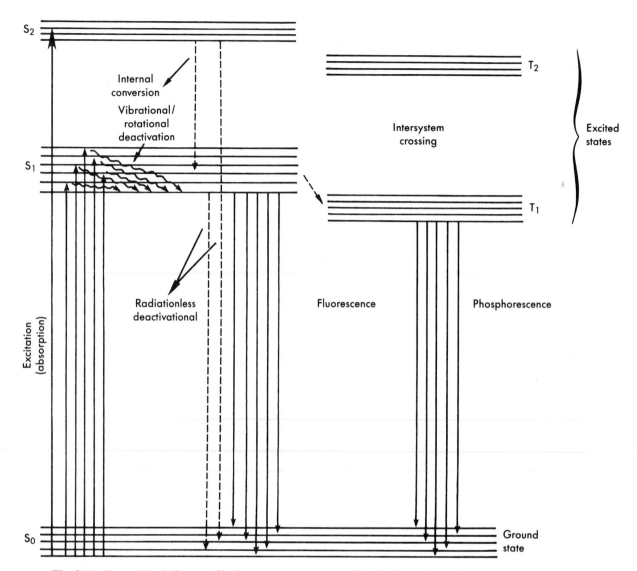

Fig. 9-1   Energy level diagram. Singlet states are represented by S_0, S_1, and S_2. Triplet states are T_1 and T_2.

low temperatures or in viscous media where these competing processes are retarded.

Molecules can also absorb chemical energy and be excited to higher electronic levels. Once in these higher electronic levels the molecules behave as if they had been excited by the absorption of light energy. When these chemically excited molecules emit light, the process is called **chemiluminescence.** A special case of chemiluminescence occurs when the chemical reaction that results in excited molecules requires an enzyme to be effective. The emission resulting from such an enzyme-catalyzed reaction is called **bioluminescence.**

Fluorometer Design

All instruments designed for measuring fluorescence use the following basic components: a light source, an excitation filter/monochromator, a sample cell, an emission filter/monochromator, and a detector. A diagram of a simplified fluorometer is shown in Fig. 9-2.

Light Source. In absorption measurements the parameter that is usually monitored and is proportional to concentration is absorbance. In fluorescence measurements, however, the emitted intensity is directly proportional to both fluorophore concentration and the intensity of the excitation beam. It is for this reason that fluores-

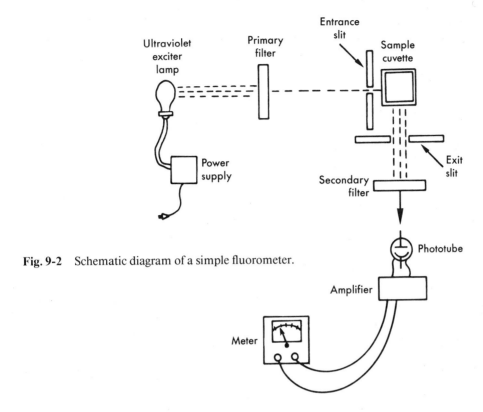

Fig. 9-2 Schematic diagram of a simple fluorometer.

cence instruments use high-intensity light sources such as mercury or xenon arc lamps. In these gas-discharge lamps electrons cause ionization and excitation of gas atoms by collision, and these excited gas atoms emit at characteristic wavelengths. Mercury lamps produce line spectra at 254, 365, and 366 nm, as well as a number of other wavelengths. Mercury vapor lamps can be modified to provide energy at other wavelengths by coating the inner surface of the lamp with a phosphor that absorbs the emitted light and reemits it at a longer wavelength. Although emission from mercury arc lamps is very intense, the presence of discrete lines is not ideal for compounds that do not have absorption bands at wavelengths coinciding with these emission lines. For this reason many instruments use xenon arc lamps, which are less intense but produce a continuous spectrum between approximately 250 nm and 600 nm. A disadvantage of xenon arc lamps is that they require a special power supply to produce a stable output. Simple fluorometer systems use mercury vapor lamps because no special power supply is needed. Because of the presence of the intense resonance lines, however, these lamps are not suitable for spectrofluorometers in which spectral scanning is required.

Excitation and Emission Filters/Monochromators. When the instrument uses filters for isolating excitation and emission wavelengths, it is called a **fluorometer**. Both interference and absorption filters have been used. The excitation filter is called the primary filter and is frequently a cutoff filter that absorbs most of the light above a certain wavelength. By selecting a primary filter that absorbs any light whose wavelength is longer than that of the excitation spectrum of the designated fluorophore, the effect of wavelength scatter that may overlap the emission spectrum of the fluorophore is minimized. The emission filter is called the secondary filter and is selected to transmit light only above a certain wavelength. In this case the filter should absorb most of the light below the emission spectrum of the fluorophore to minimize the effects of scatter. When measurements require more selective discrimination of excitation and emission wavelengths, grating monochromators are used and the instruments are called **spectrofluorometers**.

Sample Cells. In fluorescence measurements the emitted light is detected at right angles to the incident light. This is necessary to eliminate the potential interference of the excitation signal. For this reason rectangular cells are preferred, although cylindric tubes have been used. Ultraviolet light is absorbed significantly by ordinary glass. Consequently, whenever significant excitation or emission occurs in the ultraviolet region of the spectrum, quartz cuvettes, which do not have significant absorption in this region, are preferred to prevent loss of sensitivity. Moreover, if measurements are desirable in concentrated solutions, special, narrow, path-length cells may be used to eliminate an "inner filter effect" or sample self-absorption of excitation and/or emitted light. Because fluorescence instruments use such intense light sources, photodecomposition of some fluorophores can occur if extended exposure to such intense light occurs. As a result, it is important that the sample compartment have a shutter on the excitation side that can be closed whenever measurements are not being performed so that such exposure and potential photodecomposition is limited.

Detectors. Phototubes and photomultiplier tubes are required for fluorescence measurements because the fluorescence signals are generally of low intensity. Photomultiplier tubes can be sensitive to different wavelengths by varying the composition of the photocathode. Therefore for increased sensitivity a photomultiplier that is most sensitive to the emission wavelengths of the compounds to be measured should be used.

Variables Affecting Fluorescence

Analytic Variables. Light scattering of the excitation light into the detector can occur, even when the detector is positioned at right angles to the path of the incident light. It becomes a serious problem when samples are turbid, contain colloidal particles, or are contained in nonrectangular cuvettes. When the wavelength of the scattered light detected by the phototube is the same as the exciting light, it is called **Rayleigh scatter.** Even in pure solvent, however, it is possible to detect another type of scatter that is of a slightly longer wavelength than the exciting light. This scatter **(Raman scatter)** results from the chemical properties of the fluorophore,[9] and its peak intensity differs from that of the exciting light by a constant frequency (reciprocal of wavelength). Both types of scatter are most troublesome when the excitation and emission maxima of the fluorophore are close together. It can severely limit the sensitivity of a method if this type of fluorophore must be used. Careful selection of secondary (emission) filters or the use of polarized filters may be helpful in limiting the effect of scatter in these cases.

The relationship between fluorescence intensity and concentration is described as:

$$F = \Phi I_0(1 - e^{-\epsilon bc}) \text{ or } F = \Phi I_0(1 - e^{-A})$$

where F is the power of fluorescence (intensity), Φ is the quantum yield (quantum efficiency), I_0 is the radiant power of the incident light, ϵ is the molar absorptivity, b is the path length, c is the molar concentration, and $^{-A}$ is the absorbance. It is clear from this equation that although there is a relationship between fluorescence intensity and concentration, there are a number of other factors that must be considered.

The quantum yield (Φ) is a property of the fluorophore and its emission characteristics in the environment in which it is being measured. It is the ratio of the number of photons absorbed during excitation to the number emitted during fluorescence. As discussed earlier, a number of processes can contribute to the loss of energy without reemission of light. Obviously, conditions should be selected to maximize Φ if maximal sensitivity is desired.

The power and stability of the incident radiation (I_0) are also important considerations for reliable measurements because they directly affect the sensitivity and precision of the measurements.

The molar absorptivity (ϵ) describes the relative probability of excitation for fluorophores. Because emission can occur only from excited molecules, it follows that the higher the molar absorptivity, the greater the fluorescence intensity if all other variables are constant.

The path length for typical fluorescence measurements, like absorbance measurements, is 1 cm. However, for certain applications where the concentration of the sample is too high to obtain a linear dependence on concentration, shortening the path length can make the response linear. For measurements at high concentrations, front surface techniques in which excitation and emission occur only from the surface of the solution may be useful.

As an analytic technique, fluorescence obeys Beers Law only at low concentrations of fluorophore. This can best be understood by noting that the exponential in the equation above can be expanded to yield the Taylor series in the equation below:

$$F = \Phi I_0[2.3\epsilon bc - (-2.3\epsilon bc)^2/2!) - (-2.3\epsilon bc)^3/3! - \dots]$$

Therefore whenever $\epsilon bc < 0.05$, the subsequent terms of the series become negligible and the series reduces to this equation:

$$F = 2.3\Phi I_0 \, \epsilon bc$$

or

$$F = Kc$$

where K is a constant. This equation clearly demonstrates the linear dependence of fluorescence intensity on concentration when the absorbance (ϵbc) is less than 0.05. This is understandable considering that, as the absorbance increases, more and more of the exciting light is absorbed before it reaches molecules near the center of the cuvette so that they are not able to be excited. This process has been referred to as concentration quenching or self-quenching and results in less fluorescence from fluorophores near the center of the cuvette than from those near the outer walls.

Because the geometry of most instruments dictates that most of the light reaching the detector must come from the inner volume of the cells (Fig. 9-3), the fluorescence signal is easily diminished by this process.

In addition, molecules that are excited and emit photons from the center of the cell can have the light absorbed before it exits the cell and before it can be detected by the phototube if the concentration of the fluorophore is too great. In this case, however, there must be an overlap between the emission spectrum of the fluorophore and its excitation spectrum. This type of concentration quenching is called **self-absorption** and also results in a loss of linear response with fluorophore concentration. As indicated previously, if the path length is decreased, the effects of both of these processes may be reduced or eliminated without having to lower concentrations significantly.

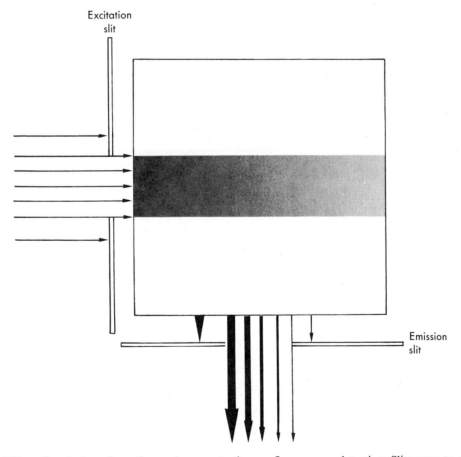

Fig. 9-3   Effect of optical configuration and concentration on fluorescence detection. Slits serve to narrow the width of the exciting light emitted and can be used to vary sensitivity. At high concentrations the intensity of light emitted decreases with distance into the cuvette because more and more of the light required for excitation is absorbed.

Finally, at high concentrations, some fluorophores can form complexes with themselves leading to excited state dimers (excimers) or form complexes with other molecules to form heterogeneous excited state complexes (exciplexes). In both instances these complexes can lead to a decrease in the fluorescence from the excited state singlet of the fluorophore and therefore result in quenching.

Chemical Variables. Perhaps the most important chemical variable to control is the presence of molecules or conditions that cause deactivation of the excited state without the emission of radiation. Any molecule that decreases fluorescence yield by such deactivation is called a **quencher,** although the term is usually reserved for nonfluorescent solutes. As indicated earlier, the actual process is called **quenching.**

There are a number of mechanisms by which this type of quenching can take palce. The simplest form that does not involve any type of direct energy transfer process is the **inner filter effect** that is analogous to the self-absorption effect previously discussed. In this case light never reaches the detector because it is absorbed by a nonfluorescent molecule that, although it becomes excited, does not reemit the radiation. A second mechanism of fluorescence quenching involves actual collisions between the excited fluorophore and other solutes so that the fluorophore's energy is transferred to the solute molecules. Again the solute molecules absorb this excess energy but do not reemit it. It is also possible to have fluorescence quenching by energy transfer even in the absence of any direct interaction such as occurs in collisional energy transfer. This can be a significant analytic problem because it is not as responsive to dilution and may require physical removal of the quencher.

Another mechanism for quenching involves the actual formation of a chemical complex (charge transfer complex) between the excited fluorophore and the quencher. In this case there is an actual electron transfer that takes place in the excited state of the complex, and the complex is deactivated through a radiationless process. In most cases the quencher is a nonfluorescent organic molecule; however, certain metal ions can form excited state complexes that result in fluorescence quenching.

Finally, molecules that facilitate intersystem crossing from the excited state singlet to the triplet state inhibit fluorescence because there is more time for radiationless deactivation processes (e.g., collisions) to occur before emission. One of the most important quenchers in this category is molecular oxygen that exists in the ground state as a triplet. Although the details of the mechanism of quenching are still unclear, it is believed to involve enhanced intersystem crossing of the fluorophore's excited singlet state to the excited triplet state. Paramagnetic transition-metal ions are also effective quenchers that probably act by enhancing the rate of intersystem crossing in the fluorophore.

Another important chemical variable that can have a significant effect on fluorescence is temperature. In general, the lower the temperature the less efficient the quenching process, particularly for the mechanisms that require intermolecular collisions or associations described previously. As a result, fluorescence intensity generally increases with decreases in temperature. For some molecules the change in fluorescence intensity can be as great as 50% with a small change (10° to 15° C) in temperature. It is therefore important to ensure that temperature changes do not occur during the measurement period. Thermoregulation of the cell compartment or cuvette itself may be necessary.

Solvent character also can affect the efficiency of fluorescence. Viscous solvents decrease the likelihood of quenching because of collisions or a complex formation in a manner similar to decreases in temperature discussed previously. Fluorophores that contain ionizable groups can be affected by the pH of the solvent. Because the fluorescence intensity from the excited states of charged and uncharged species is generally different, changes in pH affect the fluorescence intensity by altering the ratio of the charged and uncharged species. In a similar manner, some fluorophores are capable of forming hydrogen bonds with solvent or other solutes in either the ground state or the excited state. Also, these interactions generally tend to reduce the fluorescence intensity by a variety of mechanisms. Therefore solvents or other solutes that have the ability to hydrogen bond with the fluorophore should be carefully evaluated so that unexpected changes can be eliminated.

Applications

One of the major advantages of fluorescence as an analytic technique is that it is 100 to 1000 times more sensitive than absorption measurements. This is because it is a direct measurement of a signal as opposed to a ratio as is required for

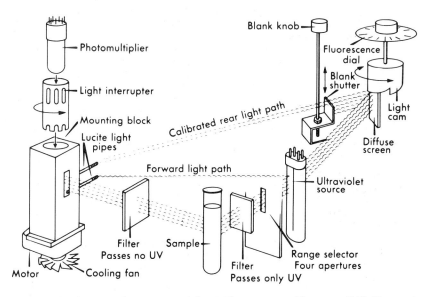

Fig. 9-4 Schematic diagram of Turner Model 111 Fluorometer. (Courtesy G.K. Turner Associates.)

absorbance measurements. For analytic applications requiring high sensitivity but for which the spectral properties of the fluorophore are known, a simple fluorometer may be the least expensive and reliable approach. Perhaps the most popular instrument in this class is the Turner Model 111 (Fig. 9-4). Model 112 has been upgraded with solid state electronics and a digital readout, but the basic design has not changed from Model 111. One of the advantages of this particular instrument is that it uses a chopper to alternately cause fluorescence from the sample and light from the light source to be detected. The light from the light source is reflected into the photomultiplier from the diffuse screen, and the blank knob is used to adjust the fraction that reaches the photomultiplier so that fluorescence from a blank sample may be a set to zero. The forward light path is included to ensure that there is always some, albeit very small, amount of light that reaches the photomultiplier tube even if nonfluorescent blanks are used. Because both front and rear paths are chopped, the output of the photomultiplier tube is an alternating current that permits drift-free amplification. The difference in intensity between the front and rear paths is presented by a servomechanism as a movement of the dial (Model 111) or as a digital signal (Model 112) and is directly related to the fluorescence of the sample. This dual-path design eliminates problems related to variations in line voltage, lamp intensity, and photomultiplier sensitivity. The instrument accepts a variety of

cuvette types (e.g, micro, continuous flow, temperature stabilized), as well as a number of filter and excitation lamp options.

Another advantage of fluorescence is that it offers increased specificity inasmuch as only molecules that fluoresce and whose fluorescence emission occurs in the wavelength region being monitored are detected in a fluorescence-based assay. In absorption measurements all molecules that absorb in the region of interest are detected and can interfere with the analysis. However, to use fluorophores effectively, it is necessary to know their spectral characteristics under the conditions desired. This information is obtained by determining the excitation and emission spectra, and a spectrofluorometer must be employed. Many models are available, some of which can automatically determine the optimal excitation and emission wavelengths (Fig. 9-5).

In chemiluminescence, light emission is caused by the excitation of molecules through a chemical reaction as opposed to photoluminescence (fluorescence/phosphorescence) in which the excitation occurs as a result of light absorption. Chemiluminescence has been used as an analytic technique to measure a number of substances because of its theoretical sensitivity particularly when compared with radioimmunoassay for measuring compounds at low concentration. For example, if ^{125}I in a typical radioimmunoassay has a specific activity of 1000 to 4000 disintegrations/minute (dpm) per femtomole then this equates to approximately 1 disin-

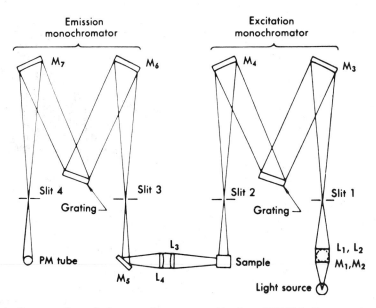

Fig. 9-5 Schematic diagram of a typical spectrofluorometer. (Aminco SPF 125; Courtesy American Instruments Co, Inc.)

tegration/600,000 labeled molecules per minute.

In contrast, chemiluminescence has a theoretical maximum of one photon detected for each molecule that undergoes the chemical reaction. In actual practice the quantum yield is more in the area of 1% (1 photon/100 molecules reacted) for chemiluminescence. Even so it is clear that chemiluminescence enjoys a major theoretic advantage. The earliest and most widely used chemiluminescent reagents were luminol or its derivatives. Luminol, as well as similar chemiluminescent reagents, had the disadvantage of requiring a catalyst or strong reaction conditions that were not suitable for some assays. In addition, if chemiluminescence is used as the label for an immunoassay, the coupling can affect light output.

Bioluminescence has theoretical advantages similar to chemiluminescence but requires the use of specific enzymes. Although enzymes have the advantage of specificity, they have the disadvantage of less stability and more limited reaction conditions. Nevertheless, both chemiluminescence and bioluminescence continue to be widely used for analyses requiring high sensitivity.

Although these general, multipurpose fluorometers/spectrofluorometers continue to be widely used, some of the most dramatic applications of fluorescence have been with fluorescence instruments that have been designed to perform a specific function (e.g., fluorescence polariza-

tion, delayed emission spectroscopy, cell analysis, or sorting).

Fluorescence polarization has recently become widely used for studying both large and small molecules. This technique requires a fluorometer capable of providing linearly polarized light to excite sample molecules. This function is accomplished by the use of a polarizing filter called the polarizer. It must also be able to detect the degree of polarization of emitted light usually in two different planes oriented at 90 degrees to each other. Again, a polarizing filter is used, but in this case it is called the analyzer. Such an instrument is called a polarization fluorometer (Fig. 9-6).

Fluorescence polarization is useful as an analytic technique because it can give information on the rate of rotation of the fluorophore in the excited state. As shown in Fig. 9-6 if a molecule absorbs plane polarized light, only those molecules whose absorption dipoles are oriented parallel to the plane of the exciting light will be excited. The excitation process is very rapid, occurring in approximately 1×10^{-15} seconds. On the other hand, reemission occurs one million times more slowly with a half-life of approximately 1×10^{-8} seconds. As a result, there is a relatively long time between absorption and reemission during which molecular rotation could occur.

If reemission were instantaneous, the emitted

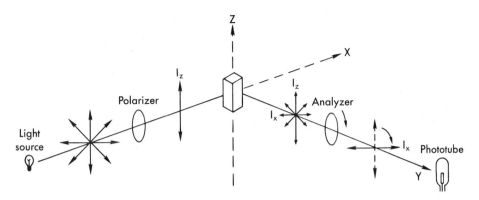

Fig. 9-6 Optical diagram of a polarization fluorometer. Light polarized in the vertical direction is absorbed by those molecules with the proper orientation. Before emission some rotation occurs so that the light emerging from the cell is partially depolarized. Measurements are taken with the analyzer oriented in the vertical direction. The analyzer is then rotated 90 degrees and measurements are taken again to determine the extent of depolarization.

light would be plane polarized with the plane of the polarized light oriented parallel to the plane of the absorption dipole. Because reemission is not instantaneous, the dipoles rotate before emission and the light is less polarized. The degree of this depolarization is directly related to the speed of rotation of the fluorophore. The more rapidly molecules rotate, the more the emitted light will be depolarized. Obviously molecular size and solvent viscosity can affect the speed at which molecules rotate in solution. Therefore large fluorophores or fluorophores attached to macromolecules would be expected to rotate more slowly. Likewise more viscous solvents would be expected to decrease the speed of rotation of a flu-

orophore. In both these instances the polarization of fluorescence would be higher than if the fluorophore tumbled more rapidly in solution because it was smaller or was in a less viscous environment. Therefore fluorescence polarization instruments have been used to measure solvent viscosity and provide information on molecular processes and to assist in detecting certain clinical conditions.

Florescence polarization has also been used to detect molecular association processes, as well as to measure binding processes. This latter technique has been used widely in the development of immunoassays for analytic and diagnostic purposes. An example of a widely used, micropro-

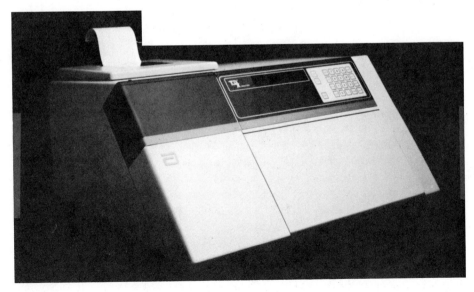

Fig. 9-7 Abbott TDX Polarization Immunoassay Analyzer. (Courtesy Abbott Corp.)

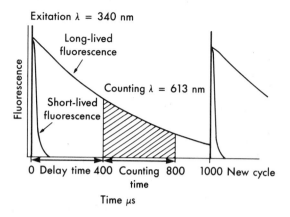

Fig. 9-8 Measurement principle from time-resolved fluorescence on the LKB Delfia Immunoassay System. The cycle time is 1 ms, and the excitation pulse lasts only 1 μs. Fluorescence measurements are delayed for 400 μs to allow background (short-lived) fluorescence to decay. (Courtesy LKB Produkter, AB, Sweden.)

cessor-controlled fluorescence polarization instrument (Abbott TDX) is shown in Fig. 9-7. One interesting innovation in this system is the use of a liquid crystal to accomplish rapid and automated rotation of the plane of the exciting light.

Another interesting analytic approach that takes advantage of the delay between excitation and fluorescence emission is called **time-resolved fluorescence spectroscopy.** The technique depends on the use of a pulsed light source and a fluorophore whose fluorescence decay time is comparatively long in relation to the decay time for the excitation pulse. The earliest instruments used special sources that could produce intense pulses with a decay time of 1 ns. By monitoring the intensity and polarization of the decay after the light source has been removed, much information can be gained about macromolecules and macromolecular binding sites. Certain lanthanide chelates have fluorescent lifetimes of 10 to 1000 μs and make it possible to use time-resolved fluorescent techniques with time gating of simpler light sources. Because natural (background) fluorescence in biologic samples has lifetimes in the 1 to 20 ns range, monitoring of lanthanide

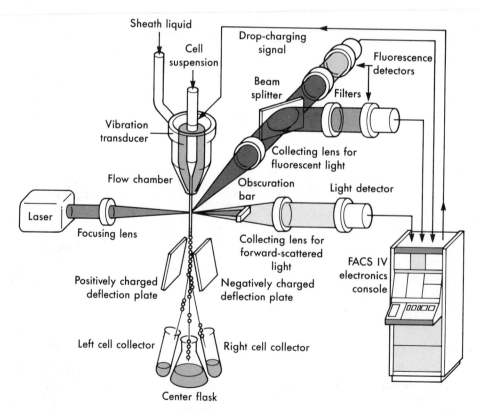

Fig. 9-9 Schematic diagram of the Becton Dickson fluorescence activated cell sorting (FACS) system. (Courtesy Becton Dickinson and Co.)

fluorescence after this background fluorescence has decayed eliminates this major limitation to sensitivity for fluorescence-based assays in biologic materials (Fig. 9-8).

Intracellular organelles and compounds can sometimes be visualized at lower concentrations by using antibodies specific to these molecules that have fluorophores covalently attached, compared with techniques that use conventional stains. This visualization requires a specially adapted microscope that allows only the light from the fluorescently labeled material to enter the aperture. Because nonlabeled materials are not visible at all, the background is very low and the technique is very sensitive. Moreover, because the fluorescent label is not visible under normal conditions, the underlying structures can be viewed by regular light microscopy to examine cellular details and correlate the distribution of the fluorescent label with these structures.

A special application of fluorescence is its use to count or physically separate certain cells from other cells. The technique uses a fluorescent label that attaches only to a particular type of cell present in a mixture. This specific labeling is frequently accomplished by using fluorescent labeled antibodies directed against some molecule on the surface of the particular cell. Different fluorophores attached to different antibodies can be used to simultaneously separate more than one type of cell. The instrument used is called a cell analyzer if it is used to determine the percentage of the various cell types. It is called a cell sorter (Fig. 9-9), if it is capable of physically separating the various cells based on the label detected. The mixture of labeled and unlabeled cells is introduced as a suspension, and the instrument monitors the fluorescence properties of individual cells as they pass through an orifice. The number of total cells and cells with each type of label are counted, and the percentage of the cell types can thus be determined. In the case of cell sorters the droplets containing the individual cells can be electrically charged depending on the label detected and then deflected electronically into different collection vessels. Cell sorters can both count the various types of cells present and physically separate them.

Review Questions

1. What are they key differences between fluorescence, phosphorescence, chemiluminescence, and bioluminescence?
2. Describe the main advantages and disadvantages of fluorometers and spectrofluorometers.
3. What are the main instrumental variables that affect fluorescence intensity, and how are they controlled?
4. What are the most important chemical variables to control in a fluorescence assay?
5. If you wished to develop an immunoassay and wanted maximal sensitivity, would you use radioimmunoassay, chemiluminescence immunoassay, or fluorescence immunoassay? Why?
6. In which way would you expect each of the following to affect fluorescence polarization from fluorophore?
   Temperature
   Molecular aggregation
   Fluorophore binding to macromolecules
   Viscosity
7. Why is it useful to utilize a fluorophore with a long lifetime for time-resolved fluorescence assays?

Bibliography

Bowie L, Carreathers S: Fluorescence polarization and the aggregation of deoxy-hemoglobin S, Anal Lett 10:835, 1977.

Dandliker WB, Kelly JR, and Dandliker J: Fluorescence polarization immunoassay. Theory and experimental method, Immunochemistry 10:219, 1973.

Diamandis EP: Immunoassays with time-resolved fluorescence spectroscopy: principles and applications, Clin Biochem, 21:139, 1988.

Dudley RF: Chemiluminescence immunoassay: an alternative to rIA, Lab Med 21:216, 1990.

Guilbault GG: Practical fluorescence, theory, methods, and techniques, New York, 1973, Marcel Dekker.

Loken MR, Gohlke JL, and Brand L: In Fluorescence techniques in cell biology, New York, 1973, Springer-Verlag.

Parker CA: Photoluminescence of solutions, Amsterdam, 1968, Elsevier.

Schroeder HR, Vogelhut PO, and Carrico RJ, et al: Competitive binding assay for biotin monitored by chemiluminescence, Anal Chem 48:1933, 1976.

Skoog DA, West DM: Principles of instrumental analysis, New York, 1971, Holt, Rinehart & Winston.

Weber G: Fluorescence techniques in cell biology, New York, 1973, Springer-Verlag.

CHAPTER 10

Electrochemistry

ANTHONY O. OKORODUDU

Potentiometric Measurement
Polarographic Measurement
Anodic Stripping Voltametry
Thermal Conductivity Measurement
Amperometric and Coulometric Measurements
Characteristics of Electrochemical Analyzers
Future Developments

The physiologic well-being of living organisms depends on a balanced control of the activity of a variety of important ions (and gases). Thus measurement of their concentrations is an important analytic function in clinical laboratory medicine. Electrochemical principles involved with the measurement of current or voltage generated because of the **activity** of specific ion species in an electrochemical cell have been used extensively for the quantitation of these essential analytes. The activity of the ionic form of the analyte is directly proportional to its concentration. Concentration can be calculated from the obtained activity using the following equation:

$$a = \gamma c$$

where:

a = activity

γ = the **activity coefficient** (the activity coefficient of each species in a solution is inversely related to the ionic strength, μ)

$\mu = 0.5(\Sigma c_i \cdot z_i^2)$; c_i = concentration and z = charge number for each species in solution

c = concentration

Use of electrochemical reactions in determining activity of ions was first applied to pH measurement, but shortly thereafter the technology was extended to include a variety of electrolytes and gases. Electroanalysis has made it possible to use very small volumes (μl) for the measurement of analytes that exist in the concentration range of 10^{-8} to 10^{-3} moles/l. Instruments that use this technique exhibit an unprecedented degree of precision, ease of operation, and a remarkably short analysis time.

This chapter will provide a general review of electrochemical principles that are widely applicable to the clinical chemistry laboratory measurements. Specifically, **potentiometric, polarographic, conductivity,** and **coulometric** techniques will be reviewed and illustrated with selected analytes. Following this general review, characteristics of some analyzers that use electroanalytic principles will be presented. The chapter will conclude with a review of new and emerging instruments in the field of electrochemistry.

Potentiometric Measurement

Nearly all conductors of electricity are metals or electrolytes with the current being carried by either electrons or ions. When current passes from metal to electrolyte or from electrolyte to metal, the type of carrier usually changes suddenly and certain interesting phenomena occur. Whenever there is an interface between the metal and ions of that metal in a solution, an electric potential is produced. This potential is called the electric potential of that metal. An electrode potential is also produced when different concentrations of an ion are separated by a membrane that is semipermeable to that ion. Nonmetallic elements such as hydrogen also have electrode potentials. It is impossible to assign a specific value to the potential of each substance because it depends on such factors as concentration and complexity of the solution and temperature, but each may be assigned a relative electrode potential using the hydrogen half-cell as 0.0 V.

$$\tfrac{1}{2}H \text{-----} H^+ + e^-$$

$$E° = 0.00 \text{ V}$$

Thus the calcium half-cell has an electrode potential of -2.87 V, and mercury has an electrode potential of $+0.789$ V.

$$\text{Ca} \text{-----} \text{Ca}^{2+} + 2e^-$$

$$E° = -2.87 \text{ V}$$

To measure an electrode potential, another voltage source (such as another metal/solution interface) is needed to measure the first against. Each of the electrodes is called a **half-cell.** The two half-cells arranged together constitute an **electrochemical cell** in which one of the half-cells maintains a constant voltage. The electrode in the half-cell with constant voltage is called the **reference electrode,** whereas the variable voltage portion is termed the **indicator electrode.** It is possible to measure the potential difference between these two electrodes and calculate the concentration of ions in the solution of the indicator (measuring) electrode (Fig. 10-1).

To clarify this concept, look at a specific measuring system. If a silver wire is immersed in a solution of silver chloride, ionization of the silver metal occurs with the formation of silver ions (Ag^+) and electrons. An electric potential now exists between the wire and the solution. If two half-cells are used, each with a silver wire or foil immersed in a different silver solution and the two solutions are connected through a meter, a differ-ence in potential can be detected between them (Fig. 10-2). Because the potential of each solution depends on the concentration of silver ions in it, the concentration of ions in one solution can be predicted if the value for the other and the difference in potential between them are known. In practice, such a system can be set up and, by calibrating it against known standards, a workable measuring system can be arrived at. A temperature difference between the two half-cells would affect the reproducibility of measurement. Other minor technical factors such as coating (e.g., protein deposit when using biologic fluids) will affect the measurements.

It is not necessary that the two half-cells contain the same materials as long as two similar potentials are produced. In fact, it is possible to devise a reference electrode that will give a very precise and reproducible potential. Using this reference electrode with a highly reliable potential, it is possible to calibrate the system with known standards and measure the concentration of the ion in question on a precalibrated scale. Fig. 10-3 illustrates a calibration scheme in which two standards are for the calibration, and the electrode slope is determined.

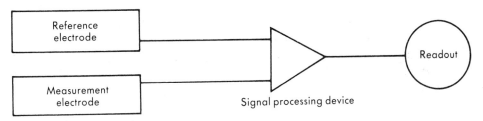

Fig. 10-1   Basic functional units of electrode system.

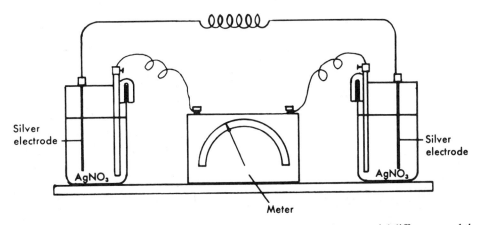

Fig. 10-2   Two silver half-cells connected through a meter. If one knows the potential difference and the concentration of silver nitrate in one half-cell, the concentration in a test solution can be calculated.

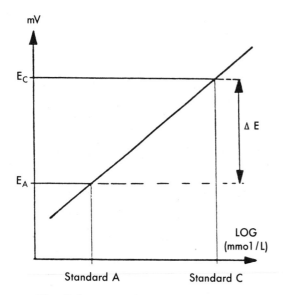

Fig. 10-3 Two point calibration scheme.

Potentiometric methods are based on the quantitative relationship between the potential of a cell as given by the following distribution of potential:

$$E_{cell} = E_{reference} + E_{indicator} + E_{junction}$$

Because the reference and junction potentials are constant, the indicator potential can be determined. The potential of the indicator (measuring electrode) can then be related to concentration.

Electrode systems used in the clinical laboratory have precalibrated readout devices that give results in concentration units. The **cell potential** is related to concentration through the **Nernst equation:**

$$E = E° + \frac{2.303\ RT}{zF} \log \frac{aox}{aRed}$$

where:

E = Electrochemical potential of an electrode

E° = Standard electrode potential (constant)

R = Molar gas constant (8.314 joules)/(mole) (°K)

T = Absolute temperature (Kelvin or K) (273° + °C = °K)

z = Number of electrons transferred in the electrode reaction

F = Faraday's constant (96,487 coulombs/mole of electrons)

a = Activity of oxidized and reduced forms

To simplify this equation, the voltage developed between the reference and measuring electrodes will be:

$$E = KT \log (C_1/C_2)$$

$$K = \text{Constant } 2.3(R/zF)$$

$(C_1/C_2) =$ If either C_1 or C_2 is known, the concentration of the unknown can be calculated from the measurement of the potential developed.

In summary, the potential of a reference electrode is a constant known potential. An indicator electrode is sensitive to the concentration of a specific component of the solution being analyzed. The potential, because of the species being measured, is obtained by finding the difference between the reference and measured potentials. By using the Nernst relationship, concentration is calculated. Different types of reference and indicator electrodes used in clinical laboratory instruments are described in this chapter.

Liquid-Liquid Junction Potential. In making an electrical connection between the reference electrode and the sample solution via a **salt bridge,** a negligible but reproducible potential is produced. This potential develops at the interface between two nonidentical solutions and is called the **liquid-liquid junction potential.** A concentrated or saturated potassium chloride salt bridge is commonly used because it provides several advantages.

Fig. 10-4 is a conceptual diagram of an enlarged section of a liquid-liquid junction. Consider the A^+ ions and the B^- ions. Initially there are none of these in the sample solution, but there is a large concentration of them in the salt bridge. These ions, following the laws of thermodynamics, will diffuse from the region of greater concentration to the region of lower concentration. Because the A^+ ions are smaller, they will diffuse more quickly than the larger B^- ions and the result will be that a small positive-negative charge difference (or potential) is established. The same process can happen with the C^+ and D^{--} ions in the sample diffusing into the salt bridge. The cumulative result, which is the liquid-liquid junction potential, can be 20 to 30 mV. This is a large value when measuring electrode potentials to a few tenths of a millivolt.

If the hydrated positive ion and the negative ion were the same size, they would diffuse at the same rate and no potential would be established. Because potassium ions and chloride ions have about the same mobilities, potassium chloride is a good compound for use as a salt bridge. This

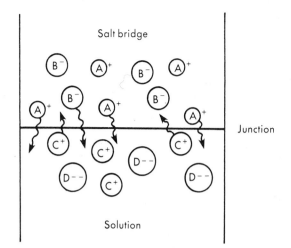

Fig. 10-4 Liquid-liquid junction.

similarlity in mobility of the ions reduces the junction potential considerably. In routine clinical analyses there is no such choice of ions in the sample solution and no control of this kind to reduce the diffusion of ions from the sample. Therefore diffusion is controlled by having a saturated potassium chloride solution in the reference electrode. This results in many ions diffusing from the salt bridge against which the sample ions must diffuse. Diffusion of ions from the sample to the junction is thus relatively negligible so that the junction potential is 1 mV or less and reproducible. Now electrode potentials can be measured to fractions of millivolts more accurately.

Reference Electrodes. A reference electrode is an electrochemical half-cell with a known constant potential against which the potential of the indicator half-cell is measured. Electrodes that generate a constant potential and can be used as a reference include the standard hydrogen electrode, the saturated calomel electrode, and the silver-silver chloride electrode. These electrodes are stable with easily reproducible half-cell potentials and have chemically stable components.

Standard Hydrogen Electrode. The standard hydrogen electrode is the international standard but is seldom used for routine work because more convenient types with reliable calibration buffers are available. Hydrogen electrodes are produced by coating a platinum electrode with platinum black (finely divided particles of platinum). Hydrogen gas at a pressure of 1 atmosphere is then bubbled around the coated platinum that is immersed in an acidic solution with H^+ activity set at unity. Although this type of electrode is quite

accurate, it is unstable and very awkward to use. This standard hydrogen electrode, by definition, has a potential of 0.00 **volts (V)** at all temperatures. It is the absolute reference half-cell used for the standardization of other reference electrodes that are present in routine clinical chemistry instruments.

Saturated Calomel Electrode. The saturated calomel electrode is a widely used reference electrode. As shown in Fig. 10-5, *A*, its function is based on the reversible reaction:

$$Hg_2Cl_2 + 2e^- \rightleftharpoons 2Hg° + 2\ Cl^-$$

The calomel electrode contains an inert element (e.g., platinum) in contact with mercury, mercurous chloride (calomel), and a solution of potassium chloride of known concentration. The saturated calomel electrode in which the solution is saturated with potassium chloride (4.2 molar (M) at 25° C), is commonly used because it is easy to prepare and maintain. If the salt concentration around the electrode is different from the salt bridge concentration, another liquid-liquid junction potential is established. For this reason the salt solution in a calomel electrode is usually saturated.

When a high degree of accuracy is desired, a 0.1M or 1.0M potassium chloride solution electrode is preferred because it reaches its equilibrium potential quicker and its potential depends less on temperature than does the saturated type. Calomel electrodes become unstable at temperatures above 80° C and should be replaced with silver-silver electrodes.

Silver-Silver Chloride Electrode. The silver-silver chloride electrode is a very reproducible electrode. Its operation is based on the reversible reaction:

$$AgCl + e^- \rightleftharpoons Ag^+ + Cl^-$$

The electrode is prepared by electroplating a layer of silver on a platinum wire and then converting the surface silver to silver chloride by electrolysis in hydrochloric acid (Fig. 10-5,*B*). The solution surrounding the electrode should be saturated with potassium chloride and silver chloride.

Indicator Electrodes. The indicator electrode system is a half-cell whose potential varies as the concentration of a specific ion in the solution changes. This change in potential is governed by the Nernst equation. The term **ion-selective electrode** (ISE) is increasingly used to describe electrodes used for measurement of ions. The ion-se-

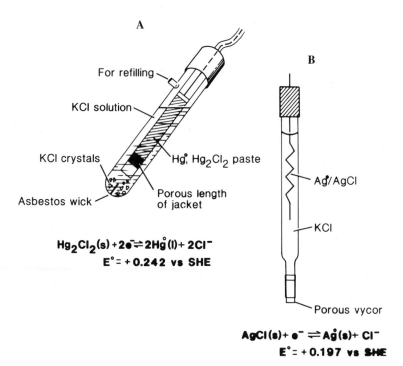

Fig. 10-5 Reference electrodes. **A,** saturated calomel electrode SCE, with asbestos wick for salt bridge junction. **B,** silver/silver chloride electrode, Ag/AgCl. (From Kaplan LA, Pesce AJ: Clinical chemistry: theory, analysis and correlation, ed 2, St Louis, 1989, Mosby-Year Book.)

lective electrode unit simply consists of a membrane separating a reference solution and reference electrode from a solution to be analyzed (Fig. 10-6). The complexity of ISE design is in the membrane formulation that determines its ionic selectivity. Several types of ion-selective indicator electrodes are described in the following section.

Glass Electrode. The glass electrode was the first and is still the most commonly used ion-selective electrode for measuring hydrogen ion activity. With certain types or compositions of

INTERNAL SOLUTION

$$M^+ X^-$$
$$\text{R} \rightleftharpoons \text{MR}^+ \quad E_{\text{memb (internal)}}$$

MEMBRANE

$$\text{R} \rightleftharpoons \text{MR}^+$$
$$M^+ X^- \quad E_{\text{memb (sample)}}$$

SAMPLE SOLUTION

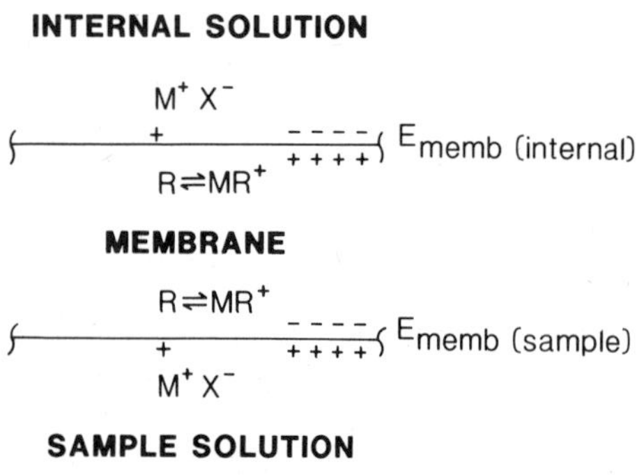

Fig. 10-6 Schematic illustration of liquid membrane ISE, where M+ represents analyte cation, and R represents neutral carrier ionophore.

glass, an electrical potential develops across a thin film of the glass when solutions of different hydrogen ion activities (concentrations) are on the opposite sides of the film. A glass electrode consists of a small bulb of special glass that contains a solution of known hydrogen ion concentration (e.g., 0.1N HCl) and an internal reference electrode, usually calomel or silver-silver chloride. The special composition of hydrated glass containing Na_2O, CaO, SiO_2, and perhaps small amounts of other ions makes the ion-exchange reaction of hydrogen at the surface of the glass possible. As a hydrogen ion combines with an oxygen ion within the lattice on the outer glass surface, a hydrogen ion leaves a binding site on the opposite surface. This combined activity on the glass surface maintains the electrical neutrality of the glass while establishing a hydrogen equilibrium and thus producing a potential. Because of the high resistance of the glass, electronic amplification is necessary for measurement of the potential.

When the glass measuring electrode and the calomel electrode (silver-silver chloride electrode) are immersed in a solution containing hydrogen ions, the small potential difference between these two half-cells is measured on a very sensitive voltmeter. When the instrument is calibrated against standards and adjusted for temperature effect, the activity of hydrogen ion (pH or negative log of the hydrogen ion activity) can be read very accurately. A very sophisticated, stable, and sensitive measuring device is required. This combination of parts is a pH meter. For convenience, both the glass measuring electrode and the reference electrode are sometimes built into a single glass housing and called a combination electrode. Combination electrodes are convenient to handle and can be used where a very small amount of fluid sample is available. No significant accuracy is lost.

The pH meter is designed to measure the effective concentration of hydrogen ions in a solution. In general, three parameters are involved in the effective concentration. The first of these is the actual molar concentration of hydrogen ions. The second is the dissociation constant of the acid, or the pKa. The third is the temperature.

Since the early twentieth century, various technicians have reported that a difference in electric potential could be measured between two solutions of different pH separated by a thin glass membrane. All the measuring devices available, however, had such a high internal resistance that the amplitude of the current produced could not be measured. Around 1930, an amplifier system was devised that allowed the pH meter, as it is now known, to be developed.

When a calomel reference electrode is used, the potential produced by hydrogen ions is quite constant, amounting to 59.15 mV/pH unit when measured at 25° C. As previously mentioned, temperature has considerable effect; each degree of temperature increase raises the cell's output by about 0.2 mV.

It is immediately apparent that there are a number of interfaces in this total pH-measuring system. The technician must assume that the potential at each of these interfaces is constant in all situations when making measurements.

If a difference in potential of 59.15 mV represents one pH unit, then a device that can measure a voltage change of 1.2 mV to indicate a change of 0.02 pH unit must be used. When the many variables, such as the phase junctions in the measuring system, the temperature effect on each of these, and variables in electrical components are considered, the technician becomes aware of how complicated this process is.

Resistance of this circuit is between 50,000 and 200,000,000 Ω. The tiny potential discussed is extremely hard to measure. For this reason a device similar to a vacuum tube voltmeter is used. Because of the high resistance of the electrode system, a circuit that will measure very high impedance is required.

When very alkaline solutions were tested with glass electrodes, it was found that pH measurements were strongly affected by the presence of sodium and other alkali metal ions. By changing the composition of the glass, this type of error could be minimized. At the same time it was found that glass electrodes could be developed that, under proper conditions, could actually measure sodium ion activity. When measuring very high pH values, some small sodium correction may be necessary. This correction is usually stated by the manufacturer.

Modern pH meters are, of course, quite different instruments. Electrode design has progressed to the point that nearly any type of configuration for any sort of use can be obtained. Very small, trouble-free combination electrodes are available for routine laboratory measurements in nearly any sort of container or condition.

Liquid Membrane Ion-Selective Electrode. Liquid membrane ion-selective electrodes have been developed that use liquid ion-exchange resins or neutral carrier electroactive substances (**ionophores**) that react selectively with specific ions. Fig. 10-6 illustrates a portion of a liquid ISE membrane. The membrane is composed of an ionophore, additives that enhance selectivity for a specific ion, and an appropriate water insoluble, nonvolatile organic solvent. The liquid electroactive substances are allowed to fill the pores of a porous membrane by capillary action or are bound by other forces, such as electrostatic action, in a membrane. The external (sample) and internal solutions then develop potentials on the surface of the electroactive substances in the membrane in much the same way that the glass membrane in a glass electrode does. The choice of ionophore is an important factor in determining the ionic selectivity of the electrode. Table 10-1 lists the composition of membrane, linearity characteristics, and possible interferences in clinical laboratory instruments. Neutral ion-carriers such as nonactin or valinomycin are used in ISEs for K^+ (Fig. 10-7), Ba^{++}, Na^+, Ca^{++}, and NH_4^+. Ca^{++}- and Mg^{++}-sensitive ISEs use phosphoric acid esters; NO_3^-, Cl^-, and other anion determinations are obtained with ISEs using membranes with electroactive substances of substituted arsonium, phosphonium, and ammonium salts.

Table 10-1 ISEs used in clinical chemistry

	Analyte	*Membrane composition*	*Linear response range (mol/L)*	*Possible interferences*
Glass	H^+	72.17% SiO_2, 6.44% CaO, 21.39% Na_2O (mol %)	$10^{-12} - 10^{-2}$	Na^+
	Na^+	11% Na_2O, 18% Al_2O_3, 71% SiO_2	$10^{-6} - 10^{-1}$	K^+, Ag^+
Solid state	F^-	LaF_3 crystal	10^{-6} — sat'd	OH^-
Liquid or polymer membrane	Na^+	Na^+ ionophore (ETH 227) 2-nitrophenylocytl ether, sodium tetraphenylborate	$10^{-3} - 10^{-1}$	Li^+, K^+, Ca^{2+}
	Cl^-	Tri-n-octylpropylammonium chloride, decanol	$10^{-3} - 10^{-1}$	OH^{-1}, Br^{-1}, F^-
	K^+	Valinomycin, dioctyladipate, PVC	$3 \times 10^{-5} - 1$	NH_4^+
	Ca^{2+}	Ca^{2+} ionophore (ETH 1001), 2-nitrophenyloctyl ether, sodium tetraphenylborate	$10^{-7} - 10^{-2}$	
	Ca^{2+}	Calcium di-(n-decyl)phosphate, di-(n-octylphenyl)-phosphate, PVC	$3 \times 10^{-5} - 1$	Mg^{2+}
	Li^+	Dodecyl methyl-14-crown-4 (ETH 1810)	$10^{-7} - 5 \times 10^{-2}$	Na^+
Gas sensors	CO_2	Combination glass pH electrode, 0.01-0.1 M $NaHCO_3$-NaCl filling solution behind silicone rubber membrane	$10^{-4} - 10^{-1}$	Organic acids
	NH_3	Combination glass pH electrode, 0.1 M NH_4Cl filling solution; behind porous Teflon gas-permeable membrane	$10^{-5} - 5 \times 10^{-2}$	Volatile amines

Modified from Meyerhoff ME, Opdycke WN: Ion-selective electrodes. In Spiegel HE, ed: Advances in clinical chemistry, vol 25, New York, 1986, Academic Press.

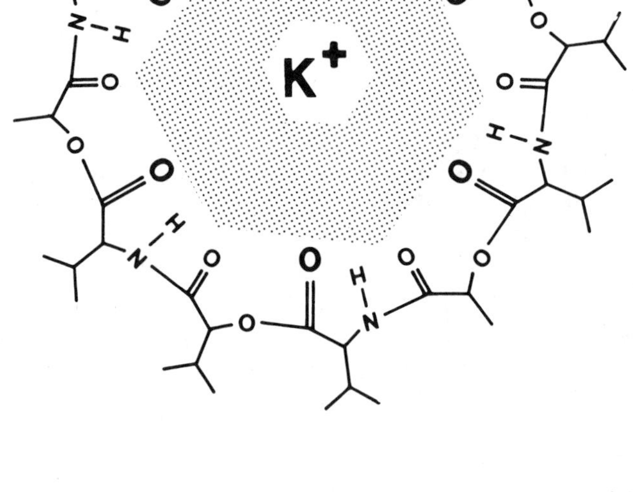

Fig. 10-7 Model of valinomycin with a hydrated K^+ in the cavity surrounded by oxygen atoms. (From Kaplan LA, Pesce AJ: Clinical chemistry: theory, analysis and correlation, ed 2, St. Louis, 1989, Mosby-Year Book.)

Precipitate-Impregnated Membrane Electrode. Once the ion-exchange mechanism of the glass electrode was established, electrochemists started to investigate ion-exchange membranes with the hope of devising an anion-sensitive electrode. In this type of electrode, a slightly soluble salt containing the anion to be measured is immobilized in a silicone rubber matrix. For example, an electrode that is to be chloride-sensitive would be constructed by forming a silicone rubber membrane that contains about 50% weight-to-weight silver chloride and silicone rubber. The silver chloride particles are generally about 5 to 10 μm in diameter and are in actual physical contact throughout the silicone rubber. Such an electrode functions because of the selective permeability of the membrane. This type of electrode can be used for measurement of anions such as chloride, bromide, and iodide.

Solid-State Electrode. The solid-state electrode is a second type of anion-sensitive electrode that functions on the same principle as the precipitate-impregnated electrode. The active membrane portion of the solid-state electrode consists of an inorganic single crystal doped with a rare earth. For example, the solid-state fluoride electrode has a crystalline lanthanum fluoride membrane that has been doped with europium (II) to lower its electrical resistance and facilitate ionic charge transport. This type of electrode has been commercially produced for Br^-, Cd^{++}, Cl^-, Cu^{++}, CN^-, F^-, I^-, Pb^{++}, Ag^+, S^{--}, Na^+, and SCN^- ion measurements.

A membrane produced by Beckman Instruments appears to be solid but is actually lipid-based in structure. The true solid membranes are crystallographic in structure, whereas the firm lipid structure is due to close spatial orientation of molecules. Lipids provide a medium in which electrostatic forces function. An ISE for K^+ consists of diphenyl ether, valinomycin, lecithin, and Nujol (mineral oil), and an NH_4^+ sensitive electrode is prepared with bromodiphyl, nonactin, lecithin, and Nujol.

Gas Electrode. In the oxygen-sensing amperometric electrode the anode and cathode are separated from the sample by a polyethylene gas-permeable membrane. A small applied potential between the anode and cathode causes an oxidation-reduction reaction with the oxygen diffusing through the membrane. A current is generated proportionately to the partial pressure of oxygen in the sample. Because oxygen diffuses instantaneously, sensor response is fast.

A Pco_2-sensing electrode is a standard glass pH electroce that has been modified to measure the concentration of carbon dioxide in aqueous solution. The electrode is placed in contact with the solution being analyzed for carbon dioxide content. Carbon dioxide can pass through a Teflon membrane because Teflon is highly permeable to the gas. After a few seconds the solution on the inside of the Teflon membrane is at equilibrium with the solution on the outside. The solution on the inside of the Teflon membrane contains sodium bicarbonate. Thus the carbon dioxide concentration has a large effect on the concentration of hydrogen ions in solution. Hydrogen ions can easily permeate a cellophane membrane that separates the reaction chamber from the glass electrode. The hydrogen ions are then detected by the glass electrode. In this way, the carbon dioxide concentration affects the pH and the pH can then be measured directly.

The technique of measuring pH has been previously discussed. Measuring Pco_2 is accomplished in the same manner, but the details of the electrode require some explanation (Fig. 10-8).

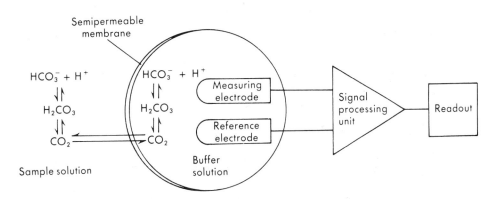

Fig. 10-8 Principle of Pco_2 electrode system.

The blood sample is separated from a combination pH electrode system by a membrane. Carbon dioxide can pass through this membrane from the blood sample into an electrolyte solution that perfuses the sensing tip of the electrode. As the carbon dioxide is absorbed by the electrolyte, carbonic acid is formed, altering the pH. This pH change is a linear function of the carbon dioxide content of the blood, and it can obviously be measured by the electronics of the pH meter on an appropriate scale. This arrangement may be called a Severinghous electrode (Fig. 10-9). The electrolyte solution perfusing its tip makes contact with both measuring and reference electrode elements. The carbon dioxide electrode in various systems may differ in physical arrangement from the electrode illustration in Fig. 10-9 but will function in the same way.

Enzyme Electrode. Enzyme electrodes have been developed to extend the application of ISEs to the measurement of nonionic compounds. In enzyme ISEs, an intermediary reaction is used to generate ions that can be directly related to the concentration of the compounds of interest. Enzymes are perfectly suited to catalyze the production of ions from a compound such as glucose or urea. Enzyme electrodes have been used specifically for glucose and blood urea nitrogen (BUN) analysis; therefore these two applications are described.

In general, an enzyme electrode is made by polymerizing a gelatinous membrane of immobilized enzyme directly over an ISE. A glucose-specific enzyme electrode (Fig. 10-10) is made by polymerizing a gelatinous membrane of immobilized glucose oxidase over a polarographic oxygen electrode. When the enzyme electrode is in contact with a glucose-containing solution, the glucose and oxygen diffuse into the immobilized glucose oxidase layer. Oxygen diffuses through a plastic membrane to the oxygen electrode where it is detected. The polarographic electrode is used to measure the oxygen consumed when glucose oxidase reacts with glucose in the sample solution. Therefore the decrease in the amount of oxygen detected by the oxygen electrode is related to an increase in the amount of glucose present. This type of electrode can also be used to detect the rate of reduction of oxygen rather than the absolute reduction and to relate it to glucose concentration.

In another approach to glucose analysis, glucose oxidase acting on the glucose produces hydrogen peroxide, which is measured by a polarographic electrode. It is the level of peroxide production, rather than the reaction rate, that is proportional to glucose concentration.

An enzyme electrode can also be used for the determination of urea. The electrode consists of a membrane containing immobilized urease over a NH_4^+-selective glass electrode. The urea in the sample diffuses into the enzyme-containing membrane where it is hydrolyzed to NH_4^+. NH_4^+ is measured by the glass electrode and is related directly to urea concentration.

Microelectrodes. Efforts are being directed to miniaturize electrodes to accommodate measurements with small amounts of solution. A creative design for a microelectrode is the combi-

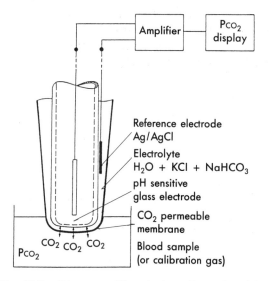

Fig. 10-9   Diagram of Severinghaus P_{CO_2} electrode. (Courtesy Instrumentation Laboratory, Inc.)

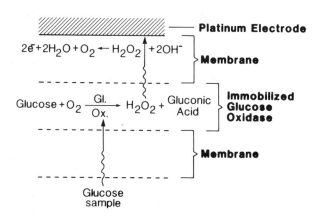

Fig. 10-10   Schematic diagram of glucose electrode. (From Kaplan LA, Pesce AJ: Clinical chemistry: theory, analysis and correlation, ed 2, St Louis, 1989, Mosby-Year Book.)

nation of ISEs with transistors. In one approach an ion-selective membrane is placed over the gate of a metal oxide-semiconductor field effect transistor (MOSFET). Such a microelectrode has been constructed with a MOSFET using a K^+-selective membrane. When the electrode is in contact with the test solution, K^+ activity at the gate results in a current drain that can be monitored and related directly to K^+ concentration. Initially, poor stability of the measured signal limited the use of this microelectrode, but the advantages of small size and direct electronic handling of the signal are incentive enough to rectify this problem. Microelectrodes are becoming more popular with improved designs that give the performance required for quantitative analysis.

Polarographic Measurement

Measurement of the **current** flowing through an electrochemical cell and the electric potential between the two electrodes while a constant external voltage is being applied is called **polarography.** Polarographic apparatus is widely used in analytic chemistry but has seldom been employed in clinical laboratory methods until recently. Measurement of the partial pressure of oxygen (Po_2) requires a different approach. The Po_2 electrode works on a polarographic principle.

The fact that nearly all conductors are metallic or electrolytic in nature was mentioned earlier. When electricity passes from a metal to a solution of electrolyte or vice versa, the type of carrier changes abruptly and either an oxidation or a reduction takes place. In the case of oxygen in solution, oxygen is reduced with the release of electrons and the current increases as a direct function of the electrons released. Hence the change in current is an analog of the oxygen concentration in the solution.

The Po_2 electrode consists of a platinum cathode surrounded by a tubular silver anode. The two electrodes are insulated from each other and make contact only through a drop of electrolyte at the electrode tip. A gas-permeable membrane holds this drop at the tip of the electrode and separates it from the blood to be measured. Oxygen in the blood diffuses across the membrane into the electrolyte where it is reduced and measured (Fig. 10-11).

The very tiny change in current sensed by the Po_2 electrode is amplified and measured by a sensitive electrometer against a reference current provided by a reference cell or Zener source. The pH meter's ammeter can be used for actually reading this signal on an appropriate scale. A polarographic electrode, often referred to as the Clark electrode, is the usual means of measuring Po_2 in the systems described here. A cutaway view of a Po_2 electrode is shown in Fig. 10-12.

Anodic Stripping Voltametry

The anodic stripping voltametric technique consists of the analyte preconcentration on the electrode followed by stripping from the electrode. A negative potential (plating voltage) is applied for a fixed period, usually 30 seconds to 30 minutes, to plate the electroactive metal ions onto the mercury electrode (Fig. 10-13, *A*). Only a fraction of the analyte is deposited on the mercury electrode during the fixed time of electroplating. Complete electroplating is time-consuming and unnecessary because the amount deposited on the mercury electrode is directly proportional to the concentration of the analyte. This preconcentration step makes it possible to measure analytes as low as $10^{-10}M$ using this technique.

After plating, the deposited metal ions are re-

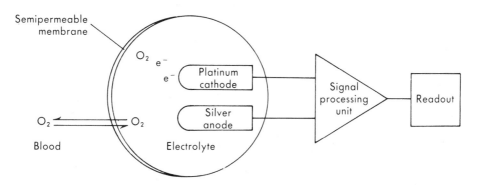

Fig. 10-11 Principle of Po_2 electrode system.

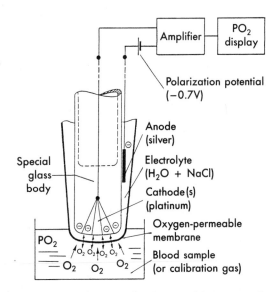

Fig. 10-12   Diagram of polarographic oxygen electrode used by Instrumentation Laboratory in its blood gas system. (Courtesy Instrumentation Laboratory, Inc.)

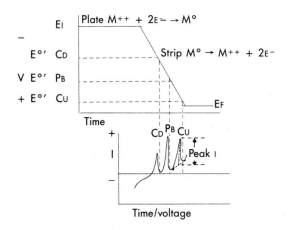

Fig. 10-13   Basic sequence of events in anodic stripping voltametry. (Courtesy ESA, Inc.)

moved from the electrode by application of increasingly positive potential. As each ion returns to solution, a sharp current peak occurs at a potential level that is characteristic for each metal. Fig. 10-13, *B* shows the current peak generated for some metals. The peak height or area is directly proportional to the analyte's concentration. By assaying standards and unknowns under identical conditions, the unknown can be identified and quantitated by peak height or area comparison.

The anodic stripping voltametric technique is used in the clinical laboratory for the quantitation of heavy metals, which include lead, copper, and chromium in blood and urine specimens. These metals can be freed from association with other biologic components of blood and urine by various digestion reagents (e.g., metexchange [marketed by Environmental Science Associates], which frees lead [Pb^{++}] for measurement).

Thermal Conductivity Measurement

Thermal conductivity detection is used for analysis of carbon dioxide in an instrument that is designated Model E 100 (Ericsen Instruments). This ingenious instrument is designed to detect only carbon dioxide by using an analytic principle. When an electric current is passed through a resistance wire, some electrical energy is lost as heat energy and thus the temperature of the wire

increases. As the wire gets hotter, resistance, in turn, increases. The heat produced is radiated into the air or surrounding gas and dissipates at a rate determined by the composition of the gas. Thus heat would dissipate more quickly in carbon dioxide than in helium. As the heat dissipates, the temperature and hence the resistance of the wire decreases. A thermal conductivity (TC) detector is a measuring device set up to sense the resistance change that occurs when the gas surrounding the resistance element changes. In most configurations the sensor is one arm of a Wheatstone bridge, which is a configuration of four resistors set up to accurately measure resistance.

In the carbon dioxide analyzer, carbon dioxide is displaced from the serum sample using lactic acid. The released gas is then forced from the reaction chamber by fluid displacement into the sensing chamber. Here the displaced carbon dioxide serves to change the relative percentage of carbon dioxide in room air, and this is sensed by the thermal conductivity detector.

The instrument is semiautomated. A 100 μl sample is required, and the test cycle requires less than a minute. The sample is injected into the reaction chamber and the cover closed. The start button is depressed, initiating a mixing sequence. Reagent fills the chamber, forcing the carbon dioxide into the TC detector. The electronic circuit converts the sensed change in resistance to mmole/L, and the result is displayed. Recycling the instrument flushes the sample and prepares the instrument for a new sample.

Amperometric and Coulometric Measurements

Amperometry deals with measurement of current at a single applied potential, whereas coulometry is concerned with measurement of charge. These techniques will be illustrated here by the coulometric method because their chemical basis is similar.

Several chloride titrators have been produced that work on the principle of **coulometry**. If a carefully controlled current is passed between two silver electrodes in an ionic solution, silver ions will be released by ionization at one electrode. If chloride ions are in the solution, these will combine with the released silver ions to produce insoluble silver chloride:

Anode electrode: $Ag \rightarrow Ag^+ + e^+$

Solution reaction: $Ag^+ + Cl^- \rightarrow AgCl$ (solid)

The chloride titrator makes use of this principle. A silver-detecting electrode and reference half-cell are included in the system to sense the excess of free silver ions when the chloride is used up. When silver is detected, the current to the silver-releasing electrode is discontinued. If the amperage of the ionizing current and the time it was flowing are known, the coulombs that passed can be calculated. Faraday's law states that the ionization produced when an electric current is passed from a metal into an electrolyte depends only on the coulombs passing through the current:

$$Q = It = znF$$

where Q is the charge passed for a finite time (t) at a constant current (I), z is the number of electrons involved in the electrochemical reaction, F is Faraday's constant, and n is the number of moles of analyte in the sample. Hence the ions of silver released by ionization, which will exactly equal the ions of chloride that were present in the solution, can be calculated.

In the clinical chemistry laboratory, a constant current coulometric assay is used for the determination of serum chloride in a fixed volume of sample. In this approach, the concentration of the unknown is calculated from the titration times for the blank (T_{blk}), standard (T_{std}), and unknown (T_{unk}) following the equation:

$[Cl^-]_{unk}$ mmol/L =
$$(T_{unk} - T_{blk})/(T_{std} - T_{blk}) \times [std] \text{ mmol/L}$$

The constant current coulometric method is needed for the determination of serum chloride in a fixed volume of serum. In this approach the concentration of the unknown is calculated from the titration times for the blank, standard, and unknown following the equation:

unknown $[Cl^-]$, mmol/L =
$$\frac{(T_{unknown} - T_{blank})}{(T_{unknown} - T_{blank})} \times (std) \text{ mmol/L}$$

Characteristics of Electrochemical Analyzers

During the 1980s, clinical chemistry laboratories experienced a rapid change of instrumentation from flame photometric and colorimetric to electrochemical-based analyzers. A search for safer, accurate, more precise, and less cumbersome ways of quantitation are among the factors that aided the rapid conversion to the electrochemical systems. Analytes such as sodium, potassium, and lithium had routinely been quantitated using the flame photometer, which is labor intensive, technologist dependent, cumbersome, and dangerous. These problems prompted many instrument manufacturers toward the use of electrochemistry. These manufacturers have sought methods of combining clinically relevant analytes that are measurable by electrochemical techniques with the formation of automated multichannel analyzers. Table 10-2 lists some characteristics of the major instruments that use electrochemical methods. These are usually multichannel systems for electrolytes or electrolytes and blood gases with or without other chemistries. Table 10-3 focuses on technical factors that have been documented to cause errors in ISE measurements. Strict adherence to the manufacturer's operation and maintenance protocol is intended to eliminate some of these factors. The analytic difference between direct ISE and flame atomic emission spectroscopy (i.e., indirect ISE) is usually handled through software manipulation in the measurement system.

Because these systems are very similar technically, the AVL 985-S Electrolyte Analyzer is presented here to fully illustrate the features of an electrochemical analyzer designed for patient care.

AVL 985-S. The AVL 985-S is a fully automatic, desktop microanalyzer with three channels for measuring sodium, potassium, and lithium by direct ion selective electrode technology (Fig. 10-14). The lithium electrode is a neutral carrier liquid membrane, and the potassium elec-

Table 10-2 Major chemistry systems that use electrochemical principles

Company	Product*	Analytes	Technology**
AMDEV/Baxter USA	Lytening	Na/K/Ca/Li/Cl	ISE
Ames USA	Seralyser	Na/K	ISE
AVL Switzerland, Austria, USA	98X-S and 99X-S	Na/K/Ca/Li Cl/TCO$_2$/pH Pco$_2$/Po$_2$	ISE
Beckman Instruments USA	Lablyte, E, and Synchron	Na/K/Ca/Li/CO$_2$/ pH/Cl	ISE
CIBA Corning USA	600 and 900 series	Na/K/Ca/Li/CO$_2$/ pH/Cl	ISE Coulometry and conductivity
DR LANGE Germany	LEA	Na/K/Cl	ISE
DuPont USA	Dimension and lyte systems	Na/K/Ca/Li/Cl	ISE
LESCHWEILER & COMPANY W. Germany	S2000 and ECO 2000	Na/K/Ca/pH Pco$_2$/Po$_2$	ISE
FRESENIUS AG FR Germany	Ionometer	Na/K/Ca/pH	ISE
HORIBA Japan	Sera-200 Series	Na/K/Ca/pH/Cl	ISE
INSTRUMENTATION LABORATORIES USA	BGE	Na/K/Ca/pH Pco$_2$/Po$_2$	ISE
IONETICS USA	Ionetics	Na/K/Ca/pH	ISE
KODAK USA	Ektachem	Na/K/Cl/CO$_2$, other chemistries	Dry chemistry
KONE Finland	Microlyte	Na/K/Ca/Li Cl/pH	ISE
MALLINCKODT USA		Na/K/Ca/pH/ Pco$_2$/Po$_2$	ISE
MEDICA USA	Easylyte	Na/K/Cl	ISE
NOVA BIOMEDICA USA	1-13	Na/K/Ca/pH Cl/ Li/Tco$_2$ Pco$_2$ Po$_2$	ISE
Pharmacia-ENI USA	Starlyte II	Na/K	ISE
RADIOMETER USA	KNA/ICA CMT 10	Na/K/Ca/pH/Cl Pco$_2$/Po$_2$	ISE and coulometry
Roche Diagnostics USA	Cobas	Na/K/Cl	ISE

*Each manufacturer has several models with different combinations of analytes.
**Sample volume ranges from 10 μL to several hundred microliters.

trode is composed of a valinomycin liquid membrane. A Na$^+$-sensitive glass electrode is used for sodium measurement. The three electrolyte electrodes are referenced to an open liquid junction flow-through calomel electrode and connected to a high input impedance voltmeter. In this flow-through arrangement, potentials generated at the different electrodes are used to calculate the relative ionic concentration of each analyte.

The throughput of the analyzer ranges from 45 samples/hour in the single measurement mode to 60 samples/hour in the automatic measurement mode. Sample types include whole blood, plasma, serum, urine, and aqueous fluids. Sodium heparin is the preferred anticoagulant for whole blood and plasma samples. At a concentration of 50 IU/mL, the amount of sodium in the anticoagulant is minimal and will not significantly alter the sodium result. For urine samples the recommended preservative is boric acid. Sulfuric acid and other organic preservatives should not be used because they interfere with the sodium and potassium electrodes. A predilution with AVL urine diluent is required for determination of urine sodium and potassium. This urine predilution step is characteristic of most ISE analyzers and serves to fix the ionic strength of the urine sample at a narrow window.

Table 10-3 General technical considerations in the use of potentiometric systems

Cause of error	Explanation
Temperature	Determination of electrode potential according to the Nerst equation is temperature dependent. Thus maintenance of a fixed and constant temperature is required in potentiometric measurement.
Interferent ions	High selectivity of an electrode for a specific ion is usually attained by modification of the ionophore and addition of various additives that reduce the electrode's selectivity for other ions. In some situations it is essential to concurrently measure the concentration of the interferent ion and correct for its effect.
Protein and miscellaneous coat on electrode	Miscellaneous components in biologic fluids change the sensitivity and selectivity by binding to an electrode surface. This problem is usually limited or eliminated by scheduled electrode cleaning (or deproteinizing) and conditioning steps recommended by manufacturers.
Loss of CO_2 and change in pH	Some ions (e.g., ionized calcium) are particularly sensitive to pH changes because of competitive binding to proteins and other complex molecules. This problem indicates a preanalytic factor that must be taken into consideration in the interpretation of results.
Ionic strength	The first equation in the chapter shows that activity coefficient (γ) of an ion depends on the ionic strength of the solution. Thus extreme changes in ionic strength (e.g., severe hyper- or hyponatremia) can affect the potentiometric measurement.
Direct vs indirect potentiometry	Direct (undiluted) measurement by ISE is concerned with ion activity in only the fluid compartment of the sample. Thus increasing the protein and/or lipid concentration introduces methodologic differences between direct ISE and indirect (diluted) ISE or the flame atomic emission spectroscopy.

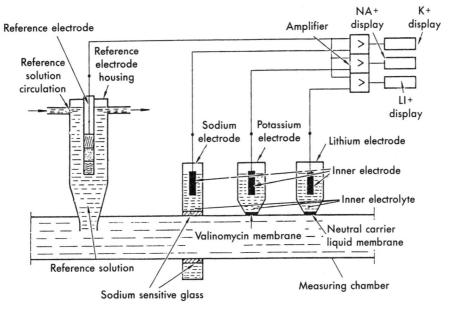

Fig. 10-14 Schematic diagram of AVL 985-S measurement system. (Courtesy AVL Scientific, Inc.)

Future Developments

Clinically acceptable ion-selective electrodes have been successfully developed for physiologically important alkali and alkaline earth cations (e.g., K^+, Na^+, Ca^{++}, Li^+, and H^+). The only relevant cation for which ISE is yet to be introduced in the clinical laboratory is magnesium. It is anticipated that the substantial efforts by various manufacturers will result in the introduction of a Mg^{++} ISE system in the mid-1990s.

To date, this technology has not been readily applied to anions because of the problems of developing ionophore-like species and electrodes with unique selectivity interactions. The inorganic anions of main interest include Cl^-, sulfate, and phosphate. Significant effort is currently in progress to improve the analytic performance of the anion selective membrane to meet clinical requirements.

Review Questions

1. _____ is an electrochemical technique that involves measurement of the current produced by chemical oxidation or reduction of an ionic species.
   A. Amperometry/coulometry
   B. Voltametry
   C. Polarography
   D. Amperometry
   E. Potentiometry

2. The measurement of hydrogen ion concentration or pH is based on the following principle:
   A. Computation from potential generated after hydrogen ions pass through a glass H^+ selective membrane
   B. Coulometric technique
   C. Amperometric technique
   D. Computation from current generated in a potentiometric assay
   E. None of the above

3. Given the following data, calculate the serum chloride concentration in mmol/L:
   Titration current: 5.9×10^{-3} amp
   Blank titration time: 16 seconds
   Titration time for a 100 mmol/L standard: 124 seconds
   Titration time for the serum sample: 128 seconds
   Serum sample volume and volume of standard titrated are 0.10 ml respectively
   A. 97 mmol/L
   B. 104 mmol/L
   C. 116 mmol/L
   D. 120 mmol/L
   E. 90 mmol/L

4. The electrode for CO_2 determination works by:
   A. Measuring a potentiometric change
   B. Measuring a change in pH
   C. Using an enzyme coupled reaction
   D. A and B
   E. Some other combination

Answers

1. A   2. A   3. B   4. D

Bibliography

Bates RG, Robinson RA: An approach to conventional scales of ionic activity for standardization of ion-selective electrodes, Pure Appl Chem 37:575, 1973.

Guilbault GG: Analytical uses of immobilized enzymes, Biotechnol Bioeng 3:361, 1972.

Heyrovsky J, Kuta J: Principles of polarography, Prague, 1965, Publishing House of Czechoslovak Academy of Science.

Lunte CE, Heineman WR: Electrochemical techniques in bioanalysis, Top Curr Chem 143:1, 1988.

Oesch U, Ammann D, and Simon W: Ion-selective membrane electrodes for clinical use, Clin Chem 32:144, 1986.

Okorodudu AO, Burnett RW, and Bowers GN: Evaluation of three first generation lithium ISE analyzers. Analytical specifications based on comparative performance, systematic errors, and frequency of random interferences, Clin Chem 36:104, 1990.

Siggaard-Andersen O: The acid-base status of the blood, ed 4, Baltimore, 1974, Williams & Wilkins.

CHAPTER 11

Electrophoresis and Densitometry

JOHN M. BREWER

Theory
Experimental
Equipment
Practice
Densitometry
Analysis and Interpretation

Electrophoresis is the separation of charged particles (compounds) based on their electrical charge. In the clinical laboratory, these compounds are usually proteins or polynucleic acids derived from blood and other biologic fluids or tissues. **Densitometry** is a procedure for quantitating and recording the pattern (**electrophoretogram**) of these separated compounds. The pattern generated from a patient sample can be compared with that from a healthy individual and thus can aid in the patient's diagnosis.

Theory

Electrical systems. In any electrical circuit the current (flow of electrons) through the circuit increases with the applied voltage. The amount of current at a given voltage is also determined by the resistance of the circuit.

Voltage = resistance × current

Specific features of electrophoresis. An electrophoretic apparatus consists of circuit that is basically water with dissolved salts. The current in this system is a flow of ions rather than electrons. Also, instead of referring to resistance, **conductivity** is more commonly expressed. In mathematic terms the conductivity of a solution is the reciprocal of its electrical resistance. Conductivity refers to the movement of charged substances (ions) rather than resistance to a solution.

When salts, such as sodium chloride, are dissolved in water, they form ions. In the case of sodium chloride these are sodium ions, each having a single positive charge, and chloride ions, each having a single negative charge. In water, these ions (and all ions) are hydrated: each ion has a cluster of water molecules, perhaps six or so, surrounding it. If a voltage is applied to the solution, the sodium and chloride ions and their clusters of water molecules will move in opposite directions (Fig. 11-1).

A voltage is applied to a solution by placing electrodes in the solution. The electrodes are connected to a source of voltage like a battery. One of the electrodes (**anode**) will be positive relative to the other (i.e., attract negatively charged ions [**anions**]), whereas the other electrode (**cathode**) will be relatively negative (i.e., attractive positively charged ions [**cations**]). The electrodes in an electrophoretic apparatus are usually made of platinum because it is a good conductor and yet is chemically inert.

Ion Movement and Conductivity. The current in an electrophoretic system consists of two flows of ions: cations toward the cathode and anions toward the anode. The number of positive and negative charges must always be equal. The conductivity of a solution is due to all the ions in the solution. The higher the ionic concentration the greater the conductivity. The conductivity increases with the ionic concentration. Some ions have more than one charge (e.g., sulfate anion has two). A mole of sulfate carries twice the charge of that of a mole of chloride. Therefore it has twice the ionic strength.

Ions with the same charge can move through water at different rates. They may be larger or more heavily hydrated and therefore carry more molecules of water. These slower ions have lower **mobilities** (i.e., they do not move as fast as other ions under a set of standard conditions, such as the same charge/concentration). The conductivity of a solution is mathematically expressed as the product of each ion's charge, its concentration, and its mobility. The sum of the products of all ions in the solution is equal to the total conductivity of the solution.

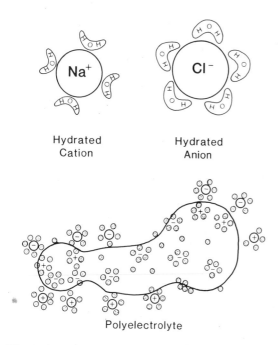

Hydrated
Cation

Hydrated
Anion

Polyelectrolyte

Fig. 11-1 Application of an electric field to a solution of ions makes the ions move. The flow of ions in both directions constitutes the current in the solution part of the electrical circuit. At the electrodes, electrons and ions are combined with and separated from each other in a process called "electrolysis" (From Kaplan LA, Pesce AJ, eds: Clinical chemistry: theory, analysis, and correlation, ed 2, St Louis, 1989, Mosby–Year Book.)

The charge of an ion depends on the pH of the solution. For example, a solution of acetate adjusted to pH 4.76 will have half the molecules protonated (to form acetic acid). Because the concentration of acetate has been reduced to one half its original value, its average charge is minus one half. It is important to understand that the fractional charges of ionic molecules are averages. At a more acid pH the fractional charge on acetate will be lower; at a more alkaline pH it will be greater. Thus the **effective mobility** of an ion can vary with pH and is related to the unit charge times the fractional (average) charge.

Macro-ions. Certain types of large ions, or macro-ions, are important clinically. Their concentrations, relative to concentrations of other macro-ions, can help in diagnosis of diseases. Biologic compounds such as proteins and polynucleic acids (DNA or RNA) are considered macroions because they are much larger than "ordinary" ions such as sulfate or chloride. Their vast size means that their mobilities are usually lower than those of small ions. As they try to move through the solution, the viscous drag on these huge ions is much greater. The viscous or frictional drag on macro-ions depends on their shape and molecular weight. A rodlike macro-ion moving sideways has more resistance than a more compact macro-ion with the same molecular weight. The frictional resistance of a macro-ion is designated by a single number called its **frictional coefficient.**

Macro-ions such as polynucleic acids/nucleotides may have many charges. At physiologic pH values (near pH 7.0) each nucleotide will contribute one negative charge; a polynucleotide, however, consisting of 20,000 nucleotides, will have a charge of $-20,000$.

Macro-ions such as proteins are more complicated in this respect because they are polymers of amino acids, some of which can be anions (like glutamate or aspartate), and some of which can be cations (like lysine, arginine, and histidine). Whether the protein will be cationic or anionic will depend on the pH, and to some extent how it is folded. However, at some pH the protein will have a net charge of zero: the average number of positive charges will equal the average number of negative charges. At this pH value the protein is **isoelectric,** and this pH is known as the protein's **isoelectric point.** Ionic compounds, like proteins whose sign of charge changes with the pH, are called **amphoteric** compounds.

The overall or net charges of different proteins will be different at a particular pH. This is because different proteins have different amino acid compositions and folding. If a mixture of proteins is placed in a solution at a pH and a voltage is applied to the solution, proteins with a net positive charge will move toward the cathode, proteins with a net negative charge will move toward the anode, and any proteins with a zero net charge will not move. At a different pH, a different group of these proteins may move toward a given electrode. Consequently, the pH at which an electrophoretic separation is carried out is important. By changing the net charge on proteins, it changes the velocities and even the directions in which they move. Therefore electrophoretic solutions are always buffered to maintain the pH.

Suppose, however, the electrophoresis is set up with a strong acid surrounding one electrode and a strong base surrounding the other (Fig. 11-2). This can be done by passing a current through the water: at the anode, oxygen is generated, leaving hydrogen ions about the electrode; at the cathode, hydrogen is produced, leaving hydroxyl ions in excess. The result is a pH gradient. If a mixture

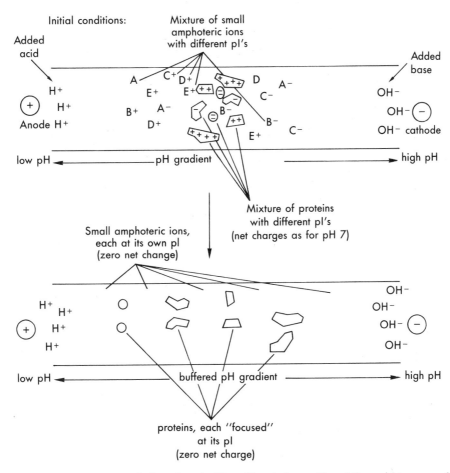

Fig. 11-2 Representation of isoelectric focusing. A pH gradient is formed by adding acid to one end of the electrophoresis channel and base to the other. In between is placed a mixture of small "amphoteric" ions. These are represented by letters; their net charge varies, depending on their position in the pH gradient. A mixture of proteins with assorted net charges is placed in the middle. A voltage is applied, with the anode at the acid end and the cathode at the basic end. The proteins and small ions move in the pH gradient according to their net charges. When they reach a pH that equals their pI, they have zero net charge and stop. The small amphoteric ions are synthesized to provide good buffering and conductivity at their pI.

of proteins with different isoelectric points is placed in the middle of the pH gradient, they would migrate to their respective isoelectric points and stop because their net charges would be zero. When substances called ampholytes are added to buffer the pH gradient, proteins will collect or focus into narrower bands. When the proteins and buffer ions stop moving, the conductivity of the solution drops to a minimum value. This technique is called **isoelectric focusing** and is discussed in more detail later in this chapter.

Fundamental Concepts Pertaining to Electrophoresis. The greater the net charge of a protein the more it is attracted toward the oppositely charged electrode and therefore the more rapidly it moves through the solution. As it moves faster,

it experiences a greater frictional drag because it must push more water molecules and small ions out of the way/unit of time. A fundamental concept of electrophoresis is that the velocity at which an ion moves depends on its net charge and the applied voltage. The greater the frictional resistance the ion encounters the lower the velocity. The "effective mobility" equals velocity of ion divided by the applied voltage, which is proportional to the charge of the ion divided by frictional coefficient of the ion (this is true of any ionic substance):

$$\text{Effective mobility} = \frac{\text{Velocity of ion}}{\text{Applied voltage}} \propto \frac{\text{Charge of ion}}{\text{Frictional coefficient of ion}}$$

Experimental

Resolution Enhancement. With electrophoresis the more the substances are separated the better. However, after they have become separated, they tend to diffuse. Over time, separated zones or bands blur and run back together. This is a major drawback of any separation procedure. There are several ways to improve separation.

Decreased Analysis Time. Performing electrophoresis in less time is easy to do; however, it can pose a major problem because of electrical heating. Applying voltage to an electrophoretic system produces a current, and passage of a current produces heat. This is called **Joule heating** and is the primary limiting factor in any electrophoretic separation. Excess heat can produce movement of solvent **(convection)**, distort flow patterns, denature macromolecules, and even melt some supporting media.

Heat production increases during electrophoresis as power or wattage is consumed and does so as a function of the current squared (I^2). The conductivity of the electrophoretic solution is also a factor. With a set voltage a greater conductivity increases the current. Because the speed of electrophoretic movement depends on the voltage applied to the solution, it is best to keep the voltage as high as possible. This means that the conductivity of the separating solution must be kept low.

The substances that are often electrophoresed are macro-ions. These charged substances will attract or repel each other depending on their charges (i.e., they will interact with each other), which is usually not desirable. The movement of each type of ion to be separated should be as independent of the others as possible. Thus, salts **(electrolyte)** are added, usually of low molecular weight, to the electrophoresis solution.

Electrolytes also carry the current (the movement of ions throughout the solution) whether or not macro-ions are present. To maximize the velocity of electrophoresis and minimize the heat produced during the analytic run, the concentration of electrolyte ions is kept to moderate values (0.05 to 0.1 M). To perform the analysis even faster, the supporting medium must be cooled. Some electrophoresis apparatuses are built so that cold water can be circulated through the apparatus; at least one uses solid state ("Peltier") cooling. Even with air cooling only, the heat dissipation is more efficient so that electrophoresis can be done in less time.

Restriction of Diffusion by Supporting Media. A **supporting medium** is generally used in electrophoresis. This is primarily because the samples to be separated are almost always denser than the electrophoretic solvent (they weigh more than an equal volume of the solvent). The samples and separated compounds would fall through the solvent and thus remix during the process. This process is called **convection** or **bulk flow.**

The supporting medium often prevents convection by supplying a matrix of fibers or polymer chains or grains that restricts the area of convection where the material is separated. (A capillary tube has the same effect. Electrophoresis can be done in capillary tubes without any supporting medium.) If the network of fibers or polymer chains is tight enough, it will offer more resistance to movement of bigger molecules. This effect is called **molecular sieving** (Fig. 11-3). It is often possible to prepare supporting media with effective pore sizes that are comparable with the effective diameters of the substances to be separated. This is especially true if they are macromolecules. Once the macromolecules are separated in the matrix, diffusion is restricted by the matrix as is electrophoretic movement.

Normally, the most important property a supporting medium must have is that it should not bind or adsorb the material being separated. Otherwise, bad tailing of zones constituting the sample's components occurs, causing overlap of separated zones.

For some applications, though, adsorption is required (i.e., such as occurs with **electroblotting**). Material that has been separated on a nonadsorbing supporting medium is electrophoresed sideways onto the adsorbent. This causes the separated material to adsorb so that separated materials cannot diffuse back together. It also concentrates the separated material in a thin layer so that it is easier to detect.

One of the major problems associated with the use of supporting media is **electro-osmosis.** This is a tendency for the solvent to move, relative to the fixed medium, when a voltage is applied. This varies from medium to medium. It is especially severe when the medium matrix is composed of charged groups. Even though the charged groups are fixed in place, ions of opposite charge are associated with them. These are small and mobile. When a voltage is applied, the small mobile ions move, carrying with them their water of hydration. This causes the solvent and any extraneous

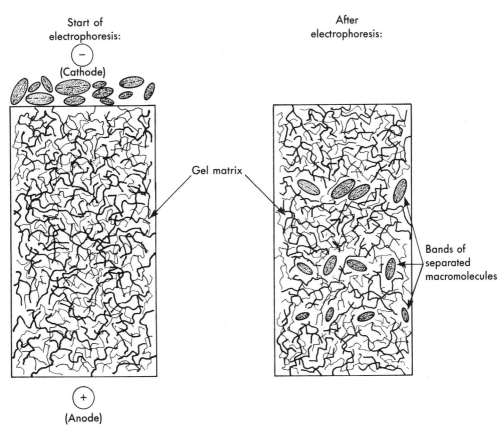

Fig. 11-3 The network or "lattice" of polymer chains in a gel can "sieve" molecules of different sizes. The network also reduces diffusion of separated molecules. If the molecules being separated have the same sign of charge and a magnitude of charge that increases with the molecular weight of the molecules, the distance they move in a given time can be used to estimate their molecular weight. This is done with proteins in SDS solutions and with DNA fragments.

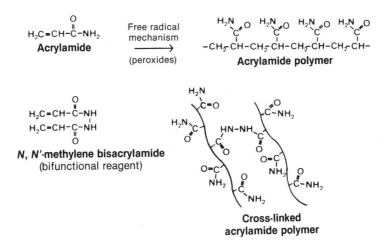

Fig. 11-4 Polyacrylamide gels are produced by polymerizing a mixture of acrylamide and a "bifunctional" (cross-linking) acrylamide derivative. The derivative shown is that in common use. The "Immobilines" have groups with pK's ranging from 3 to 9 attached to the acrylamide through the amide nitrogens. These are used in isoelectric focusing. (From Kaplan LA, Pesce AJ, eds: Clinical chemistry, theory, analysis, and correlation, ed 2, St Louis, 1989, Mosby–Year Book.)

material in the solvent, including macromolecules, to move. For example, agar consists of **agarose,** which has relatively few charged groups, and **agaropectin,** which has many. Agar gels have considerably greater electro-osmotic streaming of the solvent than do agarose gels.

Supporting media are selected for low electro-osmosis, ease and reproducibility of preparation, controllability, and suitability and homogeneity (internal consistency) of effective pore size. **Cellulose acetate,** agarose, and **polyacrylamide gels** (Fig. 11-4) are popular supporting media for clinical work.

Thinner Zones of Material. If the solution is applied in a thinner, narrow area before electrophoresis, the separated substances will form thin or narrow regions at the end of the electrophoresis thus producing a better separation (Fig. 11-5). It may be necessary to concentrate the sample(s), and apply smaller volumes. The effects of ion conductivity can be used to concentrate samples in an electrophoresis apparatus. This approach is used with isotachophoresis and disk electrophoresis.

One of two general techniques can be used to produce thinner zones of separated materials during electrophoresis. With isoelectric focusing, a shallower pH gradient and a high voltage improves separation. A shallower pH gradient requires a stronger buffering over a narrower pH range. The buffering is normally produced by "amphoteric" substances **(ampholytes).** These are separated by the manufacturer (by electrofocusing on a very large scale) and sold according to their pH range that is optimal for buffering.

These substances have been incorporated into components of a popular supporting medium, polyacrylamide gel (see Fig. 11-4). Chemically modified acrylamides can be polymerized with acrylamide. The chemically modified acrylamides have pHs that range from pH 3 to pH 9. When polymerized with ordinary acrylamide in specific amounts, the gel provides a very stable buffering system with a narrow pH range for isoelectric focusing. This can resolve proteins whose isoelectric points differ by 0.001 pH. These substituted acrylamides are called Immobilines and are sold by Pharmacia-LKB. Isolectric focusing using Immobilines is a good technique for separating abnormal hemoglobins.

The second approach is based on the fact that current in any electrophoretic channel must be constant throughout the channel. This means that the number of charges in both directions crossing any section of the channel must be the same at any given point in time. Suppose an electrophoretic channel is prepared with an ion of higher effective mobility at one end and an ion of the same sign of charge but a lower effective mobility at the other end (Fig. 11-6). Also suppose that the lower mobility ion follows the higher mobility ion to the electrode of opposite charge. If the conductivity of the solution containing the lower mobility ion is lower than the conductivity of the solution containing the higher mobility ion, diffusion will be eliminated where the two ions meet.

Because the current must be kept constant, the higher mobility ions cannot pull away from the lower mobility ions. That would create a gap, with no ions to carry the current. Therefore to keep up with the faster ion, the voltage driving the slower ion must be higher (see Fig. 11-6). If one of the slower ions diffuses into the faster ion solution, it finds itself driven by a lower voltage and therefore slows down. If a faster ion diffuses

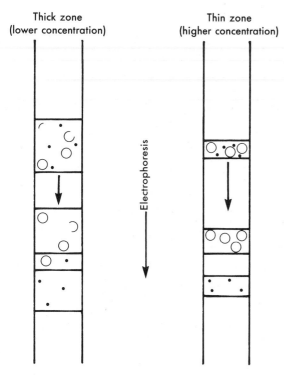

Fig. 11-5 Effect of starting zone size on resolution. A mixture of subtances shown by the open figures and the dots is electrophoresed for the same time on the same support under the same conditions. If the mixture is applied in a smaller spot ("thin zone") (i.e., as a more concentrated solution) the mixture is resolved. The mixture applied in the larger spot was not resolved, though each substance traveled the same distances as from the thin zone.

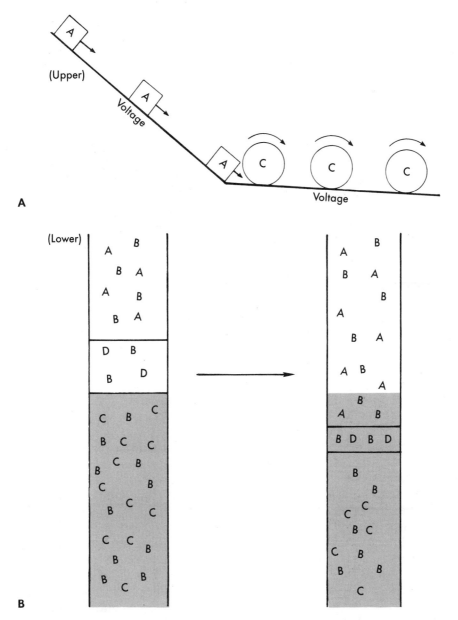

Fig. 11-6 **A,** Representation of the electrical basis of disk electrophoresis (stacking step) and isotachophoresis. A greater voltage is required to make ions of lower effective mobility (*A*'s in squares) keep up with ions of greater effective mobility (*C*'s in circles). The greater voltage is represented by the greater slope beneath the *A*'s. The *A* and *C* ions have the same sign of charge. **B,** Representation of the stacking step in disk electrophoresis and isotachophoresis. The *B* ions are of opposite sign of charge to the *A*, *C*, and *D* ions. Movement of the *A* and *D* ions into the region vacated by the *C* ion (stippled region) is accompanied by changes in ion concentration and pH. The latter is not shown. (From Kaplan LA, Pesce AJ, eds: Clinical chemistry: theory, analysis, and correlation ed 1, St Louis, 1989, Mosby–Year Book.)

back into the solution containing the slower ion, it experiences a higher voltage and thus is driven back into its own solution.

Now suppose another ion, with the same sign of charge and an effective mobility intermediate between the "leading" (highest effective mobility) ion and the "trailing" (lowest effective mobility) ion, is inserted between them. This new ion will remain sandwiched between the leading and trailing ions. In addition, diffusion where the intermediate ion and leading and trailing ions meet will be prevented for the reasons given previously.

If a mixture of ions, all with intermediate effective mobilities and the same sign of charge, were inserted between the leading and trailing ions, the same thing would happen. The intermediate ions would remain in the same zone between the leading and trailing ions. However, they would sort themselves into zones of decreasing effective mobility from front to back. Each type of ion with a unique effective mobility would form its own zone, so that these ions would be ranked or "stacked" in order of their effective mobilities, and diffusion between their zones would be prevented.

All these zones of ions must carry the same charge in the electrical circuit. If the intermediate ions are proteins, their stacked zones will probably become very thin (i.e., the proteins in these zones will become very concentrated). This is because most proteins have few charges for their size.

Most of the side chains of the amino acids found in proteins, such as alanine, glycine, valine, or serine have no charge. Furthermore, the major factor is the net charge of a protein. The effect of any negatively charged side chains of aspartate and glutamate is often neutralized by positively charged side chains of lysine, arginine, and histidine. Although a given protein at the pH of the electrophoresis may have a net charge of 10, its high molecular weight results in a low "charge to mass ratio."

Polynucleotides such as DNA and RNA have a much higher and a nearly uniform charge to mass ratio at physiologic pH values. Hence polynucleotides would not concentrate as much as proteins. A different electrophoretic separation system is used for polynucleotides.

The stacked proteins are pure and highly concentrated. If they are eluted or if their distribution is measured while stacked, the electrophoretic technique is called **isotachophoresis** (the name implies that everything is moving at the same speed). Because the stacked proteins lie next to each other, the electrophoretic system is usually set up to separate them. This is to elute them as separated zones or to analyze the pattern of separated protein zones.

If the effective mobility of the trailing ion is increased so that it is greater than the effective mobilities of the proteins, the trailing ion will move through the protein zones. These will no longer

have to move together. Each protein will migrate independently so the protein zones will tend to separate. Unfortunately, diffusion of each protein will also begin. However, because the zones were initially made so concentrated and therefore thin, the separated protein zones will still be relatively thin when the electrophoresis ends. The resolution of this technique, called **disk electrophoresis,** is greater than that of electrophoresis using a single solvent throughout the electrophoresis channel.

Effective mobilities of some ions can be changed by adjusting the pH so the average charge on the ions changes. The ion of opposite charge to the leading, trailing, and intermediate ions needs to be discussed. Such an ion must be present in a concentration equal to that of the leading, trailing, or intermediate ions to maintain "electrical neutrality." An ion of opposite charge is called a **counterion.** The effective mobility of the trailing ion can be increased by fixing the counterion concentration to an appropriate value (this can be calculated). In addition a counterion in conjunction with its "conjugate" form can serve as a buffer in the pH region that is being used. A counterion that has a conjugate form (uncharged) is used so that it does not interfere with the electrical arrangement of leading, intermediate, and trailing ions.

Examples of counterions and conjugate forms are the tris cation and tris base, or the acetate anion and acetic acid, respectively. Tris cation and tris base buffer best at pH 8.1 and acetate and acetic acid at pH 4.8. The most widely used disk electrophoretic system employs chloride as the leading ion. It is usually incorporated as a tris-chloride buffer at pH 8.9 in a polyacrylamide gel as supporting medium. The trailing ion is glycine, brought to pH 8.3 with tris. At pH 8.3, glycine has an average charge of $-\frac{1}{30}$ and thus has a very low effective mobility. The glycine solution follows the chloride as the chloride moves out of the polyacrylamide gel and subsequently encounters the uncharged tris base in the gel. The concentration of tris base is high, bringing the pH up to 9.5. The average charge on glycine at pH 9.5 is about $-\frac{1}{4}$. The glycine that moved into the more concentrated tris base solution has a greater effective mobility. It can then pass through most stacked proteins, enabling the proteins to unstack and move independently, although in thin zones.

Disk electrophoresis is usually performed with polyacrylamide gels, so the enhanced resolution provided by the stacking is combined with the re-

stricted diffusion provided by the gel. The "molecular sieving" effect of the gel can be used by itself to obtain information not only about purity of macromolecules but also about their molecular weights.

Specific Experimental Applications

Size Measurements of Proteins and Polynucleotides. Most proteins have relatively compact structures and low charge to mass ratios. If they are treated with the detergent **sodium dodecyl sulfate (SDS),** they bind about 1.4 times their own weight of the detergent and become rodlike masses with a high, uniform charge to mass ratio. The natural shape of polynucleotides is also rodlike, and when rodlike macro-ions are electrophoresed in a gel, the distance they move increases with decreasing molecular weight. In fact, molecular weights of polynucleotides and SDS-protein complexes can be estimated by how far they move relative to the position of polynucleotides or protein-SDS complexes of known molecular weight ("standards"). The resolution of electrophoresis on gels is also high enough to separate DNA fragments differing by one base (molecular weight about 330) over a total range of perhaps 300 to 500 bases. This is done when DNA pieces are sequenced.

Two-Dimensional Electrophoresis. The resolution provided by electrophoresis on a polyacrylamide gel can be increased by "two-dimensional electrophoresis." Usually, isoelectric focusing of proteins is done on a polyacrylamide gel shaped like a cylinder. This is then attached to one edge of a square, thin sheet of polyacrylamide and then electrophoresed into the sheet. If the second electrophoresis is done in the presence of SDS, separation is according to isoelectric point along one direction and according to molecular weight along the other. Over 1000 proteins can be separated in one experiment.

Immunoelectrophoresis. Sometimes diffusion of macro-ions through a supporting medium is useful. Immunoelectrophoresis techniques combine reactions between an antigen and an antibody with electrophoretic separation.

There are two groups of immunoelectrophoretic methods. The antigens may be separated by electrophoresis, usually in an agar or agarose gelatin, and then a trough is cut in the gel parallel to the direction of electrophoresis of the antigen. Antibody is added to the trough and diffuses into the agar or agarose gel. The antigens are also diffusing, and arcs of precipitate occur where relative antibody and antigen concentrations are at equivalence. The large pore size of agar and agarose gels enables relatively compact "globular" proteins to diffuse fairly readily.

Antigens and antibody can also be electrophoresed together to form "rockets." The antigens must have greater effective mobilities than the antibody. Antibodies are gamma globulins that have low effective mobilities at pH 8.6. Immunoelectrophoresis methods of this type are usually carried out in diethyl barbiturate buffers at pH 8.6. The size of the "rocket" is a measure of the antigen concentration. Precipitates between an antigen and an antibody do not diffuse because the molecular sizes of the complexes are far greater than the effective pore size of the gel.

Equipment

Electrophoresis equipment is sold by several companies. In clinical laboratories most of the equipment and consumable supplies are provided by Beckman, Helena Laboratories, and Ciba-Corning. In research laboratories Pharmacia-LKB, Bio-Rad, and Hoefer often supply reagents and equipment. There are many other firms, and most companies carry a complete line of equipment and supplies as well. Helena Laboratories, for example, offers power supplies, apparatuses for electrophoresis, reconstitutable buffers, and reagent mixtures for electrophoresis, staining and analysis, and densitometers, which are all offered separately or in an integrated package. Helena Laboratories also sells an automated electrophoresis apparatus, the REP system, which carries out the electrophoresis according to instructions programmed by the operator, stains the support medium for isozymes (isoenzymes), and scans the patterns (Fig. 11-7).

Power Supply. One of the components required for electrophoresis is a power supply that applies a voltage/current to the electrophoretic apparatus. Constant voltage, as direct current voltage, is generated to the electrophoretic apparatus via leads or cables, which are often connected to banana plugs. Some power supplies can also operate at constant current, or amperage (recommended for isotachophoresis), or constant power (recommended for isoelectric focusing). Some also allow the voltage to be applied for a preset time.

Types of Apparatus. Electrophoresis equipment is made of nonconducting materials such as glass, Lucite, or other plastic. Electrodes and electrode connections are often marked "+" and "−." They are usually at two ends or sides of the

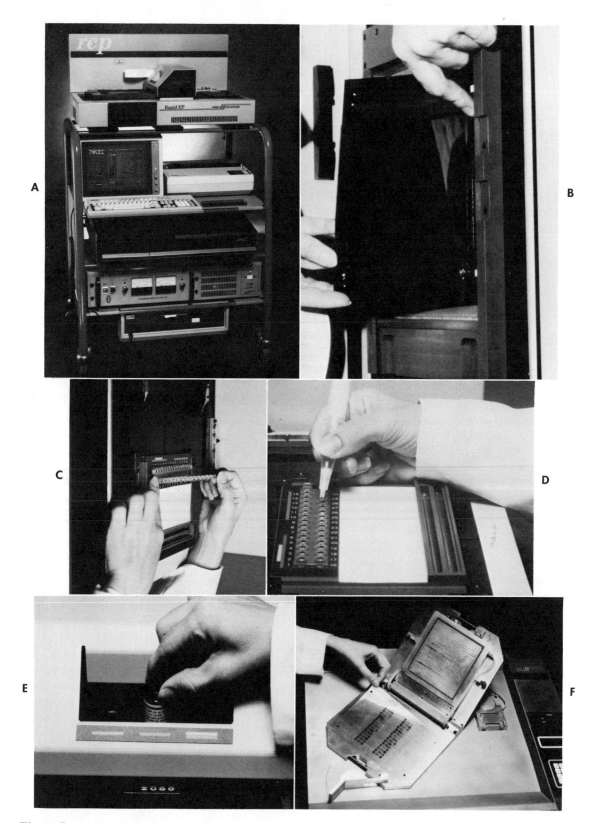

Fig. 11-7 **A,** The Helena Laboratories REP system. **B,** A sheet of plastic-backed agarose gel ("Titan Gel") is set in the chamber (upper left of instrument). **C,** Sample cups are set in the sample tray (upper right of instrument). **D,** Loading the sample cups with samples using a dispensing device. **E,** A reagent mixture, in this case for creatine kinase visualization, is placed in the top middle ("gantry") of the instrument. **F,** A stained gel in its holder in the gel processing apparatus (not shown in the upper left picture). The instrument complex includes a monitor keyboard and printer, left to right on second level down; the EDC densitometer below; the power supply and, on the lowest level, the computer. (Courtesy Helena Laboratories Corp, Beaumont, Tex.)

apparatus. Provision must be made for the supporting medium, depending on whether it is hung vertically, supported vertically, laid horizontally with or without support, and how many supports are being used.

Provisions must also be made for the electrolyte solution, often referred to as the "buffer" though it may contain other things such as SDS. These liquids may cover the supporting medium, but their main function is to conduct the current to the supporting medium while keeping the supporting medium sufficiently far away from the electrodes and their electrolysis products.

Electrophoresis can be carried out on supporting media cast in cylinders and on 1 to 20 or 30 cylinders at a time, depending on the apparatus and the experiment. The current should be increased proportionate to the number of cylinders. Electrophoresis is usually carried out with the cylinders vertical.

More often, electrophoresis is performed on flat sheets or slabs of supporting media. This is to compare the patterns produced by several samples. Each sample is placed in its own separate slot or well and then electrophoresed at the same time. These slabs can be set horizontally or vertically. In the horizontal position the slabs may need to be supported on the bottom. The upper surface may be exposed to air, in which case evaporation can be a problem. Evaporation increases the buffer concentration and conductivity of the support. If the chamber holding the support is covered, saturating the air above the support with water reduces evaporation. In some apparatuses the support is submerged in the buffer ("submarine" electrophoresis); the buffer cools the support and eliminates evaporation from it. (Submarine systems draw more current because most of the ion flow occurs via the surrounding buffer rather than through the support.) If the support is set vertically, it will probably need to be held between sheets of glass or Lucite unless it is strong enough (e.g., paper) to be hung from rods. There is no theoretic reason for preferring horizontal or vertical electrophoresis. Routine clinical electrophoresis is usually done on thin sheets of support set horizontally. The voltage depends only on the dimensions (thickness, width, and length) of the support, not on the number of samples analyzed.

Maintenance. Maintenance of the power supply is largely preventive (i.e., keeping liquids from reaching inside the chassis). Maintenance of the electrophoretic apparatus involves keeping it clean and unbroken and rinsing it and the electrodes with distilled or deionized water after each use. Avoid direct hand contact with glass or plastic plates because skin oils can contaminate their surfaces. It is important that the apparatus does not leak. Glass or Lucite equipment is easily cracked. Filling the apparatus with water and checking for leaks should be done periodically. The connecting cables need to be kept dry. They should not be bent sharply or repeatedly, otherwise the wires may break.

Practice

General Requirements. Aside from running the electrophoresis correctly, the most important criteria the operator must meet is to be able to monitor the electrophoresis in a precise manner. The same material must give the same pattern, qualitatively and quantitatively, every time. Commercial electrophoresis equipment is designed to make clinical electrophoresis as reproducible as possible.

Safety Precautions. Electrophoresis is inherently hazardous because analysis requires the use of electrical currents and conducting solutions. Therefore the same precautions used with any piece of electrical equipment should be adhered to.

Solution Preparation. The solutions used with electrophoresis must be prepared carefully. The water used to make buffers should be distilled-deionized, and the other chemicals should be of high quality. Some electrophoresis solutions are unstable (i.e., ammonium persulfate) and thus may have to be prepared fresh each day or once a week before use. Alkaline solutions with a pH of 8.0 or greater will adsorb CO_2 from the air and thus turn more acidic with time unless they are kept well sealed. Acrylamide in water slowly breaks down to acrylic acid; it also polymerizes, so the gel will have incorporated some carboxyl groups, causing an increase in electro-osmosis.

The conductivity of the prepared solutions should be reasonably accurate, but the pH of the solutions should be carefully adjusted or checked. Electrophoretic solutions (i.e., buffers) are often prepared from concentrates that are tenfold or more times the concentration of the working solutions. If this is done according to a recipe, the diluted solution will most likely have the correct pH. However, it should be checked. If the pH of the concentrated solutions must be adjusted, it is important to remember that the pH will probably shift when the concentrated solution is diluted. Thus checking the pH afterward is critical.

Preparation of Support. For reproducible results the support must be as uniform as possible. In clinical laboratories, support media such as cellulose acetate, agarose, and polyacrylamide are bought commercially. Such media are usually more uniform in electrophoretic behavior, but may vary from lot to lot or from one vendor to another. Some support media are sold with a plastic backing (Mylar) so they may be handled without tearing or breaking. Cellulose acetate is prepared for electrophoresis by soaking it in the electrophoresis buffer. This must be done carefully to avoid bubbles or blisters if the material has a plastic backing. Special soaking chambers are sometimes used. Some commercial support media may have to be washed, usually in the electrophoresis solution, before use; others are prepared with buffer already impregnated in the media. A few types have **reservoir** sections on the ends so that liquid buffers do not have to be prepared or added. Prepared supports usually have holes or indentations for alignment in the apparatus.

Although cellulose acetate is still a popular support, agarose supports tend to be used more often. Agarose appears to have superior resolving power. It is claimed that 12 to 15 proteins can be resolved from serum using agarose as compared with only five using cellulose acetate. This resolving power, however, depends in part on how these substances are manufactured.

The carbohydrate polymers—starch, agar, and agarose—must be melted and cast. Their solutions contain the electrophoresis solutions and approximately 1% carbohydrate polymer. These are heated, perhaps in an autoclave (they should be sterilized), and poured into a mold. As the solution cools, the polymer chains tangle, trapping a large volume of solution in a rigid matrix (gel). Agar and agarose can be stored in a 50°C oven in liquid form. They should not be shaken and should be poured without bubble formation, which would distort the electrophoretic pattern. For this reason, starch solutions must be degassed while hot before pouring a mold.

Polyacrylamide is essentially a plastic. It is made by adding a catalyst, usually a peroxide-like ammonium persulfate, to a solution of electrophoresis buffer and salts, acrylamide at 3% to 15%, and a dimeric acrylamide compound for cross-linking the polymer chains. The dimeric acrylamide compound is normally 3% to 5% of the acrylamide concentration. After mixing, the polymerizing solution is poured into a mold. It is then "overlaid" with water or water-saturated butanol to form a smooth, even, upper surface. Sometimes the acrylamide solution is degassed before pouring it into the mold.

Polymerization time depends mostly on the amount of catalyst added. The polymerization goes by a free-radical mechanism and is "exothermic" (i.e., heat is generated). Very fast polymerization is not good because the heat generated produces convective distortions in the polymerizing gel. This can produce distorted electrophoretic patterns. Polymerization times range from 30 minutes to 1 hour. When polyacrylamide gels have polymerized, there is a thin horizontal line that appears a few millimeters below the original top of the gel solution. Gels may be cast in plastic trays or tubes.

Preparation of Samples. The most common routine electrophoresis procedures are serum protein, hemoglobin, and isozyme electrophoretic analysis. The isozymes most often analyzed are creatine kinase (CK), lactic dehydrogenase (LDH), and alkaline phosphatase (AP). Samples of urine or cerebrospinal fluid may have to be concentrated if protein electrophoretic patterns are needed.

If the sample is to be treated with SDS, this is done before electrophoresis. After treatment, SDS, a reducing agent like mercaptoethanol, is added, then the sample(s) container is sealed, and the sample(s) is heated for 5 to 10 minutes at 100°C. This ensures that all disulfide bonds are reduced so the protein(s) can assume a rodlike shape.

Sample Application. The amount of sample applied depends on the sensitivity of the detection method. The more sensitive the detection method, the less sample needs to be applied. The volume of sample should be kept as small as possible, unless disk electrophoresis or isotachophoresis is used. For clinical work, as little as 1 µl of sample may be applied. (Electrophoresis generally uses much less material than most other clinical techniques.)

Sometimes the sample is injected into the apparatus, as with isotachophoresis, or is incorporated into the support before electrophoresis or electrofocusing. With some support media the sample is spotted onto the surface of the supporting medium. After a cellulose acetate support has been soaked in buffer, it is important that it is blotted relatively dry so that any samples applied

to the support do not run on the surface. Filter paper can be used to blot.

Sample application is very important. It is often done with a special instrument. This is to make the application as uniform as possible. Not only are the amounts of serum or whatever is being analyzed important, but the shape of the applied spot of material on something like cellulose acetate can also affect the results. (With some commercial agarose or polyacrylamide gels, holes or slots in the gels define the shape of the zone of applied material.) It is often a good idea to prime the sample applicator: apply the samples 2 or 3 times to a sheet of paper towel before setting the support in place to receive the samples. Some types of applicators can deliver several samples at once.

A "control" sample of "normal" serum, hemoglobin, or lipid must be run with the patient samples. In fact, if many samples are being electrophoresed at one time, two or three "control" samples should be set near the ends and near the middle of the row of samples. This provides a direct comparison with the patient samples and also acts as a control of the electrophoretic run.

It is important that the applicators are promptly and thoroughly cleaned after each use. Dried protein is very difficult to remove and results in improper delivery of the sample. Contamination of one set of samples with material leaching from another set because of an applicator that was inadequately cleaned is guaranteed to generate discrepant/invalid patterns.

Operation. Electrophoresis requires that the electrodes are connected appropriately so that the samples move in the right direction. For example, if protein-SDS complexes or polynucleotides are to be electrophoresed, they should migrate toward the more positive electrode (anode) because they will have a negative charge. With commercial electrophoresis equipment it is almost impossible to apply the voltage wrong.

Normally, only one parameter (i.e., voltage, current or power [wattage]), is set as a constant parameter on a power supply. The time of electrophoresis may also have to be set. The temperature is normally not considered unless the apparatus uses forced cooling.

Processing Support. Once the electrophoresis is completed, the support is usually removed and treated to visualize the separated substance. Gel supports require careful handling. Agar, agarose, and starch gels without plastic backing are brittle. They can be placed onto a flat glass plate of the

same size. Polyacrylamide gels are tougher, but they can tear. If the agarose or polyacrylamide supports have a plastic backing, they are easier to handle. However, pulling or twisting them can distort the patterns of separated proteins or lipids. Paper or cellulose acetate (with or without plastic backing) is the easiest to handle.

Some supports, used for separation of radioactive substances, are sandwiched with x-ray film in a special holder that is placed in a freezer for perhaps several days. The x-ray film is then developed. This process is called **autoradiography.** Some supports are dried before further processing, but most are stained.

Staining usually involves soaking the support in a solution of some dye that adsorbs to whatever is separated on the support. This staining solution often also contains dilute (7%) acetic acid or trichloroacetic acid. These acids precipitate proteins in the gel matrix so they do not diffuse any more. Adsorption of the dye is also increased if the proteins are precipitated. With polynucleotides, which do not diffuse very rapidly in agarose, the "dye" is ethidium bromide, which sandwiches itself between the nucleotide bases and becomes very fluorescent. In general, however, the visualization process uses colored dye. For proteins, amido black or Ponceau S are favorites for clinical work. They give blue or pink bands of protein, respectively. Amido black is generally used with agarose; Ponceau S is used primarily with cellulose acetate. For lipids or lipoproteins, fat red 7 or Sudan black B is often used. They give red or black bands, respectively.

After soaking for a few minutes up to 1 hour in the staining solution (depending on the thickness of the support), the support is washed several times in a destaining solution. Dye not bound to the separated material diffuses out of the gel into the solution. Eventually the supporting medium becomes clear except for bands of separated material, which are now colored with the adsorbed dye (Fig. 11-8). Destaining times for clinical work are kept short (about 15 minutes). Again, use of thin sheets of supporting media is important. The dye-staining process can be automated; Helena Laboratories Gel Processor apparently stains and destains gels according to a preset program.

Protein concentrations in cerebrospinal fluid and urine are normally very low and thus must be concentrated before electrophoresis or a more sensitive stain other than the conventional dye stains can be used. The "silver stain" is about 100 times more sensitive than dye stains, so it can be

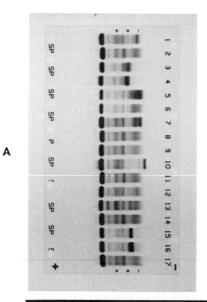

A

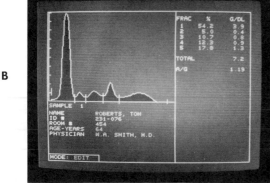

B

C

Fig. 11-8 **A,** Seventeen blood serum samples electrophoresed on agarose gel and stained with Amido Black. Note the alignment holes along two sides of the gel. The strongly stained bands closest to the "+" end of the gel plate are albumin; the immunoglobulins are at the other ("−") end. **B,** Densitometric tracing of "normal" serum protein profile. Freeze-dried normal and abnormal sera for controls are sold. **C,** Set of lactic dehydrogenase isozyme profiles. When tissue damage occurs, the amount of the isozyme (isoenzyme) associated with that tissue increases. Isozyme 1, to the left, is associated with heart muscle, and isozyme 5, to the right, is associated with liver and skeletal muscle. The fluorescence of NADH is actually observed. (Courtesy Helena Laboratories Corp, Beaumont, Tex.)

used to stain unconcentrated urine or cerebrospinal fluid samples after they are electrophoresed.

The silver stain requires treatment of the support with several solutions in succession. It resembles development of a photograph because the "color" is the silver adsorbed and reduced onto proteins. However, it can be done in the presence of light. Several companies sell kits for silver staining.

Electrophoresis is often used in the separation of multiple forms of certain enzymes called **isozymes** or **isoenzymes.** Instead of staining for protein, the gels or membranes are stained with solutions that give colored spots or bands where there is a particular enzyme activity.

Isozyme staining may simply involve treating the slab or membrane with a **chromogenic substrate** solution. This turns a visible color when the enzyme reacts with the substrate to form a colored product. Because the substrates for most enzymes have low molecular weights, they dif-

fuse rapidly. To avoid the blurring of the colored bands, the product of the reaction is often reacted with other substances to form a colored precipitate. This does not diffuse as rapidly; therefore it is stable enough for recording by photography or densitometry.

Quantitation and Recording of Results. The supporting medium can be photographed; however, for many purposes, including clinical analyses, a quantitative record of the pattern is needed. To obtain a quantitative profile of the distribution of separated substances, densitometry is done on the stained support (see Fig. 11-8). Some densitometers can measure fluorescence and adsorption, so the positions of the fluorescent bands produced by some isozymes can be recorded (see Fig. 11-8). Fluorescence measurements are often more sensitive than measurements of absorbance.

Densitometry

Densitometric measurements are absorbance measurements. A **densitometer** is a modified spectrophotometer. The modifications enable the instrument to measure and record the absorbance of the stain on a support along the support. The recording is supposed to be of concentrations of separated substances with respect to their position on the support.

Theory of Densitometry. A beam of pure or "monochromatic" light shines on a solution that absorbs some of the light. The ratio of light that passes through the solution to the original incident beam of light striking the solution is a measure of the concentration of the substance. The light that passes through the solvent (and support) alone is the "reference" value.

Apparatus. Like all spectrophotometers, the densitometer has a light source and some way of dispersing its light, sending light of different colors or wavelengths in different directions. The operator selects the wavelength of light that is most strongly absorbed by the stain used.

Some densitometers use a laser that produces red light as the light source. Laser beams are very thin but are of high intensity. Densitometers using lasers can pick up very fine details in stained gels, providing the stain absorbs the red light (most commonly used stains do).

The light is directed onto a stained support that is set on a movable carriage. The carriage may be made to move so that the light beam shines on every part of the support in turn, starting from one end and stopping at the other.

Some densitometers can only do this with single electrophoresis patterns, but others can measure supports such as two-dimensional gels or sets of electrophoresis patterns run simultaneously on a slab gel. Densitometers of this type are usually equipped with computers to handle and process all the information in slab gel electrophoresis patterns.

The light that passes through the support is measured using a phototube or photodetector. The electronic circuits in the densitometer convert the relative amounts of light transmitted by the stained substances on the support to that transmitted by the support alone. The densitometer has a recorder to make a graph of absorbance relative to position on the support.

Practice. Supports must sometimes be "cleared" (i.e., made transparent) before densitometry. Cellulose acetate supports are not transparent but are highly reflective. They are "cleared" by soaking in a solution containing methanol and acetic acid. This partially dissolves the fibers. Some commercial clearing solutions also include an elastic polymer to keep the cellulose acetate from shrinking or pulling away from the plastic backing. Commercial agarose gel supports are clear enough to be put in the densitometer after drying. They do not have to be cleared. Drying is done in a 55°C oven. Stained polyacrylamide supports can be scanned directly.

Some potential problems with densitometry are worth noting. The purpose of densitometry is to obtain a record that gives relative concentrations of separated proteins (or lipids). To do this with a stained support, the support must be soaked in the stain long enough so that the dye (or silver) bound by the proteins is proportional to the protein concentration throughout each zone of protein (or lipid). Albumin in serum is usually much more concentrated than other proteins. If the support does not soak in the stain long enough, the center of the albumin zone, where the highest concentration of albumin is, will not have taken up as much dye as it could. Consequently, the densitometric scan will show a lower albumin concentration than is actually there.

Densitometers shine light onto supports through slits of various sizes. These are usually rectangular and are selected to match the sizes of the stained bands of protein or lipid. In general it is better to select smaller slits; however, a smaller slit will transmit less light and thus give traces with a lot of "background electronic noise." However, smaller slits will give the best resolution.

The way the samples are applied to the support also affects the profile. If samples are applied so that the starting zone has an odd shape, the fine slits might show extra peaks or shoulders in a protein zone. These could be misinterpreted as separate proteins.

Electrophoresis of serum proteins followed by staining and densitometry is a semiquantitative technique. This is because different dyes stain different proteins to different extents. This is another reason why at least one "normal" control

Table 11-1 Common problems encountered with electrophoresis

Problem (symptom)	Possible cause	Possible cure
Sample on support doesn't stain	Not enough sample; SDS in support	Apply more; check sample applicator; wash support to remove SDS before staining
Sample moves wrong way	Wrong polarity for sample charge	Reverse polarity (leads); run electrophoresis at different pH
Sample does not move	Leads not connected; power supply not on; short in power supply; sample is at isoelectric point	Check voltage indicator to see if voltage applied; check leads; replace power supply; run electrophoresis at different pH
Sample bands curved	Uneven heating; sample applied as curved band	Run electrophoresis slower; check sample application
Sample bands crooked	Support is not homogeneous; sample application problem	Prepare support again carefully; try support from different source; check sample application
Sample bands "fuzzy"	Bands too wide at start; support not blotted sufficiently; electrophoresis too slow; sample is heterogeneous (like immunoglobulins)	Apply sample as thinner bands; blot support thoroughly before applying sample; run electrophoresis faster; no cure
Sample bands streak	Salt in sample; oxidation or aggregation of sample; too much sample	Remove salt; add thioglycolate to sample or run electrophoresis at different pH; apply less sample

should be electrophoresed every time with the patient samples.

Analysis and Interpretation

The physician who is treating the patient must interpret the patterns obtained. This involves comparing patterns produced by samples from patients with patterns produced by samples from "normal" or "control" (healthy) individuals. For example, certain infections and diseases produce increases in gamma globulin levels in serum. Absolute or "all or nothing" changes in specific proteins are generally associated with genetic diseases. The responsibility of the laboratory technologist is to produce accurate and consistent separation patterns. This requires attention to detail, a precise technique, and a thorough understanding of the principles of electrophoresis. Some of the common problems associated with performing an electrophoretic procedure are given in Table 11-1.

Review Questions

1. The isoelectric point of a protein is at pH 6.1. Toward what electrode, anode, or cathode will it move if it is electrophoresed at pH 8.5?
2. Toward which electrode would it move if electrophoresed at pH 3.5?

3. Electrophoresis apparatuses are now manufactured that perform electrophoresis on thinner slabs of support gels. These thinner gels are harder to work with because they are more fragile. Why use them?
4. Different proteins may have positive, negative, or zero net charges at pH 7. In sodium dodecyl sulfate (SDS) solutions most proteins have net negative charges at pH 7. Explain why.
5. Cellulose acetate strips used for electrophoresis are not supposed to be handled where the electrophoresis occurs. Why not?
6. Suppose a mistake is made in preparing an electrophoresis buffer: It is made 10 times more concentrated than the directions call for. If the voltage is set to its usual value, what is likely to happen?
7. If a polyacrylamide gel polymerizes too fast, it is likely to show a variable concentration of polymer chains in various places in the gel. How would this affect the separation pattern of a macro-ion sample?

Bibliography

Andrews AT: Electrophoresis: theory, techniques and biochemical and technical applications, ed 2, London, 1986, Oxford University Press.

Brewer JM, Ashworth RB: Disc electrophoresis, J Chem Educ 46:41, 1969.

Chen B, Chrambach A: The effect of SDS on protein zone dispersion in polyacrylamide gel electrophoresis, Anal Biochem 102:409, 1980.

Chrambach A: Recent developments in buffer electrofocusing. In Neuhoff V, ed: Electrophoresis '84, Deerfield Beach, Fla, 1984, Verlag Chemie.

Jeffreys AJ, Wilson V, and Thein SL: Individual specific "fingerprints" of human DNA. Nature 316:76, 1985.

Kaplan LA, Pesce AJ: Clinical chemistry, ed 2, St Louis, 1989, Mosby–Year Book.

Maxam A, Gilbert W: A new method for sequencing DNA, Proc Natl Acad Sci USA 74:560, 1977.

O'Farrell PH: High resolution two-dimensional electrophoresis of proteins, J Biol Chem 250:4007, 1975.

Ornstein L: Theory of disc electrophoresis, Ann NY Acad Sci 121:321, 1967.

Reynolds JA, Tanford C: Binding of dodecyl sulfate to proteins at high binding ratios: possible implications for the state of proteins in biological membranes, Proc Natl Acad Sci USA 66:1002, 1970.

Righetti PG, Gianazza, E, and Gelfi C: Immobilized pH gradients, Trends Biochem Sci 13:335, 1988.

CHAPTER 12

Chromatography

DAVID HAGE

Theory of Chromatography
Gas Chromatography
Instrumentation in Gas Chromatography
Liquid Chromatography
Instrumentation in Liquid Chromatography

Chromatography is a technique widely used in clinical laboratories for the separation and analysis of compounds. Its applications range from drug screening and confirmation to metabolic profiling. Chromatography may be defined as a separation method based on the different interactions of sample compounds with two phases: a **mobile phase** and a **stationary phase,** as the compounds travel through a supporting medium (Fig. 12-1).

A sample containing two components is applied to a column containing a solid support coated with a given chemical layer (i.e., the stationary phase). Also present in the system is solvent that is being applied continuously to the column (i.e., the mobile phase). As sample components travel through the column, they interact with the mobile phase and stationary phase to different degrees. Those interacting more strongly with the stationary phase tend to spend a longer time in the column than those preferring the mobile phase. This results in a separation of the components as they pass through the column.

The success of chromatography as a separation technique has been mainly because of the large number of mobile phases, stationary phases, and support materials available for its use. This variety allows chromatography to be used for the analysis and purification of a wide variety of compounds. Usually chromatographic techniques are classified based on the type of mobile phase they use. For example, if the mobile phase is a gas, the technique is referred to as **gas chromatography.** If the mobile phase is a liquid, the method is called **liquid chromatography.** Further distinctions can also be made based on the types of stationary phase and support materials being used. This chapter will begin with a short description of the theory behind chromatographic techniques, and then the factors that affect the ability to separate compounds will be discussed. This will be followed by a detailed discussion of the techniques and instrumentation used with gas chromatographic and liquid chromatographic methods.

Theory of Chromatography

Fig. 12-2 represents a typical chromatographic separation; the graph **(chromatogram)** shows the amount of each detectable component eluting from the column as a function of time. (This graph could also be plotted as a function of the volume of mobile phase needed to elute compounds from the column.) The time or volume it takes the mobile phase or a nonretained compound to elute from the system is referred to as the **void time (t_0)** or **void volume (V_0)** of the column. The time or volume it takes for a retained compound to elute is referred to as its **retention time (t_r)** or **retention volume (V_r).** These values are characteristic for a compound and are related to the strength with which it interacts with the stationary and mobile phase. As a result, a compound's retention time or volume can be used to determine the compound's identity. To determine the amount of the compound eluting, either the height or the area of the compound's peak is used.

The ability of a chromatographic column to separate two compounds depends on three factors: (1) the difference in the retention of the compounds, (2) the width of their peaks, or (3) the efficiency of the system. The retention of a compound can also be described by using a measurement called the **capacity factor (k').** The

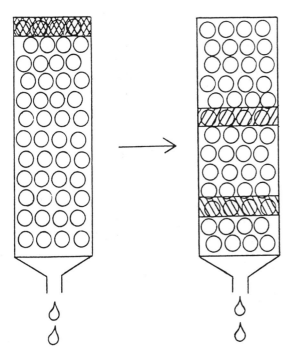

Fig. 12-1 Separation of two compounds by chromatography.

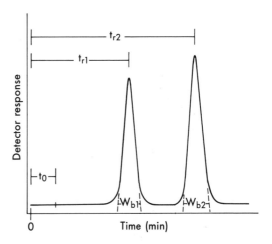

Fig. 12-2 Chromatogram for the separation of two compounds. (From Kaplan LA, Pesce AJ, eds: Clinical chemistry: theory, analysis, and correlation, ed 2, St Louis, 1989, Mosby–Year Book.)

value of k' can be experimentally determined from t_r and t_0 by the following equation:

$$k' = (t_r - t_0)/t_0$$

A similar equation can be used to determine k' from V_r and V_0. The value of k' is useful because it is directly related to the equilibrium processes involved in a compound's retention on the column. This makes it valuable in optimizing chromatographic separations.

Another parameter used to describe a compound's retention is the retardation factor (R_f). This is most commonly used in planar or thin-layer chromatography. The R_f value for a compound on a planar chromatographic support is determined by comparing the distance the compound travels from its point of application (d_r) with the distance traveled by the mobile phase in the same amount of time (d_0):

$$R_f = d_r/d_0$$

Like k', the value of R_f can be directly related to the equilibrium processes involved in a compound's retention on the chromatographic system.

The efficiency of a chromatographic system is determined by the stationary and mobile phases used in a separation, as well as the type of support in the column, the flow-rate of the mobile phase,

and many other factors. To compare the efficiencies of different chromatographic systems, one measure that may be used is the **number of theoretical plates (N)**, where

$$N = 16(t_r/W_b)^2$$

In this equation t_r is the retention time of a compound, and W_b is the baseline width of the compound's peak. The larger the value of N for a column, the greater the column's separating power or efficiency.

Another measure of efficiency that is used to compare columns of different lengths is the **height equivalent of a theoretical plate** (i.e., **H** or **HETP**). This is calculated as follows:

$$H = L/N$$

where L is the length of the column and N is the number of theoretical plates. Note that H is simply a measure of the distance along the column that is needed to generate one theoretical plate. Thus the smaller the value of H, the better the separating power or efficiency of the column. In general a good value for H is one that is ≤ 2 to 10 times the diameter of the support used in the column. Values of H greater than this represent a relatively inefficient system.

To determine how well two peaks are separated by a column, the **separation factor (α)** can be used:

$$\alpha = k'_2/k'_1$$

where k'_1 is the capacity factor of the first of a pair of compounds and k'_2 is the capacity factor of the second. Note that the separation factor measures how well two solutes are separated based only on their retention (i.e., k' values) and does not consider the effect of peak widths on the separation.

The **resolution (R$_s$)** is a second way of determining how well two peaks are separated. The definition of resolution is as follows:

$$R_s = \frac{t_{r2} - t_{r1}}{(W_{b2} + W_{b1})/2}$$

R$_s$ is useful in evaluating the quality of a separation because it considers both retention and column efficiency. A value for R$_s$ of 1.5 or greater is generally considered baseline resolution and represents a complete separation of two neighboring peaks. Values for R$_s$ less than 1.5 indicate that the peaks do have significant overlap, but even values down to 1.0 are considered adequate for most separations.

By assuming that the widths of two neighboring peaks are approximately equal (i.e., $W_{b2} \approx W_{b1}$), it is possible to relate R$_s$ directly to k', α, and N:

$$R_s = \tfrac{1}{4}\sqrt{N}\,[\alpha - 1][k_1'/(1 + k_1')]$$

This equation is useful because it shows three ways in which a chromatographic separation can be improved: (1) by increasing N (i.e., using a more efficient or longer column); (2) by increasing k' (i.e., increasing solute retention); or (3) by increasing α (i.e., increasing the selectivity of the system, or the relative retention of the second solute vs the first). The effect of changing each of these factors on the resolution of a separation is shown in Fig. 12-3. Ways of varying k' and α include changing the mobile phase or stationary phase used in the chromatographic system. N may be adjusted by changing the flow-rate, the type of support used in the column, and the column length. All of these represent experimental parameters that can be varied to obtain an optimum separation between two compounds.

Gas Chromatography

Gas chromatography (GC) has long been a popular method for separating and analyzing

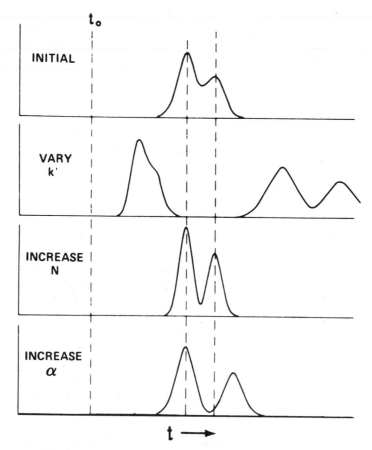

Fig. 12-3 Effect of varying K', N, and α on the resolution (Rs) of a chromatographic separation. (From Snyder LR, Kirkland JJ: Introduction to modern liquid chromatography, ed 2, New York, 1979, John Wiley & Sons.)

compounds because of its high resolving power and low limits of detection, accuracy and reproducibility, and speed. GC can be used as a separation technique for compounds that are naturally volatile or can be easily converted into a volatile form. This makes it especially useful in separating small organic molecules, including many drugs and other biologically active compounds. An example of a typical separation obtained using GC is given in Fig. 12-4.

Like other chromatographic methods, GC separates solutes based on their different interactions with the mobile phase and stationary phase. However, it differs from other chromatographic techniques in that a compound's retention in GC is determined mostly by the compound's vapor pressure and volatility, which is controlled by the compound's interaction with the stationary phase. Because the main purpose of the gas in GC is to move solutes along the column, the mobile phase in this technique is often simply referred to as the **carrier gas.** Examples of common carrier gases used in GC are hydrogen, helium, nitrogen, and argon.

Although the carrier gas does not greatly affect solute retention, the type of gas that is used is important in other ways. Factors that need to be considered in choosing a carrier gas include (1) the efficiency of the chromatographic system, (2) the stability of the column and compounds to be studied, (3) the type of detector being used, and (4) possible risks or hazards included in using the gas. Efficiency is affected by the carrier gas through changes it creates in a compound's rate of diffusion. Low molecular weight gases, such as helium or hydrogen, produce much larger rates of compound diffusion than heavier gases, such as nitrogen or argon. This is important because faster diffusion produces narrower peaks and allows faster separations. Column or compound stability can be important when using a carrier gas such as hydrogen, which can react with sample components or with the stationary phase. Detector performance must also be considered in carrier gas selection. For example, a thermal conductivity detector requires the use of hydrogen or helium, carrier gases that have thermal conductivities very different from those of most sample

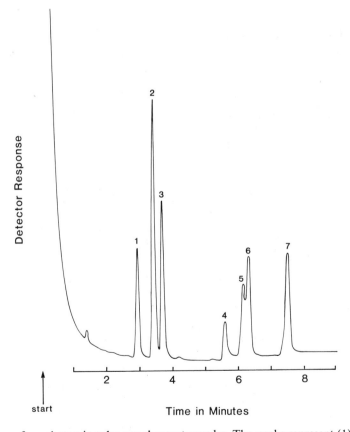

Fig. 12-4 Separation of amphetamines by gas chromatography. The peaks represent (1) D-amphetamine, (2) phentermine, (3) methamphetamine, (4) phenylpropanolamine, (5) pseudophedrine, (6) ephedrine and (7) phenmetrazine. (From Kaplan LA, Pesce AJ, eds: Methods in clinical chemistry, St Louis, 1987, Mosby–Year Book.)

components. Hazards associated with the carrier gas are important to consider when working with hydrogen, which is potentially explosive and requires special precautions in its use.

The stationary phase in GC is important because it is the main factor in determining the selectivity and retention of compounds. There are three types of stationary phases used in GC: (1) solid adsorbents, (2) liquids coated on solid supports, and (3) bonded-phase supports. If solid adsorbents are used, the separation method is referred to as **gas-solid chromatography (GSC)**. In this technique the same material acts as both the stationary phase and support material. Examples of supports used in GSC include alumina, silica, molecular sieves, and activated carbon. Although GSC was the first type of gas chromatography developed, it is currently not as widely used as other GC methods primarily because of the strong retention of many GSC columns for low volatile or polar solutes and potential catalytic changes in sample components.

Gas-liquid chromatography (GLC) is a GC technique in which the stationary phase is a liquid coated onto a solid support. Liquids used for GLC can be based on polymers, hydrocarbons, fluorocarbons, and even molten salts or liquid crystals. These liquids are typically coated onto supports prepared from diatomaceous earth, such as Chromosorb P or Chromosorb W. Over 400 liquid stationary phases are available for use in GC, but only about 6 to 12 are needed for most applications. Examples of liquid stationary phases recommended for use in GLC include dimethylsilicone, 50% phenylmethylsilicone, trifluoropropylmethylsilicone, polyethylene glycol, polyesters, and 3-cyanopropylsilicone. These stationary phases cover a wide range of polarities. Because polar compounds will be most strongly retained on a polar material and nonpolar compounds will be most strongly retained on a nonpolar material, proper selection of the stationary phase is an important factor in controlling the retention and selectivity of compounds on a GLC column.

One problem with using a liquid stationary phase in GC is that the liquid may slowly be lost from the column with time, particularly if high temperatures are being used. Loss of the stationary phase is undesirable because it contributes to the background signal of the detector and changes the characteristics of the column with time. This problem is overcome in a technique called **bonded-phase gas chromatography.** Here the stationary phase is covalently attached to the

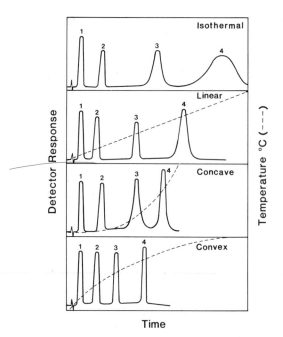

Fig. 12-5 Elution of four compounds from a GC column using isothermal elution and temperature programming with either linear, concave, or convex changes in temperature with time. (From Kaplan LA, Pesce AJ, eds: Clinical chemistry: theory, analysis, and correlation, ed 2, St Louis, 1989, Mosby–Year Book.)

support (bonded-phase support). Advantages of using bonded-phase supports are that they are more stable than liquid stationary phases and thus allow for faster, more efficient separations.

Retention of compounds can also be adjusted by changing the temperature of the column. This affects the volatility of the compounds and thus the degree to which they interact with the stationary phase. If a constant temperature is used in a GC separation, the technique is referred to as an isothermal method. If the temperature is varied with the time, the technique is called **temperature programming.** Temperature programming is commonly used in GC for samples containing a large number of different components. By proper selection of the starting temperature and the way in which the temperature is changed during the run, good resolution of both weakly and strongly retained compounds can be achieved in a minimum amount of time. An example of the use of temperature programming in GC is given in Fig. 12-5.

Instrumentation in Gas Chromatography

A schematic diagram of a typical GC system is illustrated in Fig. 12-6. A summary of commercially available GC equipment is given in Table

Table 12-1 Commercial gas chromatographic systems and detectors

Supplier*	GC/TCD†	GC/FID	GC/ECD	GC/MS	Misc. GC systems and detectors
Alltech Associates	X	X	X		
The Anspec Co.	X	X	X		X
Antek Instruments	X	X	X		X
Applied Automation	X	X			X
Applied Scientific Co.	X				
Bio-Rad Laboratories					X
Buck Scientific	X	X	X		X
Chrompack	X	X	X		X
Carlo Erba	X	X	X	X	X
Delsi-Nermag				X	
ES Industries		X	X		X
Extrel Corp.				X	
Finnigan Mat Institute				X	
Fenwal Electronics	X				
Fisons Instruments	X	X			
The Foxboro Co.	X	X			X
Gow-Mac Instrument Co.	X	X			X
Hewlett-Packard Co.	X	X	X	X	
HNU Systems	X	X	X		X
Kratos Analytical				X	
Lee Scientific		X			X
Measurement & Analysis Systems				X	
Microsensor Technology	X				
The Munhall Co.	X				
Nicolet Instrument Corp.				X	
Nuclear Sources & Services			X		
O.I. Analytical	X	X	X	X	X
PCP			X	X	X
Perkin-Elmer	X	X	X	X	
Philips Export B.V.	X	X	X		
Philips Scientific	X	X	X		X
Photovac International					X
Pi Instruments	X	X	X	X	X
Radiomatic Instruments & Chemical Co.					X
Ruska Instrument Corp.				X	
Sadtler Research Labs					X
SAES Pure Gas					X
Sensidyne		X			
Shimadzu	X	X	X	X	X
Sievers Research					X
Technical Associates					X
Tegal Scientific	X	X	X		
Trace Analytical					X
Tracor Atlas					X
Tracor Instruments	X	X	X	X	X
VG Instruments				X	
Varex Corp.	X				
Varian Instrument Group	X	X	X	X	X
Vestec Corp.				X	
Vici Metronics	X				
VICI Valco	X		X		X
Western Scientific Associates	X	X	X		X
XonTech			X		

*Data shown includes manufacturers and manufacturers/distributors listed in *Anal Chem* 62:66G, 1990.
†Abbreviations: GC = gas chromatography, TCD = thermal conductivity detector, FID = flame ionization detector, ECD = electron capture detector, MS = mass spectrometer.

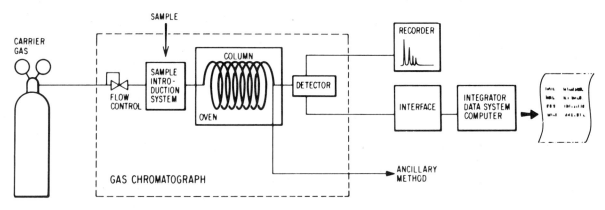

Fig. 12-6 Schematic of a typical gas chromatographic system. (From Ettre LS: Practical gas chromatography, Norwalk, Conn, 1973, Perkin-Elmer Corp.)

12-1, and an example of a commercial system is shown in Fig. 12-7. The basic design of a GC system consists of five main components: (1) a mobile phase source, (2) an injector, (3) a column, (4) a detector, and (5) a computer or recorder for data acquisition.

Mobile Phase Sources. The mobile phase source in GC is usually a standard gas cylinder, with a two-stage regulator for pressure control. The flow-rate of the carrier gas can be measured by using either bubble or thermal mass flow-meters. In some cases it is necessary to use special control devices to maintain constant flow of the carrier gas as the temperature or pressure of the system is varied. This is particularly important in systems where capillary columns or temperature-programming is being used. The carrier gas used in GC should be of high purity (i.e., >99.995% pure). If not, the chromatographic system can become contaminated thus giving rise to a loss in sensitivity and resolution. Good flow-rate and pressure control is also important in producing highly reproducible column efficiencies and resolutions.

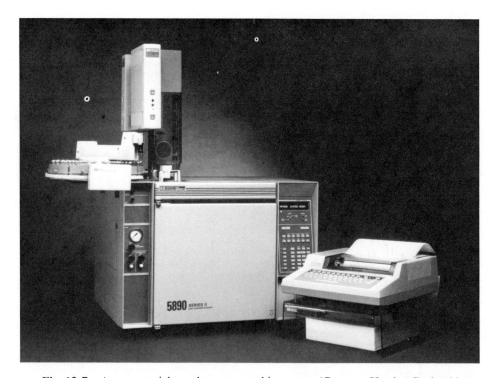

Fig. 12-7 A commercial gas chromatographic system. (Courtesy Hewlett-Packard.)

GC Injection Techniques. To inject compounds onto the GC system, either manual methods or auto-injectors can be used. For naturally volatile compounds, direct injection onto the GC system is often possible. For gaseous solutes this is done by using a gas-tight sampling valve and syringe. The valve usually has two positions; one for loading sample into the loop and one for placing the contents of the loop into the carrier gas stream. Volatile liquids or solids can also be applied directly to the GC system as long as they are dissolved in a solvent that does not overlap with their peaks or contain nonvolatile material that will deposit in the injector or column. If a packed column is being used, such compounds are injected by using a microsyringe placed into a heated injection port. As the compounds are injected into the port, they are quickly volatilized and taken by the carrier gas to the column. For thermally unstable compounds a heated injection port can be a problem in that it may cause decomposition of the sample. For these types of compounds, direct injection of the sample onto the column is sometimes used. This allows the use of a lower injection temperature.

Headspace analysis is an injection technique used for compounds that are naturally volatile but are present in a solution that also contains nonvolatile or interfering components. This method is based on the fact that volatile solutes in solution will also be present in the vapor phase immediately above the solution. By sampling this vapor phase, known as the headspace, volatile solutes can be collected and injected without interference from less volatile sample components. Headspace analysis can be performed in one of two ways: the static method and the dynamic method. In the static method, the sample solution is placed in a closed container and solute is allowed to distribute between the liquid and vapor phases at a constant temperature. After equilibrium has been reached, a sample of the vapor phase is taken and injected onto the GC system. One problem with this method is that good control of the temperature and volume of sample withdrawn is needed for reproducible results. Also, compounds with only modest volatilities may be difficult to detect by this approach. An alternative technique is the dynamic method, in which an inert gas is continually passed over or through the liquid sample, carrying with it any volatile compounds. This gas is then passed through a cold trap or solid adsorbent that collects and concentrates the volatile solutes. After collection the solutes are then removed from the trap and applied to the column. Although this technique requires more time and effort than the static method, it is also more reproducible and allows better detection of compounds with relatively low volatilities.

Sometimes the molecule of interest may not be volatile enough to use any of the injection techniques aforementioned. One approach is to derivatize the compound into a more volatile form. **Derivatization** can be used not only to increase the volatility of a compound but also to increase its thermal stability, its response on the detector, and its separation from other sample components. Most derivatization reactions used in GC can be classified into one of three groups: (1) silylation, (2) alkylation, and (3) acylation. Almost all such reactions are designed to be performed using minimal amounts of sample or reagents (i.e., 0.1 to 2.0 ml) and are typically carried out at room temperature. Some, however, do require heating at moderate temperatures (e.g., 60 to 100° C). Most of these reactions can be performed using kits that are commercially available.

Silylation is probably the most common of these derivatization techniques. This is performed by replacing active hydrogens on the compounds (e.g., R-OH, R-CO$_2$H, R-NH$_2$) with an alkylsilyl group (e.g., -SiMe$_3$). The result is that the compound is converted into a less polar, more volatile, and more thermally stable form. The most common reagent used in silylation is trimethylchlorosilane (TMS). However, a number of other silylation reagents can also be used. These include N,O-bis(trimethylsilyl)trifluoroacetamide (i.e., BSTFA) and N,O-bis(trimethylsilyl)acetamide (i.e., BSA).

The second type of derivatization, alkylation, involves the addition of an alkyl group to some active functional group on the solute. A common example is the esterification of a carboxylic acid, forming a volatile methyl ester. This is commonly performed using borontrifluoride in methanol as the reagent.

The third technique, acylation, involves the conversion of a solute into an acetate derivative. This is often used to improve the volatility of alcohols, phenols, and amine-containing compounds, or to increase their response on an electron-capture detector. Trifluoroacetic anhydride (TFAA) is a common reagent used for acylation. Another set of reagents used for this is the N-fluoroacylimidazoles. The latter group of reagents is used for compounds containing hydroxy groups, secondary amines, or tertiary amines in their structure.

Another factor that influences an injection technique for a GC system is the use of a packed column vs a capillary column. Although capillary columns are much more efficient than packed GC columns, they are also more susceptible to peak broadening when large injector volumes are used. To overcome this problem, several special injection techniques have been developed. Two common approaches are to use **inlet splitters,** and **splitless or direct injection.** In both cases the aim is to apply a narrow plug of sample to the column without causing excessive broadening of the resulting peaks in the chromatogram.

Inlet splitters are used if the compounds of interest are reasonably volatile, thermally stable, and make up between 0.001% to 10% of the sample composition. Sample is placed into the injection port and vaporized. As it leaves the injection port, only a small portion is applied to the column while the remainder goes to waste. To minimize the time that the sample spends in the injector, a high carrier gas flow-rate and high injector temperature are used. The main difficulty with inlet splitters is that solutes with different volatilities may not be divided between the column and waste streams in the same ratio. This can cause variability in the recovery of these compounds and can affect their final quantitation.

In splitless or direct injection the sample is injected along with a large volume of a volatile solvent. As this combination is applied to the column, the volatile solvent travels ahead of compounds in the sample forming a thick layer of liquid around the support material at the top of the column, which greatly increases retention of the sample components as they reach that region. This causes a narrow sample plug to form at the top of the column that helps to decrease the initial width of the sample peak on the chromatographic system.

GC Columns. The column is usually enclosed in a temperature controlled oven that is well-insulated and equipped with fans for uniform distribution of temperature. Most GC ovens allow control over a wide range of temperature (i.e., −50° to 450° C) and can be programmed to allow for a variety of temperature changes during a run (i.e., linear gradients of 0° to 30° C/min).

The column used in GC can be either a **packed** column or a **capillary column.** Packed columns are usually 1 to 2 m long, a few millimeters in diameter, and are filled with support particles coated with the desired stationary phase. Capillary, or open-tubular, columns range from 10 to 30 m in length, have inner diameters of 0.1 to 0.5 mm, and have stationary phase located only on their interior surface. Capillary columns generally have higher efficiencies and better limits of detection than packed columns, making them better for analytic applications. However, packed columns have a larger sample capacity, making them more appropriate for preparative-scale work.

GC Detectors. There are many types of detectors available for GC, but only a few are commonly used. Examples of the more common GC detectors include (1) the thermal conductivity detector, (2) the flame ionization detector, (3) the nitrogen-phosphorus detector, (4) the electron capture detector, (5) the flame photometric detector, and (6) detectors based on mass spectrometry.

The **thermal conductivity detector** (also known as a katherometer or hot-wire detector) was the first universal detector developed for GC. It measures a bulk property of the carrier gas (i.e., its ability to conduct heat away from a hot wire). This ability changes as compounds elute from the column. By detecting this change, the compounds are detected.

To detect the thermal conductivity of the carrier gas, an electronic circuit known as a Wheatstone bridge is used (Fig. 12-8). It consists of a pair of series resistors each arranged in parallel with two resistors in each leg. When the resistance of each leg of the circuit is properly bal-

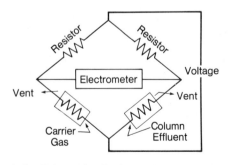

Fig. 12-8 Schematic of a thermal conductivity detector. (From Werner M, Mohrbacher RJ, and Riendau GJ: In Baer DM, Dito WR: Interpretation of therapeutic drug levels, Chicago, 1981, American Society of Clinical Pathologists.)

anced, the potential measured by the electrometer at the center is equal to zero. If the resistance of one of the legs changes, a potential is produced. This circuit is used in the thermal conductivity detector. One of the resistors in one leg of the circuit is in contact with carrier gas leaving the column (i.e., column effluent containing sample components); the second resistor from the other leg of the circuit is placed in a reference stream containing only pure carrier gas. As current is passed through the circuit, the wires in the resistors are heated. As carrier gas passes over the resistors some of this heat is removed. The extent of the heat removal depends on the carrier gas's thermal conductivity, which is influenced by its composition. As compounds elute from the column, the thermal conductivity of the carrier gas containing sample components changes differently relative to the thermal conductivity of the pure carrier gas. Thus the amount of heat removed from each resistor is also different. As the resistors heat or cool, their resistances change proportionately. The difference in the resistance between the two legs of the circuit causes the Wheatstone bridges to become unbalanced. Thus the unbalancing of the bridge is due to the difference in thermal conductivity caused by the presence of the sample components in the carrier gas. This change in resistance is measured electronically.

For a thermal conductivity detector to respond to a compound, it is necessary that the carrier gas have a thermal conductivity different from that of the sample component. Helium is the carrier gas of choice for this type of detector.

The main advantage of the thermal conductivity detector is that it is applicable to the detection of almost any compound, is nondestructive, and can be used in combination with other types of GC detectors. Some disadvantages of a thermal conductivity detector are (1) it responds to impurities in the carrier gas, (2) it is highly sensitive to changes in flow-rate, and (3) its limit of detection, which is high (approximately $10^{-7}\ M$) compared with other types of GC detectors.

The **flame ionization detector (FID)** is perhaps the most common type of GC detector (Fig. 12-9). It is also a "universal" detector capable of measuring the presence of almost any organic substance and many inorganic compounds. An FID detects compounds by measuring their ability to produce ions when burned in a hydrogen-air flame. Ions produced by the flame are collected by an electrode surrounding the flame. As

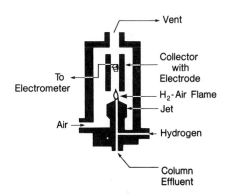

Fig. 12-9 Schematic of a flame ionization detector. (From Werner M, Mohrbacher RJ, and Riendau GJ: In Baer DM, Dito WR: Interpretation of therapeutic drug levels, Chicago, 1981, American Society of Clinical Pathologists.)

ions are produced they create a current, allowing the eluting compound to be detected.

One advantage of an FID is that it will detect essentially any organic compound. However, it will not respond to many common carrier gases or impurities such as water, ammonia, nitrogen, helium, hydrogen, and carbon dioxide. The limit of detection of an FID for organic compounds is also quite good, being approximately $10^{-10}\ M$, which is considerably lower than that obtained with a thermal conductivity detector.

A more selective type of GC detector is the **nitrogen-phosphorus detector (NPD)** or the alkali flame ionization detector/thermionic detector. The NPD is primarily used to detect nitrogen- or phosphorus-containing compounds. The NPD is similar to an FID in that both are based on the measurement of ions produced by compounds burning in a flame. However, the flame used in an NPD contains a small amount of vapor from an alkali metal such as rubidium, which greatly enhances the formation of ions from nitrogen- and phosphorus-containing compounds.

The ability of an NPD to preferentially detect compounds containing nitrogen or phosphorus makes it especially useful in the detection of organophosphate pesticides and amine-containing drugs. Like an FID, it does not detect many common carrier gases or impurities. The NPD is about 300 times more sensitive in detecting nitrogen-containing compounds and 600 times more sensitive in detecting phosphorus-containing compounds compared with an FID. It does have some response to organic compounds, but at a level typically less than that seen in an FID. Besides nitrogen and phosphorus, an NPD also has an improved response over an FID for the detection of compounds containing sulfur, halogens, and arsenic.

The **electron capture detector (ECD)** is another type of selective detector used in GC. It is a radiation-based detector that is selective for compounds containing electronegative elements such as halogen atoms. It detects compounds based on the capture of electrons by electronegative atoms in the molecule. The electrons are produced by a radioactive source, such as ^3H or ^{63}Ni, that emits beta-particles (i.e., high-energy electrons) as part of their natural decay process. As these high-energy electrons are released, they collide with the carrier gas, usually argon or nitrogen. This produces a large number of secondary, low-energy electrons. In the absence of compounds eluting from the column, a steady stream of secondary electrons is produced that goes to a collector electrode and produces a current. When a compound containing electronegative atoms elutes from the column, the compound's atoms capture some of the secondary electrons and reduce the current produced at the collector electrode. This decrease in current allows the compound to be detected.

The design of an ECD consists of a radiation source and a collector electrode. The carrier gas that is used for the production of secondary electrons in the detector is one that is easily ionized, such as argon or nitrogen. A trace amount of methane is also usually included in the carrier gas to maintain the production of secondary electrons and to create a stable detector response.

An ECD can be used to detect most compounds containing electronegative atoms, such as halogen-, nitro-, and sulfur-containing compounds. It can also be used to detect polynuclear aromatic compounds, anhydrides, and conjugated carbonyl compounds. The ECD is widely used for the determination of chlorinated pesticides, polynuclear aromatic carcinogens, and organometallic compounds. Part of the reason for its popularity is its low limits of detection (i.e., 10^{-14} *M* to 10^{-16} *M*).

Another type of selective detector used in GC is the **flame photometric detector (FPD),** which is based on the release of light from excited atoms in a flame. This detector is mainly used for the detection of phosphorus- and sulfur-containing compounds that emit light at 526 and 394 nm, respectively. The selectivity of an FPD comes from the detection of light at an emission wavelength characteristic of a given type of atom. The design of an FPD is basically the same as that of an FID, but with the addition of a spectrometer with selected filters and a photomultiplier tube for measuring light emitted by the flame. The limit of detection of an FPD for compounds with these elements may approach 10^{-14} *M*.

One additional type of detector commonly used in GC is the mass spectrometer. The resulting combination of GC and mass spectrometry, known as GC/MS, is a powerful tool for both quantitating and identifying compounds in complex samples. The GC is used to separate each compound. The mass spectrometer subsequently ionized each eluted compound into fragment ions that are then sorted according to their mass/charge ratios. This sorting procedure gives rise to graphic representation called a mass spectrum. The mass spectrum is characteristic of a given compound, and the number of ions produced is proportional to the amount of compound present. Thus GC/MS can be used for both identification and quantitation of compounds as they elute from the column. It is especially useful in confirming the presence of drugs in urine or serum, as well as identifying the presence of a wide range of other components in biologic fluids.

GC Data Recording Systems. The last component of a typical GC system is the data recording system. It can consist of anything ranging from a simple strip-chart recorder to a dedicated computer. The purpose of this device is to acquire and store data obtained from the GC detector. For many types of detectors, such as a thermal conductivity detector or an FID, a simple strip-chart recorder or integrator is adequate for most analytic applications. However, other systems, such as those using GC/MS, require a dedicated computer for managing and analyzing the wealth of data obtained by the system. Most detector manufacturers have computers and software available for processing data from their equipment, storage of data, and maintaining records for quality control of the GC system.

Liquid Chromatography

One disadvantage of GC is that it can be used only to separate compounds that are naturally volatile or that can be converted to volatile derivatives. This limits its use to about 10% to 20% of all known compounds. One way of overcoming this limitation is to use an alternative technique, liquid chromatography (LC). As already discussed, LC is a chromatographic technique in which the mobile phase used is a liquid. As in GC the stationary phase in LC can be a solid, a liquid coated onto a solid support, or a support containing a chemically bonded layer. LC was the first type of chromatography developed, but it was overshadowed by the rapid development of GC in the 1950's and 60's. Currently LC is the dominant type of chromatography and is even replacing GC in some of its more traditional applications.

The main advantages of LC over GC are (1) it can be used for the separation of any compound that is soluble in a liquid phase, (2) the use of a liquid mobile phase allows LC to be used at lower temperatures than GC thereby allowing for better separation of compounds that are thermolabile, and (3) the retention of compounds in LC depends on their interaction with both the mobile phase and stationary phase; therefore retention of solutes can be varied by changing either the type of column or the solvent passing through it. One disadvantage of LC is that it is usually less efficient, or produces broader peaks than GC. This is due to the much larger diffusion coefficients of most compounds in gases vs liquids.

Of the many types of liquid chromatography available, each type can be characterized based on its overall efficiency, or performance. The term **low-performance liquid chromatography,** or **column chromatography,** is a term used to describe LC methods that use large, nonrigid support materials that typically have particles greater than 40 μm in diameter. The use of such supports gives rise to long separations with broad peaks and poor limits of detection. The nonrigid nature of the support also means that only low pressures or flow-rates can be used to apply mobile phase to it. This is usually done by gravity flow or through the use of a peristaltic pump. Low-performance LC is also usually characterized by sample being applied to the top of an open column and by detection based on fraction collection. Because of its simple system requirements and low cost, low-performance LC is popular in sample purification and removal of interferences from samples. It is also used in some analytic applications, but this is not as common because of its low efficiency, long analysis times, and poor limits of detection.

A more efficient method is the technique of **high-performance liquid chromatography,** or **HPLC.** This method differs from low-performance LC in that it uses small, uniform, and rigid supports, usually only 3 to 10 μm in diameter.

The use of such supports produces much narrower peaks than those seen in low-performance LC and results in improved limits of detection and shorter separation times. However, to work with the smaller diameter supports, higher pressures are needed to pass mobile phase through the column. This requires the use of special pumps. Other differences between HPLC and low-performance LC are that samples are usually applied using a closed system (i.e., injection valve), and detection is typically performed on line using a flow-through detector. This makes separations in HPLC fairly easy to automate. These characteristics, along with fast analysis times and good limits of detection, have made HPLC the technique of choice for many analytic applications in the clinical laboratory. An example of a typical separation in HPLC is given in Fig. 12-10.

HPLC and low-performance LC are usually performed with columns, but supports consisting of flat beds can also be used. When these flat beds or planar supports are used in LC, the technique is called **thin-layer chromatography** (TLC). This method is particularly useful in screening a larger number of samples for the presence of a known set of compounds such as drugs or amino acids. A wide range of support materials and stationary phases are available for use in TLC. If paper is used as both the support and stationary phase in TLC, the technique is referred to as **paper chromatography.** A popular TLC commercial method that is used for drug detection is the TOXI·LAB system. It is composed of two extraction systems, TOXI·LAB A for basic/some neutral drugs and TOXI·LAB B for acidic/other neutral drugs. An unknown is identified by comparing its Rf values (and spot colors, etc.) with those of the standards.

In any of these LC methods, retention and elution of compounds in the chromatographic system will depend on how these compounds interact with both the mobile and stationary phases. To describe how solutes are retained on a column with different solvents, the terms **weak mobile phase** and **strong mobile phase** are used. The term strong mobile phase is used to describe a solvent that quickly elutes compounds from the column (i.e., produces low retention or small k' values for the compounds). This occurs if the mobile phase is very similar to the stationary phase in its chemical properties. For example, a polar solvent would be a strong mobile phase for a column that contained a polar stationary phase. In contrast, the term weak mobile phase is used to describe a

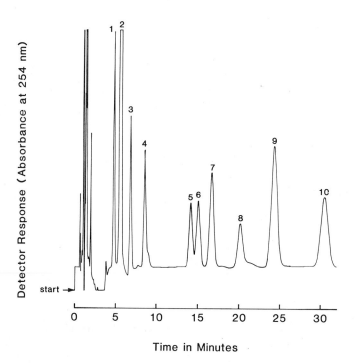

Fig. 12-10 Separation of barbiturates by HPLC. The peaks represent (1) methyprylon, (2) phenobarbital, (3) butabarbital, (4) butalbital, (5) pentobarbital, (6) amobarbital, (7) glutethimide, (8) secobarbital, (9) nitrazepam internal standard, and (10) methaqualone. (From Kaplan LA, Pesce AJ: Methods in clinical chemistry, St Louis, 1987, Mosby–Year Book.)

solvent that only slowly elutes compounds from a column (i.e., gives high retention or large k' values); this occurs if the solvent is very different from the stationary phase in its chemical properties. For instance, a nonpolar solvent would be a weak mobile phase on a column containing a polar stationary phase.

To control the elution of sample components in LC, the strength of the mobile phase can be varied during the chromatographic run. The use of a constant mobile phase composition to elute solutes is known as **isocratic elution.** Although this type of elution is simple and inexpensive to do, it does make it difficult to elute all solutes with good resolution and in a reasonable amount of time. The resolution and time of a separation can usually be improved by using an alternative approach, **gradient elution.** This is done by injecting the sample while a weak mobile phase is passing through the column and then later switching to a stronger mobile phase to elute the retained components. The change from weak to strong mobile phase can be done either in a step-wise, linear, or nonlinear fashion. Step-wise and linear gradients are most commonly used.

All techniques in LC, regardless of whether they are high- or low-performance methods, can be classified according to the way in which they separate compounds. The five most common types of LC in terms of the separation method are (1) adsorption chromatography, (2) partition chromatography, (3) ion-exchange chromatography, (4) affinity chromatography, and (5) size exclusion chromatography. Each is characterized by its own particular combination of stationary phases and mobile phases. This allows each to separate compounds through different types of chemical interactions.

Adsorption or **liquid-solid chromatography** is a technique that separates compounds based on their adsorption to an underivatized solid support. This technique is similar to GSC in that the same material is used as both the stationary phase and support material. In fact, many of the supports used in GSC are also used in adsorption chromatography. Examples of these supports include silica and alumina.

Although this was the first type of column liquid chromatography developed, it is not as widely used as other LC methods. One reason for this is that the supports used in adsorption chromatography have very strong retention of some compounds, making them difficult to elute from the column. Nonsymmetric peaks and variable retention times are also common in adsorption chromatography. However, adsorption chromatography does have a major advantage in that it is able to retain and separate compounds that can not be separated by other LC methods. A common use for this is in the separation of geometric isomers.

Partition or **liquid-liquid chromatography** separates compounds based on their partitioning between a liquid mobile phase and a liquid stationary phase coated on a solid support. The support material used in partition chromatography is usually silica coated with some liquid that is not readily soluble in the mobile phase.

There are two main types of partition chromatography: **normal-phase liquid chromatography (NPLC)** and **reversed-phase liquid chromatography (RPLC)**. Normal-phase liquid chromatography is characterized by the use of a liquid stationary phase that is polar in nature. It was the first type of partition chromatography developed but is currently not as popular as reversed-phase methods. Because NPLC has a polar stationary phase, it retains polar compounds most strongly. However, it may also be used for separating nonpolar compounds. The weak mobile phase in NPLC is a nonpolar liquid, usually an organic solvent. The strong mobile phase is a polar liquid such as water or methanol.

RPLC is the second type of partition chromatography. Its name is derived from the fact that it uses a nonpolar stationary phase, which is less polar chemically (opposite or "reversed" in polarity) from that used in NPLC. At present, RPLC is the most popular type of liquid chromatography. Its applications include the separation of a wide range of both nonpolar and polar compounds. The main reason for the popularity of RPLC is that its weak mobile phase is a polar solvent such as water. Because samples are usually applied to LC columns in the weak mobile phase, this makes RPLC ideal for the separation of solutes in aqueous-based samples such as biologic compounds. This makes it especially attractive for use in clinical chemistry. Its applications in this field have included drug confirmation, amino acid analysis, and hormone separations. It is generally the method of choice in developing any new LC analytic method for the detection of small organic-based compounds.

Although both NPLC and RPLC were originally developed using liquid stationary phases coated onto solid supports, this has the disadvantage that the stationary phase will eventually bleed from the column. This affects both the reproducibility of the separation and the overall column lifetime. To overcome this problem, bonded phases are now commonly used in both NPLC and RPLC. Typical bonded-phases used in NPLC include aminopropyl and cyanopropyl supports. Bonded-phases typically used in RPLC are octyl (C8) and octydecyl (C18) supports.

Ion-exchange chromatography (IEC) is a liquid chromatographic technique in which compounds are separated based on their charge and their different extents of adsorption onto a support that contains fixed charges on its surface. It is a relatively common technique used in the separation of charged compounds, including inorganic ions and biologic compounds such as peptides and proteins. Common applications of IEC in clinical chemistry include its use in separating amino acids, isoenzymes, and various organic ions.

There are two general types of stationary phases used in IEC: *cation exchangers* and *anion exchangers*. Cation exchangers contain negatively charged groups on their surface and are used in the separation of positively charged ions. Anion exchangers contain positively charged groups on their surface and are used in the separation of negatively charged ions. These charged groups may be attached to a variety of support materials. Cross-linked polystyrene is commonly used as the support when inorganic ions or small organic ions are to be separated. Carbohydrate-based resins, such as agarose or dextran, are commonly used when separating larger ions or biologic molecules.

Elution of solutes in IEC is controlled by adding an ion to the mobile phase that competes with sample ions for charged sites on the support. As the concentration of the competing ion increases, the sample ions elute sooner. Depending on what stationary phase and sample ion are being used, elution may also be adjusted by controlling the pH of the mobile phase. This can affect the charge on either the stationary phase or the sample ion.

Ion-pair chromatography (IPC) is a special hybrid-type of LC technique. It combines the high efficiency of RPLC with the ability to separate compounds based on their charges. IPC is usually based on the use of a standard reversed-phase column along with an ion-pairing agent in the mobile phase. The ion-pairing agent is usually a surfactant that has an ionic group at one end and a nonpolar group on the other. The purpose of the ion-pairing agent is to combine with ionic compounds of the opposite charge in the sample. The result is a neutral complex that is retained by the nonpolar stationary phase. As a result, sample ions are separated based on the types of complexes they form with the ion-pairing agent and how these complexes are retained by the column.

IPC is particularly useful in the separation of compounds that are poorly resolved by ion-exchange chromatography. Factors that can be varied to optimize a separation in IPC include the strength of the mobile phase, the concentration and type of ion-pairing agent, and the ionic strength and pH of the mobile phase. Examples of applications for IPC in clinical chemistry include its use in the separation of catecholamines and various amino acid metabolites.

Affinity chromatography (AC) is a liquid chromatographic technique that is based on the specific reversible interactions that occur between the binding of an enzyme with its substrate or the binding of an antibody with an antigen. These types of interactions are used in AC by immobilizing one of a pair of interacting molecules onto a solid support and placing it into a column. The immobilized molecule, known as the affinity ligand, can then be used as a selective adsorbent for the complementary molecule. Samples are applied to the column under conditions in which the molecule of interest will bind to the affinity ligand. Other components in the sample, because of the selective nature of this interaction, will pass through nonretained. The solute is then later eluted from the column by changing the pH or ionic strength of the mobile phase, or by applying organic solvents or competing agents that displace the analyte from the column.

The stationary phase in affinity chromatography, the immobilized ligand, is the main factor that determines what compounds can be separated by a particular affinity column. There are several types of affinity ligands, but all can be classified into one of two categories: high-specificity ligands and general, or group-specific ligands. High-specificity ligands are compounds that bind to only one or a few very closely related molecules. Examples of these include antibodies (for binding antigens), substrates (for binding enzymes), and single-stranded nucleic acids (for binding complementary strands of nucleic acids). General, or group-specific ligands are molecules that bind to a family or class of related molecules. Examples of these include lectins (for binding molecules containing sugar residues), phenylbo-

ronic acid (for binding compounds with vicinal diol groups), and synthetic dyes such as Cibacron Blue (for binding a wide range of enzymes and other proteins). Note from this list that the affinity ligand does not necessarily have to be of biologic origin. Uses of such affinity ligands in clinical chemistry include both preparative work and analytic applications. One analytic application of particular interest is the use of AC in the determination of glycosylated hemoglobins in the long-term management of diabetic patients. A commercial system, called the Column.Mate, is now available from Helena Laboratories that automates this method.

Size exclusion chromatography (SEC) is a liquid chromatographic technique used to separate molecules according to differences in their size via the different interactions of solutes with a porous support. The ability of a molecule to enter the pores of the support will depend on the molecule's size. To separate compounds in SEC, a support material is used that has a certain range of pore sizes. As solutes travel through this support, small molecules can enter the pores whereas large molecules can not. Because the larger molecules sample a smaller volume of the column, they elute before the smaller molecules. The result is a separation based on size or molecular weight.

The ideal support in SEC is a porous material that does not chemically interact with the solute molecules. In low-performance SEC a nonrigid support such as dextran, agarose, or polyacrylamide is most commonly used for aqueous samples. In high-performance SEC the support material commonly used is diol-bonded silica. In both cases the size of the pores in the support or its degree of cross-linking is what determines the size and molecular weight range that can be separated by the system. The mobile phase in SEC plays a relatively minor role and is not usually a factor in determining the retention of compounds. A common use of SEC in clinical chemistry is in the separation of large molecules, such as proteins, from peptides and other smaller biologic compounds. In research it is also used to determine the molecular weight of compounds by comparing their elution times or volumes with those obtained for known molecular weight standards.

Instrumentation in Liquid Chromatography

The instrumentation used in LC is similar in many respects to that used in GC. This again con-

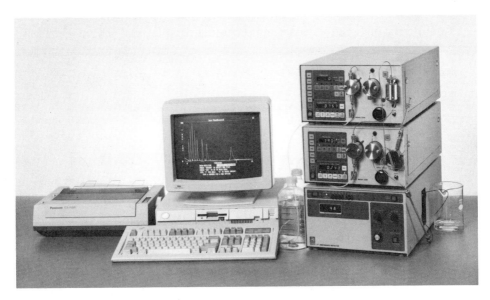

Fig. 12-11 A commercial gradient HPLC system. (Courtesy ISCO.)

sists of a mobile phase source, an injector, a column, a detector, and a means of acquiring and recording data from the detector. A typical HPLC-gradient system is shown in Fig. 12-11; a summary of other commercial systems is provided in Table 12-2. There are, however, several important differences between LC and GC equipment. For example, because LC depends on the use of liquid mobile phase, a solvent reservoir is used as the mobile phase source rather than a gas cylinder. This reservoir can consist of anything from a simple flask to more sophisticated systems with temperature control, constant mixing, and constant purging of undesirable gases from the solvent.

Liquid Chromatography Pumps. Another difference between LC and GC is that a pump is used in LC to deliver mobile phase to the system. In low-performance LC, gravity is often used as the pump. In HPLC, however, a mechanical pump is needed because more force or pressure is needed to create flow through the column. Such a pump must (1) have precise and accurate flow with no pulsations, (2) work at high pressures (typically up to 6000 psi), (3) have low internal volume, and (4) be made of materials that do not react with the solvent or its contents.

Two types of pumps commonly used in high-performance liquid chromatography are syringe pumps and reciprocating pumps. In a syringe pump, mobile phase is forced out of the reservoir at a constant flow-rate by a syringe that is slowly pushed downward by a stepper motor. This type of pump is useful for accurate work at very slow

flow-rates and delivers essentially pulse-free flow. However, it is limited by the need to periodically stop the pump and refill the solvent reservoir. Flow of mobile phase in the opposite direction is prevented by the use of check valves, which allow the fluid to travel in only one direction through the solvent chamber. Unlike the syringe pump, the reciprocating pump does not require that the solvent chamber be manually filled with mobile phase because this is automatically done as part of each pumping cycle. However, this type of pump is not as accurate as a syringe pump at very low flow-rates. Also, some pulsations in the flow-rate can occur as the pistons go in and out of the solvent chambers during each cycle.

For work using gradient elution some means of mixing two or more solvents together is also needed as part of the pumping system. This may be done either before or after the pump. **Low-pressure mixing** is a method of forming gradients in which solvents are mixed before the pumps. This is a common technique used to form gradients in low-performance LC. Low-pressure mixing can also be used in HPLC by controlling the relative amount of each solvent going into a pump through the use of a special proportioning valve. This is a relatively inexpensive means of forming a gradient in HPLC because only one pump is required. However, this technique is not very accurate at low flow-rates or when only a small amount of a particular solvent is added to the mobile phase mixture (i.e., <5% of the total composition).

Mixing solvents after they pass through the

Table 12-2 Commercial high-performance liquid chromatographic systems and detectors

Supplier*	HPLC systems†	RI detectors	Absorbance detectors	Fluorescence detectors	EC detectors
Alcott Chromatography	X				
Alltech Associates	X		X		X
American Ultraviolet Co.			X	X	
Amicon	X				
The Anspec Co.	X	X	X	X	X
Applied Biosystems	X		X	X	X
Applied Automation	X				
Autochrom	X				
Axxiom Chromatography	X	X	X	X	X
Bacharach			X		X
Beckman Instruments	X	X	X	X	
BHK			X	X	
Bioanalytical Systems	X		X		X
Bio-Rad Laboratories	X	X	X	X	X
Buchler Instruments			X		
Carlo Erba	X		X		
Chrompack	X	X	X		
Custom Sensors & Technology			X	X	
Dionex Corp.	X		X	X	X
Dorr-Oliver	X				
DuPont	X	X	X		
Dychrom	X		X	X	
EG & G PAR					X
ESA	X		X	X	X
Fisher Scientific Co.			X	X	
The Foxboro Co.			X		
Galileo Electro-Optics Corp.			X	X	
Genex Corp.	X		X		
Gilson Medical Electronics	X	X	X	X	X
Gow-Mac Instrument Co.			X		
Groton Technology			X		
Hewlett-Packard Co.	X	X	X	X	
Hitachi Instruments	X	X	X	X	X
HPLC Technology	X				
Interactive Microwave	X				X
ISCO	X	X	X	X	
Jasco	X	X	X	X	X
JM Science		X	X	X	X
Johnson Yokogawa Corp.				X	
Kontron Instruments			X	X	
Lachat Instruments	X				
LDC Analytical	X	X	X	X	
Linear Instruments Corp.			X	X	
McPherson			X	X	
The Munhall Co.	X	X	X	X	X
Nicolet Instrument Corp.	X				
Optical Technology Devices			X	X	
Oriel Corp.			X		
Perkin-Elmer	X	X	X	X	
Pharmacia LKB Biotechnology	X	X	X		X
Phenomenex	X				
Philips Export B.V.	X		X	X	
Philips Scientific	X	X	X	X	X
Quaracell Products			X		
Rainin Instrument Co.	X	X	X	X	X

Continued

*Data shown includes manufacturers and manufacturer/distributors listed in *Anal Chem* 62:71G 1990.
†Abbreviations: HPLC = high-performance liquid chromatography, RI = refractive index, EC = electrochemical.

Table 12-2 Commercial high-performance liquid chromatographic systems and detectors—cont'd

Supplier*	HPLC systems†	RI detectors	Absorbance detectors	Fluorescence detectors	EC detectors
Richard Scientific	X	X	X	X	X
Sanki Laboratory			X		
Scientific Technologies					X
Scientific Systems	X		X		
Sensorex					X
Separations Technologies	X				
Shimadzu	X	X	X	X	X
Sonntek	X	X	X	X	
Spectra-Physics	X	X	X	X	
SpectroVision			X	X	
Spectrum Scientific			X		
St. John Associates	X			X	
Sunshine Technology Corp.				X	
Tegal Scientific	X		X		X
Thomson Instrument Co.	X	X	X	X	
Timberline Instruments	X				
Tokyo Rikakikai Co.	X		X		
Tracor Instruments	X				
Varex Corp.	X		X		
Varian Instrument Group	X	X	X	X	
Vestec Corp.	X		X		
VG Instruments	X				
Viscotek Corp.		X			
Waters Chromatography	X	X	X	X	X
YMC	X	X	X		

pumps is referred to as **high-pressure mixing.** This requires the use of one pump for each solvent to be added to the mobile phase mixture. Although this method is more expensive than low-pressure mixing, it is more accurate at slow flow-rates and when small amounts of a given solvent are used in the mobile phase mixture.

Liquid Chromatography Injectors. Injection of a sample onto an LC system can be performed using either an open or closed system. An open system is the approach usually used in low-performance LC and involves placing sample directly at the exposed top of the column. Closed-system injection is the technique usually used in HPLC. This method involves injecting sample with a syringe either through a septum or into a loop on an injection valve. This is performed in a manner similar to that in GC, but with no heater in the injection port.

Liquid Chromatography Columns. As in GC, the column used in LC can be either a packed column or a capillary column. Like GC, preparative scale work in LC is typically performed using packed columns because they have a larger sample capacity. However, unlike GC, most analytic work in LC is also done using packed columns. Although capillary columns offer the same theoretic advantages in LC as in GC (i.e., narrower peaks, faster separation times, and better limits of detection), LC capillary columns must have much smaller diameters than GC capillaries before these advantages can be realized. Although work is progressing in making this possible, this is still an active area of research and such columns are not yet common in clinical laboratories.

Liquid Chromatography Detectors. The next component of the LC system is the detector. Some of the more common LC detectors used include (1) refractive index detectors, (2) absorbance detectors, (3) fluorescence detectors, (4) conductivity detectors, and (5) electrochemical detectors.

The **refractive index detector (RI)** is one of the few universal detectors available in LC. This detector measures a bulk property of the mobile phase, namely its ability to bend or refract light (i.e., its refractive index). This property varies as the composition of the mobile phase changes, such as when compounds elute from the column.

By monitoring the resulting change in the refractive index, the presence of solutes can be detected.

In a simple RI detector, light from a source is passed through a flow-cell made up of two sides: one side containing mobile phase eluting from the column and the other side containing a reference sample, usually pure mobile phase. As light passes through the cell to a photodetector, it is bent at the boundary between the two solutions if their refractive indices are different. This decreases the amount of light that reaches the photodetector and allows the presence of compounds in the mobile phase to be detected.

The main advantage of using an RI detector is that it allows the detection of essentially any compound. This makes it useful in work where the properties of the compound of interest are not yet known. This is also the detector of choice for work with carbohydrates or in the separation of polymers by size-exclusion chromatography. Some disadvantages of RI detectors are that they do not have very good limits of detection (i.e., usually 10^{-5} to 10^{-6} M) and cannot be easily used with gradient elution. To avoid baseline fluctuations with these detectors, it is also necessary that the temperature of the chromatographic system be controlled to prevent changes in the refractive index of the mobile phase with time.

The **UV/Vis absorbance detector** is another common type of detector used in LC. This detector measures the ability of compounds to absorb light at one or more wavelengths in the ultraviolet or visible range. There are three types of absorbance detectors currently available: fixed wavelength detectors, variable wavelength detectors, and diode array detectors. In a fixed wavelength detector, absorbance of the compounds in the mobile phase over only one wavelength range is monitored by the system at all times. This wavelength range is usually around 254 nm, a region in which mercury light sources have intense emission and in which many organic compounds will absorb light. A fixed wavelength detector is the simplest and least expensive of the absorbance detectors. But it is limited in terms of its flexibility and the types of compounds it can monitor.

In a **variable wavelength detector,** absorbance of eluting solutes in a single wavelength range is monitored at any given time, but this range can be easily varied over a wide spectral region. With many current instruments, the wavelengths that can be monitored range from 190 to 900 nm using a single instrument; this is achieved by adding more advanced optics to the absorbance detector, such as a grating or prism monochromator. Although more expensive than fixed wavelength detectors, variable wavelength detectors are more versatile and thus can select for a wider range of compounds (i.e., they can choose a wavelength for measurement that maximizes absorbance for a given compound but minimizes absorbance because of possible interferences from other substances in the sample). A typical limit of detection for a variable wavelength detector is 10^{-8} M.

A **diode array detector** is the third type of absorbance detector. This detector is capable of simultaneously monitoring the absorbance of eluting compounds at several different wavelengths. This is accomplished by using a series or array of photodetectors within the instrument, each of which responds to light at a different wavelength. By using such an array, an entire spectrum of a compound can be taken as it elutes from the column. Diode array detectors are currently more expensive than variable or fixed-wavelength detectors, but they do have the advantage of being able to more easily detect the presence of poorly resolved peaks. This makes them useful in confirming that a given peak represents only one eluting compound.

The **fluorescence detector** is another type of LC detector. It is more selective than either the RI or UV/Vis absorbance detectors and has lower limits of detection. As its name implies, this detector measures the ability of compounds to fluoresce, or to absorb and reemit light at a given set of wavelengths. The wavelengths absorbed and emitted in this process are characteristic of a given compound. By properly choosing which wavelengths of light are absorbed (or used to excite the molecule) and which wavelengths of emission are monitored, a signal can be obtained for the compound of interest with few or no interferences from other eluting components. The design of an LC fluorescence detector is essentially the same as a normal spectrofluorometer. This consists of a light source, a sample cell, a photodetector, and one or two monochromators for selection of the excitation and/or emission wavelengths. The main advantages of a fluorescence detector are its selectivity and its low limits of detection (i.e., its selectivity arises from the excitation and emission wavelengths used), which determine what compounds will fluoresce and be monitored; its detection limits are often in the 10^{-10} M range (because of a low background signal). Substances that can be monitored using fluorescence detectors include many drugs and their metabolites, proteins, and environmental pollutants. These detectors can also be used to detect compounds that can be easily converted to fluorescent derivatives, such as alcohols, amino acids, and peptides. Although fluorescence detectors can be used with gradient elution, extremely pure mobile phases must be used for this. This is necessary because even trace impurities can affect the background signal or quench the fluorescence of compounds eluting from the column.

A **conductivity detector** is another type of common LC detector that measures the ability of the mobile phase to conduct a current when placed in an electrical field and is dependent on the number of ions or ionic compounds present in the mobile phase. The design of a conductivity detector is made up of a flow-cell with two electrodes. These electrodes apply an electric field across the mobile phase in the flow-cell and measure the resulting current as ionic compounds elute from the column and pass through the detector.

Because conductivity detectors can be used to detect any compound that is ionic or weakly ionic, they are widely used in modern methods of ion chromatography. Limits of detection for conductivity detectors are usually around 10^{-6} M. To obtain such limits of detection, it is necessary to keep the background conductivity of the mobile phase as low as possible by using a low ionic strength mobile phase and/or by using special systems for reducing the conductivity of the mobile phase after it leaves the column.

A fifth detector used in LC is the **electrochemical detector** and is often referred to as LC/EC. Electrochemical detectors can be used to detect a wide range of compounds that can undergo electrochemical reactions (i.e., oxidation or reduction). This is commonly done amperometrically by measuring the loss or uptake of electrons from eluting compounds as they pass between two or more electrodes at a given potential difference.

One advantage of using electrochemical detectors is that they can be made relatively specific for a given compound or group of compounds by properly choosing the potential conditions at the electrodes. Examples of compounds that can be monitored by these detectors include aldehydes, ketones, aromatics, phenols, peroxides, aromatic amines, purines, and dihydroxy compounds (such as some carbohydrates). These can usually be detected at low concentrations, typically 10^{-11} M. This low limit of detection is due to the extreme accuracy with which many electrical mea-

surements, such as current, can be made.

Besides using a selective detector, the ability of an LC system to detect a compound at low concentrations can also be enhanced by derivatization. Derivatization can not only be used to improve the response of a compound on a detector, but it can also help to improve the separation of the compound from other sample components. Derivatization in LC is usually performed using either precolumn or postcolumn methods. On-column techniques are rarely used.

Postcolumn derivatization involves combining mobile phase leaving the column with a reagent that converts eluting compounds into a more easily detected form. A typical reactor used in postcolumn derivatization consists of a pump for applying reagent, a mixing tee for combining the reagent with mobile phase, and a reaction chamber. A pulse-dampener is also usually included to prevent pulsations in detector signal because of the postcolumn reagent pump. Postcolumn derivatization is useful in the detection of a wide variety of compounds. Examples of its applications include the detection of amino acids, steroids, catechols, cannabinoids, and reducing carbohydrates.

Precolumn derivatization is similar to postcolumn derivatization but involves modifying compounds in the sample before they are applied to the column. This has the advantage of being able to improve either the separation or detection of solutes. Many of the procedures used in precolumn derivatization are simple organic reactions with reagents and supplies available from chemical manufacturers. Because it does not require extra chromatographic equipment, precolumn derivatization is often less expensive to perform than postcolumn derivatization. However, it is also more difficult to automate and usually requires more time than postcolumn derivatization to perform. Care must also be taken to use a reaction that results in only one product per compound of interest. This is needed to avoid the creation of multiple solute peaks, which may contribute to a greater chance of peak overlapping and a possible loss of resolution in the separation.

Liquid Chromatography Data Recording Systems. The last component of a typical LC system is the data recording system that can consist of a strip-chart recorder, an integrator, or a dedicated computer. Although many types of detectors have relatively simple outputs and can be used with only strip-chart recorders, computer workstations are becoming popular for use with almost any type of LC system. Part of the reason for this is that they allow automatic generation of calibration curves from standards, calculation of unknown results, and even reporting of data. Many of these systems also make it possible to automate the chromatographic system. Most manufacturers of chromatographic equipment either provide such systems or use hardware and software that are already available. The best type to use for a given application is often determined by the complexity of the data to be analyzed and the computer experience of the user. If the computer system is also to be used for control of the all or part of the chromatographic system, compatibility with existing system components must also be considered.

Review Questions

1. The resolution of a chromatographic separation can be increased by using all of the following except:
   A. A longer column
   B. A stronger mobile phase
   C. A more efficient column
   D. A stationary phase with higher compound retention
2. All of the following are common derivatization techniques used in GC except:
   A. Alkylation
   B. Hydroxylation
   C. Silylation
   D. Acylation
3. All of the following are characteristic of HPLC except:
   A. Small support material
   B. Fast separations
   C. Difficult to automate
   D. Low-limits of detection
   E. Narrow peaks
4. Which of the following can be used in GC to detect a drug containing nitrogen in its structure:
   A. Thermal conductivity detector
   B. Flame ionization detector
   C. Thermionic detector
   D. Mass spectrometer
   E. All of the above

Match the following LC techniques in Column A with the types of compounds most strongly retained by them in Column B:

Column A	Column B
5. Normal-phase liquid chromatography	A. Positively-charged compounds
6. Cation-exchange IEC	B. Negatively-charged compounds
7. Reversed-phased liquid chromatography	C. Nonpolar compounds
8. Anion-exchange IEC	D. Polar compounds

9. A method of forming gradients by mixing solvents before entering the HPLC pump(s) is called "high pressure mixing."
   A. True
   B. False
10. The retardation factor (R_f value) is the ratio of the distance traveled by a compound divided by the distance traveled by the mobile phase (solvent) in a given period of time.
    A. True
    B. False
11. In size exclusion chromatography (SEC), smaller molecules will tend to elute from the column first followed by larger molecules.
    A. True
    B. False
12. An LC technique that involves the specific/reversible interaction between an immobilized molecule on a support and biologic molecules in the sample is called:
    A. Ion-pair chromatography
    B. Size exclusion chromatography
    C. Affinity chromatography
    D. Thin layer chromatography

Answers

1. B 2. B 3. C 4. E 5. D 6. A 7. C 8. B 9. B
10. A 11. B 12. C

Bibliography

Braithwaite A, Smith FJ: Chromatographic methods, ed 4, New York, 1985, Chapman and Hall.

Bowers LD: Liquid chromatography. In Kaplan LA, Pesce AJ, eds: Clinical chemistry: theory, analysis and correlation, ed 2, St Louis, 1989, Mosby–Year Book.

Grob RL: Modern practice of gas chromatography, ed 2, New York, 1985, John Wiley & Sons.

Hawkes S, Gossman D, Kartkopf H et al: Preferred stationary liquids for gas chromatography, J Chromatogr Sci 13:115, 1975.

Karger BL, Snyder LR, and Horvath C: An introduction to separation science, New York, 1973, John Wiley & Sons.

Poklis A: Gas chromatography. In Kaplan LA, Pesce AJ, eds: Clinical chemistry: theory, analysis and correlation, ed 2, St Louis, 1989, Mosby–Year Book.

Ravindranath B: Principles and practice of chromatography, New York, 1989, John Wiley & Sons.

Skoog DA: Principles of instrumental analysis, ed 3, New York, 1985, Saunders College Publishing.

Snyder LR, Kirkland JJ: Introduction to modern liquid chromatography, ed 2, New York, 1979, John Wiley & Sons.

Tabor MW: Chromatography: theory and practice. In Kaplan LA, Pesce AJ, eds: Clinical chemistry: theory, analysis and correlation, ed 2, St Louis, 1989, Mosby–Year Book.

13

Nuclear Radiation and Its Measurement

I-WEN CHEN

Basic Structure of an Atom
Nuclear Radiation and Radioactivity
Properties of Radiation and Interaction with Matter
Measurement of Nuclear Radiation

This chapter will consider the basic structure of the atom as it relates to the existence of isotope, the modes of radioactive decay associated with radionuclides commonly used in clinical laboratories, properties of nuclear radiation and its interaction with matter, principles of operation of two basic types of nuclear radiation detectors (gas-filled detectors and scintillation detectors), problems associated with nuclear radiation measurements, and the safe use and disposal of radioactive materials.

Basic Structure of an Atom

An atom is the smallest particle of an element that can exist either alone or in combination. The primary building blocks of atoms, the electron, the proton, and the neutron, are termed elementary particles. According to the planetary model of the atom developed by Rutherford in 1911, the atom consists of a central, small, positively charged body (the nucleus is composed of protons and neutrons) around which the negatively charged electrons move in defined orbits. Although the Rutherford model is oversimplified, it can be used to explain many atomic phenomena satisfactorily. The planetary model of an atom of carbon is illustrated in Fig. 13-1.

The nucleus of carbon contains six protons and six neutrons. Because complete atoms are electrically neutral, six orbiting electrons are present in the carbon atom to match the six protons in the nucleus. They move around the nucleus in a series of orbits, or shells at varying dis-

tances from the nucleus, much as the planets of the solar system travel in different orbits at varying distances from the sun. The orbits, or shells are called K, L, M, etc., starting from the innermost orbit to the nucleus. Only two electrons can be accommodated in the K shell; the L shell of the carbon atom contains the remaining four.

The physical and chemical differences between the atoms of different elements depend on the number of protons and neutrons contained in an atomic nucleus, which determines both the mass and charge of the nucleus, and the number and arrangements of the electrons, which determine the chemical properties of elements.

There are several important terms that are helpful in understanding atomic structure:

Nucleon A collective term for protons and neutrons in the nucleus.
Atomic number Z The number of protons in the nucleus.

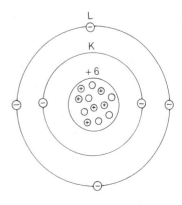

Fig. 13-1 Planetary model of carbon atom. (From Kaplan LA, Pesce AJ, eds: Clinical chemistry: theory, analysis, and correlation, ed 2, St Louis, 1989, Mosby–Year Book.)

Atomic mass number A   The total number of nucleons in the nucleus.

Neutron number, N   The number of neutrons in the nucleus.

Nuclide   A nucleus with particular Z and A numbers.

Element E   A nucleus with a given Z number.

Isotope   Nuclides with the same Z but different A numbers (various nuclear species of the same element).

Isobar   Nuclides with the same A but different Z numbers (different elements with the same atomic mass).

The atomic mass number ^{A} is represented as a left superscript and the atomic number $_Z$ is represented as a left subscript to the chemical symbol. Thus element E is written as $^A_Z E$. The most abundant, naturally occurring, stable isotope of carbon has six protons and six neutrons in the nucleus. The atomic number Z is therefore 6; the atomic mass number A is 12 (A = Z + N); and the whole atom may be written as $^{12}_6 C$. The other naturally occurring but less abundant isotope of carbon is $^{13}_6 C$, which contains seven neutrons in the nucleus. $^{12}_6 C$ and $^{13}_6 C$ are both stable isotopes of carbon, and neither is radioactive. The best-known radioactive isotope of carbon is $^{14}_6 C$, which contains six protons and eight neutrons.

Examples of other groups of isotopes of an element commonly used in clinical laboratories are $^1_1 H$, $^2_1 H$, $^3_1 H$, $^{125}_{53} I$, $^{127}_{53} I$, and $^{131}_{53} I$. $^1_1 H$ is the most abundant, naturally occurring isotope of hydrogen and has one proton but no neutron in the nucleus. $^2_1 H$ is a stable isotope of hydrogen and is known as deuterium because its nucleus contains two nuclear particles, one proton and one neutron. $^3_1 H$, called tritium, is a radioactive isotope of hydrogen, the nucleus of which is formed by a combination of a proton and two neutrons. All isotopes of hydrogen have a single circling electron and therefore have identical chemical properties; however, their physical properties are different. For example, they will have different boiling and freezing points. The tritium nucleus is unstable and will undergo radioactive transitions to become a different and stable nucleus, the nucleus of helium. The naturally occurring stable isotope of iodine is $^{127}_{53} I$. The other two isotopes of iodine mentioned here are radioactive isotopes with different numbers of neutrons in their nucleus, as indicated by their atomic mass numbers. In many cases the atomic number subscript is redundant because the atomic number

and the chemical symbol both identify the chemical species. Therefore except in some equations describing nuclear reactions, the subscript is normally omitted (such as ^{14}C, ^3H, and ^{125}I).

Nuclear Radiation and Radioactivity

The release of energy or matter during the transformation of an unstable atom to a more stable atom is termed nuclear radiation. The numbers and arrangement of protons and neutrons in the nucleus of an atom determine whether the nucleus is stable or unstable.

Nuclear Stability. There are favored neutron-to-proton ratios among stable nuclides. The ratio is equal to or close to unity for the light nuclides. When the atomic mass number exceeds 40, no stable nuclides exist with equal numbers of neutrons and protons because as the number of protons increases, the repulsive coulombic forces between the protons increase at a greater rate than the attractive nuclear force does. Therefore the addition of extra neutrons is necessary to increase the average distance between protons in the nucleus to reduce the coulombic force. For heavy nuclei the neutron-to-proton ratio is 1.5 or greater. For example, the heaviest stable isotope of lead, ^{208}Pb, has a neutron-to-proton ratio of 1:53.

Fig. 13-2 illustrates the relationship between the neutron and proton numbers of the stable nuclides. An imaginary line, called the line of stability, represented by a dashed line in the graph, can be obtained from the neutron-proton plot; the stable nuclides are clustered around this line. Nuclides deficient in protons lie below the line of stability and are unstable. Nuclides deficient in neutrons lie above the line and are also unstable. The graph also illustrates the fact that as nuclides become heavier, more neutrons are required to maintain stability.

In addition to the favored neutron-to-proton ratio, the stable nuclides tend to favor even numbers. For example, 168 out of approximately 280 known stable nuclides have even numbers of both protons and neutrons, reflecting the tendency of nuclides to achieve stable arrangements by pairing up nucleons in the nucleus.

Modes of Radioactive Decay. Unstable nuclides are generally transformed into stable nuclides by one of the radioactive-decay (disintegration) processes described in the following sections.

Decay by Alpha-Particle Emission. An alpha (α) particle consists of two neutrons and two pro-

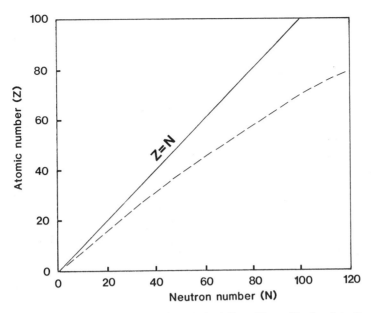

Fig. 13-2 Neutron-photon rations for stable isotopes, dashed line. (From Kaplan LA, Pesce AJ, eds: Clinical chemistry: theory, analysis, and correlation, ed 2, St Louis, 1989, Mosby–Year Book.)

tons and is essentially a helium nucleus. Heavy nuclides that must lose mass to achieve nuclear stability frequently decay by alpha-particle emission because alpha-particle emission is an effective way to reduce the mass number. The emission of one alpha particle removes two neutrons and two protons from the nucleus, resulting in the reduction of an atomic number by 2 and a mass number by 4. Very heavy radioactive nuclides that decay with alpha-particle emission are of little interest in clinical laboratories. An example of alpha-particle decay is as follows:

$$^{226}_{88}RA \rightarrow\ ^{222}_{86}Rn +\ ^{4}_{2}He \text{ (alpha particle)}$$

Decay by Beta-Particle Emission. Beta (β) particles are either negatively charged electrons (negatrons, β^-) or positively charged electrons (positrons, β^+). Proton-deficient nuclides lying below the line of stability (Fig. 13-2) usually decay by negatron emission because this mode of decay transforms a neutron into a proton, moving the nucleus closer to the line of stability. Neutron-deficient nuclides lying above the line of stability usually decay by positron emission because this mode transforms a proton into a neutron.

In beta-particle decay processes the mass number does not change because the total number of nucleons in the nucleus remains the same. Such decay processes are known as isobaric transitions. However, the atomic number increases by 1 in the negatron emission and decreases by 1

in the positron emission, resulting in a transmutation of elements (conversion of one element to another). Examples of decay by beta emission are as follows:

$$^{3}_{1}H \rightarrow\ ^{3}_{2}He + \beta^- + v \text{ (negatron emission)}$$

$$^{11}_{6}C \rightarrow\ ^{11}_{5}B + \beta^+ + v \text{ (positron emission)}$$

The **neutrino** (v) is a particle with no mass or electrical charge and virtually does not interact with matter. The only practical consequence of its emission from the nucleus is that it carries away some energy released in the decay process.

Decay by Electron Capture. In addition to the decay by positron emission, the neutron-deficient nuclides may decay by electron capture to transform a proton to a neutron. Thus the electron capture is sometimes called inverse negatron decay. It is also an isobaric transition leading to a transmutation of elements. In the electron-capture process the electron is captured from orbits closest to the nucleus (i.e., the K and L shells [K and L capture; see Fig. 13-1]). The orbital vacancy created by the electron capture is quickly filled by the electron from a higher orbit, resulting in emission of a characteristic x-ray.

Decay by Gamma-Ray Emission. In some cases the isobaric transitions previously mentioned (negatron emission, positron emission, electron capture) result in a daughter nucleus in an excited or metastable state, which means that it possesses excess energy above its minimum possible ground-state energy. Such an excited or metastable nuclide decays promptly to a more stable nuclear arrangement by the emission of gamma rays, which is electromagnetic radiation of very short wavelength:

$$^{125}_{53}I \xrightarrow[\text{capture}]{\text{electron}} {}^{125}_{52}Te^* \rightarrow {}^{125}_{52}Te + \gamma$$

Note that gamma emission is not accompanied by any change in mass number, proton number, or neutron number. This is called an isomeric transition.

Radiation Energy. In any of the radioactive decay processes mentioned previously, a fixed amount of energy is released with each disintegration. Most or all of the released energy will appear as the kinetic energy of the emitted particles or photons. The basic unit of energy commonly used in radiation is the **electron volt (eV)**. One eV is defined as the amount of energy acquired by an electron when it is accelerated through an electrical potential of 1 volt (V). Basic multiples are the kiloelectron volt (keV; 1 keV = 1000 eV) and the megaelectron volt (MeV; 1 MeV = 1000 keV = 1,000,000 eV). In general the energy of beta particles emitted from radionuclides in clinical use ranges from 18 keV to 3.6 MeV and that of gamma rays ranges from 27 keV to 2.8 MeV.

Rate of Radioactive Decay. Radioactive decay is a spontaneous process (i.e., it is not possible to predict when a given radioactive atom will decay), and the probability of decay in a large number of atoms can be given only on a statistical basis. For a sample containing N radioactive nuclei, the number of nuclei decaying at any given moment (dN/dt) can be given by the following:

$$\textbf{(A)} \qquad \frac{dN}{dt} = -\lambda N$$

In this equation, λ is the decay constant of the radioactive nuclide and the minus sign indicates that the number of radioactive nuclides is decreasing with time. Each radionuclide has a characteristic decay constant that represents the proportion of the atoms in a sample of that radionuclide undergoing decay/unit time. The decay constant, λ, is measured in units of $(\text{time})^{-1}$. Therefore the equivalence $\lambda = 0.05$ sec^{-1} means that on the average, 5% of the radionuclides are disintegrating/second. On integration of eq. A

$$\textbf{(B)} \qquad N = N_0 e - \lambda t$$

where N_o is the number of radionuclides present at time (t = 0), and e is the base of the natural logarithm. Therefore the number of radionuclides remaining after a time, t(N), is equal to the number of radionuclides at a time, t = 0 (N_0), multiplied by the factor (e − λt). This factor is the fraction of radionuclides remaining after a time, t, and is termed the **decay factor.** The decay factor, e − λt, is an exponential function of time, t (i.e., a constant fraction of the number of radionuclides present in the sample disappears during a given time interval). A given time interval is customarily expressed as a multiple of the half-life ($t\frac{1}{2}$), which is the time required for the number of radionuclides in the sample to decrease to one half its original value. The half-life of a radionuclide is related to its decay constant as follows:

$$\textbf{(C)} \qquad t\frac{1}{2} = 0.693/\lambda$$

A plot of the decay factor vs the number of half-lives elapsed, t, on semilogarithmic graph paper gives a straight line (Fig. 13-3). This straight line can be obtained by connecting two points on the curve (i.e., at t = 0, decay factor = 1.0, and at t = $2t\frac{1}{2}$, decay factor = −0.25). This graph can be used to determine the decay factor of any radionuclide at any given time, provided that the elapsed time is expressed in terms of number of radionuclide half-lives elapsed. For example, the half-life of ^{125}I is in 60 days. To calculate the residual radioactivity at 360 days, the number of half-lives elapsed must first be calculated:

$$\frac{360 \text{ days}}{60 \text{ days/half-life}} = 6 \text{ half-lives}$$

From Fig. 13-3 the decay factor at 6 half-lives is approximately 0.016. When this value is multiplied by the initial amount of radioactivity, it gives the residual activity at 360 days.

Units of Radioactivity. The average rate of decay of a sample (see Eq. A) (i.e., the average number of nuclides disintegrating per second [dps] or per minute [dpm]) is the activity of the sample and is used to determine the amount of radioactivity present in the sample.

Radioactivity is measured in **Curie (Ci)** units. One curie is defined as the activity of a sample decaying at a rate of 3.7×10^{10} dps (2.22×10^{12} dpm), which is very close to the activity of 1 gram (g) of ^{226}Ra (3.656×10^{10} dps/g). In fact, the curie was originally defined as the activity of 1 g of ^{226}Ra. The basic multiples of the curie are as follows:

1 Ci = 10^3 millicurie (mCi) = 10^6 microcurie (μCi)
   = 10^9 nanocurie (nCi) = 10^{12} picocurie (pCi)

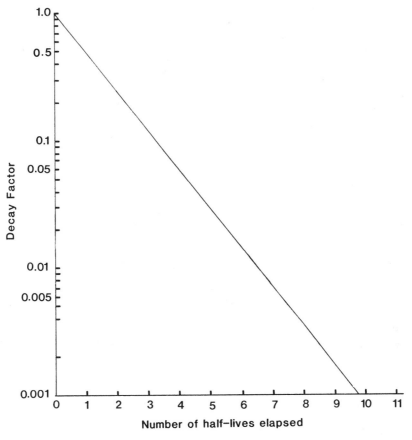

Fig. 13-3 Universal decay curve. Decay facto $(e^{-\lambda t})$ versus number of half-lives elapsed. (From Kaplan LA, Pesce AJ, eds: Clinical chemistry: theory, analysis, and correlation, ed 2, 1989, Mosby–Year Book.)

In clinical laboratories the amounts of radioactivity used are usually in the range of nanocuries to microcuries; occasionally picocurie quantities are measured. The use of Systeme International d'Unites (SI) units in radioactivity measurements has been introduced. The basic unit of this system is the **becquerel (Bq)** in which 1 Bq = 1 dps. Thus

$$1\ \mu Ci = 3.7 \times 10^4\ Bq$$

This system has not gained widespread acceptance in the United States.

In Eq. B, N_0 and N are the numbers of radionuclides present at times 0 and t, respectively. These quantities are extremely difficult to measure. However, the effects of the nuclear disintegrations can be measured more easily with use of one of the radioactive detectors to be described later in this chapter. In this way the total number of disintegrations/second occurring within the radioactive sample, or the radioactivity, at any given time can be estimated. Because the radioactivity, A, is proportional to the number of

atoms, N, Eq. B can be written as:

(D) $$A = A_0 e - \lambda t$$

Therefore the decay constant, the decay factor, and the half-life are also applicable to activity vs time.

It is often necessary to know the specific activity of a radioactive sample. This is the activity of the radionuclide/unit mass of the radioactive sample and thus is measured in microcuries/microgram, microcuries/micromole, or submultiples thereof. The specific activity of the nuclide is inversely proportional to the half-life of the radionuclide. A list of nuclides commonly used in clinical laboratories and some of their radiation characteristics are presented in Table 13-1. The specific activities of nuclides listed in Table 13-1 are calculated under the assumption that all nuclides present are radioactive (carrier free). This assumption does not always hold true. For example, the isotopic abundance of available ^{131}I preparations seldom exceeds 20 percent (i.e., only about 20% of iodine atoms present in the [131]I

Table 13-1 Radiation characteristics of radionuclides commonly used in clinical laboratories

Nuclide	Half-life	Main radiation		Specific activity*	
		Type	Energy (keV)‡	mCi/µg	mCi/µmole
^{3}H	12.3 years	β^-	18	9.7	29
^{14}C	5760 years	β^-	158	0.0044	0.062
^{32}P	14.3 days	β^-	1700	285	9120
^{35}S	87.1 days	β^-	167	42.8	1500
^{51}Cr	27.8 days	EC†	γ320	92	4690
^{59}Fe	45 days	β^-/γ	460/1099	49.1	2900
^{57}Co	270 days	EC†	γ122	8.5	480
^{125}I	60 days	EC†	γ35	17.3	2200
^{131}I	8.1 days	β^-/γ	807/364	123	16.100

From Kaplan LA, Pesce AJ, eds: Clinical chemistry: theory, analysis, and correlation, ed 2, St Louis, 1989, Mosby–Year Book.
*Carrier free.
†Electron capture.
‡Denotes the maximum energy (Emax) for the beta decay.

preparation are ^{131}I), the rest are ^{127}I (stable iodine). Therefore the actual specific activity of ^{131}I preparations is only about one fourth of the theoretical specific activity shown in Table 13-1.

Properties of Radiation and Interaction with Matter

An understanding of the properties of radiation and the mechanism of the energy loss of radiation as it passes through matter is important. The operation of every detecting device for any type of radiation depends on one or more of the particular properties of the radiation that is being measured and the interactions of radiation with matter. Further, the safe manipulation of radioactive substances requires a knowledge of the nature of radiation and its ability to penetrate matter. The harmful effects of radiation on tissues are highly dependent on the ability of the radiation to ionize matter and on the energy of the incident radiation.

The interactions of radiation with matter result in the transfer of energy from a radioactive nucleus to the surrounding material. This transfer is accomplished through processes of excitation and ionization; therefore radiation emitted from radionuclides is frequently termed ionizing radiation.

Excitation occurs when orbital electrons are perturbed from their normal arrangement by absorbing energy from the incident radiation. Ionization occurs when the energy absorbed is sufficient to cause an orbital electron to be ejected from its orbit, creating an ion pair (a free electron and a positively charged atom or molecule). This ionizing ability of radiation is best expressed by the number of ion pairs produced/unit path length (i.e., the specific ionization). Properties of various forms of radiation are presented in Table 13-2.

Particulate Radiation. Because of their relatively large mass and double charge, alpha particles produce a great deal of ionization, which causes them to lose their energy quickly in a short distance (high specific ionization; see Table 13-2). Therefore alpha particles are weakly penetrating and can be stopped completely by very thin layers of solid materials. For this reason they are less hazardous externally. However, if they get into the body, they will irradiate the tissues around them intensely, causing a serious health hazard. Alpha-emitting nuclides are seldom used in medicine.

Beta particles may be negatively or positively charged. There is no known difference between the negatron particle and the electron except for their origin. Positrons are anti-particles of electrons. The energetic negatron and positron particles also lose their energy by excitation and ionization of molecules, but because of their smaller mass and charge, their specific ionization is not as high as that of alpha particles (see Table 13-2). In general, pure beta–particle-emitting nuclides have a continuous spectrum of energy ranging from zero to a maximum of E_{max}. The term E_{max} is equivalent to the total energy available from the nuclear decay and is characteristic of each radionuclide. The majority of beta particles are

Table 13-2 Basic properties of radiation

| Radiation | Charge | Energy range | Approximate range of travel in | | Relative specific ionization* |
			Air	Water	
Particles					
α	+2	3-9 MeV	2-8 cm	20-40 μm	2500
β^-	-1	0-3 MeV	0-10 m	0-1 mm	100
β^+	+1	0-3 MeV	0-10 m	0-1 mm	100
Electromagnetic					
X-rays	None	1 eV to 100 keV	1 mm to 10 m	1 μm to 1 cm	10
Gamma rays	None	10 keV to 10 MeV	1 cm to 100 m	1 mm to 10 cm	1

From Kaplan LA, Pesce AJ, eds: Clinical chemistry: theory, analysis, and correlation, ed 2, St Louis, 1989, Mosby–Year Book.
*The number of ion pairs produced/unit path length relative to that of gamma rays.

emitted with energies of approximately ⅓ E_{max}. A portion of the energy of the beta decay process is carried away by a neutrino (v) emitted simultaneously with beta particles.

Electromagnetic Radiation. Electromagnetic radiation usually encountered in the field of medicine includes gamma ray and x-ray radiation. Except for possible differences in energy, these photons are indistinguishable and engage in the same type of interactions with matter. Unlike beta particles, electromagnetic radiation is emitted in discrete energies corresponding to the energy state transitions a nuclide may undergo when in an excited state. Because photons have no mass, are uncharged, and travel with the velocity of light, they might travel through matter for a considerable distance without any interaction and then lose all or most of their energy in a single interaction. Photons can interact with matter in several different ways, depending on their energies and the properties of the material with which they interact.

Photoelectric effect is especially important for photons with low energy (below 0.5 MeV). The photon interacts directly with one of the orbital electrons in matter (a photon-electron interaction), and the entire photon energy is transferred to the electron. Some transferred energy is used to overcome the binding energy of the electron, and the remaining energy is carried by the electron as kinetic energy, resulting in the formation of an ion pair. The ejected electron (photoelectron) in turn transfers its kinetic energy to many other electrons in its path. The photoelectric effect is especially pronounced if the atomic number of the absorbing material is high.

Compton effect or scattering occurs primarily with photons of medium energy (0.5 to 1 MeV). In this process a collision between a photon and an electron results in the transfer of only a portion of the photon energy to the electron. This interaction also results in the formation of an ion pair as in the case of the photoelectric effect. The scattered photon with reduced energy emerges from the site of interaction in a new direction. The ejected electron (Compton electron) and the scattered photon lose more energy by subsequent interactions.

Pair production occurs only with photons having energies greater than 1.02 MeV. The incident photon may interact with a strong magnetic field such as that surrounding the nucleus of an atom, and the energy of the photon may be converted to electronic mass, an electron-positron pair. The positron eventually undergoes annihilation outside the atom with the production of two 0.511 MeV photons.

Measurement of Nuclear Radiation

Nuclear radiation measurements are based on one of the principal phenomena associated with the interaction of nuclear radiation with matter (i.e., ionization and excitation of molecules within a detector). Two basic types of radiation detectors are commonly used in clinical laboratories: gas-filled detectors and scintillation detectors. This section will cover basic concepts, construction, and operation of these two basic methods of detection and measurement of nuclear radiation.

Gas-Filled Detectors. The gas-filled detector is based on the ability of nuclear radiation to produce ionization in a gas contained in the detector. Essentially, a gas-filled detector is a sealed con-

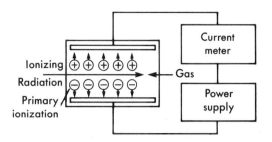

Fig. 13-4 Schematic diagram of a gas-filled detector. (From Freeman LM: Freeman and Johnson's clinical radionuclide imaging, ed 3, Orlando, Fla, 1984, Grune & Stratton.)

tainer with a positive and negative electrode (Fig. 13-4). Air, hydrogen, helium, neon, or argon is normally used in this type of detector. The positive electrode is connected to the positive side of a power supply and the negative electrode to the negative side to create a potential difference between the two electrodes. When nuclear radiation enters the detector filled with a gas, ion pairs are produced. Free electrons migrate toward the positive electrode, and positively charged gas molecules are attracted to the negative electrode. This bulk movement of charge results in a flow of current through the circuit, which is determined by an ammeter installed in the circuit. Because the amount of current produced is directly proportional to the number of ion pairs formed in the detector and because the number of ion pairs formed is dependent on the amount of energy deposited in the gas, the ammeter reading is a direct measure of the amount of energy given up by the nuclear radiation.

The ammeter reading for a given set of electrodes and for a specific gas used depends not only on the amount of ionization produced by radiation but also on the voltage applied across the electrode.

There are three main types of gas-filled detectors, classified primarily according to the voltage levels at which they operate. They are the ionization chamber, **proportional counter,** and the **Geiger-Müller (GM) counter.** Ionization chambers are generally used in radiation survey meters and dose calibrators. In the simple ionization region (about 100 to 500 volts), the voltage is sufficient to prevent recombination of ion pairs produced by radiation and all ion pairs will reach the electrodes.

A continued increase in voltage past the simple ionization region will again bring about an in-

crease in current flow into a proportional region. In this region, the applied voltage is high enough such that some of the primary electrons attain energies sufficient to produce secondary ionization and the number of ion pairs available for current conduction is increased. This process is called gas amplification. Because of this process the current flow produced by a proportional counter may be 100 to 10,000 times that produced by an ionization chamber. In general, proportional counters are relatively insensitive to electromagnetic radiation and are used primarily for counting alpha and beta radiation.

If the applied voltage is still further increased (1000 to 1500 V), gas amplification by secondary ionization occurs as in the proportional region, but unlike the proportional region, the electrons from primary ionization gain sufficient kinetic energy to produce as complete an ionization of the gas in the detector as possible. This plateau region is called Geiger-Müller region, and the flood of ions produced is referred to as an "avalanche." The minimum voltage level needed to produce an avalanche ionization is termed the threshold voltage. In the Geiger-Müller counter all radiation, regardless of energy of radiation or the number of primary ion pairs produced by radiation, will produce the same current flow and thus a Geiger-Müller counter cannot distinguish alpha-, beta-radiation and electromagnetic radiation.

Dose calibrators and survey meters are two gas-filled detectors frequently used in clinical laboratories. Dose calibrators employ ionization chambers operating in the region of simple ionization without gas amplification. They are used routinely in nuclear medicine laboratories to determine the radioactivity of radiopharmaceuticals contained in a test tube, vial, or syringe.

Survey meters are widely used for general room monitoring, locating sites of contamination, and evaluating the handling and disposal of radioactive materials. Geiger-Müller detectors are often used in survey meters because of their high sensitivity as a result of their high operating voltages (about 1000 V). They are available in various configurations depending on the specific application. A common configuration is that of a sealed, gas-filled cylindric end window tube with a central wire serving as the positive electrode and the cylinder wall serving as the negative electrode.

An inert gas such as argon with a small amount of halogen quenching gas is normally

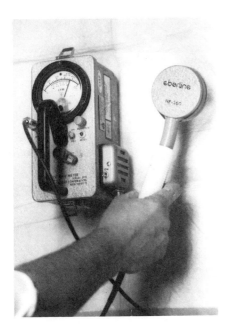

Fig. 13-5 Survey instrument used to detect location and relative amount of radioactivity. System is usually based on a Geiger-Müller counter. (From Bernier, DR et al: Nuclear medicine technology and techniques, ed 2, St Louis, 1989, Mosby-Year Book.)

used in sealed Geiger-Müller tubes. Because of the high operating voltage the primary ionization of gas molecules produced by nuclear radiation entering the Geiger-Müller tube will proceed to ionize the entire gas. Absorption of energy by the quenching gas momentarily stops the avalanche of ionization. Current pulses are produced by this alternating ionization-quenching sequence and are recorded on a rate meter in units of counts/time, exposure/time, or they can be converted to audible sound by a ticking device. Fig. 13-5 shows a survey instrument employing a Geiger-Müller counter.

Scintillation Detectors. Scintillation detectors are the most commonly used detectors in clinical laboratories. Scintillation counting is based on the principle that a charged particle (alpha or beta) entering the detector or an electron excited in the detector after an interaction with an incoming photon (gamma ray) will dissipate its energy within the scintillator contained in the detector by various processes of interaction mentioned previously. A portion of the energy absorbed by the scintillator is emitted as photons in the visible or near-ultraviolet region of the electromagnetic spectrum.

Scintillators or fluors are substances capable of

converting the kinetic energy of an incoming charged particle or photon into flashes of light (scintillation). There are two type of scintillation detection methods: solid crystal scintillation and liquid scintillation.

Crystal Scintillation Detectors. The most commonly used fluor for detecting gamma radiation by scintillation is a single crystal of sodium iodide containing small amounts of thallium (about 1%) as the activator. Fig. 13-6 is a block diagram of the common types of thallium-activated sodium iodide crystal scintillation detectors. The crystal is usually in the shape of a well, and the sample to be counted is allowed to sit in the well. The sodium iodide crystal is very hygroscopic. It is encapsulated in a metal (such as aluminum) to prevent it from absorbing atmospheric moisture, except for one face, usually the bottom face of the crystal well. This part of the crystal well is covered by a transparent material such as Lucite and is optically coupled to the transparent face of a photomultiplier tube.

A gamma ray emitted from the sample placed in the crystal well is highly penetrating and therefore can pass through the glass or plastic wall of the test tube containing the radioactive sample and enter the crystal. As the gamma ray passes into the crystal, it produces excitation or ionization (i.e., the electrons are moved from the valence level to the conduction level in the crystal). The electrons in the conduction level are in an energetically unstable state and will fall back to the valence level, giving off light photons in the process. This process of light emission termed fluorescence or phosphorescence will not occur in a crystal of pure sodium iodide at room temperature. In the presence of thallium impurities, "luminescence centers" are created in the crystal. These centers trap the excited electrons, and light photons are released from the crystals as the excited electrons return to the valence level. About 20 to 30 light photons are produced for each kiloelectron volt of energy absorbed. Because the sodium iodide crystal is hermetically sealed in an aluminum can and because alpha and beta particles can be absorbed by the aluminum, crystal scintillation detectors are generally used for detection of x-rays and gamma rays.

The photons pass through the transparent crystal and strike the photocathode of the photomultiplier tube, causing a release of electrons from the cathode. The energy required to release one photoelectron from the photocathode is about 300 to 2000 eV.

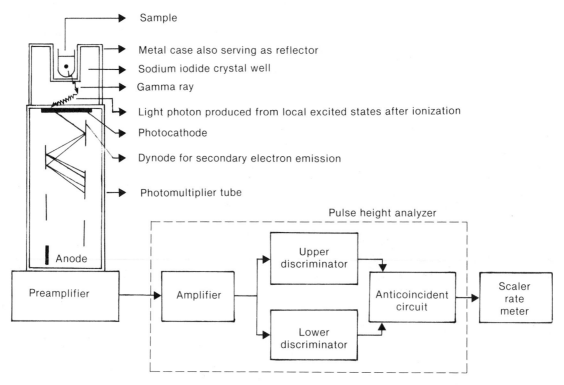

Fig. 13-6 Block diagram showing principal components of typical crystal scintillation counter. (From Kaplan LA, Pesce AJ, eds: Clinical chemistry: theory, analysis, and correlation, ed 2, St Louis, 1989, Mosby–Year Book.)

In addition to the conversion of the light photons emitted by the fluor into a pulse of detectable electrons, the photomultiplier also amplifies the minute amount of current produced from the photocathode to a level that can be effectively handled in conventional electronic amplifier circuits. This is achieved by a process of electron multiplication. As illustrated in Fig. 13-6, a series of metal plates, termed dynodes, are spaced along the length of the photomultiplier tube. The dynode surface is coated with a material capable of emitting secondary electrons when struck by an accelerated electron. Each dynode is maintained at a potential voltage higher than the preceding one. The initial photoelectrons are accelerated toward the first dynode and strike it to produce secondary electrons, which are then accelerated toward a second dynode. About three or four electrons are released from the dynode for each striking electron. This process is repeated until an amplification of about 10^8 is achieved.

The current output of the photomultiplier tube is amplified, and the resulting voltage pulse is shaped for optimal counting by conventional electronic circuitry such as that shown in Fig. 13-6. The preamplifier reduces the distortion of the electrical signal produced by the photomultiplier tube. The preamplifier output is further amplified by the amplifier to give a voltage of up to 10 V.

The function of the pulse-height analyzer is to sort out the pulses according to their pulse height and to allow those pulses within a restricted range (the photopeak) to reach the rate meter for counting. This is accomplished by means of **discriminators.** A lower discriminator sets the lower limit, and an upper discriminator sets the upper limit of the energy range to be counted. The lower discriminator excludes all voltage pulses below the lower limit; the upper discriminator excludes voltage pulses above the upper limit. The energy interval represented by the difference between the two discrimination levels is called the window width. Only the pulses with energy in the preset discriminator window pass through the anticoincident circuit and are counted because the anticoincident circuit will transmit a pulse arriving at its input from the lower discriminator only if there is no pulse arriving from the upper discriminator at the same time. This mode of operation is termed differential counting. The discriminators can also be set to count every pulse that exceeds the setting of the base control. This mode of operation is termed integral counting. In some counters the discriminator controls consist of a lower level discriminator, termed the base control, and the window-width control. The value of the base control and the window width gives the upper level of the energy window selected.

It is important to note that the magnitude (height) of the output pulse (an analog voltage pulse) of the photomultiplier tube is proportional to the intensity of light photons produced in the crystal by a gamma ray and hence to the gamma ray energy deposited in the crystal, whereas the number of voltage pulses/unit time is related to the activity of radioactive samples being analyzed. Each radionuclide has a characteristic spectrum of energies (pulse height), as noted earlier.

Beta particles produced during the beta decay processes give a continuous energy spectrum, whereas photons produced by the gamma decay have a discrete and specific energy value (see Table 13-1). This specific energy value would appear in the gamma ray energy spectrum as a single vertical line at that energy level corresponding to the energy of the emitted gamma ray if the

crystal scintillation detector used were perfect. In reality, however, the intensity of light produced in the crystal and transmitted to the photocathode, the number of electrons ejected from the photocathode, and the number of electrons collected at the anode for each total absorption interaction in the crystal detector are slightly different.

These differences produce a bell-shaped curve (photopeak) instead of a single vertical line (Fig. 13-7). All gamma ray emitting nuclides have their own characteristic photopeaks in their energy spectra that are very useful in the identification of such radionuclides. The width of the photo peak is dependent on the quality of the detector used; the better the detector, the less spread out the photo peak.

Fig. 13-7 shows an energy spectrum of ^{125}I. As described previously, the nuclide ^{125}I decays into ^{125}Te by electron capture with the emission of 35 KeV gamma rays by the excited state of the ^{125}Te daughter nuclide and 27 and 31 KeV Te x-rays. The photopeak at about 28.5 KeV is attributable to the single-photon detection of the two x-rays and the 35 KeV gamma rays, whereas the photopeak at about 56.8 KeV is due to the coincident

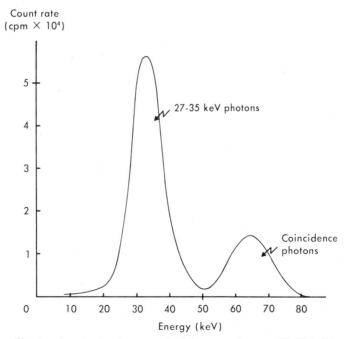

Fig. 13-7 Spectrum of ^{125}I, showing the dominant peak of the x-ray photons (27-35 keV) and the apparent energy recorded in the detector when two photons happen to cause a scintillation simultaneously (coincidence photons). (From Thorell JI, Larson SM: Radioimmunoassay and related techniques: Methodology and clinical applications, St Louis, 1978, Mosby–Year Book.)

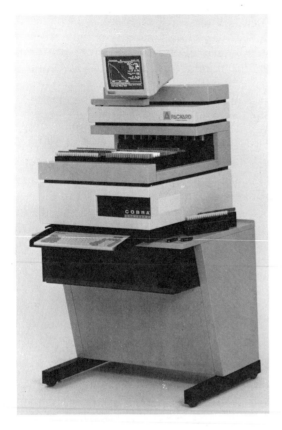

Fig. 13-8   Cobra Model 5005 Automatic Multidetector Gamma Counter. (Courtesy Packard Instrument Co.)

summing of the two x-rays or one x-ray and the 35 KeV gamma ray. The 56.8 KeV photopeak is called the **coincidence photopeak** and is the result of emission of coincidence pair of photons during the ^{125}I decay processes (i.e., the emission of two photons within the resolving time of the detector). Both photons of the pair are detected by a high efficiency sodium iodide crystal detector and are recorded as a single event with a pulse height equivalent to the sum of the energies of the two photons.

This unique energy spectra is used to determine the counting efficiency for ^{125}I of some solid scintillation analyzers without the use of a standard of known disintegration rate. This technique is known as the coincidence method. In the energy spectrum of ^{125}I the total number of counts in the coincidence peak relative to the number of counts in the photopeak depends primarily on the efficiency of the detector. Higher efficiency increases the probability of both photons of the coincident pair being detected. Therefore

detector efficiency and hence the actual activity of the radioactive sample can be determined from the number of counts in each of the two peaks according to the following equation derived by Eldridge:

$$dpm = \frac{(P + 2C)^2}{4C}$$

where *P* is the number of counts (cpm) in the photopeak, *C* is the cpm in the coincidence peak, and *dpm* denotes the disintegration/minute of the sample. P and C can be obtained by counting the sample twice, once with discriminators of the pulse height analyzer set for the photopeak and once with discriminators set for the coincidence peak.

Counting efficiency of a detector is the ratio of the number of counts recorded (cpm) to the number of photons produced in the radioactive sample during a certain time (dpm). Therefore

Counting efficiency (%) =
$$\frac{cpm}{dpm} \times 100\% \text{ or } \frac{p + c}{dpm} \times 100\%$$

Note that the only data needed for the determination of counting efficiency are p and c.

A scintillation detector equipped with two or more pulse-height analyzers (multichannel analyzers) can be used to simultaneously count two or more radionuclides, either in the same sample or in different samples, provided that there is sufficient energy difference between them so that a certain portion of the energy of one radionuclide can be detected free from the second radionuclide. For example, the major photopeak of ^{125}I occurs at 27 keV and that of ^{131}I occurs at 364 keV. In addition to the 364 keV photopeak, a minor ^{131}I photopeak occurs at 32 keV. For counting a mixture of these two isotopes, one analyzer channel, A, is centered at 27 keV and the other channel, B, at 364 keV, with the window width of about 20 to 40 keV. Channel B gives the true count for ^{131}I because ^{125}I does not contribute counts to channel B. Counts from channel A, however, represent the sum of the true counts for ^{125}I and the ^{131}I spillover. The extent of the ^{131}I spillover can be estimated by counting the pure ^{131}I standard in both channels.

Crystal scintillation counters equipped with multiple detectors are used primarily in the clinical laboratory performing radioligand assays including radioimmunoassays (RIA). These assays involve counting of a large number of radioactive samples. With the use of a multidetector instrument, the total assay counting time can be reduced considerably. A crystal scintillation counter equipped with 48 detectors has been developed to facilitate the radioligand assay procedure. However, it is absolutely necessary to make sure that all detectors in such counters perform in an equivalent fashion. Crystal scintillation counters of this type are usually also equipped with a built-in computer for on-line processing of assay results (Fig. 13-8).

Radioligand assays are extremely time-consuming and labor-intensive. They require not only a large number of pipetting steps but also a strict control of assay times and conditions. Therefore the precision of many manually performed radioligand assays has been relatively poor compared with other clinical laboratory assays. Only the Concept-4 Radioassay Analyzer and the Automated Radioimmunoassay Systems (ARIA-II and ARIA-HT) are still in use in a relatively limited number of laboratories.

Liquid Scintillation Detectors. Liquid scintillation detectors are primarily used for counting beta–particle-emitting radionuclides such as ^{3}H, ^{14}C, and ^{32}P. Unlike that of gamma photons, the penetration of negatron particles is so short that they cannot penetrate the wall of the sample container for interaction with crystal scintillators. In liquid scintillation counting the sample is dissolved or suspended in a solution or "cocktail" consisting of a solvent such as toluene, a primary scintillator such as 2,5-diphenyloxazole (PPO), and a secondary scintillator such as 1,4-bis-2 (5-phenyloxazolyl)-benzene (POPOP) (Fig. 13-9). The beta particles from the radioactive sample dissolved in the scintillation cocktail ionize and excite the molecules of the solvent. The excitation energy is transferred to the primary scintillator, which emits light photons when the excited electrons return to the ground energy level. The wavelength of light emitted by the primary scintillator is frequently too short (about 350 to 400 nm) for efficient detection by the photocathodes of photomultiplier tubes. The secondary scintillator absorbs the photons emitted by the primary scintillator and reemits them at a longer wavelength (about 340 nm). Thus the secondary scintillator is also termed a **wavelength shifter.** However, the modern photomultiplier tubes are sensitive to the wavelength of the primary scintillator. The secondary scintillators are used today primarily for more effective transmission of the energy from the beta particle to produce light flashes especially when a large amount of

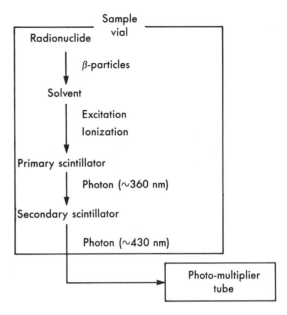

Fig. 13-9 Initial scintillation processes in a liquid scintillation analyzer.

color-quenched sample is placed in the scintillation solution. Problems related to quenching will be discussed later in this chapter.

The operating principles of solid crystal scintillation analyzers and liquid scintillation analyzers are basically the same except for the difference in initial scintillation detection. A typical arrangement of the principal components of a liquid scintillation counter is shown in Fig. 13-10. The light photons produced in the sample vial are detected and amplified by the photomultiplier tubes in the same manner as for the crystal scintillation counter. In the liquid scintillation detector, however, a second photomultiplier tube, a coincident circuit, and a summation circuit are incorporated to eliminate the electronic noise associated with the photomultiplier tube and to improve counting efficiency for low-energy beta-particle emitters.

Noise pulses are random events, and the probability of two photomultiplier tubes producing noise pulses simultaneously is relatively small. In contrast, the beta particle produces a burst of photons and two photomultiplier tubes will receive photons almost simultaneously. The output pulses from each photomultiplier tube are fed into a coincident circuit to check if a pulse from one photomultiplier tube is accompanied by a corresponding pulse from the other within the allowed time interval (termed the **coincidence re-**

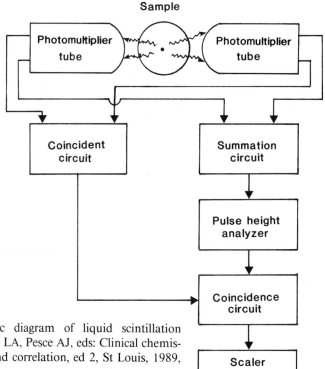

Fig. 13-10   Schematic diagram of liquid scintillation counter. (From Kaplan LA, Pesce AJ, eds: Clinical chemistry: theory, analysis, and correlation, ed 2, St Louis, 1989, Mosby–Year Book.)

solving time, usually about 20×10^{-8} second). Pulses within the resolving time produce a coincident signal that is electrically sent to the coincident gate. Most noise pulses do not meet the coincidence resolving time requirement and are excluded. The summation circuit is incorporated to sum all coincident pulses to obtain the true pulse height. The summed coincident pulses are amplified, sorted, and counted in a manner similar to that for the crystal scintillation counter.

In liquid scintillation counting, proper energy transfer cannot occur unless the sample is in contact with the scintillation solution to give a colorless, transparent, homogeneous solution. Some radioactive samples are not soluble in the scintillation solution, and so it may be necessary to add one or more substances to obtain a homogeneous scintillation mixture. Solubilizers such as methylbenzethonium chloride (Hyamine 10X) are used to facilitate dissolution of the sample in the scintillation solution, or jelling agents such as aluminum stearate are used to enhance the counting efficiency by stabilizing the sample suspension in liquid scintillators. Many commercial liquid scintillation cocktails of nonpolar media (toluene or xylene) contain some type of surfactant such as the tritons (polyoxyethylene ethers and other surface-active compounds) to main-

tain aqueous samples in colloidal suspensions so that the aqueous samples can be counted at high efficiency. Nonvolatile, radioactive materials are also counted on solid supports such as filter paper disks or glass fibers immersed in a scintillation solution. The disadvantage of this counting method is the relatively low counting efficiency because of impurity quenching.

Quenching is basically a process that results in the reduction of the overall photon output of the sample. Impurities present in the radioactive sample may compete with the scintillators for energy transfer (i.e., the energy is lost to a non–light-producing process). This phenomenon is termed impurity quenching (chemical quenching). Water in aqueous samples or a support medium such as a filter disk may cause impurity quenching. Colored substances such as hemoglobin may absorb the light photons produced by the scintillation process before they can be detected by the photomultiplier tubes, or they may change the wavelength of the light photons to a value not suitable for efficient detection by the photocathodes of photomultiplier tubes. This phenomenon is called color quenching. Quenching in liquid scintillation counting is detected and corrected by efficiency determination. The efficiency of the measurement is defined as the ratio of the observed counts/minute (cpm) to the absolute units of disintegrations/minute (dpm):

$$\text{Efficiency} = \frac{\text{cpm}}{\text{dpm}}$$

Because the quenching characteristics of each sample are different, the efficiency must be determined for each sample. By knowing the counting rate (cpm) and the counting efficiency of a sample, the absolute radioactivity (dpm) of the sample can be calculated. Several methods for efficiency determination have been developed, but only those most frequently used are discussed.

Efficiency Determination. *Internal standards,* one of the oldest methods, is the most accurate for efficiency determination when properly carried out. In this method the sample is counted before and after the introduction of a calibrated standard of the measured radionuclide. The difference between the count rates before and after the spike, divided by the calibrated activity of the spike in disintegrations/unit time, is termed the counting efficiency. The disadvantages of this method are the time-consuming manipulation of the sample and the loss of sample for recount after the introduction of the spike.

The sample-channels ratio method is based on a downward shift of the pulse-height spectrum of the photon as a result of the quenching-induced decrease in the pulse height of many energetic decays (Fig. 13-11). The degree of the shift is related to the extent of quenching or counting efficiency and is expressed by the change in the ratio of the sample counts obtained from two different discriminator window settings (channels). As shown in Fig. 13-11, one channel is usually set to measure the entire isotope spectrum (L_1 to L_3) and the second channel is restricted to only a portion of the spectrum (L_1 to L_2). In this method, channel ratios (L_1 to L_2 to L_1 to L_3) of a set of artificially quenched standards of known efficiencies are determined and plotted against counting efficiency to obtain a quench curve. The efficiency of any unknown sample can be determined from its channel ratio and the quench curve. This method requires no additional sample manipulation, unlike internal standardization, and is suitable for handling a large number of samples through automation. This method, however, may result in large errors in highly quenched samples or samples with low count rates.

Unlike the internal standard method, the known activity in the external standards method is provided by an external source of gamma ra-

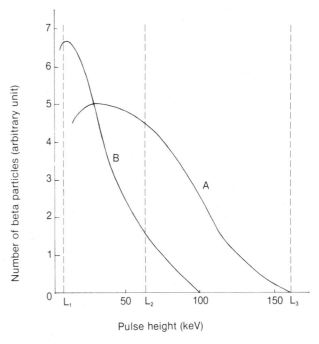

Fig. 13-11 Unquenched, **A**, and quenched, **B**, pulse-height spectra of ^{14}C. L_1 to L_2 denotes discrimination levels. (From Kaplan LA, Pesce AJ, eds: Clinical chemistry: theory, analysis, and correlation, ed 2, St Louis, 1989, Mosby–Year Book.)

diation, such as ^{226}Ra, placed at a fixed position adjacent to the sample vial. The external gamma ray source generates electrons through the Compton collision process in the scintillation solution. The Compton electrons transfer energy to the solution and cause scintillation in the same way as beta particles do in the scintillation medium. The energy spectrum produced by Compton electrons is also affected by the presence of quenching materials, as in a typical beta-particle spectrum.

The sample is counted twice, once in the absence of and once in the presence of an external standard. As in the sample-channels ratio method, a set of quenched standards of known efficiencies is used to obtain a correlation curve between the sample-counting efficiency and the count rate of the external standard. The counting efficiency of a sample can be determined from the count rate of the external standard counted with the sample and from the correlation curve. The external standard method has become an integral part of almost all modern liquid scintillation detectors.

Another problem encountered in liquid scintillation counting is **chemiluminescence,** the production of light photons by a chemical reaction between the sample material and the solute or solubilizer added to the scintillation solution. Chemiluminescence gives rise to single photons and can be excluded by the coincident circuit of the liquid scintillation counter. However, when chemiluminescence reactions are of sufficient intensity, non–beta-particle coincident pulses may be generated that interfere with the beta-particle scintillation counting. The chemiluminescent effect will eventually disappear, but this may take several hours or longer, especially at low temperatures. Chemiluminescence can be monitored by repeated counting of the sample. Some modern instruments are capable of automatically monitoring and correcting for the chemiluminescent effects.

As with crystal scintillation counting, mixed-isotope counting is possible with a liquid scintillation counter with multichannel analyzers. A common example of dual-label counting involves a mixture of tritium, with a maximum beta-particle decay of 18.6 keV and ^{14}C, with a maximum beta-particle decay of 156 keV. Fig. 13-12 shows a computer-aided benchtop liquid scintillation analyzer manufactured by Packard Instrument Co. This instrument has a sample capacity of either 408 standard vials (20 ml) or 720 small vials (7 ml glass vial or microfuge tube) and is equipped with a built-in computer for controlling all aspects of operations of liquid scintillation analyzers, including sample change, spectral analysis, quenching correction, and performance monitoring.

Counting Statistics. Because radioactive decay is essentially a random process, it is unlikely that successive measurements on a given sample will result in the same number of counts. However, radioactive decay obeys a Poisson distribution. The Poisson distribution density formula can be applied in the calculation of the precision of measurement at a given count rate. If a single measurement of total counts, N, is made, then precision of this measurement in terms of the percent coefficient of variation (%CV) can be estimated to be as follows:

$$\%CV = \frac{\sqrt{N}}{N} \times 100\%$$

For example, at a total count of 100, CV = 10%; at 1000, CV = 3.2%; at 10,000, CV = 1%. This approximation is applicable only when the background count is negligible compared with the sample count. When significant background

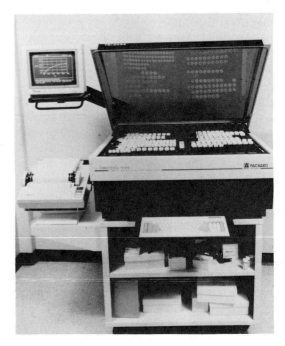

Fig. 13-12 Tri-Carb 1900 CA Liquid Scintillation Analyzer. (Courtesy Packard Instrument Co.)

counts are present, the formula for the standard deviation of a difference must be used:

$$\%CV = \frac{\sqrt{N + B}}{S} \times 100\%$$

where B is the background count and S is the sample count (N − B). Thus a total count of 100 in the presence of a background count of 10 gives the following:

$$\%CV = \frac{\sqrt{100 + 10}}{100 - 10} \times 100\% = 11.7\%$$

Precision can be increased by prolonging the counting time, but a 1% CV (i.e., 10,000 counts) is satisfactory in most applications.

Radiation Health Safety. Although the quantity of radioactivity handled in the clinical laboratory is usually very small, a basic knowledge of radiation safety is vital to every laboratory worker who has frequent contact with radioactive substances because the biologic effects of long-term exposure to very low doses of ionizing radiation are still largely unknown and may prove to be hazardous to health.

Radionuclides commonly used in the clinical laboratory are either beta-particle emitters, such as ^{14}C and ^{3}H, or gamma-ray emitters, such as ^{125}I and ^{57}Co. Both forms of radiation produce their biologic effects by producing ionization and excitation along their paths in the tissue. However, beta radiation is less penetrating than gamma radiation; thus beta-particle emitters are considered to be more hazardous in terms of internal radiation and less hazardous in terms of external radiation than gamma-ray emitters. Therefore the primary concern with beta-particle emitters is to prevent the entry of radioactive materials into the body through inhalation, ingestion, or absorption by the skin; with gamma-ray emitters other factors such as shielding, exposure time, and exposure distance are also important when considering radiation safety.

Regular monitoring of both personnel and work areas is an important radiation safety procedure. It is necessary to periodically measure the radiation exposure doses of personnel to ensure that radiation doses received are below the recommended limits. The following three basic units are used to measure radiation exposure and dose.

The **roentgen (R)** is a unit of x-rays or gamma rays and measures the quantity of ionization produced by photon radiation in a given sample of air. One R equals that quantity of photon radiation capable of producing one electrostatic unit of either sign in 0.001293 g of air.

The **radiation absorbed dose (rad)** is a measure of local energy deposition/unit mass of material irradiated by any ionizing radiation. One rad is equal to 100 ergs of absorbed energy/gram of absorber.

The **roentgen equivalent, man (rem)** is that dose of ionizing radiation causing the same amount of biologic injury to human tissue as 1 rad of x-ray, gamma ray, or beta-particle radiation. In the case of alpha radiation, the dose in rems equals the dose in rads multiplied by 20 because only 0.05 rad of alpha radiation is needed to produce the same biologic effects as 1 rad of x-ray, gamma ray, or beta-particle radiation. The recommended maximum permissible dose to the whole body is 0.5 rem/year for the general public and 5 rems/year for radiation workers.

Film badges are probably the most commonly used and cost-effective way of monitoring personnel. The photographic film becomes progressively optically dense when exposed to ionizing radiation and thus may be used to monitor the radiation dose received by the wearer. Because most clinical laboratory personnel working with radioimmunoassays routinely handle ^{125}I-labeled compounds, it is advisable to monitor possible accumulation of radioactive iodine in the thyroid glands. Arrangements should be made to have the radioactive content of each worker's thyroid measured at least twice each year or after each radioiodination experiment. It is necessary to keep all records of radiation exposure of all workers handling radioactive materials for at least 5 years. Each laboratory should have a portable radiation detector, such as a portable Geiger-Müller survey meter, to monitor radioactivity in an area in which radioactive materials are routinely handled. Monitoring of beta radiation usually requires taking samples of the work area with swabs and using a liquid scintillation counter to determine the presence of radioactivity.

Internal radiation exposure is controlled only by preventing the entry of radioactive materials into the body. This requires strict adherence to the general rules for radiation safety. Mouth pipetting of radioactive materials should never be done. All persons working in radioactive areas must wear the designated protective clothing (a standard laboratory coat is satisfactory in a clinical laboratory involved in radioimmunoassays) and disposable gloves. Radioactive materials must be properly labeled, stored, and used only at specially designated areas. Work involving the possible generation of volatile, radioactive substances, such as radioiodination, should be performed in an exhaust hood. The working surface should be covered by a layer of disposable absorbent material. In addition to the proper operating technique, cleanliness and good housekeeping are essential to prevent and minimize the spread and buildup of contamination.

Persons contaminated by radioactive materials should be quickly decontaminated to prevent the possible transfer of radioactivity to internal organs by absorption through the skin. Facilities for decontamination, such as a shower and an eyewash station, should be available in each laboratory. Absorbent materials should be used to remove spilled radioactive material. The contaminated area should then be scrubbed with soap and water. It is a good practice to cover the contaminated area immediately with a piece of paper to prevent spreading of the radioactivity to other parts of the laboratory.

The radioactivity level of the radioactive waste materials generated in clinical laboratories involved in radioimmunoassays is usually very low, but such radioactive waste material should still be disposed of according to the guidelines established by the Nuclear Regulatory Commission (NRC) of the United States. Some states (NRC agreement states) are approved by the NRC to regulate the use, safety, and disposal of radioactive material in the state, provided that the regulations are more restrictive than the NRC regulations. Therefore it is important to be familiar with the state regulations on radioactive materials if the laboratory is located in an NRC agreement state.

Review Questions

1. In which of the following modes of radioactive decay is a neutron transformed into a proton?
   A. Negatron emission
   B. Positron emission
   C. Alpha decay
   D. Electron capture
   E. Gamma ray emission

2. Because of their lack of charge and mass, which of the following nuclear radiation is most highly penetrating?
   A. Positron
   B. Negatron
   C. Gamma ray
   D. Alpha particles
   E. Neutron

3. The stability of the nucleus of an atom depends on:
   A. Number of neutrons in the nucleus
   B. Number of electrons in the atom
   C. Neutron-proton ratio
   D. Number of protons in the nucleus
   E. Energy states of orbital electrons

4. From the following list of nuclides, pick out those that are isotopes and isobars:
   $^{125}_{53}I$, $^{1}_{1}H$, $^{3}_{1}H$, $^{3}_{2}He$, $^{125}_{52}Te$, $^{131}_{53}I$

5. The definition of the roentgen is based on the ionization of:
   A. Water
   B. Air
   C. Nitrogen gas
   D. Helium gas
   E. Muscle tissue

6. The basic function of a photomultiplier tube is to convert _____ to _____.
   A. X-rays; photons
   B. γ-rays; photons
   C. Photons; electrons
   D. Electrons; photons
   E. None of the above

7. If the voltage applied to the electrodes of an ionization chamber is not sufficient:
   A. The ion pairs formed by the radiation will recombine before reaching the electrodes
   B. The radiation cannot produce ionization in the chamber
   C. Spontaneous discharge will take place
   D. Gas amplification will occur
   E. None of the above

8. A gamma scintillation counter registered 1.6×10^6 cpm for a mock ^{125}I standard having one microcurie (2×10^6 dpm) of radioactivity. What is the efficiency of this counter?
   A. 80%
   B. 16%
   C. 32%
   D. 8%
   E. 40%

9. Sample-channels ratio technique is used to:
   A. Check the stability of a liquid scintillation counter
   B. Calibrate the pulse height analyzer of a gamma counter
   C. Calibrate the amplifier output of a gamma counter
   D. Make quenching correction in liquid scintillation counting
   E. Detect chemiluminescence in liquid scintillation counting

10. The amount of light emitted by the sodium iodide crystal in a gamma counter by a radioactive sample is proportional to the:
    A. Diameter of the crystal
    B. Amount of energy deposited in the crystal by the radioactive sample
    C. Thickness of the crystal
    D. Radioactivity of the sample
    E. All of the above

Answers

1. A 2. C 3. C 4. $^{1}_{1}H$ and $^{3}_{1}H$, $^{125}_{53}I$ and $^{131}_{53}I$ are isotopes; $^{3}_{1}H$ and $^{3}_{2}He$, $^{125}_{53}I$ and $^{125}_{52}Te$ are isobars, 5. B 6. C 7. A 8. A 9. D 10. B

Bibliography

Chen IW: Isotopes in clinical chemistry. In Kaplan LA, Pesce AJ, eds: Clinical chemistry: theory, analysis, and correlation, ed 2, St Louis, 1989, Mosby–Year Book.

Links JM: Instrumentation. In Bernier DR, Christian PE, Langan JK et al, eds: Nuclear medicine technology and techniques, ed 2, St Louis, 1989, Mosby–Year Book.

14

Osmometry

ANDREW MATUREN
ROBERT A. WEBSTER

Osmolality
Colligative Properties and Osmometry
Freezing Point Depression Osmometry
Vapor Pressure (Dew Point) Osmometry
Colloid Osmometry

Osmolality

Molality is a term used to describe the concentration of a solution and is defined as the number of moles of solute/kilogram of solvent (water). The related term, **osmolality,** is the number of moles of particles of solute/kilogram of water, without regard for the mass, size, diversity, or ionic activity of the particles. The relationship between molality and osmolality depends on the number of particles into which a molecule of the solute dissociates. For example, a 1 molal solution of glucose is also a 1 osmolal solution because the glucose molecule does not dissociate into smaller active particles. A solution that is 1 molal in sodium chloride is 2 osmolal because the sodium chloride will dissociate into sodium ions and chloride ions. Furthermore, a solution that is 1 molal in glucose and 1 molal in sodium chloride is 3 osmolals because osmolality depends only on the number of particles of solute/kilogram of water.

Osmometry as used in the clinical laboratory is a measurement of the osmolality of an aqueous solution such as serum, plasma, or urine; it measures the concentration of the total of all ions and molecules present. In biologic fluids of clinical interest a few small molecules and ions are the major contributors to the osmolality of the fluid. In normal serum these are the electrolytes, glucose, and urea. Larger molecules such as proteins are present in serum in much higher concentrations in terms of weight/volume, but because of their high molecular mass and the fact that they

do not dissociate into smaller particles, the number of particles of protein is much lower than the number of particles of sodium, for example. The concentration in serum of those particles that are the major contributors to serum osmolality is highly regulated in the normal healthy individual, and the osmolality of serum may therefore be calculated if the concentrations of these particles are known. One convenient formula for the calculation of serum osmolality requires knowledge of the concentrations of sodium, glucose, and urea in mmol/L:

Calculated serum osmolality (mOsm/kg

(A) $\quad H_2O) = 2 \times Na^+ + Glucose + Urea$
$$\text{(mmol/L) (mmol/L) (mmol/L)}$$

This formula expresses the concentration of the particles in the International System of Units (SI units) of mmol/L. Another formula used in many American laboratories (Holmes Formula) expresses glucose and urea concentrations in historical units of mg/dL, and these analytes must then be corrected by a factor that is the molecular mass of the analyte divided by 10 (the latter to convert dL to L):

Calculated serum osmolality (mOsm/kg

(B) $\quad H_2O) = 2 \times Na^+ + \dfrac{Glucose\ (mg/dL)}{18} +$
$$\text{(mmol/L)}$$
$$\dfrac{Urea\ (mg/dL)}{2.8}$$

In these formulas the sodium concentration is multiplied by a factor of 2 to include the osmotic effect of the corresponding anion particles, mainly chloride and bicarbonate. The serum osmolality may also be measured in the laboratory using one of the techniques of osmometry to be described later in this chapter. When the measured osmolality, which reflects the osmotic effect of all particles in solution, is compared with the calculated osmolality that reflects only electrolytes, glucose, and urea, the difference is the **osmolal gap:**

(C)

$$\begin{aligned} \text{Osmolal gap (mOsm/kg H}_2\text{O)} = \\ \text{Measured osmolality} - \\ \text{(mOsm/kg H}_2\text{O)} \\ \text{Calculated osmolality} \\ \text{(mOsm/kg H}_2\text{O)} \end{aligned}$$

The average osmolal gap in the normal individual is 0 to 10 mOsm/kg H_2O. When the osmolal gap of serum exceeds this range, the presence of small particles other than electrolytes, glucose, or urea in serum, in amounts sufficient to affect the measured osmolality, is suspected. The most common substances that affect the osmolal gap in this manner are alcohols, such as ethanol, and ketones present in diabetic ketoacidosis.

In the case of urine there is no formula for the calculation of osmolality because the number and type of small particles excreted in urine may vary so widely. Osmometric measurement of urine in the clinical laboratory is an assessment of the kidney's ability to concentrate the urine (i.e., conserve body water while excreting a concentrated solution of small particles including urea, creatinine, phosphate, ammonia, and excess electrolytes).

Measurement of serum or urine osmolality in the laboratory provides valuable clinical information in many situations. In serum the measured osmolality compared with the calculated osmolality provides information toward the detection of unmeasured small particles in serum. Measured osmolality in serum is also used to follow treatment of fluid and electrolyte imbalances (e.g., postsurgical and trauma patients), diabetes, renal failure, and burns. In urine the measured osmolality is used to assess the concentrating ability of the kidney. The clinical usefulness of serum and urine osmolality measurement has fostered the availability in the clinical laboratory of relatively simple and accurate instrumentation for osmometric measurements.

Colligative Properties and Osmometry

As osmotically active particles are added to a solution and the osmolality of the solution increases, four other properties of the solution are also affected. These properties are called the **colligative properties** of the solution because they can be measured and mathematically related to each other and to the osmolality. These properties are osmotic pressure, boiling point, freezing point, and vapor pressure. As the osmolality of a solution (i.e., an aqueous solution such as serum or urine) is increased (1) the osmotic pressure of the solution increases, (2) the boiling point is elevated (i.e., the solution boils at a higher temperature than pure water), (3) the freezing point is depressed (the solution freezes at a lower temperature than pure water), and (4) the vapor pressure is depressed (essentially a solution containing particles is less prone to evaporate at a given temperature than is pure water at the same temperature).

Osmometry in the clinical laboratory uses the measurable changes in the colligative properties of solutions that occur as particle concentration in the solution increases. Before a discussion of the operation principles of clinical laboratory osmometers, it is first necessary to define the colligative properties in further detail.

Osmotic pressure is the hydrostatic pressure required to stop the diffusion of a solvent (e.g., water) through a semipermeable membrane from a region of lower solute concentration to a region of higher solute concentration. Fig. 14-1 shows the effect of osmotic pressure in a U-shaped tube, the two halves of which are separated by a membrane permeable to water but not to solute particles. A solution of solute in water is placed on the left side of the membrane, and pure water is placed on the right. The solute molecules on the left cannot move across the membrane, but water molecules from the left side can move to the right in an attempt to equilibrate the "concentration" of water across the membrane. This will have the effect of diluting the solute and also increasing the volume on the left side of the membrane. The increase in volume on the left side creates an increased hydrostatic pressure on the membrane that will eventually stop any further net increase in water volume on the left side. If the membrane does not break from this pressure, an equilibrium will be maintained between water flowing from right to left (along the concentration gradient of the water), and water being forced from left to right by increased hydrostatic pressure on the left. This hydrostatic pressure is called the **osmotic pressure.** The osmolality of a solution such as serum or urine can be determined from the measurement of the osmotic pressure in a system where the sample is placed on one side of a membrane in a sealed system and pure water or a solution of known osmolality is on the other side. In practice, however, it is not convenient to determine osmolality by osmotic pressure measurements carried out in this manner; osmotic pres-

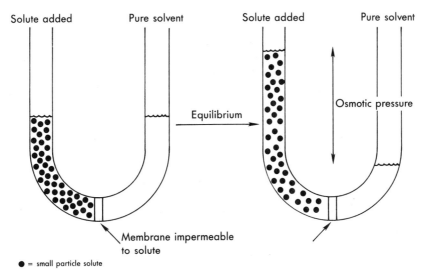

Fig. 14-1 Osmotic pressure. The two sides of A are separated by a membrane that is permeable to solvent but not to solute particles. At equilibrium (B), osmotic movement of solvent to the solute side has increased the hydrostatic pressure on the left side and decreased it on the right. This pressure difference across the membrane is the osmotic pressure.

sure measurement is used in the clinical laboratory only in a specific form of osmometry that measures **colloid osmotic pressure** or **oncotic pressure.** The principle of this form of osmometry will be discussed later in this chapter.

Vapor pressure is the pressure exerted by the vapor, or gaseous, phase of a solvent when in equilibrium with the liquid state of the same solvent. The molecules of solvent on the surface of a liquid are in constant motion, and some of these molecules escape (i.e., evaporate) from the surface of the liquid into the atmosphere above the surface, forming a gaseous phase above the solvent's liquid phase. If solute particles are added to the liquid, some of the solute molecules will occupy the surface layer of the liquid, and by their presence in the liquid, effectively decrease the concentration of the solvent in the liquid phase. When this happens, solvent molecules tend to remain in the liquid phase and there is less evaporation or movement of solvent into the vapor phase. Thus at a given temperature the addition of solute particles to a solution decreases the vapor pressure above the solution. This concept is illustrated in Fig. 14-2.

Related to vapor pressure is the concept of **dew point,** which is the temperature at which the molecules of solvent in the vapor phase, at a given pressure, will condense to re-form a liquid. The greater the solute concentration in a solution, the lower the water vapor pressure above the solution

will be. At a lower vapor pressure in a closed space, there will be fewer water molecules in the vapor phase above a solution and the decrease in temperature necessary for these water molecules to recondense into a liquid (i.e., reach the dew point) will be greater. Measurement of the depression in temperature necessary to reach the dew point in the vapor phase above a solution is the principle of **vapor pressure depression osmometry,** which will be described in further detail later in this chapter.

Freezing point is the temperature at which the liquid phase and the solid or crystalline phases of a solution exist at equilibrium. Added solute molecules interfere with the interactions of solvent molecules in a solution thus lowering the temperature necessary for formation of the solid phase. One osmol of solute in water lowers the freezing point of a solution 1.86° C below that of pure water. Freezing-point depression osmometry is the most common method of measurement of osmolality in the clinical laboratory.

Boiling point is the temperature at which the vapor pressure above a solution equals the atmospheric pressure. Addition of solute to a solution decreases the vapor pressure above a solution thus increasing the temperature that is necessary to bring the vapor pressure up to the temperature of the surrounding atmosphere. Boiling point elevation is not a practical means of measuring the osmolality of a biologic fluid be-

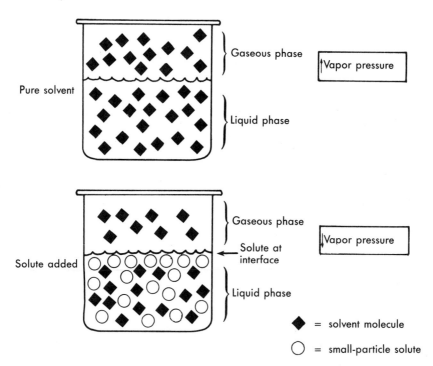

Fig. 14-2   Decrease in vapor pressure in the gaseous phase above a solvent is seen when a small-particle solute is added to the solvent.

cause proteins in the sample tend to coagulate at higher temperatures, changing the composition of the sample. Boiling point elevation is not used in osmometric measurements.

Freezing Point Depression Osmometry

Freezing-point depression osmometry, or cryoscopy, measures the particle concentration (os-

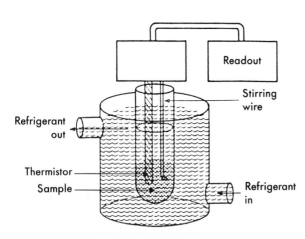

Fig. 14-3   Functional diagram of a freezing-point osmometer. (From Coiner D: Basic concepts in laboratory instrumentation, ASMT Education and Research Fund, Inc., 1975-1979.)

molality) of a solution by measuring the freezing point of the solution relative to the freezing points of standard sodium chloride solutions of known osmolality. Fig. 14-3 displays a diagram of the functional components of freezing-point osmometers available from several instrument manufacturers. A freezing-point osmometer consists of a sample chamber that contains a stirrer and a **thermistor,** or an electronic temperature-sensing device, that is connected to a readout calibrated in mOsm/kg H_2O. The sample chamber is either in contact with an electronic cooling device or can be lowered into a refrigerator chamber containing antifreeze. The design of the sample chamber and the method of cooling vary among instrument models and manufacturers.

The sample is placed in the sample chamber with the stirrer and the thermistor immersed in the sample. The sample in the chamber is rapidly **supercooled** (i.e., the temperature of the sample solution falls below its freezing point). During the supercooling phase in a freezing-point osmometer, the solution may reach a temperature of $-5°$ to $-7°$ C. When a solution is cooled rapidly, it may not crystallize even though its temperature is below the freezing point. In a supercooled solution of this nature, crystallization (freezing) may be initiated by adding a crystal or a particle

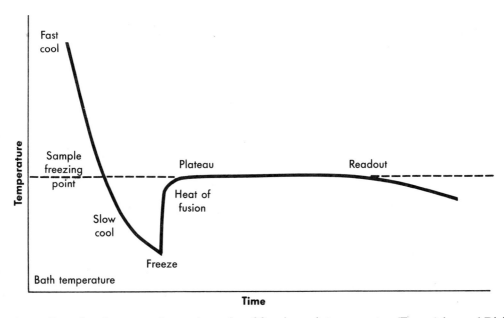

Fig. 14-4 Uniform freezing curve: thermodynamics of freezing-point osmometry. (From Advanced Digimatic Osmometer Model 3 MO User's Guide, Advanced Instruments, Inc., Needham Heights, Mass.)

of impurity to the solution or by agitating the solution. When the solution in the sample chamber reaches a temperature several degrees below its freezing point, the sample is agitated with the stirrer to initiate freezing. As ice crystals begin to form, heat is released from the solution during the freezing process. This heat is called **heat of fusion.** The rate of release of heat of fusion by the formation of ice crystals rapidly reaches equilibrium with the rate of removal of the heat of fusion by the cold temperature of the sample chamber. This equilibrium temperature, which is the **freezing point** of the solution, stays constant for several minutes once it is reached.

The thermistor immersed in the sample is made of semiconductor metals that have less resistance (i.e., become better electrical conductors) as the temperature rises. The resistance of the thermistor rises as the solution is supercooled, then drops as the temperature rises with release of heat of fusion, and then reaches a plateau when the freezing point or equilibrium point is reached. The temperature at the plateau, in terms of thermistor resistance, is detected by a Wheatstone bridge circuit in the readout device. Results are displayed in units of mOsm/kg H_2O when the instrument has been calibrated with solutions of known osmolality (e.g., sodium chloride solutions). Fig. 14-4 uses a graph of temperature change over time to illustrate the events in osmometric measurement by freezing point de-

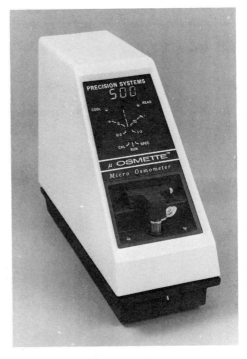

Fig. 14-5 Precision Systems Micro Osmette. (Courtesy Precision Systems, Inc.)

Table 14-1   Characteristics of clinical osmometers*

Manufacturer	Model	Technique†	Sample size (μL)	Precision‡	Measurement time (sec)
Advanced Instrument, Inc. (Needham Heights, Mass.)	3D11	FP	200	1.5%	50-70
Fiske Associates, Inc. (Needham Heights, Mass.)	OS	FP	250	1.5%	90
	OR	FP	50		30
Precision Systems, Inc. (Sudbury, Mass.)	5002	FP	200	1.5%	180
	μOsmette	FP	50		
Wescor, Inc. (Logan, Utah)	5100C	VP	8	2.8%	90
Instrumentation Lab, Inc. (Lexington, Mass.)	186	COP	300	—	90
Wescor, Inc. (Logan, Utah)	4100	COP	300		

From Kaplan LA, Pesce AJ, eds: Clinical chemistry: theory, analysis, and correlation, St Louis, 1989, Mosby–Year Book.
*All models are manually loaded with sample and have automated measurements and reporting. Variations in sample size, automated sampling, and printing are available.
†*FP* = Freezing-point depression; *VP* = vapor pressure; *COP* = colloid osmotic pressure.
‡From College of American Pathologists survey.

pression. Table 14-1 lists several application characteristics of currently available freezing-point osmometers. Two examples of freezing point osmometers are the Precision Systems Micro Osmette and Osmette II (Figs. 14-5 and 14-6).

Vapor Pressure (Dew Point) Osmometry

As described previously, the vapor pressure of the gaseous phase of a solvent above a solution is decreased as the osmolality of the solution increases. As vapor pressure decreases, the number of water molecules in the gaseous phase in a

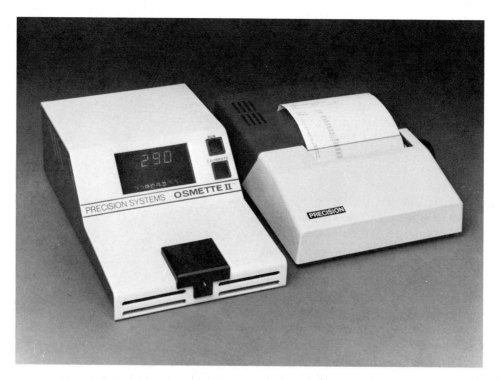

Fig. 14-6   Precision Systems Osmette II. (Courtesy Precision Systems, Inc.)

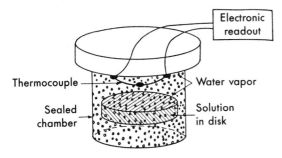

Fig. 14-7 Functional diagram of a vapor pressure osmometer. (From Coiner D: Basic concepts in laboratory instrumentation, ASMT Education and Research Fund, Inc., 1975-1979.)

closed space above the solution decreases. A reduced number of water molecules in the gaseous phase requires a greater reduction in temperature before the dew point temperature, at which water condenses into a liquid, is reached. The only commercially available vapor pressure osmometer actually measures dew point depression, which is an explicit function of vapor pressure depression, as an indicator of the osmolality of the sample solution.

Vapor pressure (dew point) depression osmometry is the passive process using relatively simple instrumentation. It differs from freezing point depression osmometry in that during a dew point depression measurement the physical state and temperature of the sample itself is not changed. A vapor pressure osmometer (Fig. 14-7) consists of a sealed chamber containing a **thermocouple.** A thermocouple (Fig. 14-8) consists of strips of two dissimilar metals, joined together at one end and attached to a voltmeter at their separate ends. A thermocouple exhibits two inde-

pendent electrical phenomena called the **Peltier effect** and the **Seebeck effect.** Both of these are used in dew point depression measurements.

The Peltier effect is observed when an electrical current is passed through the two metal strips. Because of their different properties, one metal junction will heat and the other will cool. The Seebeck effect is seen when, in the absence of an electrical current, the temperature of the joined end of the two metal strips increases. The change in temperature causes one of the metals to attain a positive charge relative to the other at the ends attached to the voltmeter, which can be calibrated to measure the temperature change.

In a dew point depression measurement the sample is placed on a solute-free disk that is sealed into the chamber containing the joined end of the thermocouple. The chamber is sealed, and the vapor pressure and temperature of the gaseous phase in the space above the specimen rapidly come to equilibrium. At this point the thermocouple, via the attached voltmeter, measures the temperature of the specimen and sets this temperature as the reference point on "blank" for the measurement. A current is then passed through the junction of the thermocouple, cooling it via the Peltier effect to a temperature well below that at which water from the gaseous phase will condense into liquid droplets on the surface of the metal junction. At this point, the current is stopped.

Analogous to the heat of fusion described previously for the freezing-point osmomter is the **heat of condensation** observed in this system, which is the heat produced when water molecules from the gaseous phase condense to form a liquid. When the current across the thermocouple is turned off, heat of condensation causes the tem-

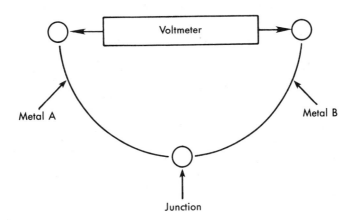

Fig. 14-8 Functional diagram of a thermocouple as used in a vapor-pressure osmometer.

perature of the junction to rise, eventually equilibrating with the warmer temperature of the chamber. This stable temperature, at which condensation and evaporation are at equilibrium, is the dew point temperature and is sensed by the voltmeter as a stable plateau via the Seebeck effect. The difference between this temperature and the basal temperature of the chamber recorded earlier is the dew point depression and is read out in mOsm/kg H_2O when the instrument is calibrated with solutions of known osmolality. The temperature changes that occur over time in a dew point osmometry measurement are shown in Fig. 14-9.

The only commercially available clinical vapor pressure osmometer (Wescor 5500, Wescor, Inc., Logan, UT) is described in Table 14-1 and is shown in Fig. 14-10. In clinical applications it is important to note that the vapor pressure or dew point osmometer cannot be used in detection of volatiles (e.g., ethanol) in serum by osmolal gap determinations; clinically encoun-

tered concentrations of ethanol may actually cause an increase rather than a decrease in the vapor pressure or dew point above the sample thus producing an erroneously low serum osmolality result.

Colloid Osmometry

The last clinical application of osmometry to be discussed in this chapter is called **colloid osmometry** or **oncometry** and, of the several principles discussed, relates most closely to the changes in osmotic pressure seen with changes in particle content of solutions. It also differs from freezing point and vapor pressure osmometry in that its clinical application is entirely different.

As discussed previously, macromolecules such as proteins contribute very little to the serum osmolality (only about 1 mOsm/kg H_2O) measured by freezing point or vapor pressure osmometers. This is due to their high molecular mass, large particle size, and tendency not to dissociate into smaller particles. Molecules such as proteins, with a mass of 30,000 daltons or greater, are called **colloids,** whereas particles of lower mass are called **crystalloids** (e.g., glucose or urea) if they are uncharged and **ions** (e.g., sodium or chloride) if they are charged. Although crystalloids and ions are the major contributors to total serum osmolality, it is sometimes clinically use-

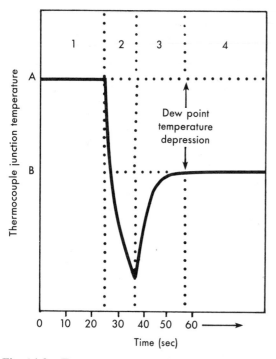

Fig. 14-9   Temperature changes occurring in vapor-pressure depression (dew point) osmometry. **A,** Reference-point (starting) temperature. **B,** Dew point temperature. 1. Sample equilibration time. 2. Maximum thermocouple cooling. 3. Increase to dew point (heat of condensation). 4. Dew point equilibrium. (Modified from 5500 Vapor Pressure Osmometer, Wescor, Inc., Logan Ut, 1988).

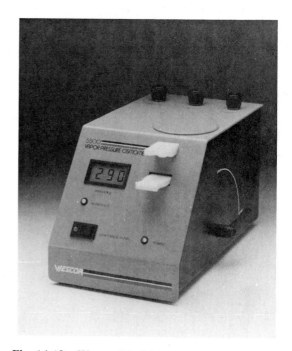

Fig. 14-10   Wescor Model 5500 Vapor Pressure Osmometer. (Courtesy Wescor, Inc.)

ful to know the contribution that serum proteins alone make to the serum osmolality. The clinical usefulness of this measurement, called **colloid osmotic pressure** or **oncotic pressure,** lies in the fact that proteins in serum (particularly albumin) tend to attract water molecules and thus hold fluid within the circulatory system. When serum protein concentration is decreased, the colloid osmotic pressure is decreased and there is increased likelihood toward the development of edema or accumulation of fluid in the extracellular space. Measurement of serum colloid osmotic pressure is useful in guiding intravenous fluid therapy to prevent the development of edema, particularly pulmonary edema.

The instruments available for measurement of colloid osmotic pressure use an operational principle very similar to the description of osmotic pressure presented earlier in this chapter and illustrated in Fig. 14-1. The colloid osmometer consists of a sample chamber and a reference chamber separated by a membrane that is permeable to water, crystalloids, and ions but is impermeable to colloids. Serum or other fluid containing protein is placed in the sample chamber. The reference chamber contains a reference saline solution and is in contact with a pressure transducer that has been calibrated in units of mm Hg using a mercury manometer.

Before measurement of a serum specimen the reference saline solution is placed in the sample chamber and in the reference chamber. There is no net movement of particles across the membrane, and the transducer registers no pressure change. When serum is placed in the sample chamber, the saline from the reference chamber flows by osmosis into the sample chamber, increasing the hydrostatic pressure on the sample side and creating negative pressure on the reference side. The maximum pressure change occurs at about 90 seconds after introduction of the serum sample and then begins to decrease as macromolecules begin to move to the reference side. The colloid osmotic pressure reading of the sample in mm Hg is taken at a maximum rather than an equilibrium point. Characteristics of the two commercially available clinical colloid osmometers are listed in Table 14-1.

Review Questions

1. When a mole of glucose is added to a kilogram of water, which of the following changes occur in its colligative properties?
   1. The boiling point is decreased
   2. The osmotic pressure is increased
   3. The vapor pressure is increased
   4. The freezing point is decreased
      A. 1, 2, and 4
      B. 2, 3, and 4
      C. 2 and 4
      D. 1 and 2
2. The colligative property generally measured by a clinical laboratory osmometer is the:
   A. Osmotic pressure
   B. Freezing point
   C. Dew point
   D. Vapor pressure

Use the following information to answer no. 3 and 4.

A patient, brought to the emergency room, has the following laboratory results:
Sodium = 140 mmol/L
Glucose = 80 mg/dL
BUN = 6.0 mg/dL
Osmolality = 316 mOsm/Kg H_2O

3. The calculated osmolality on this patient using the Holmes formula is:
   A. 186
   B. 267
   C. 286.5
   D. 316
4. The "osmolal gap" suggests that this patient may be suffering from ethanol intoxication or ingestion of some other volatile substance.
   A. True
   B. False
5. The tendency for a solution to remain in the liquid state when cooled below its normal freezing point is called:
   A. Supercooling
   B. Heat of fusion
   C. Fast cooling
   D. Heat of condensation
6. The method of osmometry used in the clinical laboratory that truly measures a change in osmotic pressure is which of the following?
   A. Freezing point osmometry
   B. Vapor pressure osmometry
   C. Colloid osmometry
   D. Dew point osmometry
7. The temperature sensing device in freezing point osmometry is a:
   A. Thermocouple
   B. Stirrer
   C. Thermistor
   D. Manometer
8. The particles that have the greatest effect on the colloid osmotic pressure of serum are:
   A. Electrolytes
   B. Crystalloids
   C. Glucose
   D. Protein

9. Which of the following are true statements regarding vapor pressure osmometry?
   1. The physical state of the sample is not changed during measurement
   2. Cannot be used in the detection of volatiles
   3. During measurement, a plateau is seen due to heat of fusion
   4. The specimen remains liquid during supercooling
      A. 1, 2, and 4
      B. 2, 3, and 4
      C. 2 and 4
      D. 1 and 2

Answer Key:

1. C   2. B   3. C   4. A   5. A   6. C   7. C   8. D   9. D

Bibliography

Advanced Digimatic Micro-Osmometer Model 3MO, User's guide, Advanced Instruments, Inc, Needham Heights, Mass, 1988.

Alpert NL: Osmometers. In Alpert NL, ed: Clinical instrument systems, vol 7, no. 8, Macor Publishing, New York, 1986.

Barlow WK: Applications of osmometry, Am Lab, 18(11):124, 1986.

Corner D: Analytical techniques and instrumentation. In Bishop ML, Duben-Von Laufen JL, and Fody EP, eds: Clinical chemistry: principle, procedure, correlations, Philadelphia, 1985, JB Lippincott.

5500 Vapor Pressure Osmometer, Wescor, Inc, Logan Ut, 1988.

Freier EF: Osmometry. In Tietx NW, ed: Textbook of clinical chemistry, Philadelphia, 1986, WB Saunders.

Kaplan LA: Measurement of colligative properties. In Kaplan LA, Pesce AJ, eds: Clinical chemistry: theory, analysis, and correlation, ed 2, St. Louis, 1989, Mosby–Year Book.

Lee LW, Schmidt LM: Elementary principles of laboratory instruments, ed 5, St Louis, 1983, Mosby–Year Book.

Steinrauf MA: Osmometry. In Hicks R, Schenken JR, and Steinrauf MA, eds: Laboratory instrumentation, ed 2, Hagerstown, Md, 1980, Harper & Row.

15

Nephelometry and Turbidimetry

LARRY E. SCHOEFF

Principle
Detection of Scattered Light
Instrumentation
Limitations
Refractivity

Principle

Interaction of Light with Particles. To understand the principle of nephelometric or turbidimetric assays, the concept of **light scattering** must first be examined. When a collimated (i.e., parallel, nondivergent) beam of light strikes a particle in suspension, some light is reflected, some is scattered, some is absorbed, and some is transmitted. **Nephelometry** is the measurement of the light scattered by a particulate solution. **Turbidimetry** measures light scatter as a decrease in the light transmitted through the solution.

In considering nephelometry the question of how light is scattered by a homogeneous particle suspension must be examined. Three types of scatter can occur. If the wavelength, λ, of light is much larger than the diameter of the particle ($d < 0.1\lambda$), the light is symmetrically scattered around the particle, with a minimum in the intensity of the scatter occurring at 90 degrees to the incident beam, as described by Rayleigh (Fig. 15-1, *A*).

If the wavelength of the incident light is much smaller than the diameter of the particle ($d > 10\lambda$), most of the light appears to be scattered forward because of destructive out-of-phase backscatter, as described by the Mie theory (Fig. 15-1, *B*).

If, however, the wavelength of the light is approximately equal to the size of the particles, more light appears scattered in a forward direction than in a backward direction (Fig. 15-1, *C*), as described by **Rayleigh-Debye scatter.**

One of the most common uses of light-scattering analyses is the measurement of antigen-anti-

body reactions. Because most antigen-antibody complex systems are heterogeneous with particle diameters of 250 to 1500 nm and the wavelengths used in most light-scattering analyzers are 320 to 650 nm, the scatter seen is essentially Rayleigh-Debye, with the blank scatter being primarily described by Rayleigh scatter. Therefore the ability to detect light scatter in a forward direction ($\theta = 15$ to 90 degrees) would lead to greater sensitivity for nephelometric determinations. Such is the case in the newer rate and laser nephelometers.

Detection of Scattered Light

Turbidity. Turbidity is a measure of the reduction in the light transmission caused by particle formation, and it quantifies the residual light transmitted (Fig. 15-2). The instrumentation required for turbidity measurements ranges from a simple manual spectrophotometer available in most laboratories to a sophisticated discrete analyzer. Because this technique measures a decrease in a large signal of transmitted light, the sensitivity of turbidimetry is limited primarily by the photometric accuracy and sensitivity of the instrument. Instruments used for turbidimetry can be used for many other assays, such as enzyme assays and those assays based on color development.

Nephelometry. Nephelometry, on the other hand, detects a portion of the light that is scattered at a variety of angles (Fig. 15-3). The sensitivity of this method primarily depends on the absence of blank or background scatter because the instruments are detecting a small increment of signal at a scatter angle on a supposedly black or null background. Ideally no light is detected in the absence of a scattering species, and so subsequent scatter in samples is measured against this black background. The signal is magnified by the use of a photomultiplier so that the detection range is increased. However, such measurements

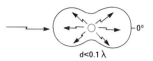

A   SMALL PARTICLES
-LIGHT SCATTERED SYMMETRICALLY
BUT MINIMALLY AT 90°   (RAYLEIGH)

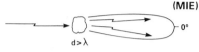

$d < 0.1 \lambda$

B   VERY LARGE PARTICLES
-LIGHT MOSTLY SCATTERED FORWARD
(MIE)

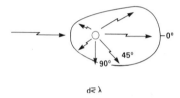

$d > \lambda$

C   LARGE PARTICLES
-LIGHT SCATTERED PREFERENTIALLY
FORWARD   (RAYLEIGH-DEBYE)

$d \gtrsim \lambda$

Fig. 15-1   Effect of particle size on scattering of incident light in a homogeneous solution. (From Gauldie J: In Kaplan LA, Pesce AJ, eds: Nonisotopic alternatives to radioimmunoassay, New York, 1981, Marcel Dekker.)

TURBIDIMETRY

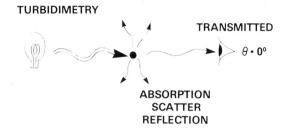

TRANSMITTED

$\theta = 0°$

ABSORPTION
SCATTER
REFLECTION

Fig. 15-2   Schematic diagram of turbidity measurements. θ, Angle of detection. (From Gauldie J: In Kaplan LA, Pesce AJ, eds: Nonisotopic alternatives to radioimmunoassay, New York, 1981, Marcel Dekker.)

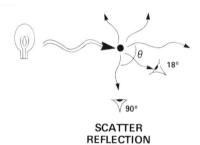

SCATTER
REFLECTION

Fig. 15-3   Schematic diagram of nephelometric measurement. θ, Angle of detection. (From Gauldie J: In Kaplan LA, Pesce AJ, eds: Nonisotopic alternatives to radioimmunoassay, New York, 1981, Marcel Dekker.)

require the committed use of a **nephelometer,** which has limited use in other assays.

Instrumenation

Components. A schematic layout of the basic components of a nephelometer is shown in Fig. 15-4. Typical systems consist of a light source, a collimating system, a wavelength selector such as a filter (the last two items are unnecessary with laser light sources), a sample cuvette, a stray light trap, and a photodetector.

Light Source. Fluoronephelometers such as the Technicon instrument use a medium-pressure mercury-arc lamp as a light source, which serves both for nephelometry and fluorometry. The relatively high intensity light and short-wavelength emission bands make this a good source. Other light sources range from simple low-voltage tungsten-filament lamps and light-emitting diodes to sophisticated low-power lasers. Lasers have become a viable light source for the measurement of immunoglobins and other specific proteins. They produce stable, highly collimated, and intense beams of light (typically 1

milliradian divergence) that require no additional optical collimators as do other light sources. The sophistication of laser nephelometers (e.g., the Hyland PDQ) to achieve broad range linearity with antigen/antibody complexes is primarily attributable to the light source employed.

LASER is an acronym for Light Amplification by Stimulated Emission of Radiation. Its applicable significance as a light source for spectroscopic analysis of materials was well established in the research laboratory, especially in the area of analysis called Raman spectroscopy, which involves altering the frequency and phase of light scattered by material in a suspended medium. A portion of light scattered from a laser beam passing through a transparent sample has its frequency lowered (Stoker lines) or raised (anti-Stoker lines) by the molecular vibration frequencies of the material of the sample. Light scattered from the needlelike laser beam can be conveniently focused on the entrance slit of a

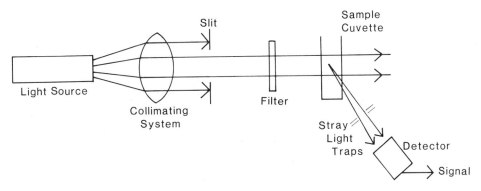

Fig. 15-4 Schematic of basic components of a nephelometer.

spectrometer, which can then measure the displacements of these Raman lines. Because of the high light intensity that can be achieved in a monochromatic laser beam, a substantial increase in sensitivity (the ability to detect weak light scattering) has been achieved over previous conventional instruments. A basic understanding of laser technology is essential for appreciating the inherent characteristics that make lasers ideal light sources for nephelometric techniques.

Conventional nephelometers employ ordinary light sources such as incandescent lamps or mercury vapor tubes. The light waves emitted from these light sources are incoherent and omni-directional. However, laser light is coherent and uni-directional and travels in a very thin, collimated beam that is monochromatic and extremely intense.

A typical helium-neon laser lamp, such as in the Hyland PDQ laser nephelometer, consists of a slender glass, plasma tube (Fig. 15-5, *A*) that surrounds both a glass laser core and high energy pumping electrode. The glass plasma tube and core are filled with free helium and neon (both in a gaseous state). A fixed mirror positioned at the rear of the laser tube is fully reflective. Another mirror at the front of the tube is partially reflective. When the electrode is charged electrically, the helium atoms are excited to a high energy state, and by collision, they transfer this energy to the neon atoms (Fig. 15-5, *B*). This is possible because by coincidence, the excited state of the helium atoms coincides exactly with the excited state of the neon atoms. In turn, the excited neon atoms randomly emit photons. When interaction between these atoms occurs, the neon atoms are now capable of amplifying light by stimulated emission (Fig. 15-5, *C*). Although some of the photons escape, many, whose initial direction co-

incides with the axis of the tube, will bounce back and forth between the end mirrors many times, stimulating many other atoms to emit photons with each phase resulting in an amplification. Because one of the mirrors is slightly transparent, a portion of the light bouncing between the mirrors

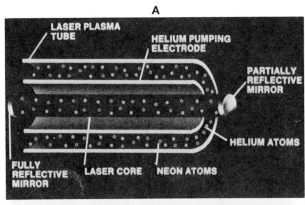

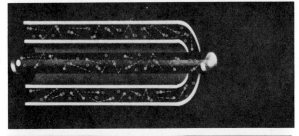

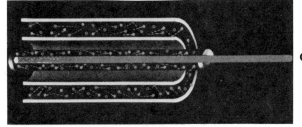

Fig. 15-5 *A*, He-Ne laser tube. *B*, He excitation and He-Ne collision. *C*, Ne emission and amplification.

will leak out slowly at first, and then become faster and stronger through the partially transparent mirror, to emerge as the laser beam.

In optical systems using laser light, another example of which is the Behring Auto Laser LN, it is easier to reduce stray light, which contributes to background scatter, and to mask the transmitted beam thus allowing measurement of forward scatter. The increase in light intensity achievable with lasers also results in an improvement of signal-to-noise ratio, but this is limited somewhat by detector saturation. The high degree of collimation and the single energy level (monochromatic) of this light make it ideal for light scattering techniques. Disadvantages of laser sources include cost, safety problems, and the restricted availability of limited fixed wavelengths.

Because particle size may continually change during the course of reaction analysis, as during immune precipitate formation, light scatter at a single wavelength may change whereas the average light scatter over a number of wavelengths remains relatively constant. The Beckman Auto-ICS System employs a broad-band filter for selection of a wavelength region from a normal tungsten lamp source to overcome this problem, which is obviously more acute in rate methods when the size of the particle is changing rapidly.

In all cases the photodetector system must be matched to the wavelength or wavelengths of the scattered light, that, for nephelometry and turbidimetry, corresponds to the incident light wavelength or wavelengths.

Angle of Detection. Because particles the size of antigen-antibody complexes appear to scatter light more in the forward direction, there is an increased signal-to-noise ratio as the detector is placed nearer the transmitted path (0 degrees). Fig. 15-6 shows the magnitude of the difference expected in an IgG-anti-IgG system.

The blank signal, described best by Rayleigh scatter (see Fig. 15-1 *A*), is not as affected by an

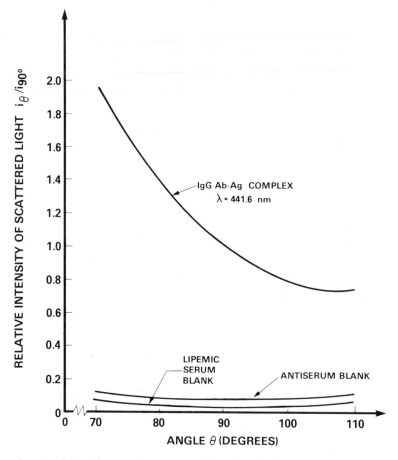

Fig. 15-6   Effect of angle of detection on the apparent light-scattering intensity for IgG/anti-IgG reaction products. Effect on serum blank and lipemic blank. (From Kusnetz J, Mansberg HP: Optical considerations: nephelometry. In Ritchie RF, ed: Automated immunoanalysis, part 1, New York, 1978, Marcel Dekker.)

Table 15-1 Automated clinical instruments available for light-scattering analysis

	Technicon AIP	Hyland PDQ (OISC 120)	Behring Auto laser LN	Beckman Automated ICS	Reaction rate analyzer*	Centrifugal fast analyzer†
Nephelometer (N) (angle) or turbidometer (T)	N (90°)	N (31°)	N (5°-12°)	N (70°)	T	T
End-point (E) or kinetic (K) analysis of reaction	E + blank	E + blank	E + blank	K	K or E	K or E
Light source (wavelength, nm)	Mercury arc (357 nm)	Laser (632.8 nm)	Laser (632.8 nm)	Tungsten lamp (400-550nm)	Variable: ultraviolet to 700 nm	Variable: ultraviolet to 700 nm
Samples/hour	120	120	120-240	30-50	20-40	300
Reaction time	10 min	1 hour	1 hour (no PEG)	30 sec	1-2 min (kinetic)	1-2 min (kinetic)
Other type of analysis	++	+	+		+++	++++

Modified from Deverill I, Reeves WG: J Immunol Methods 38:191, 1980. PEG = Polyethylene glycol. Plus sign indicates ability of instrument to perform other measurements in addition to light-scattering analysis.

*For example, those by Abbott TDx Turb. (Irving, Tex.)

†For example, Roche (COBAS Bio) (Nutley, N.J.)

altered angle of detection. Thus although most early nephelometers detected light scattered at 90 degrees for reasons of manufacturing ease, which limited low-angle measurement capability, the detection of forward light scatter theoretically should provide greater sensitivity. The newer instruments tend to operate with lower detection angles, optimized in many cases to give the highest signal-to-noise ratio for the particular instrument's optics. Several of the systems listed in Table 15-1 detect forward light scatter and possess the increased sensitivity expected. Obviously, detection at 0 degrees is not possible because of the high intensity of the transmitted beam, but some laser-equipped fast analyzers using a mask to block the transmitted beam are able to operate at very low angles. Instruments employing low-angle detectors tend to have greater sensitivity than the 90 degree type of instruments. If the angle of detection in a nephelometer is set at 90 degrees, as in older instruments, then the scattered light is referred to as **"Tyndall light,"** named after the physicist who worked with this principle.

Applications. There are numerous clinical applications for turbidimetry and nephelometry. Various microbiology analyzers use turbidity measurements to detect and compare over time the amount of bacterial growth in broth cultures. Turbidimetry is routinely used to measure the degee of antibiotic sensitivity from such cultures. In coagulation analyzers turbidity measurements are employed to detect fibrin clot formation in the cuvette wells. Turbidimetric assays have long been used in clinical chemistry to quantitate protein content in biologic fluids, such as urine, cerebrospinal fluid, and body cavity fluids.

Currently the single greatest use of nephelometry is the measurement of antigen-antibody complexes that are formed in the popular enzyme immunoassay techniques for various constituents. Some analyzers use a nephelometric principle to assay enzymes that act on particulate substrates. Specific blood cell counters use light scatter detection to distinguish different types of blood cells.

An example of a popular rate nephelometer is the Beckman Array 360 Protein/Drug System (Fig. 15-7), a fully automated, random access instrument dedicated to detecting antigen-antibody complexes by light scatter measurement. The analytic module contains sample and reagent carousels, a fluid transport system, the optics, and a data reduction processor. Samples are loaded onto a 40-position carousel where appropriate dilutions are automatically prepared by the instrument. Reagents are located on a 20-position antibody wheel and used with the appropriate buffers and diluents stored on the analyzer. The pick-up and delivery of sample and reagent are performed by two robotic arm pipettes, which incorporate precision step motors to provide accurate dispensing and positioning. Analysis is performed by two identical rate nephelometers within the analyzer, which operate independently and thereby improve throughput. Selected tests can be programmed to run on one or the other optical unit, as user preference and calibration needs dictate.

The Array measures light scatter to determine

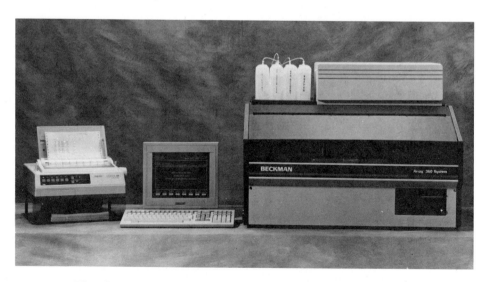

Fig. 15-7   Array 360 system (Courtesy Beckman Instruments, Inc).

the rate of formation of insoluble immunoprecipitation products resulting from a specific antigen (protein to be measured) combining with a specific antibody to that antigen. Formation of complexes increases for a fixed amount of antibody relative to the amount of antigen present. The instrument has the ability to monitor that optimal reaction proportions are being maintained. Three measurement points are distinguished from the reaction curve: (1) baseline scatter before reactants are introduced, (2) initial scatter caused by adding diluted sample only to the measurement chamber, and (3) the resulting scatter as immune complexes develop after addition of antibody to the sample (antigen). Eventually maximum scatter will equate to an end point.

The Array allows random access testing of many specific proteins, such as apolipoproteins, immunoglobulins, and prealbumin, and therapeutic drugs, such as theophylline.

Limitations

Turbidimetry vs Nephelometry. Although the principle of nephelometry—detection of a small amplifiable signal on a black background—should lend this method high sensitivity, the sophistication and specifications of the instruments available do not achieve this goal. Turbidimetry—detection of a small decrease in a large signal—should be limited in sensitivity; however, current instruments have excellent discrimination and can quantify small changes in signal, thereby allowing turbidimetric measurements to achieve high sensitivity.

Turbidimetry and nephelometry have similarities to absorption spectrophotometry, and many sources of interference and errors are common to all these systems. Many techniques that can be used to minimize absorption interferences (see Chapters 7 and 8) are also applicable to turbidimetry and nephelometry. Because of the uniqueness of nephelometric measurements, especially in the case of antibody-antigen reactions, some specific applications are discussed in the following sections.

Choice of Wavelength. Basic light-scattering theory predicts that the intensity of scattered light increases as shorter wavelengths of incident light are used. Most immunologic assay reactions employ serum protein reactions requiring the choice of a wavelength at which neither the proteins nor colored serum components absorb appreciably. Because proteins absorb strongly below 300 nm

and serum has an absorption peak at 400 to 425 nm because of porphyrins, instruments tend to operate in the 320 to 380, or 500 to 650 nm range. Reduction of the protein concentration by dilution will decrease background absorption. Most immunochemical reactions measured by nephelometry use high-affinity antibodies that allow for large dilutions of protein and consequent improvement of sensitivity.

Comparison of Sensitivity. Sensitivity in nephelometers is largely controlled by the amount of background scatter from sample and reagents. Because background scatter can be high relative to specific scatter, instruments do not reach their full potential of sensitivity. This limitation, coupled with the higher wavelengths generated in laser instruments, accounts for the fact that laser instruments show no great increase in sensitivity over conventional nephelometers.

Sensitivity in turbidimetric measurements depends on the ability of the detector to resolve small changes in light intensity. Using low wavelengths and high-quality spectrophotometers with their high-precision detection systems, sensitivity in turbidimetry is usually adequate for many measurements and in many cases compares well with nephelometry. Theoretically, with additional refinements, nephelometry ultimately should provide higher sensitivity than turbidimetry.

End Point vs Kinetic Analysis. Examination of light scattered as a function of time, after there is mixture of an antibody and antigen, shows that after an initial delay there is an almost linear increase in scatter followed by a slower attainment of plateau scatter. The secondary reaction occurs much more slowly than the first because larger particles form and begin to flocculate, and they distort the scatter intensity seen at forward angles. Both turbidity and nephelometry measurements behave in this manner.

There are two basic ways of measuring light scatter caused by this reaction: end point analysis and rate analysis. End point analysis requires blank (reagent) determinations and a reasonable amount of elapsed time before final measurement. Fig. 15-8 shows the forward scatter developed at 70 degrees in a rate nephelometric analyzer. Comparing the two graphs, the differences between an end point analysis (blank value vs reading at t = x) and a rate or kinetic analysis (increase in scattered intensity over a set time interval) can be seen. The kinetic approach, which electronically subtracts any blank signal, does not

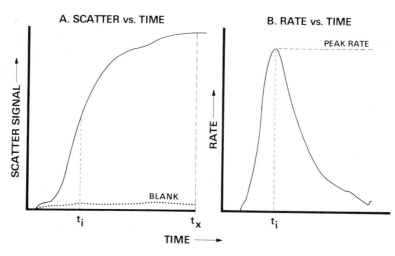

Fig. 15-8 Kinetic analysis of light scattering. *Curve A,* Intensity of scattered light signal vs time; *curve B,* rate of change of scattered light signal vs time.

require a separate reagent blank to be run. Both kinetic and end point analysis can be applied equally to turbidimetry and nephelometry.

Summary. Both turbidimetry and nephelometry are nonabsorptive techniques based on radiation scattering photometry. Factors that affect both types of measurements include: (1) the size and shape of the particles, (2) the intensity and wavelength of the incident light, and (3) the refractive index, or difference in speed of light passing through both the suspended medium and the suspended particles.

In turbidimetry a particulate substance in suspension blocks or reflects a portion of the incident light, resulting in decreased transmitted light that is directly proportional to the substance's concentration. The chosen wavelength for analysis is different from the one that the test substance normally absorbs, and light detection is the same direction as the incident beam. In general, turbidimetric measurements tend to have less sensitivity at low concentrations than do nephelometric measurements.

Nephelometry differs in that light scatter from the particulate substance is measured at some angle, preferably less than 90 degrees, from the incident beam of light. The angle of predominant scattering varies according to particle size and wavelength of light. The monochromatic incident light is usually of short wavelength in the near ultra-violet range. The intensity of scatter is proportional to the number of particles in suspension. The two types of nephelometric assays—endpoint and kinetic—depend on whether photometer readings are taken at the end

of, or during, formation of particulate complexes. Nephelometric measurements tend to have better sensitivity at low concentrations than turbidimetric measurements. A comparison of several commercially available light-scattering devices and some of their features is given in Table 15-1.

Refractivity

Principle. When a beam of light impinges on a boundary surface, it can be reflected, absorbed, or, if the material is transparent, pass into the boundary and emerge on the other side. When light passes from one medium into another, the path of the light beam will change direction at the boundary surface if its speed in the second medium is different from that in the first (Fig. 15-9). This bending of light is called **refraction.**

Because the degree of refraction of a light beam depends on the difference in the speed of light between two different mediums, the ratio of the two speeds has been expressed as the index of refraction, or **refractive index.** The relative ability of a substance to bend light is called **refractivity.** The expression of a refractive index, n, is always relative to air with the convention that n of air = 1. The measurement of the refractive index is the measurement of angles because the light is bent at an angle proportional to the relationship of n in the medium through which the light is passing:

$$\frac{n}{n_1} = \frac{\sin \theta}{\sin \theta_1}$$

The refractivity of a liquid depends on (1) the wavelength of the incident light, (2) the temper-

Fig. 15-9 Schematic illustrating bending of light when it passes from a medium of one density into a medium of a different density, with an angle of deflection, θ^1.

Fig. 15-10 Schematic of an Abbé refractometer. (From Shugar GJ, Shugar RA, and Bauman L: Chemical technicians ready reference book, New York, 1973, McGraw-Hill.)

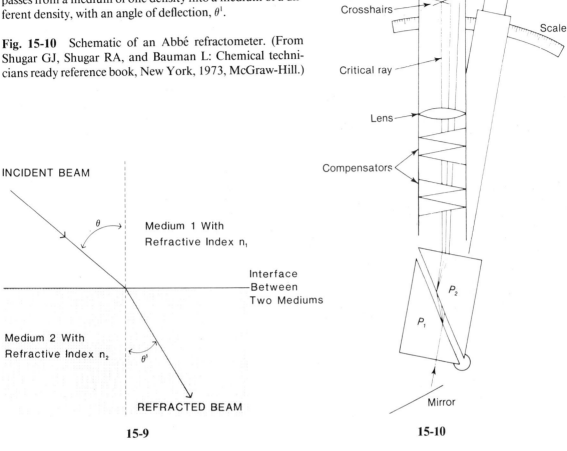

15-9

15-10

ature, (3) the nature of the liquid, and (4) the total mass of solid dissolved in the liquid. If the first three factors are held constant, the refractive index of a solution is a direct measure of the total mass of dissolved solids.

Instrumentation. Most clinical refractometers are based on the Abbé refractometer (Fig. 15-10), marketed by American Optical Corporation. This refractometer consists of two prisms and a series of lenses. Light passes through the first prism where the light beam is dispersed. The dispersed light passes into and through the thin layer of the liquid sample where it is refracted. The light beam passes through a second prism where the light is again dispersed and on leaving is again refracted. The boundary at the edge of the refracted light beam is aligned perpendicularly to the scale on which serum protein concentrations or specific gravity can be read. The scale for reading serum protein (g/dl or g/L) is established by calibration of the instrument against a "normal" serum solution.

This type of refractometer is extraordinarily simple, having no moving or electrical parts. Therefore it is easily reproducible, measuring protein with a precision of $\pm$ 1% and an accuracy of $\pm$ 1 g/L. The sample size is 50 μl.

More complex refractometers are used to monitor column effluents for high-performance liquid chromatography (HPLC) analysis.

Applications. Refractometry has been applied to the measurement of total serum protein concentration. The assumption of this analysis is that the serum matrix (i.e., the concentration of electrolytes and small organic molecules) remains essentially the same from patient to patient. Because the mass of protein is normally so much greater than the mass of other serum constituents, small variations of these other substances have no significant effect on the refractive index of serum. Refractometers are calibrated against normal serum, and total protein concentrations are read directly from a scale.

Refractometry is also used to estimate the specific gravity of urine samples. The refractive index is linearly related to the total mass of dissolved solids and thus to specific gravity. This remains valid over most of the range normally encountered for urine (i.e., up to 1.035 g/ml).

When the concentration of small molecular weight compounds or particulate matter greatly increases, positive interference results. This interference occurs in the presence of hyperglycemia, hyperbilirubinemia, azotemia, lyophilized samples, and hyperlipidemia. Hemolysis will also result in false-positive values for total serum protein.

Review Questions

1. Define turbidimetry and nephelometry. What do these two techniques have in common? How are they different?
2. Which technique—turbidimetry or nephelometry—has the greatest sensitivity at low concentrations of the substance being measured?
3. Why have lasers become the most popular type of light source for current use in nephelometers?
4. Name two clinical applications of turbidimetry and of nephelometry.
5. Why are forward angle nephelometers preferred over 90 degree angle instruments?
6. Identify three factors that can affect both turbidimetric and nephelometric measurements.
7. The measurement of angles of bending light by a substance through a medium and the proportional relationship between the two expresses the substance's _____.
8. What is the most common use of refractometers in the clinical laboratory?

Bibliography

DeCresce R: Array protein system, Lab Med 18(1):47, 1987.

Deverill I, Reeves W: Light scattering and absorption developments in immunology, J Immunol Methods 38:191, 1980.

Gauldie J: Principles and clinical applications of nephelometry. In Kaplan LA, Pesce AJ eds: Nonisotopic alternatives to radioimmunoassay, New York, 1981, Marcel Dekker.

Glover F, Gaulden J: Relationship between refractive index and concentration of solutions, Nature 200:1165, 1963.

Kaplan LA, Pesce AJ: Clinical chemistry: theory, analysis, and correlation, ed 2, St Louis, 1989, Mosby–Year Book.

Kusnetz J, Mansberg H: Optical considerations: nephelometry. In Ritchie R: Automated immunoanalysis, part 1, New York, 1978, Marcel Dekker.

Meloy T: Today's education. What should you know about the laser? Sept, 1968 p 61.

Ritchie R, ed: Automated immunoanalysis, parts 1 and 2, New York, 1978, Marcel Dekker.

Rubini M, Wolf A: Refractometric determination of total solids and water of serum and urine, J Biol Chem 225:868, 1957.

Schawlow AL: Laser light, Sci Am, 219:120, 1968.

CHAPTER 16

Gas Chromatography— Mass Spectrometry

SHERWOOD C. LEWIS
ROBERT H. WILLIAMS

The origin of mass spectrometry lies in the work of Sir J.J. Thomson, the discoverer of the electron. His later finding of the isotopes of neon led his student, Francis W. Aston, to develop the first device able to separate atoms of different masses. Thus Aston, using this "mass spectrograph" subsequently was able to prove that most elements exist as mixtures of isotopes. Although these notable achievements were attained in the early part of this century, it was not until the 1940s that mass spectrometers were made available commercially. Even then, their complexity and high cost assured their relatively limited use and certainly placed them out of the reach of most clinical laboratories. By 1975 to 1980, however, major advances in electronics, high vacuum technology, and computer development had brought about drastic changes in mass spectrometry instrumentation. It was now possible to produce far simpler, reasonably priced, and more reliable mass spectrometers. Today many clinical laboratories have added this type of instrumentation to their complement of analytic tools. No longer should the principles and techniques of mass spectrometry be foreign to the clinical laboratorian.

Principles of Operation

Mass spectrometry is based on the principle of ionization of molecules and their subsequent fragmentation when impinged on by a suitable source of energy. When the energy is controlled and unvarying, the ionization and fragmentation processes are reproducible. The resulting pattern of fragment masses and their relative abundances yield the characteristic mass spectrum of the molecule producing the fragments.

Several types of energy sources have been employed for producing the ionization of molecules within the mass spectrometer. Most commonly used, however, is a beam of electrons whose energy is sufficient to bring about ionization and fragmentation of a parent molecule. This is referred to as **electron-impact ionization.** The reactions involved are illustrated in Fig. 16-1. Important features of these reactions should be noted:

1. Ionization produces a positively charged **molecular ion** whose mass is that of the neutral parent molecule. Many compounds do not yield an unfragmented molecular ion. The resulting mass spectrum of such a compound will be devoid of an ion whose mass is characteristic of the molecular weight of that compound.
2. Fragmentation results in a variety of **fragment ions** of different masses.
3. Positively charged, neutral, and negatively charged ions may be produced by the ionization process. (Most mass spectrometers employed in clinical applications make use

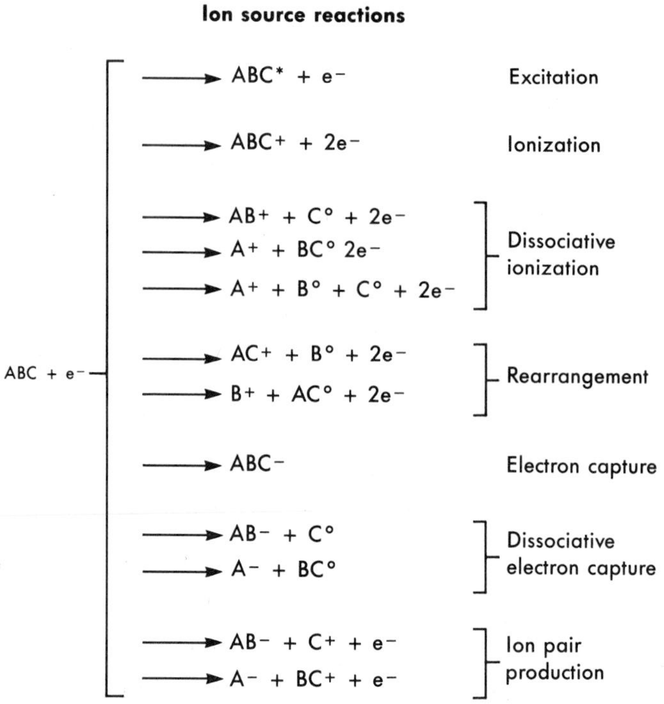

Ion source reactions

Fig. 16-1 Reactions that occur in the ion source of a mass spectrometer. (Courtesy Finnigan MAT.)

of the information associated with the positive ions generated.)

Instrumentation—Mass Spectrometer Components

The typical mass spectrometer is composed of several sub-units, each performing a necessary function in the production (and in some cases the identification) of the mass spectra of compounds being analyzed. Each of these sub-units will now be described.

Inlet System. The **inlet** system provides a means of admitting samples to the mass spectrometer. When the mass spectrometer is used as part of a combined **gas chromatography/mass spectrometry (gc/ms)** arrangement, the inlet represents the interface between the gas chromatograph and the mass spectrometer. As such it must allow passage of the volatile compounds separated by the gas chromatograph into the **ion source** region of the mass spectrometer where ionization and fragmentation will occur. It is necessary for the inlet to be heated to maintain the sample in the vapor state. It also must accommodate the atmospheric pressure of the gas chromatograph column's exit with the high vacuum condition required for operation of the mass

spectrometer. To do so, the inlet provides a means of stripping away most of the carrier gas while allowing the sample's component molecules to enter the ion source.

The inlet system may include a means of introducing solid samples to the ion source (**direct probe analysis**). In this case a sample can be presented to the inlet system of the mass spectrometer in solid form, vaporized by the heated inlet system, and introduced to the ion source.

It is possible to interface the mass spectrometer to other sources of sample (e.g., a high-performance liquid chromatograph). When this is done, the essential function of the inlet system remains the same: separation of sample molecules from the carrier medium and presentation to the ion source.

Ion Source. Ionization and fragmentation of sample molecules occur in the region of the mass spectrometer known as the **ion source**. This region, maintained at high temperature and vacuum (typically 10^{-4} to 10^{-6} torr), provides conditions for vaporized sample molecules to be ionized.

In the electron impact mode of ionization a heated filament is the source of the electrons that bombard the sample molecules. Reproducibility of the fragmentation pattern is assured by using an electron energy, measured in electron volts (eV), which is fixed at the desired level (usually 70 eV). The degree of fragmentation also depends on the temperature of the ion source. For this reason the ion source temperature must be considered when comparing mass spectra of unknown compounds with reference spectra.

Although electron ionization is perhaps the most commonly used form of ionization, several other means of ionizing the parent molecule being analyzed are available. One such technique is **chemical ionization** whereby the ionization of sample molecule is brought about by the introduction of a reagent gas into the ion source. The reagent gas becomes ionized by the electron beam. The reagent gas ion then reacts with sample molecules, ionizing them with little fragmentation resulting. This "soft" form of ionization yields mass spectra with great molecular ion abundances. Such spectra are useful in deducing the molecular weight of unknown compounds.

Chemical ionization can also be of particular effectiveness in distinguishing between compounds having similar electron impact mass spectra. Such is the case with methamphetamine and phentermine, which are structural isomers. Their gc retention times and electron impact spectra are nearly identical, making their identification as separate entities nearly impossible by most gc/ms protocols. However, the chemical ionization spectra (using methane as the reagent gas) of these two compounds are sufficiently different that they can be clearly differentiated. Examination of the chemical ionization spectra for the two compounds reveals a prominent ion at m/z 133 in the spectrum of phentermine that is absent in the spectrum of methamphetamine (Fig. 16-2).

Another means of ionizing sample molecules is that of **fast atom bombardment.** In this mode, sample in solid form is bombarded with a beam of atoms such as argon. This results in the ionization of molecules with some fragmentation also occurring. The technique has had particular success in the analysis of large biomolecules but is not employed in systems commonly used for clinical or forensic purposes. The same can be said for various other types of soft ionization techniques that include **field desorption ionization** and **desorption chemical ionization.** Both types are useful in the analysis of thermally labile or low-volatility molecules because the molecules are desorbed from a surface in the ionic form and then subjected to mass analysis.

Mass Analyzer. Ions produced in the ion source, representing the parent molecular and fragment ions, must be sorted according to their masses. (More correctly, it is the **mass-to-charge ratio (m/z)** of these ions that is actually distinguished during mass analysis.) However, most ions are singly charged and the resulting spectrum of masses represents singly charged ions and their relative amounts or **abundances.** The mass analyzer must be able to separate the ions based on their differing masses and present them to a suitable detector. Mass analyzers have most commonly been the **magnetic sector** type or the **quadrupole** type. In the magnetic sector device ions that enter the analyzer have been accelerated out of the ion source by the application of a very high voltage. Under the influence of a magnetic field ions of different mass-to charge ratios are deflected according to the equation: $m/z = H^2R^2/2V$ where m is the mass of the ion, z is its charge, H is the magnetic field strength in gauss, R is the radius of the curved path of the deflected ion, and V is the voltage applied to accelerate the ions out

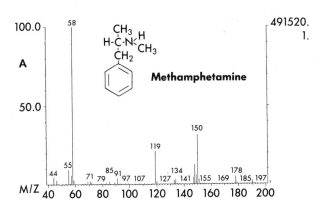

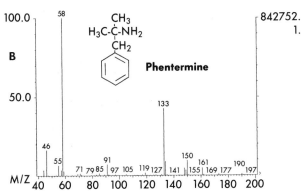

Fig. 16-2 Use of chemical ionization (CI) to produce full-scan mass spectra to differentiate **A**, methamphetamine from **B**, phentermine (obtained with methane reagent gas). (Courtesy Finnigan MAT.)

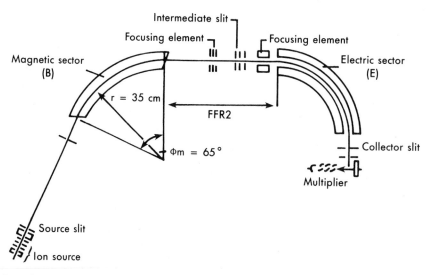

Fig. 16-3 Diagram of a high resolution double-focus mass spectrometer. (Courtesy Finnigan MAT.)

of the ion source. Ions of a given m/z ratio selectively exit the magnetic sector as the magnetic field strength, H, is varied. Alternately, the magnetic field may be held constant and the voltage changed to achieve selection of ions allowed to exit the magnetic sector. A mass analyzer employing a single magnet to focus the ions yields low resolution of the ions of different masses. To increase resolution, an electrostatic field can be placed in tandem with the magnetic field, allowing additional focusing of ions (Fig. 16-3). Such **double-focus mass spectrometers** are not often used for routine clinical purposes as they are quite expensive and provide more than the resolution needed for compound identification and quantitation in a clinical setting.

The quadrupole is a very popular type of mass analyzer used in a large number of today's mass spectrometers. The basic features of the quadrupole analyzer are seen in Fig. 16-4. With application of selected direct current (DC) and radiofrequency (RF) voltages to the two pairs of metallic rods, only ions of specific mass/charge ratio can pass undeflected to the exit end of the rods where they are then detected. All other ions have unstable trajectories along the path of the rods and are deflected toward the rods, never reaching the detector. By continuously and repetitively varying or "ramping" the voltages applied to the rods, it is possible to generate the complete mass spectrum of ions sequentially making their way through the quadrupole.

A frequently used variation of quadrupole-based mass spectrometry is **selected ion monitor-**

ing **(SIM),** known also as **mass selective detection (MSD).** In this mode of operation the voltages applied to the quadrupole are not ramped in a continuous fashion. Instead they are sequentially set to values specific for select ions to be detected. Only certain key characteristic ions are monitored rather than a complete mass spectrum of a compound. By "dwelling" only on these ions, it is possible to increase the system's sensitivity when very low concentrations of the compound are presented to the mass spectrometer. This increase in sensitivity, however, is ob-

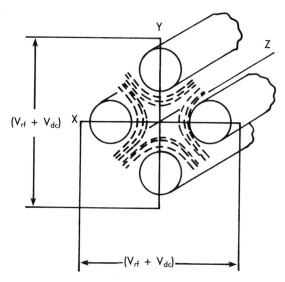

Fig. 16-4 Schematic of a quadrupole mass analyzer showing the quadrupole rods and the applied voltages. (Courtesy Finnigan MAT.)

tained by sacrificing the opportunity to examine a full mass spectrum.

A newer form of mass analyzer that is now in widespread use is the **ion trap detector.** Actually a three-dimensional variant of the quadrupole, the ion trap functions both as an ion source and mass analyzer. In design and construction it is a very simple device (Fig. 16-5). Three electrodes in the form of a ring and two end caps compose the source and analyzer combination. Ions produced in the cavity provided by the ring and end caps are trapped there until selectively ejected as the scanning radio-frequency voltage on the ring electrode is varied. These ejected ions are then detected by conventional means.

A major advantage of the ion trap detector is its ability to acquire full-spectrum data at very low sample concentrations. This greater sensitiv-

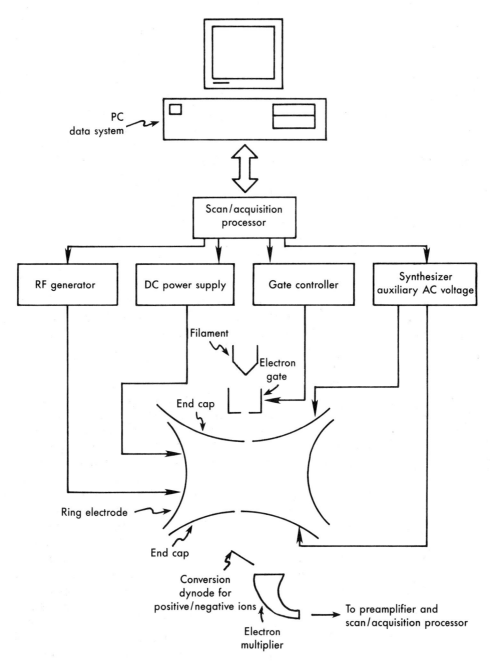

Fig. 16-5   An ion trap detector and associated components form a complete ion trap mass spectrometer. (Courtesy Finnigan MAT.)

ity allows compound identification based on a complete mass spectrum of the unknown. At such low sample concentrations a quadrupole-based system would have to operate in a SIM mode with little or no opportunity for unequivocal identification.

It should be appreciated, though, that the full-scan capability, whether achieved by ion trap or quadrupole analysis, has a potential disadvantage when compared to SIM. Contaminant substances will contribute to the mass spectrum of the compound of interest, degrading the purity of that compound's spectrum. On the other hand, with SIM there is a more selective ability to focus on those ions characteristic of the compound of interest, thereby filtering out contaminant ions.

The unique operating characteristics of the ion trap detector have led to interesting and useful opportunities for improving on its basic capabilities. For example, by applying a supplemental RF voltage to the end cap electrodes of the ion trap (known as axial modulation) the trap can store more ions without saturation of the trap because of space-charge effect. This results in greater sensitivity, resolution, and reproducibility of spectra. Latest generation ion trap-based mass spectrometers take advantage of this axial modulation enhancement.

Although complete mass spectra of molecules can be obtained using the ion trap, it should be recognized that it is also possible to operate the trap in a mode that emulates SIM. When doing so the voltages are set to allow only ions of a selected mass to exit the trap at a given time. A subtle difference exists between this **multiple ion detection (MID)** mode and a quadrupole's SIM. Sensitivity is increased in true SIM operation through increased dwell time in monitoring a selected ion. The MID monitors the chosen ion over a time period no greater than would be the case in full-scan acquisition. Fig. 16-6 compares the basic components of a quadrupole mass spectrometer with that of an ion trap model.

Ion Detector. Frequently the detection of ions separated by the mass analyzer is accomplished by an **electron multiplier.** Ions impacting the multiplier's primary surface, the first dynode, trigger a release of secondary electrons. A cascade of electrons occurs similar to that in a photomultiplier detector of photons. This results in an amplification, or gain, of about a million-fold for each ion reaching the detector. Additional circuitry associated with the electron multiplier permit the recording and display of the ions that have reached the detector via the mass analyzer. Another type of detector is the **ion-photon conversion** detector. Here, ions leaving the mass analyzer strike a phosphor that then emits a photon for each ion that hits the phosphor. A conventional photomultiplier then registers these photons with further amplification occurrring in the usual fashion.

Data System (Computer). The **data system** is an indispensable part of any modern mass spectrometer. It controls the multiple operating parameters of the spectrometer's sub-units. It also receives, stores, and manipulates the vast quantity of information produced during the acquisition of even a single mass spectrum. The importance of the data system in this latter function can be appreciated even more when it is considered that a typical gas chromatograph/mass spectrometer run may contain many chromatographic "peaks" whose mass spectra must be analyzed.

Beyond the essential functions already mentioned, the data system has another potent capability. Built-in libraries of reference spectra for known compounds can be searched by the system's computer and compared with an unknown spectrum obtained during a run. Thus it is possible to match up an unknown spectrum with a reference spectrum found in a library of thousands of spectra. Such a search and match can be completed in seconds, making this feature one of the most impressive aspects of the data system's operation.

All of the data system functions can be given added power and flexibility by the use of specially developed software that simplifies instrument operation, compound identification, and quantitation. Two such packages are the "Witness" software of Finnigan MAT, San Jose, California, and the "Target" software designed by THRU-PUT Systems, Inc. of Orlando, Florida. The Witness program, developed exclusively as GC/MS drug testing software, provides for initial setting of operating parameters and subsequent processing of samples for drug identification and confirmation. Target software creates a user-friendly interface that enhances processing of samples and reporting of results, greatly simplifying these tasks for the operator. Some similarities exist between the two products with regard to enhancement of the built-in data systems. Both can be customized for specific GC/MS methods and provide a forensic audit trail. However, the Witness compound identification routines are based on full-scan mass spectra whereas the Target sys-

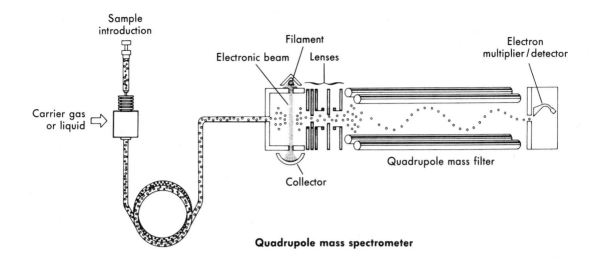

Quadrupole mass spectrometer

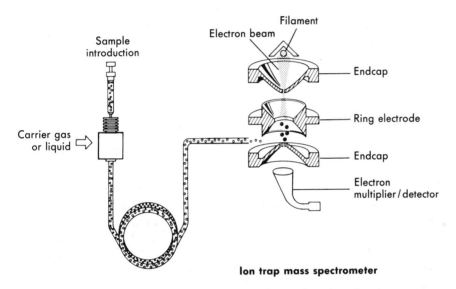

Ion trap mass spectrometer

Fig. 16-6 Comparison of the basic components of a quadrupole and an ion trap mass spectrometer. (Courtesy Finnigan MAT.)

tem uses the ion ratios from SIM analyses. Both systems are discussed in greater detail later in this chapter.

Vacuum System. It is necessary to maintain a very high vacuum (10^{-5} to 10^{-7} torr) in the mass spectrometer's inlet, analyzer, and detector regions. In the inlet, if it represents an interface to a gas chromatograph, the sample must be introduced to the mass spectrometer devoid of most of the carrier gas. Various technqiues are used to accomplish this stripping away of carrier gas and consequent enrichment of sample molecules. These techniques incorporate devices such as the **jet separator** or the **membrane separator,** and in some instruments, an **open-split interface.**

Within the ion source itself, ionization and collision-free transit of the formed ions depend on a condition of high vacuum. For similar reasons the mass analyzer also is maintained at high vacuum. Finally, at the elevated temperature required for its operation the detector would be destroyed quickly if subjected to pressures approaching atmospheric.

Vacuum systems for mass spectrometry use either **oil diffusion pumps** or **turbomolecular pumps.** The oil diffusion pump uses hot oil vapor streaming at high speed over a series of baffles to create a high vacuum. A turbomolecular pump contains a series of vanes rotating at ultra-high speed to evacuate a volume to which the pump's inlet is connected. For either type of pump to function, a forepump is required to reduce the system's pressure to less than 0.1 torr before operating the diffusion or turbo type pumps.

Production of Mass Spectra

The following discussion is limited to a description of electron-impact mass spectrometry.

Tuning and Calibration. By whatever means a sample is introduced to it, the mass spectrometer's basic operational mode is the same for each analysis. Before running samples it is necessary to tune and mass-calibrate the spectrometer. Tuning assures that the gain, electron energy for ionization, resolution, and sensitivity are adjusted for generation of spectra of maximum quality. Tuning may be performed automatically by the computer, although most systems permit manual tuning by the operator. Thus a "customized" tuning can be achieved to obtain maximum sensitivity, albeit with some loss of resolution.

Calibration is performed by mass analysis of a calibration compound and tuning the spectrometer to yield the correct m/z values known to exist for the major ions of the calibrating compound. As with the tune function, most instruments are designed to perform the calibration automatically.

Acquisition and Display of Mass Spectra. During a mass analysis, repetitive mass scans of short duration (0.5 to 2 seconds) are made and a mass spectrum is acquired as the result of each scan. Hence it is possible to collect several complete mass scans during the brief residence time of a given molecular species in the ion source. With each scan the detector's output and the data system's manipulation of that output combine to create a mass spectrum showing each ion and its intensity (abundance) in graphic form (Fig. 16-7). The horizontal axis of the mass spectrum represents the m/z values in **atomic mass units (amu).** The vertical axis is a scale of the ion intensities.

Several important features of a mass spectrum can be seen in Fig. 16-7. The ion of greatest abundance (in this case at 82 amu) in a mass spectrum is known as the **base peak.** The abundances of all other peaks in the spectrum are normalized with respect to the base peak. It is therefore common to refer to the "relative abundance" of the different ions with the base peak ion representing 100%.

Sometimes an ion fragment will be seen at a m/z value that represents the molecular weight of the compound and thus is referred to as the molecular ion. In Fig. 16-7 a prominent molecular ion is seen at 303 amu. The ions other than the molecular ion are those referred to as **fragment ions.** These are the ions resulting from molecular fragmentation in the ion source. When examined by the experienced mass spectrometrist these may be used to help identify the structure of the parent molecule.

Another type of ion, formed by bond breakage and migration of atoms within the molecule, may be present in the mass spectrum. These **rearrangement ions** can be useful identifiers of certain functional groups within the molecule.

It is important to note that if nonvolatile compounds are to be introduced to the mass spectrometer via the gas chromatograph they must first be derivatized. It is important that the compound of interest is not only volatile, but also stable during the GC/MS process. Otherwise many

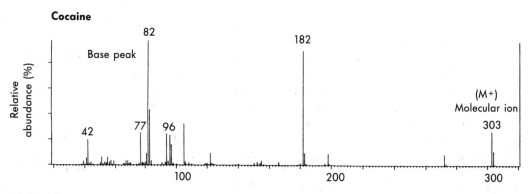

Fig. 16-7 Mass spectrum of an organic compound of clinical interest. The molecular ion (303), base peak ion (82), and other significant fragment ions are seen in the spectrum. (Courtesy Finnigan MAT.)

degradation products can be formed, giving rise to unwanted fragmentation patterns, especially with the high temperatures encountered during GC/MS analysis. **Derivatization** provides for increased volatility and often stability of a compound thus making it more amendable to gc/ms analysis.

It is also important to note that with derivatization the fragment ions will be obtained from the derivatized molecule rather then the native molecule. Mass spectra libraries often contain the spectra of both derivatized and native molecules.

Compound Identification from Mass Spectra—Library Searches

One of the greatest strengths of mass spectrometry is its ability to make a nearly unequivocal identification of organic molecules. The unique "fingerprint" patterns of the mass spectra of these molecules permit such identification to be made. However, to take advantage of this strength it is necessary to have access to a voluminous data base of known reference spectra. Such data bases are available. When included as part of the mass spectrometer's computer, they are accessible as part of the utility programs for making searches of these "libraries." It then becomes a simple matter for the mass spectrometer operator to compare an unknown spectrum obtained during a run with those in the library. Libraries may vary in size from relatively small user-created listings of compounds of particular interest to that user (such as a drug/metabolite library) to extremely large libraries. An example of the latter is the Environmental Protection Agency-National Insititutes of Health (EPA-NIH) library, containing approximately 50,000 entries.

A number of different algorithms have been devised for conducting mass spectral searches. The search and match process requires little more than a few keystrokes and several seconds of search time.

Full Scan Spectra. The result of a library search conducted to identify an unknown component in a sample subjected to GC/MS analysis using full-scan mass spectra is depicted in Fig. 16-8. In this example the search is based on the Finnigan INCOS library search algorithm that uses the information obtained from a full-scan spectrum. The spectrum may or may not contain the molecular ion. The upper spectrum is that of the unknown compound, whereas the lower spectrum is that of the library compound most closely

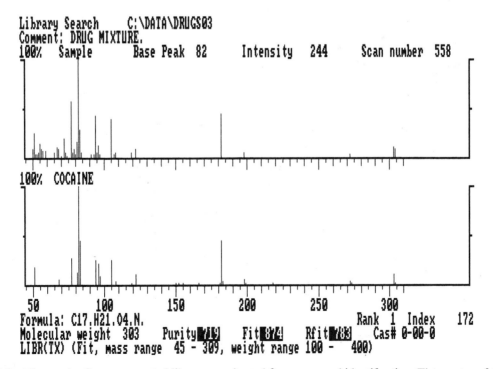

Fig. 16-8 The result of a mass spectral library search used for compound identification. The spectra of the unknown compound and the library compound most closely matching it are displayed, along with information describing the quality of the match.

matching the unknown. The quality of fit is indicated by the values for "purity," "fit," and "reverse fit." Values of 1000 would represent a perfect matching of every ion in the unknown spectrum with those in the library spectrum. Such perfect matches are rarely seen because of differences that exist from instrument to instrument. (This approach is similar to that used by the Finnigan MAT Witness software that is discussed in greater detail later in this chapter.)

Selected Ion Monitoring. Another approach to compound identification that is quite common to many laboratories that are performing drug analysis by GC/MS is based on selected ion monitoring (SIM). The SIM mode provides a convenient means of confirming the presence of a drug and its quantity. Figs. 16-9, 16-10, and Table 16-1 illustrate the basic approach to SIM analysis. Fig. 16-9 shows the full scan spectra of the dimethyl derivative of 11-nor-Δ-9-tetrahydrocannabinol-9-carboxylic acid (THC-COOH), the major metabolite of (−)-trans-Δ-9-tetrahydrocannabinol (THC) or marijuana. Three ions are chosen for analysis of the unknown drug and

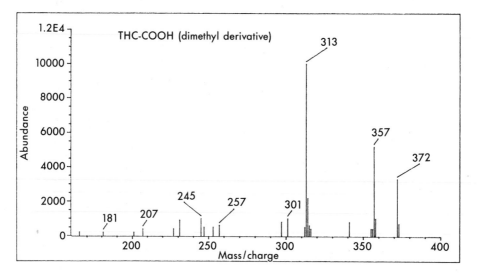

Fig. 16-9   Mass spectrum of the dimethyl derivative of THC-COOH showing major ions (313, 357, 372) chosen for selected ion monitoring. (Courtesy Hewlett Packard.)

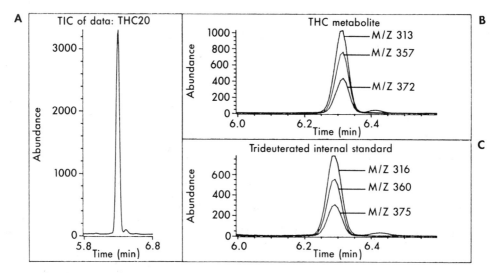

Fig. 16-10   Total ion chromatogram. (**A**), extracted chromatograms for THC-COOH (**B**), and internal standard (**C**), used for selected ion monitoring.

Table 16-1 SIM ions for THC-COOH and the trideuterated internal standard

	Metabolite	Internal standard
Quantitation ion	313	316
Peak qualifier #1	357 (71%)	360 (71%)
Peak qualifier #2	372 (35%)	375 (35%)

Courtesy Hewlett Packard.

internal standard, one for quantitation and the remaining two for confirmation. The latter two ions are called the **qualifier ions or peak qualifiers.** The ions for this example are given in Table 16-1 with the percentage (shown in brackets) representing the relative intensities of the qualifying ions compared with the quantitating ions.

Fig. 16-10, *A* depicts the total ion chromatogram (TIC) for the dimethyl derivatives of THC-COOH and the internal standard, which appear as coeluting peaks. To analyze the data from each compound, the individual ion chromatograms are retrieved from the TIC and then each chromatogram is integrated separately (Fig. 16-10, *B* and *C*). The system is standardized by performing a multipoint calibration. This procedure establishes a linear response for a chosen level of detection for the analysis (Fig. 16-11). Each point represents the response of a TCH-COOH standard relative to the internal standard. A positive result is reported only if the confirming (selected)

ions are found at the proper retention time and in the proper response relative to the quantitated ion (ion ratios). The appropriate retention time is established by the procedure including the type of derivative used during analysis. Usually a retention window is established that dictates the allowable limits for an acceptable retention time. The same holds true for the ion ratios. For those laboratories that are engaged in drug testing in the workplace, these limits are often established by a federal agency such as the National Institutes for Drug Abuse (NIDA). This is especially true if federal employees or employees of those companies that are federally regulated (i.e., power companies regulated by the Nuclear Regulatory Commission [NRC]), are being tested for abuse of drugs.

Basic Approaches to Quantitative Analysis of Compounds

Regardless of the initial approach to identification of a compound (i.e., full scan vs SIM analysis), the ability of the mass spectrometer to selectively monitor specific ions (the SIM mode) gives the instrument a capability for quantifying a substance. However, before a compound can be quantitated and analyzed by the mass spectrometer it first must be isolated by the gas chromatograph. Great selectivity and sensitivity are achieved by this combination. Following chromatographic separation the spectrometer can be used to monitor a selected ion or several ions

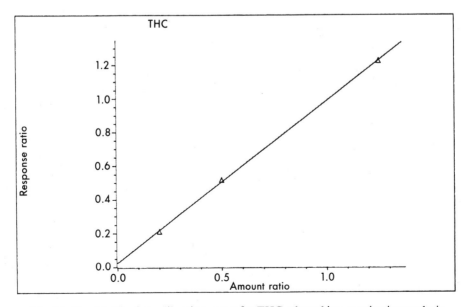

Fig. 16-11 Multipoint calibration curve for THC selected ion monitoring analysis.

known to be characteristic of the compound. Greater selectivity and sensitivity are gained if these ions are of high mass values because ions of lower mass are more likely to be common to many different molecules.

Calibration can be based on the use of external standards, or internal standards can be used that have the same advantages as when employed in other quantitative methods. Unique to mass spectrometry, however, is the use of isotopically labeled internal standards. When atoms that are stable isotopes are incorporated into the standard of the analyte, the standard is chemically and physically the same as the analyte. When added to the sample before analysis, it behaves identically to the analyte throughout processes of extraction, concentration, and chromatography. The standard differs from the analyte only in its mass and can be distinguished as such by the mass spectrometer (see Fig. 16-10 *B* and *C*). Fragments of the parent molecule containing the isotope are measured as are fragments of the natural analyte. Ion ratios of the labeled internal standard ions to those of the analyte are used to determine the quantity of the analyte in the sample.

As with an automated library search and identification of unknown compounds, the quantitation process is easily conducted by most mass spectrometers. Here again the data system has the built-in capacity to carry out the calculations required to accurately quantify many analytes of interest to the clinical chemist or toxicologist. Some of these data systems, which were alluded to in a previous section, are described in greater detail in the following sections.

GC/MS Data Systems Used in Clinical Laboratories

WITNESS System-Finnigan MAT. The criteria used for compound confirmation using this system are based on data generated by a GC/MS using the full scan mode. Figs. 16-12 and 16-13 represent a typical reporting format produced by the Witness System using amphetamines as an example. The top scan in Fig 16-12 illustrates a typical total ion chromatogram (TIC) for a standard mixture of methanolic phenethylamine carbethoxy derivatives. An arrow is pointing to the compound that represents amphetamine. The scan below indicates the total amount of ion current contributed by the compound of interest or in this case, amphetamine, and is proportional to the amount of compound present. The third scan is a full scan mass spectrum of amphetamine found in the standard mixture denoted above in the TIC. This scan is compared with the scan toward the bottom of the report that represents the full scan mass spectrum of amphetamine found in the reference library for identification and confirmation.

Below the mass spectra scans is a set of numbers. The important ones to note are the actual retention time (Act RT), which is compared with the expected retention time (Exp RT), the percent difference (% Diff) if any, and the fit (which was mentioned to earlier during the discussion related to compound identification). For the compound to be identical to one in the library using this format, the retention time must be identical (or within an acceptable range) and the fit must meet the criteria set by the operator. When the retention times are within limits and the fit is equal to 1000, there is unequivocal evidence that two compounds are identical. The two compounds not only have identical fragmentation patterns but also the relative intensities of the ions are similar. As the fit decreases from 1000, so does the probability that the two compounds are identical albeit they may be similar. The format shown in Fig. 16-12 is used to determine if the operating conditions of the instrument are correct and that it has been standardized correctly. If all criteria have been met (the standard has been correctly identified), the program will denote the status as "PASSED." If the criteria have not been met because of improper calibration, reagent deterioration, loss of vacuum, etc., the status will read "FAIL."

With the Witness system, a fit in the range of 800 to 850 or above is generally considered acceptable for confirmation. However, each laboratory should determine the minimum confidence level or fit that is acceptable. Fig. 16-13 represents a typical confirmation report. In this example, a minimum fit of 700 is deemed acceptable although the actual fit is 908 for the internal standard and 986 for amphetamine. In additon to fit criteria the program also compiles additional data in a user-friendly format, such as comparison of TIC scans and individual ion chromatograms, comparison of mass spectra and retention times, linearity data, and quantitative results, that helps in the identification of compounds. The program also determines the status of the analytical run; if the criteria are met for confirmation the program prints the status as "POSITIVE," if not, it prints it as "NEGATIVE."

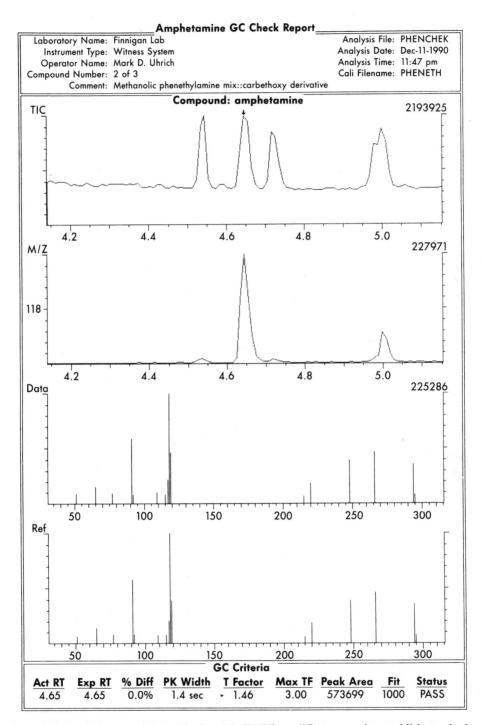

Fig. 16-12 A GC Check Report using the Finnigan MAT "Witness" System used to establish standard conditions of the GC/MS system for a particular compound. (Courtesy Finnigan MAT.)

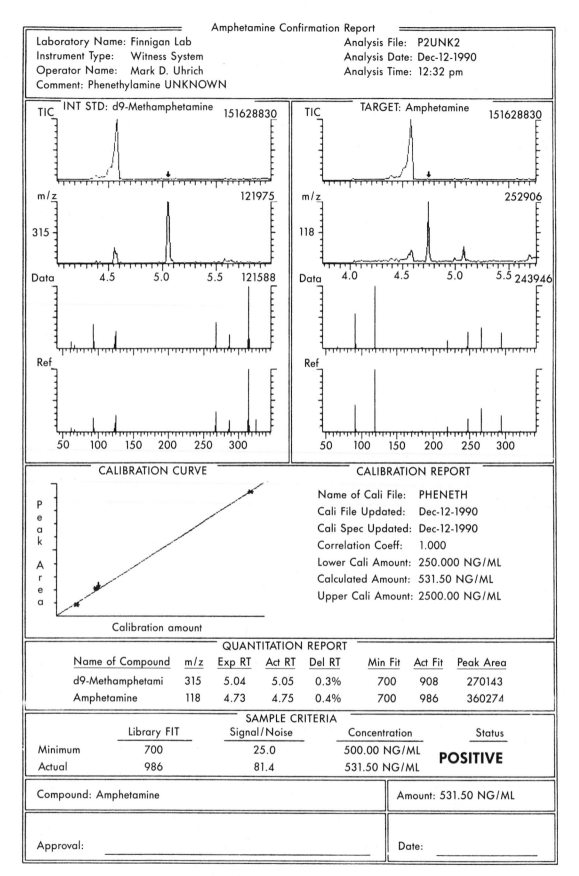

Fig. 16-13 A confirmation report using the Finnigan Mat "Witness" System showing TICs, mass spectra, calibration information, and criteria for a positive sample. (Courtesy Finnigan MAT.)

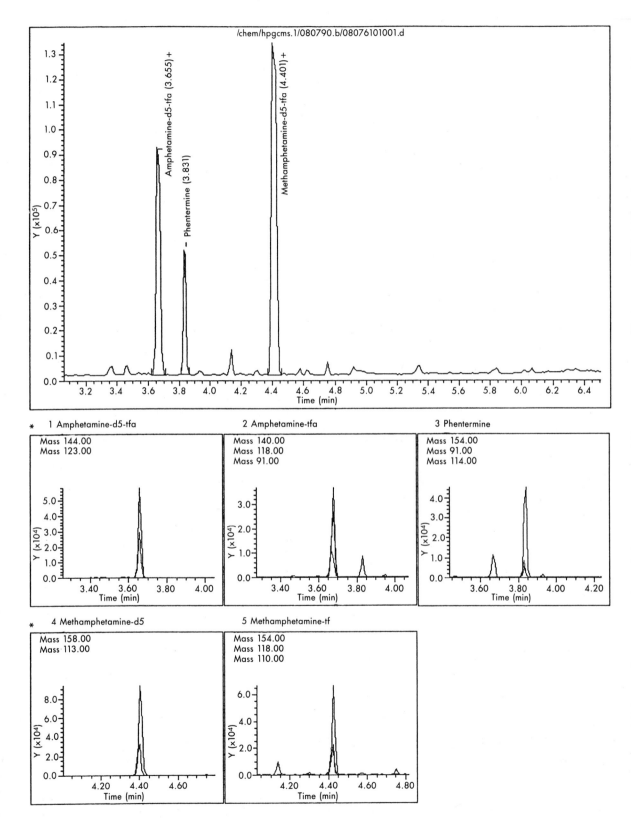

Fig. 16-14 A typical GC-MS chromatogram and extraction of individual ions and relative intensities using the THRU-PUT Systems "Target" software. (Courtesy THRU-PUT Systems, Inc.)

The Finnigan MAT Witness system also provides other key operating information such as instrument status, quality control plots, and quality assurance information using its data management system. All this information in combintion with its check and confirmation reporting format provides the necessary documentation required for forensic/medico-legal work.

THRU-PUT Systems TARGET Drug Report. This software package also provides a user-friendly format for drug analysis and has several features that are similar to the Witness system. However, the main difference is that selected ion monitoring (SIM) is primarily used. THRU-PUT Systems offers several reporting formats. Fig. 16-14 is an example of one type of report that generates a typical chromatogram and extracts the individual ions and relative intensities as overlays. Note that for each compound, the selected ions are identified in the upper left-hand corner. The plots represent these ions and overlap because they have the same retention time. The peak height displays the relative ion intensities for each fragment and can be used to calculate ion ratios for a given compound.

Fig. 16-15 is an example of a tabular report generated by the TARGET software for confirmation and quantitation of drugs, in this case the sympathomimetic amines. It provides essential information such as retention times, selected ions that have been monitored and their individual ion currents, concentration data, acceptable (tar-

```
        Thru-Put Systems Environmental and Drug Testing Laboratories

                        sympathomimetic amine quantitationss
        Data file: /chem/hpgcms.i/080790.b/08076101001.d
        Lab. Id. :
        Inj Date : 07-AUG-90 12:37:40          Tune Date:
        Operator : joey jacob                  Inst ID: hp
        Smp Info :
        Comment  : non-NIDA specimen report
        Method   : /chem/hpgcms.i/080790.b/amps2.m
        Meth Date: 24-Oct-1991 15:30 target
        Cal Date : 07-AUG-90 12:37:40          Cal File: 08076101001.d
        Als bottle: 61                         Calibration Sample, Level: 1
        Dil Factor: 1.000                      Target Version: Target  2.00
        Integrator: HP RTE                     Compound Sublist: all.sub
        Rpt Date : 24-Oct-1991 15:36           Sample Type: WATER
```

				CONCENTRATIONS				
				ON-COL	FINAL			
RT (REL RT)	MASS		RESPONSE	(ng/mL)	(ug/L)	TARGET	RANGE	RATIO
* 1 amphetamine-d5-tfa						CAS #:		
3.655(1.000)	144		67528	1000	1000			100.00
3.655(1.000)	123		30156			35.73-	53.59	44.66
2 amphetamine-tfa						CAS #:		
3.677(1.006)	140		36642	500	500			100.00
3.677(1.006)	118		30286			66.12-	99.18	82.65
3.666(1.003)	91		13549			29.58-	44.37	36.98
3 phentermine						CAS #:		
3.842(0.873)	154		56843	500	500			100.00
3.831(0.870)	91		9223			12.98-	19.47	16.23
3.831(0.870)	114		5368			7.55-	11.33	9.44
* 4 methamphetamine-d5-tfa						CAS #:		
4.401(1.000)	158		123711	1000	1000			100.00
4.401(1.000)	113		40784			26.37-	39.56	32.97
5 methamphetamine-tfa						CAS #:		
4.423(1.005)	154		73901	500	500			100.00
4.423(1.005)	118		26541			28.73-	43.10	35.91
4.423(1.005)	110		25557			27.67-	41.50	34.58

Fig. 16-15 An example of a tabular report of GC-MS data (i.e., retention times, ion intensities and ratios, and compound concentrations) generated by the THRU-PUT Systems "Target" software. (Courtesy THRU-PUT Systems, Inc.)

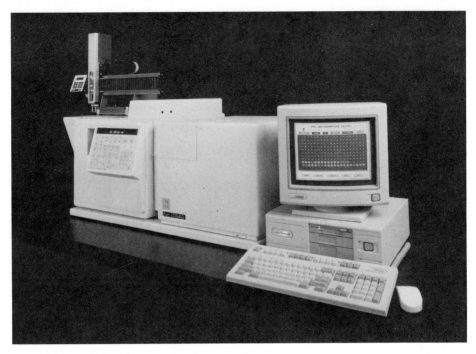

Fig. 16-16 Finnigan MAT ITS40 integrated GC/MS/DS combining an ion trap mass spectrometer with a Varian Model 3400 gas chromatograph. (Courtesy Finnigan MAT.)

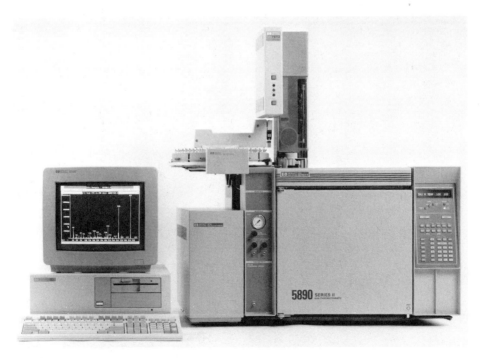

Fig. 16-17 Hewlett Packard Model HP5971A MSD with HP5890 Series II gas chromatograph and HP Vectra PC data system. (Courtesy Hewlett Packard.)

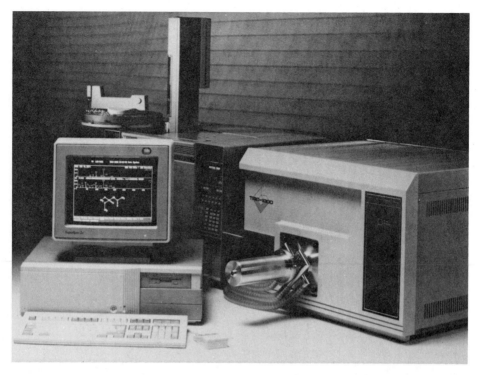

Fig. 16-18 VG MASSLAB Model VG Trio-1000 Benchtop GC/MS system with an LC/MS option. The quadrupole-based analyzer uses an ion-photon conversion type of detector. (Courtesy Fison Instruments.)

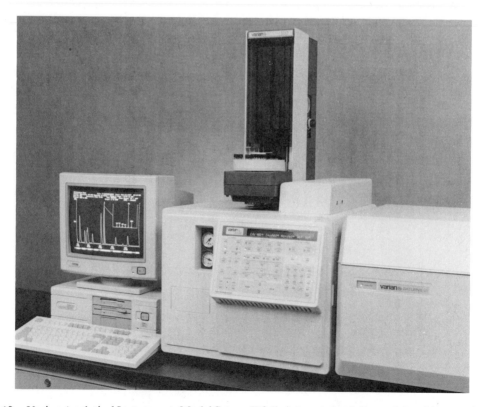

Fig. 16-19 Varian Analytical Instruments Model Saturn II fully integrated-axially modulated-ion trap benchtop system GC/MS. (Courtesy Varian Analytical Instruments.)

get) range for ion ratios, and the actual ion ratios generated during the analytic run. As with all SIM analyses, to confirm the presence of a particular compound, the retention time and ion ratios of the unknown sample must meet certain criteria. Many clinical laboratories use TARGET Software in conjunction with the UNIX System and Hewlett Packard's Model 5971A MSD to perform confirmatory drug testing.

Mass Spectrometers for Clinical Use

In recent years there have been a number of instruments introduced that are of a price range, size, and simplicity that make them suitable for use in the routine clinical or toxicology laboratory. Such instruments are often of the bench-top variety and require the usual in the way of power and other utilities. The box at the left is provided as a representative sampling of currently available bench-type analyzers, which are shown in Figs. 16-16 to 16-19, and should not be taken as a truly complete compilation of all instruments. In each case the instrument's manufacturer and a brief description of features are given.

Review Questions

1. Which of the following does not occur in the ion source of a mass spectrometer?
   A. Fragmentation
   B. Rearrangement
   C. Formation of negative ions
   D. Formation of positive ions
   E. Ion-photon conversion

2. In a mass spectrometer set up for electron impact ionization the ion source pressure is approximately:
   A. 10^{-5} torr
   B. 1 atmosphere
   C. 10^{-1} torr
   D. 10^{-10} torr
   E. None of the above

3. Common types of mass analyzers used in lower-priced spectrometers are:
   A. Magnetic sectors
   B. Quadrupoles
   C. Ion traps
   D. A and B
   E. B and C

4. For quantitative use, selected ion monitoring, compared with full scan monitoring, has the advantage of being:
   A. More selective
   B. More sensitive
   C. Faster
   D. More specific
   E. B and D

5. The base peak in a mass spectrum is that ion that
   A. Has the highest m/z ratio
   B. Has the greatest abundance
   C. Has the lowest m/z ratio
   D. Corresponds to the molecular weight of the molecule
   E. Has the lowest abundance

Mass Spectrometers in Clinical Use
QUADRUPOLE MASS SPECTROMETERS

Hewlett Packard—5971 MSD
   Modes: EI, CI
   Oil diffusion pump
   Mass range: 10 to 650 amu
   SIM mode: 20 groups of 10 ions
   Mass selective detector
   "Target" software: requires HP UNIX system upgrade

Delsi Nermag Instruments—Automass 150
   Modes: EI, CI
   Two turbomolecular pumps
   Mass range: up to 1000 amu
   Negative ion monitoring
   Ion-photo conversion detector

Fisons Instruments—VG Trio-1000/VG MASS-LAB
   Modes: EI, CI
   Turbomolecular pump
   Mass range: 2 to 1000 amu (standard)
              2 to 2000 amu (optional)
   HP 5890A Gas Chromatograph
   Ion-photo conversion detector
   Optional HPLC interface

ION TRAP MASS SPECTROMETERS

Finnigan MAT—ITS40
   Modes: EI, CI
   Turbomolecular pump
   Mass range: 10 to 650 amu
   Axial modulation
   Varian Gas Chromatograph
   "Witness" software

Finnigan MAT—ITD
   Modes: EI, CI
   Turbomolecular pump
   Mass range: 10 to 650 amu
   Accommodates several types of gas chromatographs

Varian Instruments—Saturn II
   Modes: EI, CI
   Turbomolecular pump
   Mass range: 10 to 650 amu
   Axial modulation
   Varian Gas Chromatograph

SIM = selected ion monitoring, EI = electron impact, CI = chemical ionization, HPLC = high performance liquid chromatography

6. The ions that are used in selected ion monitoring to confirm the presence of a compound are called the:
   A. Quantitation ions
   B. Peak qualifiers
   C. Base peaks
   D. Molecular ions
7. The "Target" software is generally used to provide graphic and tabular reports derived from full-scan GC/MS analysis.
   A. True
   B. False
8. For a compound to be reported as positive using selected ion monitoring (SIM), the confirming ions must have a value within a given range that is acceptable for:
   A. Retention time
   B. Quantitation
   C. Ion ratios
   D. A and C
9. The purpose of derivatizing a sample is to make the compound:
   A. More water soluble
   B. Less nonpolar
   C. More volatile
   D. Less thermolabile
   E. C and D
10. The term "fit" as applied to full scan GC/MS refers to how close an unknown spectrum matches a reference spectrum.
    A. True
    B. False
11. The advantage of the ion trap mass spectrometer compared with the quadrupole mass spectrometer is its ability to acquire full-scan spectrum data at very low sample concentrations (increased sensitivity).
    A. True
    B. False

Answers

1. E   2. A   3. E   4. B   5. B   6. B   7. B   8. D
9. E   10. A   11. A

Bibliography

Deutsch DG, ed: Principles, uses and applications of analytical toxicology, New York, 1989, John Wiley & Sons.

Dunham L: GC/MS Confirmation of THC, MSD Application Brief, Pub No. 23-5953-8069, Avondale, Pa, 1987, Hewlett-Packard Company.

Jones LV: Mass spectrometry. In Curry AS, ed: Analytical methods in human toxicology, part 1, Weinheim (Fed Rep of Germany), 1985, Verlag Chemie GmbH.

Karasek FW, Clement RE: Basic gas chromatography–mass spectrometry. Principles and techniques, Amsterdam, 1988, Elsevier.

Pfleger K, Maurer H, and Weber A: Mass spectral and GC data of drugs, poisons and their metabolites, parts I and II, Weinheim (Fed Rep of Germany), 1985, VCH Verlags-gesellschaft mbH.

AUTOMATION IN THE CLINICAL LABORATORY

CHAPTER 17

Definitions, Concepts, and Approaches

MARGUERITE QUALE

Preanalytic Considerations in Automation
Analytic Factors in Automation
Postanalytic Considerations in Automation

Automation is becoming more complex and increasingly necessary for the efficient operation of today's laboratory. Automation is generally achieved through instrumentation that mechanizes all or most of the manual steps in a process or procedure. Some degree of automation has been present in the clinical laboratory for many years but in limited settings. Clinical chemistry automation began with such instruments as the Technicon Autoanalyzers. Hematology automation began with the earlier versions of the Coulter Counters. During the past seveal decades the fields of general chemistry and hematology have seen a rapid proliferation in types and manufacturers of instrumentation from the early days. Recently several manufacturers have been able to automate some assays used in microbiology and with the recent advent of new technologies that have been used to develop monoclonal antibodies, automation in immunochemical assays has become a reality.

The driving forces behind this interest in automation are as many and varied as the instrumentation that has appeared in the marketplace. Manufacturers have also responded to the physician's desire to bring laboratory testing to the patient, rather than use the traditional system in which the patient comes to the laboratory. Physician Office Laboratories (POL) have increased with the introduction of small, easy-to-operate bench analyzers. Surgical and critical care units have demanded immediate laboratory results, particularly in situations in which patient risk is high, such as trauma and organ transplant units.

The demand for home testing has also increased. This has been made possible with the development of portable instrumentation and/or electrode systems that can monitor a patient's status directly. This is changing the traditional concept of a laboratory. The good side of bedside testing is that physicians have test results available immediately for monitoring patients and thus can respond to life-threatening situations much faster. The downside of bedside testing is that often the quality of the results suffers because nonlaboratory staff often do not understand the concept of quality assurance and its practices. This has led in some degree to the newest federal regulations that all laboratories must face.

Laboratories have received bad press concerning the quality of patient results, particularly in the areas of cholesterol and pap smear testing. Cholesterol testing is being done everywhere, often by nonlaboratory staff with minimal or no training. Only laboratories engaged in interstate testing or receiving Medicare payments have been regulated under the Clinical Laboratory Improvement Act of 1967 (CLIA '67). These regulations have been the standard for laboratory testing. They also have served as the guidelines for accrediting agencies such as the Joint Commission for Accreditation of Healthcare Organizations (JCAHO) and the College of American Pathologists (CAP) for inspection of laboratories. Congress has responded to the public's concern over accurate laboratory results with the Clinical Laboratory Improvement Amendents of 1988 (CLIA '88). CLIA '88 changes the scope and complexity of the CLIA '67 standards significantly. Under CLIA '88 all laboratories doing human testing are regulated, including POL and satellite laboratories. This means that all laboratory settings performing human testing must conform to the quality assurance measures that help to maintain the quality of laboratory results and health care. These regulations have also increased the requirements for the evaluation of any instrument or test method that is introduced into the laboratory. Many of the nontraditional laboratories are not familiar with the procedures for reviewing an instrument's performance.

Another force that is causing an increase in laboratory automation is the ever declining reimbursement by Medicare and Medicaid and other factors that focus on controlling the rapidly increasing costs of medical care. The largest component in medical costs is personnel. Hospital administrators are faced with the necessity to control costs to match declining income and often look at lowering personnel costs as a means to decrease expenses. Laboratories, once considered profit generating areas, are now labeled as cost centers. Thus laboratories face the same demands to cut personnel. This can only be achieved, without affecting the quality of laboratory work, by increasing the productivity of the staff. Automation is one answer to performing manual, repetitive, time-consuming steps that can occupy a large portion of a technologist's time. Automation thus allows the technologist to perform other tasks such as evaluating test results or introducing new tests for which automation does not exist.

Immunologic techniques have increased the ability to automate some areas of the laboratory that in the past did not lend themselves to automation. For example, many traditional radioimmunoassay methods are being replaced by a wide variety of nonisotopic methods. Serology tests, such as C-reactive protein (CRP), can be measured by such methods as nephelometry. The sensitivity and specificity of these antigen-antibody reactions has led to the development of new tests for diseases that in the past could only be evaluated by a physician via monitoring a patient's response to treatment. New technologies have allowed many of these immunologic reactions to be automated.

The reasons for increased automation have been briefly discussed. The remainder of this chapter will describe the general concepts that underlie automation and provide the necessary criteria that needs to be evaluated when considering automation for a laboratory setting.

Quality assurance concepts provide for three natural divisions of the testing process: preanalytic, analytic, and postanalytic steps in a test method. The preanalytic portion consists of all the steps necessary to provide a patient specimen for testing. The analytic portion is the actual testing of the specimen. The postanalytic steps encompass a variety of procedures related to what happens to the patient results. Quality assurance in a hospital setting looks at all aspects of patient care from the time the patient is admitted until the patient is discharged. The laboratory's involvement in quality assurance begins with the physician who will order a test, proceeds through the steps that are involved in carrying out that test request, and even includes what the physician will do with the results of that test. Automation plays an important role in this process by helping to reduce human error, increasing the speed and reliability of the results, and increasing the availability of tests.

Preanalytic Considerations in Automation

The preanalytic portion of the testing process is often taken for granted by the technologists who perform patient specimen testing. However, it is probably the most important aspect of the entire testing process. For example, if a specimen for a particular test is not drawn from the correct patient, or the specimen integrity is questionable, it does not matter if the test results are accurate or how fast they are received by the physician. Automation at this stage of the process is not traditionally perceived as automation of the laboratory. However, it does play a significant role in the quality of laboratory testing and is the beginning of how successful automation can be in the analytic process. Fig. 17-1 outlines the steps involved in patient testing and the preanalytic steps that occur.

Laboratory testing would not exist without the first step of the preanalytic stage. If physicians did not order laboratory tests, there would be no need for a laboratory. However, many of the problems that exist with laboratory testing originate at this point. The physician can order the wrong test, fail to order a needed test, order the test for the wrong time, or as commonly occurs, order more tests than are actually needed. All of these are costly errors because hospital reimbursement, particularly with Diagnostic Related Groups (DRG), does not provide for patient hospitalization longer than necessary or for patient testing that is not warranted. Computerization plays an important role throughout the testing process and makes possible much of the automation that exists today. It helps to alleviate many of the problems often associated with this stage of the preanalytic process. Information can be included in a computer system that helps to identify tests that are associated with a diagnosis or a disease state. By reviewing test orders in a computer system,

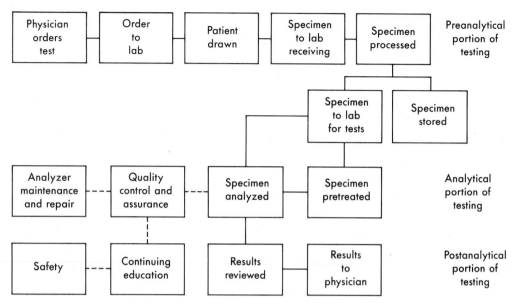

Fig. 17-1 Outline of the steps involved in patient testing.

physicians can note tests that have already been processed, review results as they become available, and become aware of reference ranges or flags that can point out abnormal results that can aid them in the diagnosis or treatment of their patient. The computer can also be the first step in notifying the laboratory that a test order exists. Orders can be directly transmitted to the laboratory across an interface between the laboratory and hospital computer, including printing labels and assigning accession numbers. This direct transfer of information will decrease the number of incorrectly ordered tests and alert the phlebotomist that a patient sample needs to be drawn. For tests that may be run only once or twice a week, a technologist can check for test orders that are being drawn and delay a run to include these new patient specimens. A computer system makes it easier to check on duplicate orders and may decrease the number of times that a patient sample needs to be drawn by allowing the phlebotomist to coordinate different sets of test orders, especially when several physicians may be treating the same patient.

Once the patient sample has been obtained, there are a number of different ways for the sample to reach the laboratory. The least efficient and most costly is a human transport system. If the phlebotomist is expected to carry the specimens to the laboratory, testing may be delayed because of the number of patient samples that need to be drawn. In institutions where a number of differ-

ent health professionals may be collecting specimens, the individual transporting the specimen may be a nurse or doctor whose time would be better spent attending to the patient.

Pneumatic tube systems provide a mechanical means of sending these specimens to the laboratory. These systems are fast, can deliver individual specimens as they are drawn, and allow the phlebotomist to continue drawing other patient samples without delaying specimen receipt by the laboratory. Pneumatic systems, however, limit the size of the specimen that can be sent. Also in cases where the specimen contains known blood-borne agents, they are not suitable because breakage of the specimen container may spread the agent. Another drawback of a pneumatic system is that transport routes are not easily changed because its tracks are built into walls or tunnels.

Another way to transport specimens is to use a robotic system that may be computer programmed to follow a specific route or may follow a magnetic strip on the floor. This method of transport would allow larger specimen containers, such as those that are used for collection of 24-hour urine specimens to be transported, or permit large numbers of specimens to reach the laboratory. This type of system makes it easier to change current transport routes or add to existing routes as areas are remodeled or new ones are constructed.

Once samples have arrived in the laboratory, specimens must be prepared for testing. This preparation may be minimal as with testing done on whole blood such as arterial blood gases and blood cell counts. However, most testing is performed on serum or plasma. Most of this specimen processing is currently done manually; however, robotic systems do exist and are in limited use in some institutions. This will be an area of increasing interest as these systems are refined because the steps in specimen processing are time consuming. Also there are many safety concerns such as those related to Acquired Immunodeficiency Syndrome (AIDS) and hepatitis that need addressing during specimen processing.

The use of **bar codes** with laboratory instrumentation, as a means of specimen identification, is becoming increasingly popular. A bar code is a means of encoding information into a series of bars of various widths and color intensities. For clinical laboratories this information can include patient demographics, test order information, and the computer assigned accesssion number. Ideally, a bar code label would be generated at the patient's bedside by scanning the arm band before the phlebotomist draws the specimen. This would allow for positive patient identification at the collection source and thus would eliminate incorrectly labeled specimens and decrease the number of incorrectly drawn patient specimens. Less ideally, these bar codes could be generated at the specimen processing area and subsequently be placed on the collection tubes or aliquot tubes. However, the latter approach can still lead to incorrectly labeled tubes.

Automation in the preanalytic steps is generally limited by the computer capabilities of an institution. However, with the development of robotics, many of the time-consuming manual steps during this stage will become automated, thus providing laboratory personnel with additional time to perform patient testing.

Analytic Factors in Automation

The analytic portion of patient testing is the area of the laboratory that lends itself most readily to automation. Automation in the clinical laboratory is becoming increasingly more complex, involving instruments that have larger test menus and the capability of handling a higher volume of patient samples. Because of newer technologies there is an increased number of tests that have been automated. Traditional laboratory methods are becoming obsolete as manual assays from many laboratory disciplines are being replaced with ligand assays that have be-

come automated. In the past, automation was confined to the chemistry and hematology laboratories. However, most sections of the laboratory currently have some type of automated instrumentation. Physicians are also demanding that results be made available sooner, particularly in acute care settings. With the advent of POL instrumentation physicians have also become more aware of faster turn-around-time for patient results.

Laboratory Characteristics. Probably the most important concept in laboratory automation is that each laboratory is a unique entity and that there is no ideal instrumentation. Each laboratory must thoroughly evaluate its needs, the physician needs, technologist capabilities, space and environmental conditions, and workflow and workload before and during instrument acquisition. Although subsequent chapters will discuss in detail specific laboratory instrumentation that is currently available for the various laboratory disciplines, there are basic attributes and characteristics of automated instruments that should be considered regardless of the tests that are being performed or the location of the laboratory. The box below contains a list of some of these characteristics that the laboratory manager or director should consider when purchasing an instrument.

Test Menu. One of the first decisions that must be made is the type of **test menu** that is desired. The test menu is a list of the analytes or tests that a laboratory would like to be able to provide for patient testing. For example, in a hematology laboratory the test menu might include a complete blood count and a differential and reticulocyte count. In immunology the test menu might include a C-reactive protein, rheumatoid factor, and antithyroid antibodies. In larger institutions where laboratory sections are separate entities, the test menu will depend on how tests have been allocated. For example, hepatitis testing may be found in immunology, chemistry, or immunohematology. In smaller institutions, POLs, or sat-

---

Laboratory Characteristics to Evaluate Before Instrument Consideration

Test menu desired
Laboratory workload
Laboratory workflow
Need for walk-away capability

ellite laboratories, the instrumentation desired may need to do a more varied test menu, crossing traditional laboratory boundaries.

When test menus are considered, the laboratorian needs to consider not only the test that is currently required but also must try to project future testing needs. It may take as long as 1 to 2 years for a new test to be become available for an instrument. Manufacturers will provide a list of currently available tests and tests that are being developed. In some cases the technology employed by an instrument may limit the test menu and thus the availability of future tests that are desired by the laboratory. Currently the line of instrumentation that has test menus that are rapidly changing are the automated immunoassay analyzers. The tests that have been developed for these analyzers are those analyses that in the past were only available by radioimmunoassay techniques (such as hormones and tumor markers). If the laboratory serves a fertility clinic, the availability of such hormones as estradiol may be a deciding factor in purchasing an instrument. Large cancer centers would concentrate on tumor marker availability, as well as the manufacturer's commitment to new markers as they are discovered.

Workload. The next factor that must be considered is the laboratory's **workload.** Workload is the number of test results that are generated by a laboratory during a given time period. Laboratory sections that predominantly perform low volume or specialized tests, such as hormones, will have a small workload. Chemistry laboratories, on the other hand, generally have a large workload because of tests such as glucose, renal and liver function tests, and electrolyte profiles are commonly and frequently ordered. Smaller laboratories will often have a combination of low- and high-volume tests. This variety of tests that a laboratory performs is referred to as the **test mix.**

The workload of an automated instrument is determined by its throughput or number of test results/hour or higher. The throughput on large general chemistry analyzers may be 500 to 700 test results/hour. However, an immunoassay analyzer, which does lower volume testing, may only perform 100 to 150 tests/hour, yet still be considered highly productive.

Workflow. Another factor that should be evaluated is the **workflow** of the laboratory. Workflow is the way in which laboratory tests are processed. For example, a critical care laboratory will run all tests immediately. At the opposite end of the spectrum is the reference laboratory that runs the majority of its testing once a day in large batches. Most laboratories have a mixed workflow: a small group of stat tests that are run as they are received. The largest portion of their testing, which is routine, is processed either in large batches or, more often, is dictated by the needs and expectations of their physicians. In the latter case a laboratory must decide if the same instrument will be required to do both stat and routine testing. If the decision is made to purchase different instruments, then the test methodologies must be shown to be compatible. This decision may limit the instrumentation that is available.

Walk-Away Capabilities. The next aspect to consider is the need for walk-away capabilities of the instrumentation. **Walk-away capability** is the ability of the operator to program the instrument and then leave the instrument to perform other tasks while the instrument processes the tests. This is affected by two factors: the sample and reagent capacity of the instrument and staffing.

Reagent capacity is the number of different reagents that can be stored on an analyzer at any time. This storage capacity is determined by the number of available reagent slots, on board reagent stability, and storage requirements (i.e., refrigeration). Analyzers that have small reagent capacities or use reagents that cannot be stored on the analyzer until the expiration date will require more operator intervention as reagents will need to be removed or changed at the end of each run.

In high-volume laboratories the sample handling capabilities will also affect the walk-away capabilities. Most large-volume analyzers can store a large number of reagents on board and are only limited by the number of samples that can be placed on the analyzer. Special preparation steps, such as those that are required for high density lipoprotein (HDL) analysis, will also limit the amount of time the operator can spend away from the analyzer. Another extra step that is often part of sample processing is the need to make dilutions. Dilutions are required when a test result exceeds the linear limits of the instrument (as often happens with enzymes). Some analyzers, such as the Baxter Paramax, have the ability to make on-board dilutions; other analyzers decrease the need for dilutions by extending the linear limits for the tests.

The number of available personnel will also affect the need for walk-away capabilities. The

smaller the laboratory staff, the greater the need for the staff to run more than one instrument at a time or to be able to do other tasks such as required paperwork or answer the telephone.

Instrument Characteristics. Once the laboratory's needs such as workload, workflow, and test menu are determined, the next step is to investigate the instrumentation that is available to determine the characteristics of each and ascertain which ones will meet the needs of the laboratory. These characteristics can then be divided into three classes: essential, important, and unnecessary. Each laboratory director must set the specifications for the instrumentation for the laboratory. The analyzers that meet most of these characteristics can then be evaluated further. Preliminary investigation into the type of instrumentation that is available can occur via current journal articles, exhibits at meetings, journal advertisements, and textbooks. Specifications for each instrument can be acquired by contacting the instrument manufacturer. The box below lists the characteristics that should be considered when selecting an automated instrument.

Bar Codes. Bar coding is becoming increasingly important for many institutions as a means of providing positive sample identification, particularly if it is available from the first stages of sample collection. A patient sample with a bar code can also provide a way for the analyzer to recognize the tests required for the sample. This will help to decrease the number of tests that the operator may inadvertently fail to program, which can cause a delay in the availability of test results. It will also save operator time by allowing the operator to place the sample on the instrument and then walk away.

Bar codes are also appearing on many reagent packages. Thus analyzers that can read bar codes are able to recognize the reagent that is being loaded, the lot number, the expiration date, and the calibration curve that is needed for that particular lot of reagent. Federal regulations and good laboratory practice require that each new lot of reagent be checked before use. Bar codes provide a means to warn the operator that a calibration is needed before analyzing patient samples.

There are a variety of bar codes available (i.e., Codabar, Code 19, and Code 39). Some analyzers can use only one type of bar code, and if the laboratory computer system is not capable of printing the bar code that is required, then a separate bar code printer is necessary. This will increase the purchase price of the instrument, as well as add an extra step in specimen processing. Some instruments, such as the Beckman Synchron CX7, are capable of reading a variety of bar codes at any time. This may be desirable in institutions that do a large volume of reference laboratory testing and receive an assortment of bar coded samples. Some of the smaller analyzers do not have the ability to read the bar codes on board the instrument. However, many provide a wand that will read the patient sample for identification and then provide a list of tests that have been bar coded for test selection.

Bar codes can make sample handling easier, more efficient, and reduce the errors in both patient identification and the testing process. They may help increase laboratory productivity by decreasing operator intervention time with the analyzer and thus increase the walk-away capacity.

Primary Tube Sampling. Another aspect of sample handling that requires consideration is the way in which a sample is introduced to the testing process by the analyzer. With increasing safety concerns pertaining to the transmission of AIDS and hepatitis, the ideal analyzer would sample directly from the **primary tube** without removing the stopper. Hematology analyzers have been among the first to provide this option, but only one automated chemistry analyzer, the Baxter Paramax, currently has this capability. However, an instrument with this option should also be evaluated for the tube size that it will accept and its ability to recognize an unacceptable sample.

One advantage of **primary tube sampling,** when combined with bar coding, is the ability to load samples onto the analyzer and then allow the analyzer to process the samples while the operator is free to perform other tasks. However, the number of different sample sizes the analyzer will

---

Features Available for Automated Laboratory Instruments

Ability to use bar codes
Primary tube sampling
Sample processing features
   Batch
   Random access
   Discrete
   Continuous flow
Measuring devices
Mixing methods

accept without special handling or without removing the stopper can be a limiting factor. This may be important particularly in institutions with a large pediatric or neonatal population (the samples drawn are generally much smaller than those for adults). Special handling of smaller samples decreases the productivity advantages of this feature, and the need to remove the stopper eliminates the safety advantages.

The second aspect to consider is if the analyzer can recognize an unacceptable sample. For hematology analyzers, which require whole blood, the analyzer should be able to warn the operator of partially clotted samples. For analyzers that require serum, the presence of fibrin in the sample can cause short sampling or clogged probes. In either situation the reliability of patient results would suffer or the results could be delayed if the analyzer did not warn the operator of the unacceptable sample.

Many of the newer automated analyzers are capable of addressing this problem, which allows the primary tube to be placed directly on the analyzer without the stopper. Although this does not answer safety concerns, it does aid productivity by eliminating the need to aliquot the specimen into sample cups. This feature allows for positive sample identification if bar codes are available.

Sample Processing. The next aspect to consider is how the analyzer processes samples. Four concepts need to be discussed in this section: **batch, random access, discrete** and **sequential** or **continuous flow.** The first two describe how the test requests are programmed. Batch analyzers run the same test or tests on all samples in a run. A random access analyzer allows the operator to choose the tests to be performed on each sample independently from all other samples. Whether batch or random access processing will meet the needs of the laboratory will depend on the number of samples that are processed, the number of different tests that are processed, and if the use of profiles is encouraged. Batch analyzers lend themselves well to profiling if the variety of tests requested for each patient is limited. If a different group of tests is ordered on each patient, then batch analyzers may perform a large number of unnecessary tests that will increase the cost of testing. This will occur when a batch analyzer that runs a panel of tests, such as Technicon SMAC System, runs the entire panel, whether requested or not, on all samples. Random access analyzers provide much more flexibility in patient testing but increase the operator's time in programming the samples as the requests for each sample must be programmed separately. However, bar coding can provide this information and thus alleviate this problem. When these tests are programmed manually, the risk of missing a test increases also, particularly as the number of tests desired for a sample increases. Some analyzers do provide the flexibility to offer either batch or random access processing. Many larger institutions will have one batch analyzer to run profiles (or dedicate an analyzer for batch testing) but will limit the hours of day this instrument is in operation; they will have a second, random access analyzer to process stat testing and routine test requests during the time the profiling analyzer is not in operation. With this situation, however, the director must make sure that the results produced by each analyzer are compatible or that the results of one analyzer can be adjusted to match the results of the other.

The last two concepts, discrete and sequential, refer to how the analyzer provides a reaction environment for the test. A discrete analyzer processes the test reaction in an environment that is separate from the other test reactions that are occurring. These analyzers provide a variety of receptacles in which the sample and reagents are mixed and the reaction occurs. Most use cuvettes; however, some provide their own unique reaction container: a dry film slide such as found with the Kodak Ektachem analyzers, a "boat" as seen with the PB Diagnostics' Opus, or a "baggy" as used with the Dupont ACA systems. Some of these containers contain the reagents, and only the specimen needs to be added. Other instruments add both the reagents and the specimens.

A sequential or continuous flow analyzer pumps reagents through the system continuously, introducing samples at regular intervals and segmenting the flow to separate one specimen from another. An example of a continuous flow analyzer is the Technicon SMAC System. These instruments may be best used as profiling instruments as they perform as batch analyzers, running the same tests on all samples.

Measuring Devices. Another feature of an automated instrument that should be considered is the measuring device that is used. The methods that are used for measurement use a wide variety of principles such as spectrophotometry, fluorometry, electrochemistry, reflectance, chemiluminescence, and nephelometry. These principles have been discussed in earlier chapters. However, the principle of measurement that is employed does affect the performance of an analyzer. Some methods tend to be affected by interfering substances, whereas others influence the sensitivity or linear range of the instrument. Spectrophotometry, depending on the wavelengths employed by the instrument, can be highly affected by hemolysis or lipemia. Some instruments use different wavelengths (differential spectrophotometry) to eradicate any interferences. Many of the traditional isotopic techniques, such as radioimmunoassay (RIA) tests, have not been converted to immunoassay methods until now because earlier nonisotopic methodologies could not provide sufficient sensitivity. However, newer methods of measurement, such as chemiluminescence and fluorescence polarization, can provide adequate sensitivity and thus have been able to replace many of the isotopic methods.

Mixing Methods. Once reagents and samples have been added, they need to be mixed to complete the reactions and to provide a uniform appearance for the detection devices. A variety of methods are employed to ensure adequate mixing. The Technicon continuous flow analyzers use the principle of inversion via mixing coils, the Dupont ACA analyzers use mechanical vibration, and centrifugal analyzers use the outward movement that is induced by centrifugal force. Although the type of system may not be a deciding factor in the choice of an analyzer, an instrument that does not provide adequate mixing will generate inconsistent results and therefore be eliminated during the selection process.

Performance Characteristics. The available features on each instrument can help to narrow down the large assortment of analyzers to just a few analyzers that still can potentially meet the needs of the laboratory. The next step is to evaluate the performance characteristics of each instrument. These characteristics are listed in the box below. Good laboratory practice has always dictated that laboratorians to understand the capabilities and limitations of a given test method. CLIA '88 standards have provided these same standards in writing. These new federal guidelines are forcing laboratories to provide more detailed information about the performance characteristics of all test methods and, on demand, make them available to all clients. However, these guidelines do not dictate any level of performance. As long as acceptable proficiency testing is maintained, the decision is left up to the laboratory.

Manufacturers are expected to provide performance characteristics for their instrumentation. However, these must be verified in the laboratory's own setting and with the patient population that the laboratory serves. Many companies will provide the technical staff to evaluate these characteristics. This may be a determining factor in instrument selection as verification of instrument performance is a time-consuming process (particularly for analyzers with large test menus).

Linearity. The **linearity** of a method is the range over which patient results can be reported without manipulating the sample (i.e., using a dilution). The linear range is generally defined by the values of the highest and lowest calibrators that are available for a particular instrument. This linear range must be verified periodically, usually at least once a year. A large linear range will mean fewer dilutions of patient samples and therefore save the operator time and provide a faster turn-around-time for results. One problem with a large linear range is that the target value of quality control material is often of insufficient magnitude that it cannot be used to evaluate the upper end of the range. Consequently a special control material may have to be used periodically to verify these ranges. This will add to the cost of a test.

Sensitivity. The **sensitivity** is the lowest value that can reliably be detected by a method without providing a false positive result. For many general chemistry tests the sensitivity is not generally an area of concern because the concentration of many analytes in a patient's serum is sufficiently high. However, for analytes that exist in very low quantities, such as some hormones, the sensitivity of the method may be a deciding factor in the choice of an automated analyzer. For example, sensitivity is an important issue when the lower limits of the analyte can be of diagnostic value (i.e., a low human chorionic gonadotropin [hCG] level, which may be indicative of an ectopic pregnancy, or a low thyroid stimulating hormone

---

Performance Characteristics of an Analyzer to Be Evaluated

Linearity
Sensitivity
Specificity
Accuracy
Precision
Stability
Carryover

[TSH] for the differential diagnosis of hyperthyroidism).

Specificity. The **specificity** is the ability to measure only the analyte requested. Some methods will measure not only the analyte requested, but also another analyte that will react with reagents in the test system. When this occurs, the physician may make an inaccurate diagnosis based on a falsely elevated result. One common example of a test that may be nonspecific is the alkaline picrate method for the measurement of creatinine. There are many interferences in this method; however, most chemistry instruments currently employ it for the measurement of creatinine. Some however, try to minimize the effect of the interfering substances by increasing the temperature of the reaction (e.g., the Beckman Synchron CX7). Another method for measuring creatinine, which could be used to eliminate the interferences commonly found in the alkaline picrate method, is an enzymatic method, such as that employed by the Kodak Ektachem analyzers.

When an analyzer is evaluated, the methods employed must be carefully examined or evaluated for specificity. Although an analyzer may not be rejected for one nonspecific method, the laboratory must be aware of the limitations of its methods to better aid the physician with evaluating results that do not appear consistent with a diagnosis.

Accuracy and Precision. The **accuracy** of a method is its ability to determine the true or actual value of an analyte. Standards used on an instrument should be traceable to recognized agencies such as the National Bureau of Standards. It is much easier to obtain pure standards for inorganic compounds than it is for biologic compounds, particularly hormones. Methods used on an analyzer should be traceable or compared with reference methods. Some reference methods, such as glucose oxidase for glucose, are easily automated; others, such as the Abell-Kendall for cholesterol, are not. These concerns are becoming more self-evident with the new CLIA regulations as target values will be used to decide if proficiency testing will be acceptable.

Precision is the degree of reproducibility of a method. Precision is reflected in the coefficient of variation (CV) of the method. The smaller the CV, the more precise the method (the standard deviation divided by the mean times 100). A lower precision is desirable as it will allow the physician to readily determine if a patient value

has actually changed, thus allowing a better evaluation for treatment of the patient.

One approach to the evaluation of instrument precision and accuracy before the actual verification of the manufacturer's in-house claims is to look at CAP survey results. CAP will provide the means, standard deviations, and coefficients of variation for most of the instruments and their analytes in tabular form, which makes it easier to compare the performance of different instruments. They will also provide target values for the various analytes that can be tested. One problem often encountered with CAP specimens, however, is that the specimens are lyophilized, which can produce matrix effects with some analyzers (i.e., Kodak Ektachem 400 or 700). These matrix effects will make it appear that the analyzer is inaccurate compared with the assigned target value even though it is not. In these cases the manufacturer may request that peer group comparisons be used.

Stability. The **stability** of all components of an instrument system is another important feature to consider. These components include reagents before use, reagents in use, calibration curves and, in some cases, analyte stability. **Shelf life** is the term used to define reagent stability before use and can be as short as 1 month or longer than 1 year. A longer shelf life is desirable as each new lot of reagent must be evaluated against the old reagents. This evaluation process increases the cost of testing. New lots must be calibrated, quality control (QC) must be verified, and if the QC range has shifted, a patient correlation may need to be performed.

Once reagents are opened and placed in the analyzer, "on-board" stability generally decreases, sometimes significantly. Some reagents require refrigeration for extended stability that the analyzer may not be able to provide. Some reagents are composed of two components that need to be mixed and once combined are not as stable as the individual components. Evaporation or contamination can also decrease on-board stability of the analyzer's reagents. Reagents that must be discarded before they are used up will increase the cost of testing.

Stability of calibration curves also has an effect on cost. Calibrators and subsequent controls increase the number of nonpatient tests that must be added into the cost analysis of each test. Some analyzers need to be calibrated several times a day; others can go 6 months without recalibration.

In a few instances, "analyte" stability may need to be considered. Some analytes are temperature labile, and refrigerated sample compartments are desirable, particularly for large runs. Evaporation is a concern, especially when sample processing areas are large. This is particularly important as sample size decreases.

Carryover. Another concern when evaluating performance is **carryover.** Carryover occurs when a previous sample or reagent contaminates successive tests in a run, causing the next sample to have an aberrantly higher or lower result. Carryover is most notable when analytes occur in extremely high quantities such as with hCG levels during the course of pregnancy or with enzymes. Carryover of reagents could also occur in systems that reuse cuvettes that are insufficiently washed after each testing cycle.

Miscellaneous. There are several other factors that should be considered before the acquisition of any piece of laboratory equipment. These factors include environment, maintenance/service, quality control, and training.

Environment. The environment of a laboratory may limit the ability to acquire some instruments because construction would be required before its installation. Most instruments have a temperature and humidity range that is optimal for its operation. Certain areas of the country such as the south and southwest may be affected by these extremes.

The electrical requirements also need to be evaluated. Most instruments, particularly those controlled by computers, require a dedicated line, or a voltage stabilizer, to maintain a constant current. Space restrictions may dictate whether a benchtop or floor model analyzer will be acquired by the laboratory. If a liquid chemistry system is being considered, there must be an adequate water supply and drainage. Satellite laboratories may find that a dry reagent system would better suit their needs because the water supply may be inadequate or drains may not be available.

Maintenance/Service. Another factor to consider before acquiring an instrument is its maintenance and downtime. This can most easily be accomplished by contacting a laboratory that has the instrument and has a workload similar to the laboratory where the instrument will be used. Maintenance time will generally be the time the analyzer is not in use, thus potentially delaying patient results. Daily and weekly maintenance may add significantly to the time the operator

cannot process patient samples. If only one analyzer is available and a large portion of the work is stat samples (such as that found in an operating room laboratory), the maintenance requirements may need to be minimal. Monthly or quarterly maintenance may also take a considerable amount of time, particularly if an analyzer has a lot of tubing or a large waterbath area that must be periodically changed.

Downtime is the time that an analyzer is unavailable for testing because of periodic maintenance or reasons pertaining to troubleshooting. Maintenance is generally scheduled and can be planned for times when the work volume is slower. Troubleshooting, however, is not planned downtime and may occur at the busiest time when the analyzer is needed the most. Downtime can be estimated by contacting other laboratories that are using or have used the analyzer in question. A salesperson can usually provide a list of customers that laboratory personnel can contact who will share their experiences. It is also worthwhile to contact a laboratory that is no longer using the analyzer to ascertain the reasons for removing the analyzer.

Another aspect to consider that is related to maintenance and troubleshooting is the service provided for the instrument. The hours that service personnel are available, the quality of the service personnel, the speed of response when problems occur, the cost of the service through a service contract or as a request, and the service training for laboratory personnel are all important aspects to consider. Any time an analyzer is nonfunctional, the quality and turnaround time for patient results can be affected. This becomes even more more important when there is no backup analyzer.

Quality Control. Another important consideration in selecting an analyzer may be the ability of the instrument to monitor, store, and calculate QC. The operational functions of a clinical laboratory that pertain to QC can occupy a considerable amount of operator time. The QC rules used by many laboratories have become more complex since the development of Westgard multirule formulas. An analyzer that can warn the operator when control values are out of range may be important particularly if unskilled personnel are performing the testing. Even if skilled personnel are employed, the time required to document QC can be considerable, particularly on analyzers with a large test menu. Most instruments have the ability to at least store and calculate simple QC formulas such as mean, standard deviation, and coefficient of variation. Some will even provide Levey-Jennings charts to visually show shifts and trends. The time that the instrument can save in reference to the overall quality control program can be important.

Training. One last feature to consider may be the training the manufacturer will provide during and after installation. Most manufacturers will train one operator before installation. This individual might be expected to train all other laboratory employees, write the procedure manual, set up the QC aspects of the analyzer, and perform the instrument evaluation. This can be an enormous task for one person to accomplish. However, many manufacturers will provide technical personnel to help with all or some of these installation tasks. With large laboratory staffs this might be a deciding factor between two analyzers that appear to be equally acceptable.

Postanalytic Considerations in Automation

Once an analyzer is generating patient results, the laboratory must then deal with these results. As in the preanalytic stages of patient testing, automation is relegated predominantly to the computerization that is available in the institution. Physicians may receive patient results in a variety of ways: from a computer screen, a paper copy, a phone call, or a combination of these three. The fastest of these is through a computer system. In many laboratory settings the patient results can be transmitted directly from the laboratory instrumentation, to the laboratory computer system, and then to the hospital computer system (a process called **uploading**). One of the major advantages of this, aside from speed, is the decrease in clerical errors that can occur when a human operator must transcribe results manually. The laboratory may also want instrumentation that can process test requests directly from satellite computer terminals at nursing stations, the emergency room, and clinics (a process called **downloading**). When investigating an analyzer, the capability to interface (unidirectional and/or bidirectional) with the laboratory and/or hospital information system may be important.

In addition to the way a physician receives routine results, the laboratory must be concerned with a method of notifying a physician of critical or panic value results. The CLIA '88 regulations require that special notification procedures be in place for these critical results. Most laboratories currently notify physicians of these results by telephone, a procedure that is time consuming and frustrating particularly during off shift hours and weekends. A computer system that has the capability to print these results on a special printer or with a warning sound could significantly decrease the time spent in making telephone calls, without jeopardizing the availability of these results to physicians. Facsimile (Fax) machines are also used in some institutions as a means of notifying physicians of stat or critical results.

Conclusion

This chapter has reviewed some basic concepts in laboratory automation that will serve as a foundation for the chapters that follow. These subsequent chapters will describe in detail specific analyzers that are available to the various laboratory disciplines. It is important to note that each laboratory is unique. If automation is to aid the laboratory in increasing speed and reliability of patient results while decreasing costs and allow the best use of operator time, the needs of the laboratory must be thoroughly understood. Therefore manufacturers need to produce instrumentation that meets those needs. Such analyzers need to be carefully chosen and evaluated. It is also important to be aware of the regulations that will affect the choice and introduction of an instrument into the laboratory. Laboratory settings are becoming more diverse. Laboratory boundaries are changing, and new technologies are emerging. Clinical instrumentation is rapidly changing to meet the challenges of laboratory medicine. Automation is beginning to move beyond the realm of simply testing a patient sample. It is beginning to encompass the entire testing process from order generation through use of test results. It is up to each laboratory to choose its instrumentation carefully to maintain and improve the quality of patient care.

Review Questions

1. Personnel costs are not a factor in the desire to automate the clinical laboratory.
   1. True
   2. False
2. Advances in immunology have aided in the automation of tests that were difficult to automate in the past.
   1. True
   2. False

3. The test menu is a combination or variety of tests offered by a laboratory.
   1. True
   2. False
4. Service need not be considered when selecting an instrument.
   1. True
   2. False

Choose the best answer for each of the following questions.

5. The number of test results that a laboratory will generate over a period of time is known as:
   A. Workflow
   B. Carryover
   C. Workload
   D. Workload recording
6. Bar codes can be used for the following purposes:
   A. Identify reagents
   B. Test programming
   C. Identify interferences
   D. A and C
   E. A and B
7. The ability to process only the analytes requested is called _____ testing.
   A. Continuous flow
   B. Discrete
   C. Sequential
   D. Random access
8. A mode of testing by which samples are processed independently of all others is called _____ analysis.
   A. Sequential
   B. Discrete
   C. Batch
   D. Random access
9. The ability of a test to measure only the analyte requested is referred to as its _____.
   A. Linearity
   B. Sensitivity
   C. Specificity
   D. Precision
10. The parameter that refers to the reproducibility of a method is called _____ and is usually measured by a statistic called the _____.
   A. Accuracy, coefficient of variation (CV)
   B. Precision, standard deviation (SD)
   C. Linearity, range
   D. Precision, coefficient of variation (CV)
   E. Accuracy, mean

Answers

1. F 2. T 3. F 4. F 5. C 6. C 7. D 8. B 9. C 10. D

Bibliography

Kaplan LA, Pesce AJ, eds: Clinical chemistry: theory, analysis, and correlation, ed 2, St Louis, 1989, Mosby–Year Book.

CHAPTER **18**

Automation in the Chemistry Laboratory

JACK A. MAGGIORE
ROBERT H. WILLIAMS

Instrument Classification
Common Chemistry Analyzers

During the past 10 years the clinical laboratory has experienced great innovations in the automation of chemistry analyzers. Analyzers are faster and easier to use. Methods are more precise, sensitive, and specific. Still, many of the same principles are found in today's instruments that appeared in earlier models. Manufacturers have worked toward automation with "walkaway" capabilities and minimal operator intervention. This has allowed technologists to perform additional technical functions such as manual procedures and quality assurance duties. Nevertheless, some of the first automated chemistry analyzers are still found in many clinical laboratories. Many serve as backup instruments to the newer and higher volume analyzers of today. This chapter will focus on some of the automated chemistry analyzers found in today's clinical laboratories.

Instrument Classification

Automated clinical systems are all classified according to their mode of operation. The earliest automated systems were strictly **batch analyzers** that performed one analysis on individual specimens. Although the analysis was automated, the rate at which tests could be performed was limited in many cases to the speed of an experienced technologist performing the test manually. Many of today's benchtop analyzers such as the COBAS-BIO use a batch approach. A batch analyzer will frequently employ both **sequential** and **discrete** techniques. Specimens are often sam-

pled from a carousel and are subsequently analyzed in the same sequence. Analysis is likely to occur in discrete or individual cells or cuvettes. Not all sequential and discrete analyzers are classified as batch instruments. The Beckman ASTRA 8 is one such example; it samples sequentially and then performs isolated analyses in a discrete fashion. But because the ASTRA is capable of performing more than one assay/sample during an analytic run, it is not classified as batch. Instead an operator may choose which assays are to be performed thus classifying the ASTRA as a **selective analyzer.**

Continuous flow analyzers, such as the Technicon Chem I$^+$, process each specimen in the same manner. Samples are automatically tested for all available chemistries regardless of the tests requested. Continuous flow analyzers are best suited for laboratories that have a high volume of multiple-test profiles.

Centrifugal analyzers use cuvette cells in the form of rotors. Reagent and sample are mixed via centrifugal force that is generated as the rotor turns. Most centrifugal analyzers are also classified as sequential and discrete. The COBAS-BIO is an example of a centrifugal analyzer that uses strictly batch analysis. The Instrumentation Laboratory Monarch, however, because of its unique design, has **random access** capabilities.

Random access analyzers are the most commonly encountered systems. The random access feature allows operators to program a variety of tests, profiles, or combinations of both on any given number of specimens in any order at any time. Random access analyzers are obviously all considered selective, with most employing discrete analyses as well. The **throughput** of a random access analyzer is determined not by the reaction times of the analyses but by the time required for mechanical movements and optical measurements. The throughput of a batch analyzer is directly proportional to its reaction time.

When an analyzer performs all programmed analyses on one specimen before commencing the sampling on a subsequent sample, the instrument is classified as **specimen oriented.** The Olympus DEMAND is one such system that is also considered random access.

Common Chemistry Analyzers

The Abbott Spectrum EPx. The Abbott Spectrum EPx (Fig. 18-1) is capable of performing tests as a batch, STAT, random access, and **tandem access** analyzer. Tandem access is a unique feature of the EPx that allows the operator to program the assays to maximize the rate at which patient tests are completed. In a batch mode the **walk-away capability** of the analyzer allows an operator to run up to 2400 tests without any intervention. STAT samples may be programmed at any time. Samples may be scheduled or programmed onto the EPx by downloading information through a specimen bar code, entering the sample identification number (SID), or entering the patient identification number (PID). The EPx is capable of laser scanning and reading most common bar codes. Carousels are designed to accept 5, 7, and 10 ml sample tubes. The sample probe senses the liquid level of a specimen to alert the operator against short sampling. The Teflon tip of the probe minimizes **carryover.** The sample volume ranges from 1.25 to 10 μl. The EPx will flag the results when analyte concentrations fall

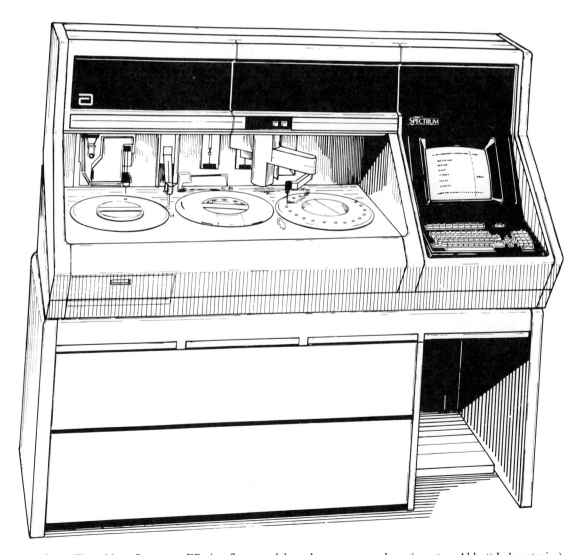

Fig. 18-1 The Abbott Spectrum EPx is a floor model random access analyzer (courtesy Abbott Laboratories).

outside the linear range of the analyzer. The operator has the option to use the **autodilute** feature or to manually dilute the specimen for reassay.

Communication with the analyzer is accomplished through a touch-screen color monitor and a keyboard. Calibration data, quality control (QC) results, Levey-Jennings charts, maintenance schedules, and workload recording data are stored by the on-board data management system.

The optical system has the capacity to read 16 wavelengths from 340 to 660 nm simultaneously for performing polychromatic, bichromatic, or monochromatic analyses. The EPx uses photometric analysis for general chemistry and enzyme tests and an ion-selective electrode (ISE) **module** for electrolytes. Photometric analysis occurs within a glass cuvette that is automatically washed by the analyzer for reuse.

All reagents are liquid and are stored on-board the Spectrum EPx. The reagent carousel is divided into four sections: three are refrigerated and one is kept at room temperature. A total of 31 reagent positions are available/carousel plus three electrolyte assays. Reagent containers are bar coded with the reagent name and lot number.

Liquid level sensors are also employed by the Spectrum EPx to monitor and inventory reagent supplies. The operator is alerted when reagent supplies are in short supply. The Spectrum EPx can be **bidirectionally interfaced** with a variety of laboratory computer systems. To assist operators in troubleshooting, the EPx contains a built-in modem that allows direct communication to technical support staff.

The Baxter Paramax 720ZX. The Baxter Paramax 720ZX (Fig. 18-2) is a random access analyzer capable of processing approximately 650 tests/hour. The unique features of the Paramax include dry tablet reagent technology, sealed disposable reaction cuvettes, and Closed Container Sampling.

Closed Container Sampling eliminates the need to uncap and recap tubes. A special cannula called a *S*ampling *T*hrough *A R*ubber stopper (STAR) enters the collection tube. A second liquid-sensing probe gains access through the STAR probe into the collection tube and aspirates the sample. The STAR probe does not touch the specimen nor does it bore a visible hole into the stopper. The design of this probe causes a semicircular cut into the rubber stopper, and the elastic nature of the stopper reseals the cap. To in-

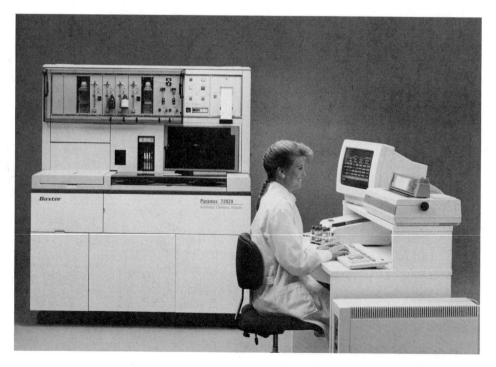

Fig. 18-2 The Baxter Paramax 720 ZX is a high-throughput, random access analyzer (courtesy Baxter Healthcare Corp.)

itiate the sampling process, a bar code-labeled collection tube or suitable adapter is loaded into a sample loading carousel. Each sample loading carousel holds 48 tubes, divided into 12 coded sectors. The computer tracks the sample tube location from loading to unloading. A standard 10 ml collection tube may be used directly; other sizes may be used with special sampling adapters. Microsampling is possible through the use of a microcup inserted into an alternate tube made specifically for the Paramax. Most bar code labels are compatible with the Paramax, which is also equipped to print bar code labels. Primary sample identification through bar code labeling is the only means of specimen identification by the analyzer; thus bar codes are required on all specimens. STAT sampling is accomplished by loading samples directly onto the sample carousel thus bypassing the loading carousel.

Most assays require no operator intervention when a result is higher than a set linear limit. The Paramax autodilutes specimens by aspirating less sample volume. The instrument then corrects for the dilution factor and prints both the original and rerun values.

The Paramax uses dry reagent tablets (for common chemistries and enzymes), which have a shelf life of 18 months when stored at refrigerator temperatures. On-board stability is between 10 and 90 days. Reagent dispensers are bar coded and may be placed in any location on the reagent carousel. More than one reagent dispenser from the same lot number may be loaded as the Paramax automatically begins using a new dispenser when needed.

Electrolytes including lithium are performed by ISE. The ISE reagents are in a liquid form and require the use of an on-board syringe pump. The Paramax has six syringe pumps in all; one for the ISE reagent, one for adding the diluent to dissolve the tablets, two for sampling and diluting, and two for the other available liquid reagent systems that are **"user defined"** methods (immunoassays, therapeutic drugs, and drugs of abuse).

Calibration for all analytes is required monthly unless a new lot number is placed into use, major maintenance is performed, or QC dictates such a need. A two-level comprehensive calibrator is available for 18 analytes, with other analytes requiring separate calibrators.

The Paramax cuvette supply is a continuous spool of 2000 plastic reaction cells. The cuvette track moves the cuvettes through a 37° C water bath at a speed of one position every 5 seconds,

or 720 movements/hour. To minimize the biohazard risk to the operator, the used cuvettes are heat-sealed.

The plastic cuvettes receive a reagent tablet followed by diluent. The cuvette passes through an ultrasonic device to dissolve the tablet. A photometric reading is taken to ensure that the tablet is fully dissolved. This serves as the reagent blank. If the Paramax obtains an acceptable blank reading, the cuvette advances to receive the sample. Additional diluent is dispensed to bring the total volume in each cuvette to 300 μl. A sample blank is created by dispensing specimen and diluent into a second cuvette. This allows for corrections for hemolysis, icterus, and lipemia. There are eight photometric read stations to monitor the reaction. Bichromatic measurements are made through seven interference filters.

The Paramax can be bidirectionally interfaced. QC and workload recording programs are used by many Paramax sites and are user-programmed. A built-in modem helps to track the instrument status and assists with advanced, technical troubleshooting.

The Baxter Paramax Model 720 and Model 520. The Paramax Model 720 differs from the 720ZX in that it has a 32 position reagent carousel rather than 48. The 720 also does not have a capability to assay lithium via ISE. The Paramax Model 520 has a throughput of 520 tests/hour and has features similar to the 720 except that it cannot perform ISE tests.

The Beckman ASTRA 8. Although the Beckman ASTRA (or Synchron AS 8) (Fig. 18-3) was introduced in the early 1970s, it is still found in many clinical laboratories today. The word "ASTRA" is an acronym for *A*utomated *ST*at and *R*outine *A*nalyzer. The Beckman ASTRA is a discrete, selective, sequential analyzer. Most laboratories use ASTRAs for moderate to high volume routine panel testing. Typically, seven or eight channels are used by a laboratory to include electrolytes, renal function tests, and glucose.

The analyzer consists of an assay compartment that houses the analytic modules (a unique feature of the instrument), an electronics compartment that houses the circuit boards, a microprocessor with disk-operated system, the keyboard, a video display unit, and a sampler. The sample carousel has 40 positions, 38 for samples and 2 for calibrators.

Specimens are added to sample cups and then placed on a carousel. The operator programs the analyzer through a keyboard and can choose to

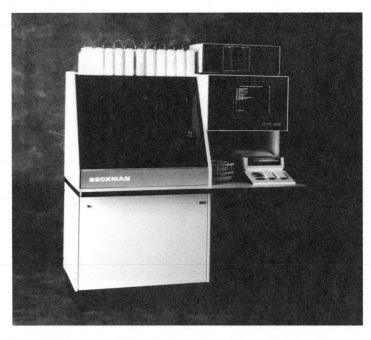

Fig. 18-3 The Synchron AS 8 system (ASTRA) is a selective, discrete, sequential analyzer with replaceable analytic modules (courtesy Beckman Instruments, Inc.).

run the ASTRA in one of three modes: the basic mode: specimens are assayed on all channels; the program mode: one assay/combination of assays are programmed for an individual specimen; and the STAT mode: immediate interruption for specimens of higher priority. On completion of STAT specimens, the ASTRA automatically returns to the previous testing without further operator involvement.

The throughput time of an eight-test panel on the ASTRA is approximately 1 minute. In the basic mode the throughput is 480 tests/hour. Results are displayed on a video display unit (VDU) and printed on an instrument tape or other printer substitute. The VDU is also the communicative link between the instrument and the operator; malfunctions, calibration data, and diagnostic instructions are displayed.

The sample volume for most individual assays is 15 μl; an eight-test panel requires approximately 150 μl including **dead volume.** The sampling mechanism of the ASTRA is two probes that move as a single unit. When the probes move into the sampling position, a test of conductivity occurs first to detect missing cups or insufficient samples. Motor-driven syringes aspirate the specimen plus two air bubbles that act to minimize cross-contamination. The dual probes move from the sampling area into the analytic section

of the ASTRA. Following a rinse of the outside of the probes, the probes separate and each simultaneously dispenses a specific volume of specimen into the appropriate reaction chambers. The dual probe design reduces the throughput time of the analyzer.

All the test modules are calibrated to run one assay except the ISE module, which runs sodium and potassium simultaneously. Three or four peristaltic pumps move the reagents into the reaction cup, sip excess reagent, and then drain the chamber following the completion of measurement. A typical module is diagrammed in Fig. 18-4. If a module fails, the ASTRA system allows for a rapid replacement of the unit with a spare.

Twenty-three assays are available for use on the ASTRA. This menu includes enzymes, electrolytes, and common chemistries. Six assays use an electrochemical principle, the rest are spectrophotometric. Reagents are liquids; some assays, such as creatinine, require mixing of two components to form the reagent that is used on the analyzer. Most assays are calibrated once every 8 hours; glucose and some enzymes, however, are calibrated every 2 hours.

The software features include the programming and storing of normal ranges for serum and spinal fluid and storing QC ranges for up to 10 controls. When a patient or QC result falls out-

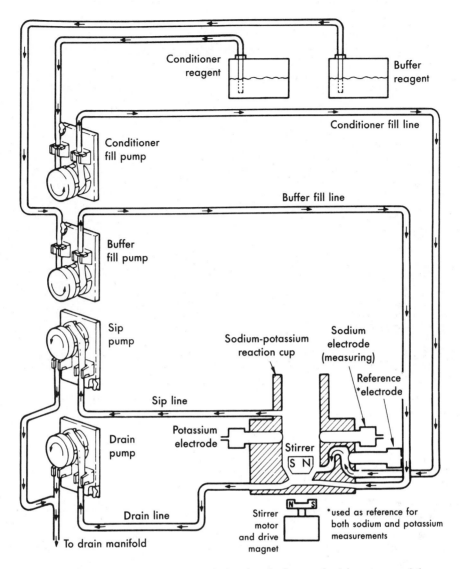

Fig. 18-4 A typical ASTRA module is diagrammed, showing the four peristaltic pumps and the reagent pathway (courtesy Beckman Instruments, Inc.).

side the preset limit or the linear range, the ASTRA will flag the result. If a glucose level exceeds the linear range, the ASTRA can autodilute the sample by aspirating half of the required sample volume. The dilution is then corrected for when the result is displayed. This software feature is known as ORDAC, which stands for *Over Range Detection And Correction.* The ASTRA can also be **unidirectionally interfaced.**

The Beckman Synchron CX3. The CX3 (Fig. 18-5), employs many of the same assays and technologies as the Beckman ASTRA. Like the ASTRA, the CX3 is used for moderate to high volumes of electrolyte panel testing. Programming is random access; the operator is able to per-

form panels, profiles, individual tests, or any combination within the same run, STAT or routine. The CX3 is able to sample directly from primary sample tubes for faster processing. The sample carousel can accommodate as many as 80 specimens using disposable specimen cups or a variety of primary tubes. The throughput of the CX3 is as high as 600 tests/hour using BUN, glucose, and creatinine in a panel. Typically, an uninterrupted run of 75 specimens of an eight-test profile will result in a throughput of 540 tests/hour. The test menu consists of calcium, sodium, potassium, chloride, CO_2, glucose, BUN, and creatinine. Glucose and BUN are rate technologies, creatinine and calcium are colorimetric, and so-

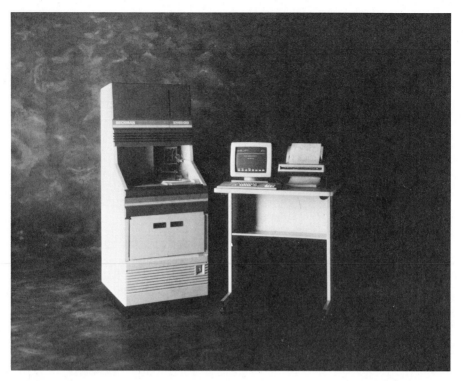

Fig. 18-5 The Synchron CX3 system is a random access analyzer suited for moderate to high volume electrolyte panel testing (courtesy Beckman Instruments, Inc.).

dium, potassium, CO_2 and chloride are performed by ISE.

The CX3 reagent system is similar to the ASTRA, except the reagents for the former are concentrated and there are a number of major technical changes. Chloride, which uses amperometric titration on the ASTRA, is an ISE system on the CX3. Calcium and creatinine are analyzed using bichromatic optics, and the reaction for creatinine occurs at 41° C. Both of these changes help to reduce the effects of potential interferences. Two-point calibrations are required once every 8 hours for all tests.

The sampling mechanism is centralized and rotates from the specimen carousel to the dispensing locations by using the arc motion of the single-arm sample probe. This eliminates the need of a transport mechanism. The modular design has two peristaltic pumps/channel. The sample mechanism is equipped with a liquid-sensing probe that automatically adjusts to the sample height of evacuated tubes. This feature helps to eliminate some of the problems encountered with small sample volumes. The specimen requirements are the same as the ASTRA in terms of sample volume and dead space.

The software features of the CX3 include programming for 8 trays of 80 specimens, storing results for 800 samples, monitoring 5 control ranges, use of Westgard rules, monthly and cumulative summaries, plotting Levey-Jennings charts, and monitoring of reagent inventory. The CX3 also has bidirectional interfacing.

The Beckman Synchron CX4 and CX5. The Synchron CX4 Clinical System is a rapid, random access analyzer. Its intended purpose is to complement a STAT electrolyte analyzer in a moderate to high volume clinical chemistry laboratory. The Synchron CX5 is essentially the same analyzer as the CX4, but has an additional capacity to perform electrolyte analyses by ISE. Like the CX3, both instruments can be bidirectionally interfaced and are able to perform panel and profile testing, single tests or combinations, and STAT testing. The software capabilities of both instruments are also similar to the CX3.

Both the CX4 and CX5 Clinical Systems have a test throughput of 525 tests/hour. Tests are prioritized by the analyzer to maximize throughput by analyzing those tests with the longest incubation times first. The sample volume for photometric chemistries vaires from 3 to 25 μl, whereas

ISE chemistries require 60 μl for the four-test panel (Na, K, Cl, CO_2). About 100 Beckman and "user-defined" assays are available and include the common chemistries and enzymes, urine chemistries, therapeutic drugs, drugs of abuse, and immunoglobulins. The user may select 24 tests on-board for use on the CX4 and 28 tests on the CX5.

Sampling may occur from either the primary tube or from specimen cups. A laser bar code sample scanner is also a feature of both the CX4 and CX5. Specimen sectors have replaced the carousel and are capable of holding 120 specimens. The 12 sectors hold 10 specimens and are shuttled to the various sampling stations. The sample probes are equipped with a liquid level sensor to monitor the sample and reagent condition. Carryover is minimized with a two-step wash action of the sample probe. The ORDAC autodilution option may be used for any or all tests at the discretion of the user.

All reagents are liquid, require no dilution or preparation, and are packaged as three-compartment cartridges that are bar coded. Most reagents are refrigerated and have an on-board stability of 30 days. Both the CX4 and CX5 have an automatic inventory tracking system that provides reagent status reports and warns when a reagent is in low supply or is outdating. Most chemistries need to be calibrated every 2 weeks or as the reagent lot number changes.

The spectrophotometric tests use an extensive cuvette system. The 80 glass cuvettes of the CX4 and CX5 are automatically washed, dried, tested, and reused without system interruption. The instrument will notify the operator if a cuvette needs to be replaced. The requirements for the automated cuvette-washing system is 9 L of deionized water/hour and thus a suitable drain system is required.

The Beckman Synchron CX7. The features of the CX3 and the CX4 have been combined in the Beckman Synchron CX7 (Fig. 18-6), which has a comprehensive test menu: 80 tests are available including thyroid tests and specific protein analyses. The analyzer has a STAT capability with a 1 minute response. The maximum throughput is 825 tests/hour when running uninterrupted electrolyte profiles concurrently with routine chemistry panels.

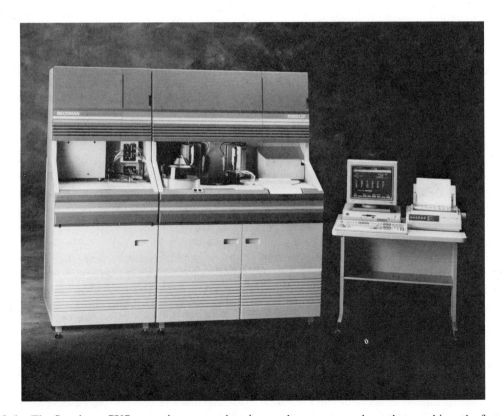

Fig. 18-6 The Synchron CX7 sysem is a comprehensive random access analyzer that combines the features of the CX3 and the CX4. (Courtesy Beckman Instruments, Inc.).

The analyzer is actually two systems under the control of a single computer control unit. The left side of the analyzer (Fig. 18-6) is designed to perform STAT analyses in a very similar fashion as the Synchron CX3. This section analyzes electrolytes including CO_2 and calcium, BUN, creatinine, and glucose, all which have a 1 minute turnaround time. The right side of the analyzer (Fig. 18-6) performs all remaining assays, much like the Synchron CX4. Most reagents are liquid and packaged in bar coded three-pot containers. The on-board stability of the reagents ranges from 30 to 42 days. The CX7 has 32 positions for reagents: 24 refrigerated and 8 at room temperature. It also has a reagent level sensor that provides updates on remaining available tests in a given cartridge.

Sampling occurs from a central location with specimens set into sectors. The CX7 system can sample specimens directly from primary tubes of various sizes including a 2 ml microtube or from disposable sample cups. The sample capacity is 63 samples, or 9 sectors of 7 tubes. Before sampling, the instrument can program up to 420 samples (sector mode). The minimum sample volume varies from 3 μl (glucose) to 60 μl (four-test electrolyte panel). The ORDAC autodilution option is available for most chemistries.

Bar coding is another enhancement of the CX7. Specimen bar codes are scanned by an on-board laser that recognizes four different bar code symbologies. The operator may intermix bar coded tubes, sample cups, and/or microtubes within the same run or even the same sector. The operator always has the option of entering identification or test request information from the system keyboard, as well as the option of running the analyzer with or without the bar code reader. When the system is in the bar code/read sample mode, sampling automatically occurs without the need for manual programming because the host computer performs all required programming (known as host computer discrete downloading).

Concurrent calibration is one of the unique features of the CX7. Because all assays, with the exception of electrolytes, are duplicated in the system, calibrations may be performed without the need to stop running specimens and without the need for instrument downtime. Most assays need to be calibrated every 90 days, as QC dictates, or as lot numbers change. Enzymes require no calibration on the system, but new lot numbers and new shipments of enzyme reagents need to be verified before use.

A pulsed xenon lamp is the main light source for the colorimetric tests. The optics system uses 10 filters spanning from 340 to 700 nm. Like the CX4 and CX5, the CX7 contains 80 reusable glass cuvettes. Washing the cuvettes requires 13 L of deionized water/hour.

The 80-megabyte hard drive stores up to 10,000 patient results, 2000 sample programs, and 32,000 QC data points. The hard drive also stores reagent inventory, workload recording data, and calibration information. Other software features include the reporting of up to 40 calculated parameters, as defined by the operator.

The Kodak Ektachem 700 Series. The Ektachem 700 is a random access analyzer that uses dry-reagent film technology. Thin coats of reagents are impregnated onto thin layers of plastic film and are mounted into a slide (Fig. 18-7, *A* and *B*). The Ektachem 700 is optimally suited to perform in a laboratory with moderate to high test volumes. The series of Ektachem 700 analyzers may be configured in one of three capabilities: the Ektachem 700S analyzer designed for enhanced STAT testing; the Ektachem 700P analyzer designed for simple profile testing; and the Ektachem 700XR analyzer that combines STAT testing and profiling for colorimetric, enzymatic, and electrolyte assays. The systems are identical in terms of sampling, programming, calibration, reagents, and basic principles. These general features are discussed below.

Sampling occurs through an apparatus called the **proboscis.** The proboscis is a positive-displacement pump in the metering tower that aspirates aliquots of specimens and dispenses uniform volumes of specimens onto reagent slides. Specimens may be sampled directly from a variety of sizes of evacuated tubes or from sample cups of varying sizes. There are 10 locations/sample tray, with four programming quadrants available, giving a total of 40 possible specimen locations.

The proboscis is equipped with a pressure sensor that can detect specimens clotted with fibrin (causes increased pressure), or if insufficient sample or no sample exists (causes decreased pressure). Each sample uses an individual disposable tip that eliminates specimen carryover. The design of the pierceable cap acts to minimize sample evaporation and helps to remove any excess fluid from the metering tips. Ten μl are required for all analyses, except enzymes, which require 11 μl.

The various layers of a typical Ektachem colorimetric and potentiometric slide are illustrated

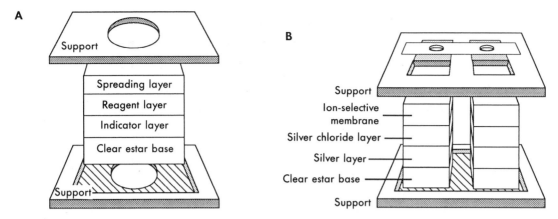

Fig. 18-7 A typical Kodak Ektachem, **A,** colorimetric slide and **B,** potentiometric slide illustrating the various layers (courtesy Eastman Kodak Co.).

in Fig. 18-7, *A* and *B*. In a typical colorimetric slide (Fig. 18-7, A), the first layer is known as the **spreading layer.** This layer meters sample by uniformly dispersing the drop of specimen over the entire surface of the slide, traps large and interfering molecules, and serves as a white reference background. The fluid diffuses through the spreading layer to the **reagent layers.** These layers provide buffer, supply enzyme catalysts, act as barriers, and change pH as needed. The dye layers develop color proportional to the concentration of the analyte. Clear ESTAR acts as a base and allows for reflectance measurements. Polyethylene support layers hold coated chemistry elements in place. A typical potentiometric slide is shown in Fig. 18-7 B. Sample size and electrolyte reference fluid are metered simultaneously for each slide. A paper bridge provides a fluid to fluid interface and forms two electrical half-cells. The ion selective layer makes the slide specific for the analyte. The ions make contact with the AgCl/Ag layers. Clear ESTAR acts as a rigid support as with the colorimetric slides. Two pairs of electrometer contacts pierce the Ag/AgCl layer and then measure the potential difference between two half-cells. Polyester support layers hold the coated chemistry elements in place in a manner similar to the colorimetric slide. Regardless of the methodology one slide is used/assay and then is discarded.

All Ektachem 700 series analyzers have an option known as positive sample identification (PSID). This option allows the Ektachem to read specimen bar codes placed onto specimen tubes or microsample adapters. Bidirectional interfacing eliminates the need for manual sample programming. All specimens may be programmed

through the use of a touch-screen monitor as panels or individual tests in a batch or random access mode. STAT sampling occurs immediately on the completion of the sample that is currently being metered.

The reagents are packaged in bar coded cartridges of 18 or 50 slides/pack. Most cartridges require refrigerator storage, with a few requiring long-term storage in the freezer. Slide supply number 1 houses both the colorimetric and potentiometric slides; slide supply number 2 houses the rate or enzymatic slides that require a special desiccant to control the relative humidity (Fig. 18-8). The Ektachem systems monitor slide volumes and display the remaining available tests through a special option. When fewer than six tests are remaining, the Ektachem will alert the operator through a displayed alarm on the CRT.

When the operator initiates sampling, slides are dispensed from the cartridges and loaded onto a device called a **slide metering block.** These six slide blocks are attached to a distributor that moves the slides from the slide supplies to the sample metering stations (see Fig. 18-8). At this position, the slides receive their appropriate volume of specimen. The first incubator encountered by the clockwise rotation of the dispensors is the colorimetric incubator. This incubator has a capacity of 27 slides; additional slides are loaded as space is available. Slides are removed from the 37° C colorimetric incubator and are placed into a reflectometer. Colorimetric assays all use endpoint reactions requiring approximately 5 minutes. Readings are taken every 12 seconds until reaction endpoint is determined.

The enzymatic assays use kinetic reactions and move to the rate incubator (see Fig. 18-8).

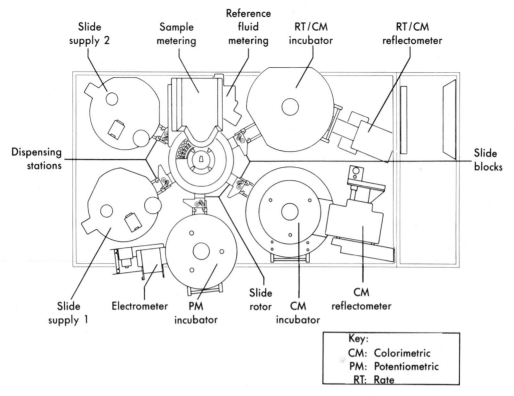

Fig. 18-8 The major components of the Kodak Ektachem 700 system (courtesy Eastman Kodak Co.).

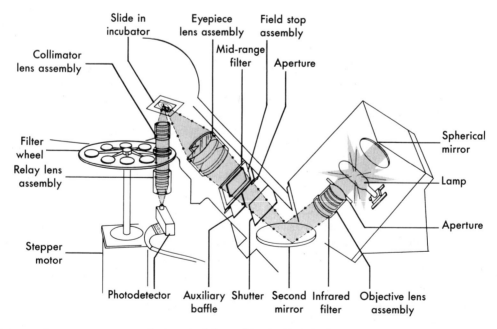

Fig. 18-9 Reflectance photometry is the principle used by the Kodak Ektachem to quantitate all enzymatic and colorimetric tests (courtesy Eastman Kodak Co.).

The rate incubator has 24 slide positions. A reflectometer reads the rate slides in situ. Fifty-four readings are taken during the 5 minute incubation to determine enzyme activity through rate algorithms.

A third incubator receives the potentiometric slides (see Fig. 18-8). These slides are maintained at 25° C and are monitored by an electrometer. Electrolyte determinations take approximately 3 minutes. Following completion of all analyses, slides are removed from the incubator and discarded into disposal boxes.

Calibration is required every 6 months, as lot numbers change, or as QC dictates. Linearity is performed on all assays annually. Because the pure white background is essential to reflectance readings, a white reference test should be performed before calibrations.

All Kodak Ektachem systems use a principle known as **reflectance photometry** (Fig. 18-9). The design of the reagent slides makes it impractical for light to shine directly through the medium, as is the case when cuvettes are used. Instead, light is reflected off the shiny base of colorimetric and kinetic slides into a light detector. The radiant energy from a quartz-halogen lamp is collimated and passes through an infrared filter. The energy, in the form of heat, is directed to the slide. The reflected radiant energy is passed through a filter and is detected. The difference between the light reflected off a pure white source (the white reference) and the light reflected from a reacting slide is proportional to analyte being measured. Results are transmitted to the instrument's printer, as well as to the interfaced computer system.

The software features include configuring of special reports, selecting a variety of calculated parameters, performance of diagnostic and troubleshooting techniques, storing selective test panels, and maintenance of QC data. Data may be printed in Levey-Jennings format to generate monthly, quarterly, or annual reports.

The Ektachem 700S and 700P. The Ektachem 700S analyzer is capable of performing only colorimetric and electrolyte assays. Twenty-eight assays are available. The throughput is slightly enhanced because electrolyte assays are performed in 3 minutes rather than 5. The Ektachem 700P analyzer performs only colorimetric and kinetic assays. This configuration is designed for an Ektachem to run alongside an electrolyte analyzer, or to accompany a second, full-service Ektachem, such as a 700XR. Thirty-one assays compose the test menu of the 700P. Both the 700S and 700P can be upgraded to a full test menu.

The Ektachem 700XR. The Ektachem 700XR is the full-capacity analyzer of the 700 series. Its configuration includes use of all incubators; therefore it has the capability to perform all 35 methodologies currently available from Kodak. The 700XR is equipped with an automatic sample management system that improves sample tracking. The Ektachem Model 700XR analyzer C series (or 700XRC) (Fig. 18-10) has an enhanced throughput up to 750 tests/hour and a color touch-screen monitor. The enhanced software package of the 700XRC provides storage of 8000 patient results, the capability to select age and sex normal ranges, additional calculated parameters, and calculation of workload recording data.

The Kodak Ektachem 500. The Kodak Ektachem 500 analyzer is a random access analyzer designed for laboratories with low-volume testing. The throughput of this analyzer is 300 tests/hour. Many of the same features previously mentioned for the Ektachem 700XR apply to the 500 as well. The main difference is the size of the analyzer; the colorimetric and rate incubators have been modified and combined into a single incubator.

The Kodak Ektachem 250. The Kodak Ektachem 250 (Fig. 18-11) is a smaller random access analyzer that is designed for the lower-volume laboratories with limited space. All of the same dry-reagent slide methodologies can be performed on the 250. There are some physical changes to the analyzer. The sample trays have been replaced by sample "traps" that are moved into and out of the metering area. The sample metering tower has been replaced by an internal sampling mechanism. The throughput of the Ektachem 250 is approximately 250 tests/hour. Other features unique to this new model of Ektachem include ability of the analyzer to scan and read reagent cartridge lot numbers via bar codes, a single incubator that accomodates all three types of reagent slides, and the ability to perform on-board dilutions. This analyzer, like all other Kodak analyzers, may be linked to a bidirectional computer interface.

The DuPont ACA III. The DuPont ACA III (Fig. 18-12) is a discrete, selective analyzer with a maximum throughput of 50 tests/hour. It is often used in laboratories to perform tests of small volume or in larger laboratories to perform specialty assays not available on other higher throughput

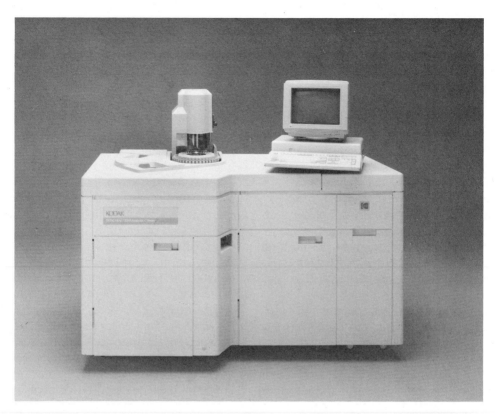

Fig. 18-10 The Kodak Ektachem 700XR Analyzer C Series is a high throughput, random access instrument using layered dry-slide technology (courtesy Eastman Kodak Co.).

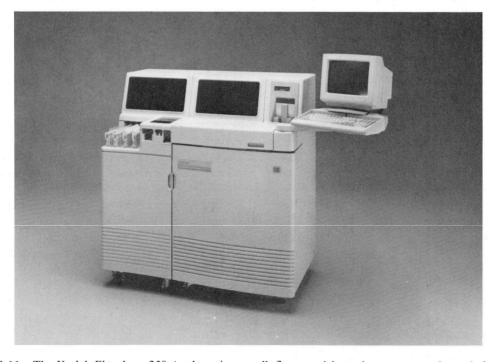

Fig. 18-11 The Kodak Ektachem 250 Analyzer is a small, floor model, random access analyzer designed for lower-volume laboratories (courtesy Eastman Kodak Co.).

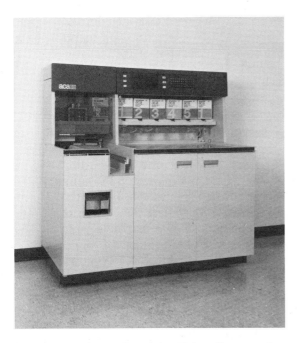

Fig. 18-12 The DuPont ACA III is a discrete, selective analyzer, capable of performing a wide array of assays (courtesy E.I. du Pont de Nemours & Co., Inc.).

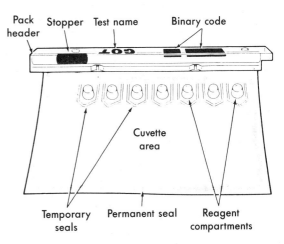

Fig. 18-13 A typical ACA binary-coded reagent pack (courtesy E.I. du Pont de Nemours & Co., Inc.).

analyzers. ACA stands for *A*utomated *C*linical *A*nalyzer; a unique feature of this instrument is the reagent pack. For every assay, the required reagents are prepackaged into plastic **binary coded packs** that also function as the cuvette (Fig. 18-13).

Specimens are aliquotted into plastic specimen cups and are attached to an identification card. The operator pencils in the patient identification and demographics. The specimen is loaded onto the ACA III followed by one or two reagent packs. The operator pushes the OPERATE button to start the sampling process. The sampling needle is flushed with diluent and then moves to the specimen cup for aspiration. During this time the ACA reads the binary code on the reagent pack and has determined the required volume of specimen. The sample volume is fairly large for most assays; most enzyme analyses require 200 to 500 μl, whereas most therapeutic assays require 20 μl. To reduce the dead volume to 20 μl (from 100 μl), small microsample adaptors are available.

A positive-displacement pump aspirates sample and buffer and dispenses them through a rubber hub found in each reagent pack. The reagent pack is then pushed onto a chain that carries the pack through the various stations of the analyzer. The first two positions are for 37° C incubation of

the specimen and buffer. The chain moves the pack into an area known as the **breaker-mixer.** The reagents are in seven separate compartments of the pack. The breaker-mixer breaks the first four compartments to release the contents. Reagent, buffer, and specimen are mixed through the agitating motion of the breaker-mixer. After three incubation positions a second breaker-mixer breaks the remaining compartments and again mixes the contents of the pack. The chain moves the pack into the photometer position. The color of the reaction is read, and the result is printed and displayed. The chain indexes one additional time to drop the sealed reagent pack into a biohazard waste receptacle. This entire process takes approximately 7 minutes.

The methods are measured bichromatically with the exception of those assays requiring two packs, where a blank is used. Reagent packs are kept refrigerated until used. Calibration is required when the pack lot number changes, major troubleshooting or maintenance is performed, or as QC dictates. The buffers and diluents are packaged into 1 L boxes that are stored on-board the analyzer at room temperature.

The 80 assays that are available cover a broad spectrum of analyses, including coagulation factors, thyroid function tests, therapeutic drugs, specific proteins, immunoglobulins, and drugs of abuse. An ISE module is available to perform sodium and potassium analyses. The analyzer may be unidirectionally interfaced.

The DuPont ACA IV. The DuPont ACA IV is a discrete bench-top analyzer that employs the same test methodologies as the ACA III. The throughput is 76 tests/hour. The sampling mechanism is similar to the ACA III except the sampling needle is not accessible to the operator during the sampling process, a safety feature. Bar coding of sample cups eliminates the need for manually writing in patient identification information. A simple keypad serves as the programming center of the entire system. The instrument status is displayed on a VDU to the operator in the form of **icons,** or symbols that depict the current activity. The internal components of the ACA IV differ from the ACA III in that there are four chain-indexing stations rather than seven.

The test menu of the ACA IV is almost identical to the ACA III because the two analyzers use the same reagent packs and calibrators. The ISE module, however, is not available, so sodium and potassium analyses are not possible on the ACA IV. Calibrations on the ACA IV may be performed concurrently with patient samples to eliminate unnecessary instrument downtime. For most assays, calibrations are required every 3 months or as lot numbers change.

The DuPont Dimension. The DuPont Dimension (Fig. 18-14) is a discrete, random access analyzer that can be used to analyze electrolytes, routine chemistries, therapeutic drugs, enzymes, and special chemistry tests including urine applications. Thirty seven tests are available. The maximum throughput of the analyzer is up to 200 ISE tests and 200 photometric tests/hour. The unique features of the Dimension include the Flex reagent cartridges, ultrasonic probe mixing, and blow-molded Surlyn film cuvettes.

Programming of patient and sample data is via a keyboard. Specimen is aliquotted into a disposable sample cup, capped with an evaporation-preventing lid, and placed on the sample wheel. A function key on the keyboard is pressed to initiate processing. Two sample wheels contain 60 positions for loading of sample cups; one wheel may be placed onto the analyzer while a second is being programmed. Sample volume is generally 10 to 12 μl. However, some assays require 2 μl or as much as 60 μl. If ISE tests are requested, the ISE sample probe aspirates the required volume of specimen into the ISE electrode stack assembly. STAT sampling may be initiated at any time; a minimum of five STAT positions is always available.

Processing of specimens for photometric tests initiates the formation of reaction cuvettes. They are blow-molded from a special plastic ionomer resin film known as Surlyn (the plastic used in the

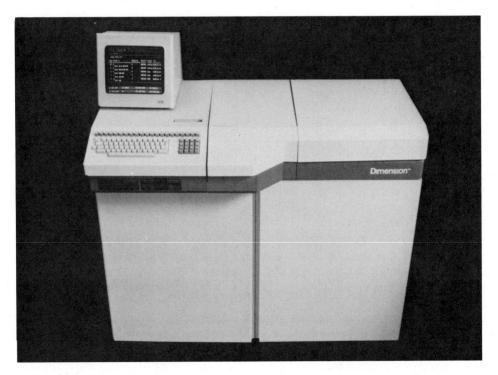

Fig. 18-14   The DuPont Dimension is a discrete, random access analyzer that forms cuvettes on-board (courtesy E.I. du Pont de Nemours & Co., Inc.).

ACA reagent packs). It is loaded onto the instrument as a cartridge that contains two rolls of film capable of forming 12,000 reaction cuvettes. The cuvette is read in an empty state to ensure optical clarity. Then a photometric sample arm aspirates the specimen from the sample cup and dispenses it into a newly formed cuvette.

The reagents of the Dimension are packaged into bar coded containers called Flex cartridges. Each contains up to six wells of lyophilized reagents. The number of tests/cartridge is method dependent. The photometric reagent probe pierces the seal of one of the cartridge wells and hydrates the reagent. The Dimension updates the reagent inventory following each series of tests. The refrigerated reagent storage wheel has 45 storage spaces where the reagents are stable for up to 30 days unopened or 5 days once hydrated. Following reagent hydration, the system dispenses it into the cuvette and ultrasonically mixes the specimen and reagent. After incubation, multiple absorbance readings are taken by a photometer that is capable of reading between 290 and 700 nm. Before completion of the reaction, the cuvette is sealed on top and then is cut and dropped into a biohazard waste container. The calibration stability of most assays is 2 to 3

months. Two lot numbers of the same reagent with their respective calibration curves may be stored on-board the Dimension at the same time; it automatically uses the appropriate curve as reagents are placed into use. The Dimension may be bidirectionally interfaced.

The Instrumentation Laboratory Phoenix. The IL Phoenix (Fig. 18-15) is a selective bench-top analyzer with an eight-test menu. The Model 900 performs urea nitrogen, creatinine, calcium, sodium, potassium, chloride, and total CO_2 testing, whereas the model 905 measures total protein in place of CO_2. The Phoenix processes up to 75 samples/hour with a maximum throughput of 600 tests/hour when performing the eight-test panel. All assays are completed within 2 minutes.

The required volume to perform any or all of the four electrolytes by ISE is 20 μl, 16 μl for the glucose/urea, 18 μl for creatinine, and 42 μl for total CO_2. The sample cup has a dead volume of 25 μl.

An operator uses a touch-pad and color monitor to enter the PID, identifies a cup position, and then selects which tests to run. The sample tray consists of two removable rings. The outer ring holds 40 specimen cups; the inner ring holds four STAT specimens or five calibrators. The sy-

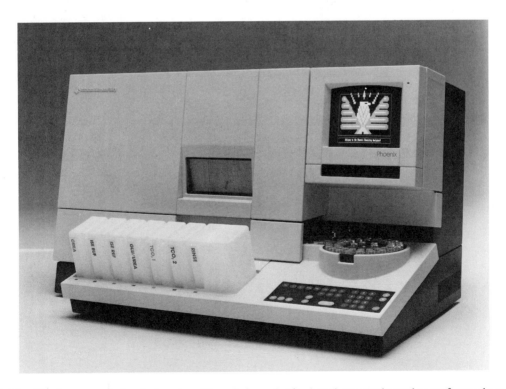

Fig. 18-15 The Instrumentation Laboratory Phoenix is a selective bench-top analyzer that performs electrolyte panel testing (courtesy Instrumentation Laboratory).

ringe sampler is attached to a robotic arm. The syringe aspirates and dispenses samples into the various test channels. There is no sample-sensing device on the probe, so the operator needs to be cautious of short or clotted specimens. The linearity of all assays, except CO_2, is extended through a software feature known as ALEX (automatic linearity extension). This feature automatically reruns the out of range analytes by aspirating half the sample volume thus giving a twofold dilution.

The Phoenix uses liquid reagents packaged in 500 ml, color-coded, plastic containers that are stored at room temperature. The reagent containers are self-tapping, thus neither a reagent probe nor reagent pump is required. This design allows use of the entire volume of the reagents because they are loaded upside down and thus drain

without dead space. The operator is alerted with a display message when fewer than 10 tests are available. Calibration is recommended to be performed every 8 hours.

A unique feature of the IL Phoenix is the solid-state fluidics system, consisting of compact acrylic blocks with interconnecting channels to replace tubing elements found in other fluidics systems. The test channels of the Phoenix are the system's analytic modules (Fig. 18-16). Samples and reagents flow through the acrylic blocks and are mixed. The reagent lines, sample lines, and mixing chambers are molded into the block. This design minimizes the amount of tubing found in other analyzers and the specimen and reagent volume/assay.

The most original test channel is the glucose/urea module that employs a technique known as

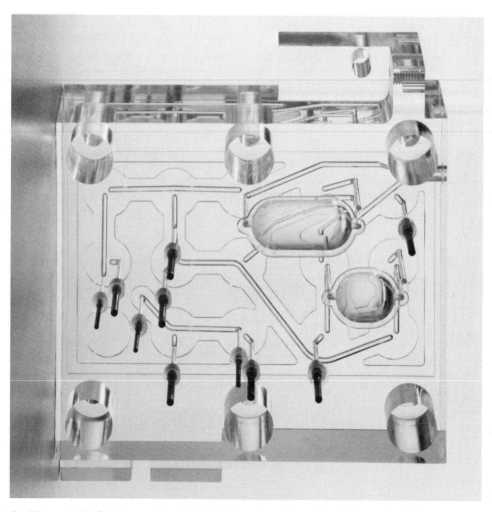

Fig. 18-16   The analytic fluidics module of the IL Phoenix replaces the tubing and coils found in many other systems (courtesy Instrumentation Laboratory).

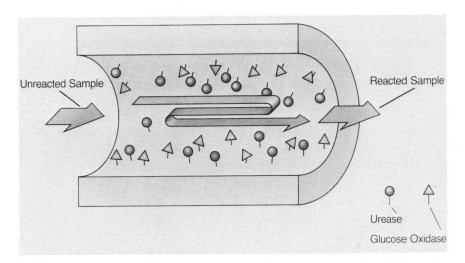

Fig. 18-17 Coimmobilization is a technique used by the IL Phoenix. Glucose and BUN are simultaneously measured by the same analytic module, in which urease and glucose oxidase are bonded to a nylon coil (courtesy Instrumentation Laboratory).

coimmobilization. Both glucose oxidase and urease are bonded to a nylon coil that feeds into an electrode chamber. Glucose is determined by measuring the decrease in oxygen as it is converted to glucuronic acid and hydrogen peroxide; urea is hydrolyzed by urease to produce ammonia that is read by an ISE. The schematic of this analytic channel appears in Fig. 18-17.

The Phoenix can be interfaced unidirectionally. The software features include quality control data storage and statistics, printing of Levey-Jennings charts, the use of Westgard's multirules, and the tallying of tests to prepare workload data.

The Instrumentation Laboratory Monarch.
The IL Monarch (Fig. 18-18) is a centrifugal analyzer that is capable of performing random access functions. Older models of centrifugal analyzers were classified as strictly batch instruments. The unique feature of the IL Monarch is the analyzer's ability to automatically change the cuvette wheels to run a variety of assays simultaneously. This function is analogous to programming a jukebox to select and play records. When electrolytes are included in a multitest panel, the throughput of 600 tests/hour is possible.

There are four areas of the Monarch: the pipette arm, the analysis compartment, the fluidics module, and the optics unit. The pipette arm, composed of two stainless steel pipette tips, moves between the sample, reagent, wash bath, and loader table positions. A coil at the bottom of the coils heats the fluids before they are dispensed. Pipette tips are cleaned between each aspiration to eliminate the effects of carryover. The syringe module transfers samples and reagents to the 39 cuvette rotor and ISE analyzer cups (spin cups). The sample volume requirements range from 2 to 20 μl for photometric analyses and 30 μl for ISE tests. There are 44 numbered positions on the sample ring, 38 of which are available for patient samples; the remaining 6 are reserved for calibrators and an electrolyte activator solution.

The analysis unit has three main functions: sending the rotors (cuvette wheels) into the loading area, positioning them for analysis, and removing them for disposal (Fig. 18-19). The feed stack of rotors holds 24 cuvette wheels that are stored on top of each other. Two sensors alert the operator when eight (or fewer) rotors are available or when the discard stack contains 24 rotors. The rotors are prepackaged in stacks of 16 for easier manual loading. To prevent evaporation, a cover is placed over the rotor while it is spinning to mix the contents. The Monarch is capable of producing up to 39 analyses on one rotor in 3 minutes. The unique feature of this centrifugal analyzer is the rotor. Light of a selected wavelength is directed through a grating monochromator. The beam of light passes through the cuvette position from the top through the photomultiplier tube at the bottom. Potentiometric analyses are performed when a diluted sample passes through ISEs.

The reagent containers for the Monarch are wedge-shaped bottles referred to as "boatILs" (Fig. 18-20), which are bar coded thus allowing the operator to place them in any position on the

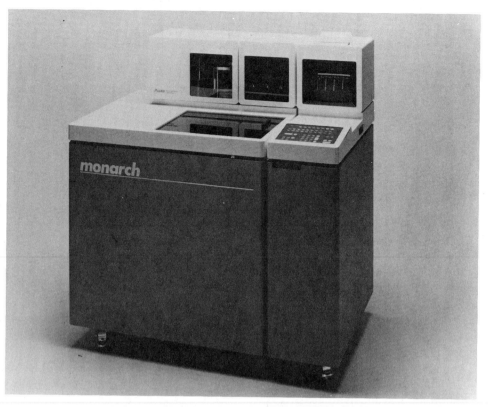

Fig. 18-18 The Instrumentation Laboratory Monarch is a centrifugal analyzer with random access features (courtesy Instrumentation Laboratory).

reagent carousel. The reagent volumes are monitored by a level sensor. Most boatILs contain 20 ml of reagent (75 tests). The on-board reagent stability is 7 to 12 days.

The system performs a series of checks before rotor loading is initiated including necessity of calibration, presence of a sample cup in each of the requested positions, the volume of diluent, and the amount of waste.

STAT specimens may be added to the Monarch as they arrive. STAT requests are run in a patient-priority (or specimen-oriented) mode.

The test menu is fairly extensive and includes enzymes, common chemistries, electrolytes, special chemistries, immunoglobulins, and urine and spinal fluid applications. Because the Monarch employs an "open-reagent system," other vendor's reagents may be used on the system, thus expanding the menu to include therapeutic drugs and drugs of abuse.

The software features include on-board storage of calibration curves, user-defined assay programmability, storage of 38,000 test and QC results, and tracking of reagents and supplies used,

including disposable materials. Bidirectional interfacing is also available.

The Olympus DEMAND. The Olympus DEMAND (Fig. 18-21) is a random access analyzer that is specimen oriented (i.e., every test requested on each sample is performed before the next specimen is sampled). The throughput of the DEMAND approaches 40 tests/hour, or 600 when the ISE module is used. The DEMAND is suited for laboratories with small to medium test volumes. The unique features of the analyzer include disposable rectangular cuvettes and concentrated liquid reagents.

Samples are aliquotted into disposable plastic cups and are placed onto a numbered serpentine chain (greater than 100 positions) that is enclosed in a high-humidity chamber to limit the effects of specimen evaporation. Positions on the chain are color-coded to indicate where calibrators or controls should be placed. When the instrument reads these color codes, it automatically begins to run a calibration or analyze a control. The operator requests patient tests through the instrument's keyboard and CRT. The specimen is as-

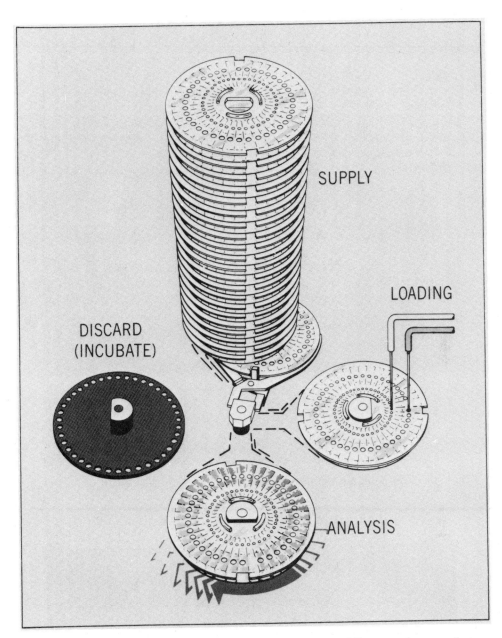

SUPPLY

LOADING

DISCARD
(INCUBATE)

ANALYSIS

Fig. 18-19 The analysis unit of the IL Monarch showing the stations of the rotors (courtesy Instrumentation Laboratory).

signed a specific position on the chain. Operators may preprogram profiles of 2 to 23 tests; up to 8 profiles may be stored on the analyzer's floppy disk. STAT testing is initiated via the keyboard as soon as the current sample has been processed; results are available in 10 minutes.

The reaction cuvettes of the DEMAND are rectangular and disposable. Up to 1000 cuvettes can be loaded, which are fed onto a 72-position rotating reaction ring. This reaction (cuvette) ring circulates through a 37° C water bath and in-

dexes every 9 seconds. As one rotation is complete, used cuvettes drop through a chute into a biohazard waste disposal bag.

The sample volumes vary from 5 to 25 μl and are metered by a positive-displacement syringe. To minimize the effects of specimen carryover, the sample probe is flushed with deionized water. A second wash station washes the probe internally and externally.

The liquid, concentrated reagents are packaged in 18 ml vials. They are stored on-board the

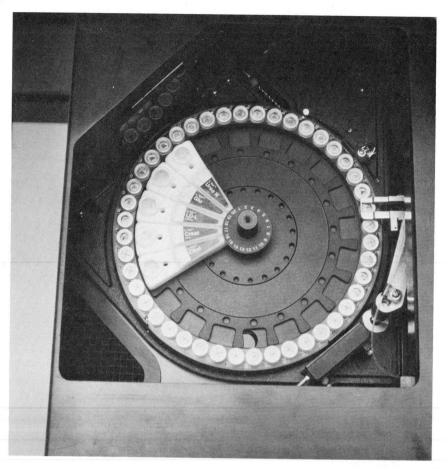

Fig. 18-20   The bar-coded reagent cartridges used on the IL Monarch are called boatILs (courtesy Instrumentation Laboratory).

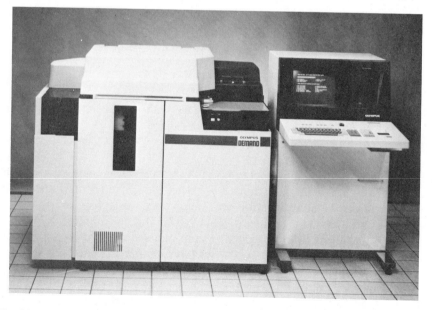

Fig. 18-21   The Olympus DEMAND is a specimen-oriented, random access analyzer suited for mid-sized laboratories (courtesy Olympus Corp.).

analyzer in a refrigerated compartment and are stable for 5 days. Each reagent vial can produce 300 assays. The reagent concentrate is automatically diluted threefold with prewarmed, deionized water.

A single lamp directs a monochromatic beam of light through 1 of 10 filters. The 15 fixed-photometer stations, located around the outer circumference of the cuvette turntable, obtain light signals through these filters every 9 seconds. Biochromatic readings may be selected and programmed correction for serum blanks to compensate for potential interferences because of lipemia, icterus, and hemolysis.

The software features include storage of modifications of test parameters, storage of patient and quality control data, evaluation and printing of Levey-Jennings plots, and a report-writing utility program. The system may be interfaced unidirectionally or bidirectionally.

The Olympus REPLY. The Olympus REPLY is a random access system that is capable of running 600 tests/hour. Many of the same features of the DEMAND are also seen in the REPLY (Fig. 18-22). The same disposable, rectangular cuvettes are used in the system as are the liquid, concentrated reagents. The enhancements given

to the REPLY include primary tube bar coded sampling, improved STAT sampling, and an expanded test menu.

The sample loader of the REPLY is only a slight modification of the DEMAND. Samples are similarly placed on a continuous serpentine chain of interlocking holders (Fig. 18-23). Up to 100 samples may be loaded onto the REPLY, which accommodates both sample cups and primary collection tubes. The REPLY is equipped with a laser bar code reader. Although an operator may load STAT specimens while the chain is moving, the STAT/QC turntable is an easier way to program STAT requests. However, it is not equipped with a bar code reader. Consequently, all STAT samples require manual programming.

Certain assays require two different reagents designated as R1 and R2. Most of the assays requiring the use of a second, or R2 vial, are the therapeutic drugs, drugs of abuse, and thyroid assays. Like the DEMAND, the REPLY automatically dilutes the concentrated reagents with warmed, deionized water. The REPLY uses a reagent inventory system that measures the remaining reagent and calculates the available tests. An audible alarm alerts the operator when a user defined level is exceeded.

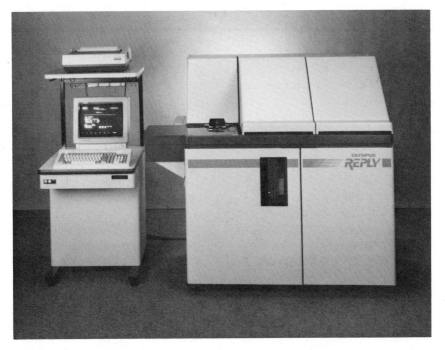

Fig. 18-22   The Olympus REPLY is a random access analyzer that employs many of the same features as the DEMAND. The REPLY has an expanded test menu and the capability of sampling from primary collection tubes (courtesy Olympus Corp.).

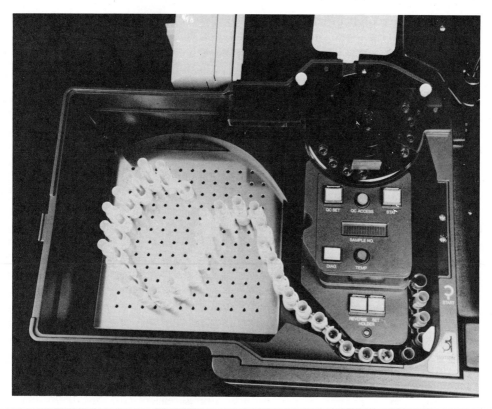

Fig. 18-23 The serpentine chain of specimens is a feature unique to the Olympus REPLY (courtesy Olympus Corp.).

Calibration is required every 30 days for most photometric assays or as a new reagent lot number is started. The operator needs to determine the frequency and the replicates of calibration and whether a full calibration or partial calibration is needed. The REPLY recognizes solutions in yellow, color-coded specimen holders as calibrators. After calibration the calibration data and curve are displayed and stored. The ISE module is automatically calibrated every 8 hours with one standard run after every sample.

The cuvette and photometer unit of the REPLY are very similar to that of the DEMAND, where more optical readings than necessary are performed with the computer discarding the unnecessary absorbances. The only difference is that a dry incubator bath has replaced the water bath. The water requirements for the system are approximately 10 L/hour (for reagent dilution and probe washing).

The software features of the REPLY include storage of reagent inventory and calibration data and use of the Westgard multirule format for QC. Also, because the REPLY is an open-reagent system, the software permits the operator to select

the calibration parameters for reagents from other vendors. The REPLY may be interfaced bidirectionally or unidirectionally.

The Olympus AU5000 Series. The Olympus AU5000 series is a family of high-speed analyzers suited for large hospital laboratories or reference laboratories that perform a high volume of patient profiles. The mode of operation of the AU5000 is classified as discrete, selective, and sample-based. The series consists of the AU5021, AU5121, AU5031, AU5131, AU5041, and AU5061 and ranges from a throughput of 100 samples/hour (2700 tests to 27 types of analyses) for the AU5021 using two separate modules to a throughput of 300 samples/hour (7800 tests to 26 types of analyses) for the AU5061 using six separate modules. The AU5061 has a maximum throughput of 1300 tests/hour if an optional flame photometer is used to run electrolytes (Na, K, Cl). Some of the models are capable of analyzing drugs of abuse as well. The model 5021 is shown in Fig. 18-24.

All analyzers in the series are classified as discrete; each test is performed separately in a quartz glass cuvette. The 192 glass cuvettes are automatically washed, dried, and reused by the analyzer. They are test-dedicated (i.e., only one type of analysis is performed in each cuvette during the life of the cuvette). This eliminates the possibility of cross-contamination between reagents. Test results from any given cuvette are available approxiately 8½ minutes after the addition of a sample. Cuvettes are incubated in a dry, 37° C environment to eliminate the need to clean and maintain a water bath. A deionized water supply up to 90 L/hour is required (for the AU5061) to wash the cuvettes.

All specimens are introduced to the system by 10-position color-coded racks that are fed by a rack feeder (30 position). The black racks are for priming and contain no samples, the white racks are for running routine patient samples, and the red racks are for STAT samples. The AU5000 analyzers are capable of sampling from primary collection tubes or from disposable cups. The average sample volume is approximately 6 μl/test (less than 200 μl for a 27-test chemistry profile). The instruments are equipped with bar code readers and can be bidirectionally interfaced. If bar codes are not used, the operator must load the specimens in the order they are programmed to avoid identification errors. The proper sequence of the racks must also be monitored because the rack number is not encoded. If a STAT sample needs to be processed, a button is pushed to back the routine sample racks out of the sampler. STAT results are available in approximately 15

minutes. Once STAT sampling is complete, the analyzer automatically resumes sampling of routine racks.

Some reagents are prepared by the manufacturer; others need to be reconstituted. Olympus reagents are stable on-board for an average of 12 days. The system's computer updates the reagent inventory when new reagents are added. Calibrations are required each time the instrument goes through a start-up procedure or when reagent lot numbers are changed. The software features of the systems include customized, chartable patient reports, diagnostic troubleshooting programs, reagent inventory, and storage of 4200 patient sample results.

The Roche Diagnostics COBAS-BIO. The COBAS-BIO is a discrete, batch, centrifugal analyzer. This table top system (Fig. 18-25) uses 30 discrete, disposable reaction cuvettes that are assembled onto a rotor. The cuvette rotor trays are manually loaded by the operator as needed. Specimens are transferred into disposable plastic cups and loaded onto the circular specimen tray. The sample cups are capped with a pierceable snap-top that prevents evaporation. The test menu of the COBAS-BIO is fairly broad because many assays that use one or two reagents may be programmed for use on the system. Many laboratories use the COBAS-BIO as a batch analyzer for enzymes and esoteric assays. The maximum throughput is 400 results/hour.

A test is numerically selected from the key-

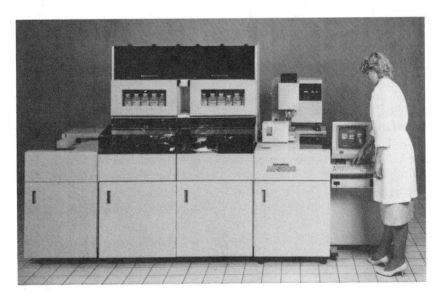

Fig 18-24 The Olympus AU5021 is a large, discrete system suited for commercial laboratories. The maximum throughput of this analyzer is 2700 tests/hour (courtesy Olympus Corp.).

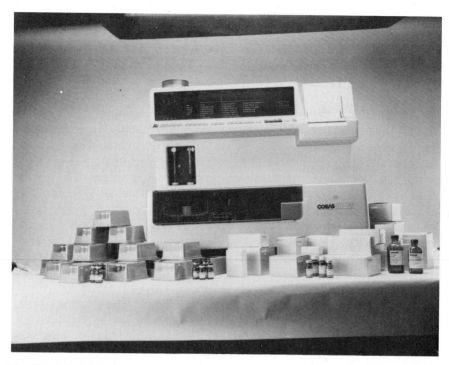

Fig. 18-25   The COBAS-BIO is a bench-top, batch, discrete, centrifugal analyzer (courtesy Roche Diagnostic Systems).

board on the control panel of the analyzer. Only one test may be run at a time. The operator selects the analytic mode as well (i.e., either fixed-point or kinetic). The specimen cups may be placed in one of two positions. When cups are in the down position, specimens will be sampled. If specimens are placed in the up position, no aspiration takes place. This feature gives a degree of selectivity to the analyzer to run a different batch of tests on the same tray of specimens. The minimum sample volumes vary from 2 to 80 μl depending on the test. Specimen carryover is minimized through the instrument's ability to partition an air bubble between the sample and a column of deionized water. The sample is washed out and diluted accordingly as the deionized water is delivered.

The reagents for the COBAS-BIO are loaded onto a storage tray that is loaded onto the analyzer when the assay is to be run. The reagent dispensing system requires the use of a disposable tip that is changed whenever a new assay is to be run.

The photometric readings on the COBAS-BIO are taken through the longitudinal axis of the cuvette well. The optical path length of the light

beam depends on the volume of the dispersed fluids and the geometry of the cuvette.

The microprocessor tracks the fluid volumes, linearity, substrate depletion, and electronic noise. Computer messages are displayed to the operator for assistance in instrument troubleshooting. The system may be interfaced unidirectionally.

The Roche Diagnostics COBAS MIRA. The COBAS MIRA (Fig. 18-26), is a patient-directed, random access, bench-top analyzer. The COBAS MIRA is capable of performing a wide variety of assays, including immunoassays, routine chemistries, electrolytes, and special chemistries. The analyzer has a throughput of 140 tests/hour. Individual tests, profiles, or combinations for each specimen are programmed through a keypad. The maximum sample capacity is 90 patients/run. Up to 26 customized panels may be preprogrammed into individual keys on the alphanumeric keypad, which speeds the manual programming process. The COBAS MIRA automatically repeats tests and performs dilutions when results exceed a programmed linearity limit. Calibration for most Roche assays is required monthly or as reagent lot numbers

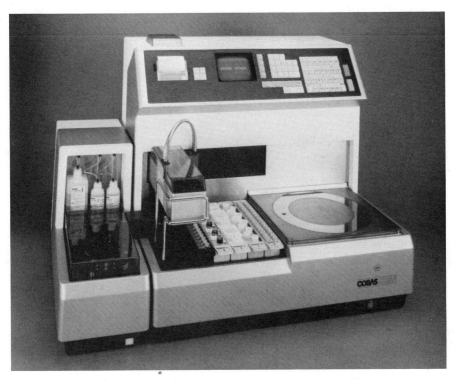

Fig. 18-26 The COBAS MIRA is a random access, bench-top analyzer capable of performing a wide variety of assays (courtesy Roche Diagnostic Systems).

change. The ISE module is automatically calibrated every 4 hours.

The system has an on-board reagent capacity for 15 three-reagent chemistries. The reagents are supplied by Roche for general and special chemistries. The thyroid assays and therapeutic drug monitoring reagents are supplied by Syva and are specially packaged for use on the COBAS MIRA system.

The optics system consists of 72 disposable cuvettes that are manually loaded by the operator as 6 racks of 12. This is the limiting feature of the walk-away capability of the system: once 72 assays are run, an operator must reload additional cuvettes. The instrument will signal the operator when additional cuvettes are needed. The COBAS MIRA continuously performs photometric checks to alert the operator to a variety of errors, such as substrate depletion, antigen excess, reagent integrity, and deterioration of electrode slope range.

The software features include cumulative QC data maintenance, generation of Levey-Jennings plots, storage of calibration curves, and self-diagnostic checks that aid in troubleshooting. The system can also be bidirectionally interfaced.

The Roche Diagnostics COBAS MIRA S. The COBAS MIRA S is very similar to the COBAS MIRA. One enhancement is the throughput of 204 tests/hour when an ISE is used for electrolyte testing. Another improvement over the COBAS MIRA is its ability to load and process 300 cuvettes at one time: a major improvement in the walk-away capabilities of the system. The COBAS MIRA S can also scan bar codes to simplify programming and provide positive sample identification. Bar coded profiles on a special program card can also be set up when a bidirectional interface is not available. The reagent system has also been improved via an on-board reagent cooling system that keeps reagents fresher and more stable. Finally, the test menu has been expanded to include Syva EMIT drugs of abuse testing that are useful.

The Roche Diagnostics COBAS FARA and FARA II. The word "FARA" is an acronym for *F*lexible *A*utomation for *R*andom/Robotic *A*nalysis. The COBAS FARA (Fig. 18-27), is a centrifugal analyzer that combines the sophisticated optical system of the COBAS-BIO and a sampling

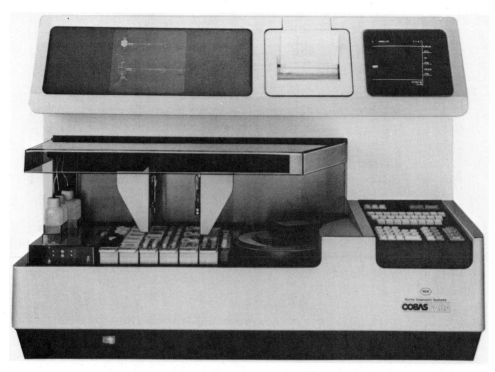

Fig. 18-27   The COBAS FARA is a centrifugal analyzer that combines the optical system of the COBAS-BIO and the sampling mechanism of the COBAS MIRA (courtesy Roche Diagnostic Systems).

mechanism similar to that of the COBAS MIRA. In combining the features of these two instruments, Roche Diagnostics has introduced an analyzer with a test throughput of 400 tests/hour, an expanded test menu, and an improved STAT sampling mechanism.

The COBAS FARA is equipped with a high-capacity flexible rack system. The rack system accommodates up to 150 patient samples or 50 reagents plus 10 calibrators and controls. Racks are identified with binary coding to ensure positive sample and reagent identification. The sample cups have attached caps that minimize evaporation and preserve the sample integrity.

A microprocessing unit controls the movements of the pipetting arms that move independently of each other. This feature permits simultaneous electrolyte and photometric determinations therefore increasing analyzer throughput. The pipettors are also equipped with fluid detectors to ensure that sufficient sample and reagent are available for analysis. The microvolume pipetting capability provides a sampling range of 0.1 to 95 μl. The COBAS FARA, like the COBAS MIRA, provides sample autodilution when an analyte concentration exceeds the linear limit of an assay.

The COBAS FARA uses an alpha-numeric keypad for programming. The operator may program individual tests, test profiles, or any combination of assays or profiles. Up to 104 routine and 26 STAT tests are available on the COBAS FARA, including electrolytes, routine chemistries, special chemistries, and immunoassays. Many reagent assays are available through Roche; however, being an open-reagent system other vendor's reagents may be substituted.

The cuvette rotors are disposable and resemble the rotors used on the COBAS-BIO. Thus the horizontal design of the optics system gives absorbance readings independent of liquid volume. The COBAS FARA allows the operator to select between endpoint and kinetic spectrophotometry and turbidimetry.

The software features of the system include on-board QC, rapid self-diagnosis, plots of absorbance readings vs time, and automated calibration. The system may be bidirectionally or unidirectionally interfaced.

The Roche Diagnostics COBAS FARA II. The COBAS FARA II system has many of the same features as the original COBAS FARA system. The major enhancement given to this system is

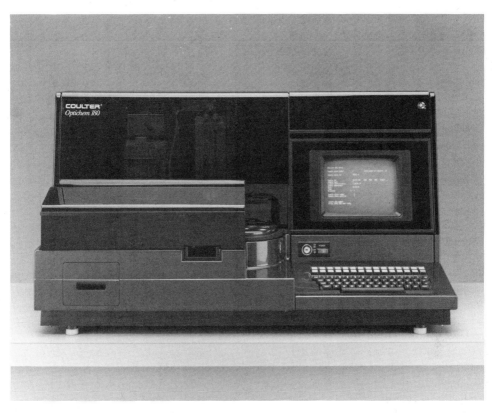

Fig. 18-28 The Coulter OptiChem 180 system is a bench-top, random access analyzer that can perform routine and esoteric assays (courtesy Coulter Electronics, Inc.).

the ability to perform fluorescence polarization (FPIA) therapeutic drug assays.

The Coulter OptiChem 180. The Coulter OptiChem 180 (Fig. 18-28) is a routine, STAT bench-top clinical chemistry analyzer that is suited for smaller, low-volume laboratories. The maximum throughput of this selective, discrete, random access system is 180 test results/hour. Despite its small size, the Coulter OptiChem 180 has features found in many larger systems including a flexible test menu of 100 assays, autodilution and rerun for analytes exceeding the dynamic range, and a comprehensive computer software package. The test menu is quite extensive, and to broaden the testing possibilities, the instrument uses an open-reagent system, so many user-defined assays and test parameters may be programmed. Applications for drugs of abuse testing, therapeutic drug monitoring, immunoassays, and many common chemistries are available.

The keys on the keyboard are labeled with individual test names and profiles. Tests may be ordered in a batch mode if so desired. The Coulter

OptiChem has a STAT interrupt capability; STATs may be programmed and manually added at any time.

Sampling occurs through a robotic arm that is equipped with a level-sensing probe to avoid errors caused by short sampling. The operator is alerted if the sample volume is too low. The probe is automatically washed and cleaned between sampling to minimize the effects of specimen carryover. The water requirements for the probe washing assembly are minimal: only 2.5 L/day with no external plumbing. The minimum sample volume for most tests is less than 10 μl (range 2 to 100 μl). The sample plate accommodates 84 sample cups. This plate is cooled to minimize the evaporation of the samples.

The majority of the reagents of the Coulter OptiChem are liquid and ready to use. The reagent tray of the analyzer has an on-board capacity of 24 reagents. Like the sample plate, the reagent tray is also cooled to minimize evaporation and increase the stability of the reagents. The calibration frequency is determined by the operator.

The Coulter OptiChem 180 uses a discrete

analysis principle. Samples and reagents are dispensed into a single cuvette cell that is incubated and measured. The disposable multicell cuvette contains 12 of these individual cells. Up to 30 of these multicell cuvettes may be loaded into the system, allowing a walk-away capability of 120 tests.

The Coulter OptiChem system has an integrated module for measurement of electrolytes. Direct ISEs are used to measure sodium, potassium, and chloride in serum, plasma, or urine. The ISE module is self-calibrated every 2 hours.

The Coulter OptiChem can be bidirectionally interfaced. Software features include on-line QC data management for 31 days of values, calculated parameters, storage of 1500 patient results, self-diagnostic instrument checks, and workload recording statistics.

The Boehringer Mannheim/Hitachi 705. The Hitachi 705, introduced in 1981, is a discrete, random access, multichannel analyzer (19 different tests) that is suited for use in mid-sized laboratories. The throughput of the system is 180 tests/hour, or up to 300 when running electrolytes with the ISE accessory.

Any combination of the 19 different tests may be randomly selected on each sample. Following programming, specimens are positioned in the sample carousel that houses 40 sample cups in the outer ring and has a 30 coded-position inner ring for calibrators, controls, a reagent blank, and STAT requests. STATs may be placed on the carousel at any time during a run.

The pipetting of sample occurs by motor-driven, positive-displacement syringes. The reagent pipettes are equipped with a liquid level sensor that detects the absence of or insufficient quantities of reagent. The probe also permits monitoring of reagent volumes. The reagents are housed under a transparent cover to minimize evaporation. The reagent storage area consists of two compartments. The refrigerated compartment houses 20 reagent containers for up to 10 assays. The second reagent compartment is at room temperature; it accommodates 12 reagent containers for 6 assays.

The samples and reagents are dispensed into the reaction disk that contains 48 discrete cups in 6 removable sectors of 8 wells. The reaction disk sits in a water incubation bath set at 37°, 30°, or 25° C. The optical source is positioned in the center of the circulating disk with light emissions passing through the reaction cups to a bichromatic spectrophotometer. The ISE unit is found in the center of the sample carousel. All assays must be calibrated daily.

The reaction cup-rinse unit, positioned over the reaction disk, is a seven-probed apparatus that aspirates the waste and subsequently washes the cups. Distilled water is then added to establish a blank absorbance reading. After this water is aspirated, the cups are reused. Water requirements for washing are 100 L/hour.

One of the unique features of the Hitachi 705 is its ability to correct for icterus, lipemia, and hemolysis using the spectral characteristics of these interferents for semiquantitation. The user determines when to use this feature and how to correct for these common interferences.

The computer of the Hitachi 705 receives the operating parameters from a cassette tape. This tape also stores all test results for one day plus the QC data for the day. QC ranges are processed daily along with calculation of the mean and standard deviation.

The Boehringer Mannheim/Hitachi 704. The Hitachi 704 (Fig. 18-29) is a selective, random access analyzer that is suited for optimal performance in a medium-sized hospital. It may be used as a primary analyzer, specialty analyzer, or complementary analyzer to a larger system. The measurement is classified as discrete because individual reaction cells are employed by the system.

The 704 is considered to be a second-generation 705 analyzer because many of the same features of the 705 are incorporated into the design and principles of the 704. The throughput is slightly enhanced with a maximum of 360 test results/hour. This is mainly attributed to the 90-position sample disk, the 40-position reagent disk, and the efficiency of the new floppy-disk software. Programming the Hitachi 704 is essentially the same as the 705. The sample pipettor is equipped with liquid level detectors for accurate aspiration of specimen from 1 to 20 μl. After each sample the probes are washed and flushed to eliminate carryover and to increase precision.

Reagents are loaded onto a 40-position disk with storage for a 20-test menu. Twenty additional assays may be added on a second tray, giving a total on-line menu of 40 assays. Twin reagent kits are available commercially that permit the analysis of two assays in the same cuvette. The Hitachi 704 can also perform specialty tests, such as thyroid assays, immunoglobulins, therapeutic drug monitoring assays (TDMs), and drugs of abuse in urine (DAUs). The system is

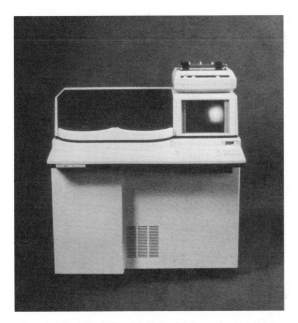

Fig. 18-29 The Hitachi 704 with its enhanced computer software is considered by many to be a second generation of the Hitachi 705 (courtesy Boehringer Mannheim Corp.).

classified as an open-reagent system because Syva reagents may be used. The calibration is automatic and is performed weekly, monthly, or as needed. The ISE assembly is calibrated daily.

The photometric system of the Hitachi 704 is essentially the same as the 705, with the biggest change seen in the cuvette-washing unit. Only 6 L of water/hour are required; the water feeds into an internal reservoir from an external system. The optical mode may be selected by the user as monochromatic or bichromatic, depending on the anticipated interferences. The system may be unidirectionally interfaced with a variety of laboratory computer systems.

The Boehringer Mannheim/Hitachi 717. The Hitachi 717 is a discrete, selective, random access analyzer that is used as a main chemistry analyzer in medium-sized laboratories or as a complementary analyzer to larger analyzers in large laboratories. The analyzer is capable of performing 35 tests on-line with a maximum throughput of 750 tests/hour. The design of the analyzer is strikingly similar to the Hitachi 704 including the open-reagent system/test menu. There are some enhancements that increase the efficiency of the system.

The system is equipped with a bar code reader for positive sample identification. Primary collection tubes may be directly loaded onto the 110-position sample carousel, or specimens may be aliquotted into sample cups. Manual programming may be used with the operator using the keyboard and loading the specimens in a sequential fashion. Up to 1000 patients may be programmed, with the enhanced data disk capable of storing 1000 sequence numbers.

Autodilution and/or rerunning of specimens is user-defined for a variety of parameters (i.e., abnormally elevated sample values, or values exceeding the instrument's analytic range). Dilutions are performed by aspirating smaller volumes of sample with the same amount of reagents.

The reagent system of the Hitachi 717 consists of two identical refrigerated reagent carousels, each holding 32 reagent containers. The containers are not bar coded so the position of the reagents must be manually programmed. Although two containers for the same assay can be loaded on the Hitachi 717, it does not automatically begin using the second reagent bottle when the first container is low or empty; this must be initiated through the operator. A locking cover fits over each reaction disk to minimize evaporation.

Most assays require daily calibration; only seven assays are calibrated monthly. Concurrent calibration is a feature of the system; control samples are analyzed immediately after a calibration for verification. The cuvette system consists of 120 semidisposable cuvettes that are automatically washed by the cell rinse unit. This unit requires 20 L of deionized water/hour that feeds into an internal reservoir.

Software features of this system include QC data management, graphical representation of QC in Youden or Levey-Jennings plots, and bidirectional interfacing.

The Boehringer Mannheim/Hitachi 736 Systems. The Hitachi 736 systems are selective, discrete analyzers suitable for commercial and high-volume laboratories. The features of the Boehringer Mannheim/Hitachi 736 systems are similar to those seen in previous Hitachi models, only larger and faster. The two models of the Hitachi 736 are the 736-50 (processes 300 samples/hour with a maximum throughput of 8100 tests/hour) and the 736-30 (processes 150 samples/hour for a test throughput of 4050 tests per hour). The 736-50 consists of six analytic units that perform four photometric tests each and an ISE module that contains two sets of electrodes. The 736-30 has three analytic units (each performing

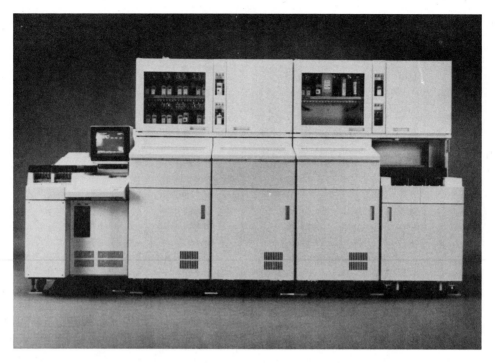

Fig. 18-30 The Hitachi 736-300 system, with its maximum throughput of 4050 tests/hour, is suited for laboratories performing large volumes of panel testing (courtesy Boehringer Mannheim Corp.).

eight photometric tests) and an ISE module (Fig. 18-30). Optimally, the Hitachi 736 systems are used as profile analyzers, with a repeated group of tests run on a large number of patients. Although the systems are true random access analyzers, they are sample based. This means that a fixed number of samples are run/hour (either 300 or 150 maximum). Most other analyzers are test oriented, which means that the maximum throughput depends on the tests that are programmed not the number of specimens.

The Hitachi 736 systems can sample from primary sample tubes or specimen aliquot cups. They use a color-coded rack system for identification of samples: black for calibrators, ivory for controls, gray for routine samples, and red for STATs. STAT sampling is made possible by placing the specimen as near as possible to the rack carrier. The typical turnaround time for a STAT is 15 minutes. Thirty racks fit into a sample tray, and two trays may be loaded onto the analyzer. The systems are equipped with bar code readers to scan both the samples and the racks and are capable of being bidirectionally interfaced.

Each unit has a pair of positive displacement syringes that are driven by stepper motors. Liquid-level sensing devices ensure sufficient sample

volume. Each analytic unit also has 192 nondisposable cuvettes that rotate through a temperature-controlled water bath. The cuvettes are washed and dried in one of four wash stations in each unit.

The daily start-up of the analyzer includes reagent priming that requires 15 minutes and 3.6 ml of reagent. Other daily maintenance includes instrument checks, calibration, and QC testing. The required maintenance time average 60 minutes; much of this maintenance time is automated and unattended.

The 27-test menu of the Hitachi 736 consists of routine chemistries, electrolytes, and enzymes. Because of this "limited" test menu most laboratories back up the 736 systems with a low-volume analyzer that is capable of performing automated esoteric assays. The software features of the Hitachi 736 systems include storage of 4000 sample results and 30 day on-line QC data management.

The Boehringer Mannheim/Hitachi 747 Systems. There are two models that make up the Hitachi 747 series; they are the 747-100 and the 747-200. Both are discrete, selective, random access analyzers that are suited for large, high-volume laboratories. The 747-100 system (Fig. 18-

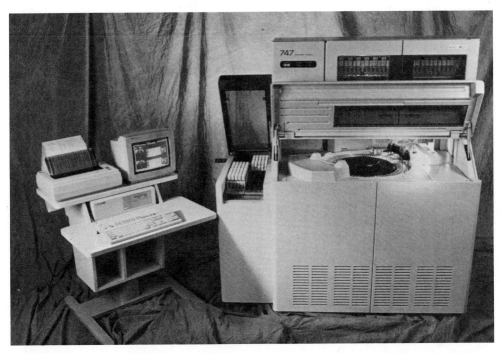

Fig. 18-31 The Hitachi 747-100 system combines a high test throughput with the capability of performing routine and esoteric assays, DAUs, TDMs, and specific proteins (courtesy Boehringer Mannheim Corp.).

31) is capable of analyzing 150 samples/hour with a maximum test throughput of 3300/hour. The throughput of the 747-200 is 6600 tests/hour. Unlike the 736 systems, the 747-100 is a single analytic unit with a single, 480-position cuvette wheel. The 747-200 essentially has two analytic units. The 747 systems have a broader test menu than the 736 system and are equipped with a high-speed graphics printer.

Many characteristics of these systems are similar to the 736 series, such as the use of 5-position multicolored sample racks, the walk-away capability of loading 150 samples/run, the cuvette washing system, primary tube sampling, and bidirectional interfacing.

In the Hitachi 747-100, sampling occurs through four positive displacement syringes that are equipped with liquid level sensors. These pipettors are capable of accurately aspirating and dispensing between 1 and 20 μl. When test results are out of the analyzer range for an assay, autodilution may be programmed.

The reagent storage refrigerated area of the Hitachi 747-100 houses up to 64 reagent bottles. Each assay uses two reagents, giving an on-board capacity of 32 assays plus three ISEs. One reagent of each assay acts as an assay blank. The feature of the 747 systems that automatically places

newly loaded reagent bottles into use is known as Insta-Link. This feature is a cost-saving device that helps laboratories use the full-packaged volume of reagents. The expanded test menu of the 747 systems includes urine screens for drugs of abuse, therapeutic drug monitoring, thyroid tests, and specific proteins. The daily start-up procedure is made easier through the AIM function (*A*uto *I*ntegrated *M*aintenance). This function improves the walk-away capability of the analyzer during the unassisted maintenance and internally tracks the maintenance sequence of the system.

The software enhancements of the 747 systems include workload-recording data management, on-line quality control data for 10 levels of control with Levey-Jennings charts, and the storage capacity of a combined 20,400 routine and STAT samples.

The Technicon CHEM 1⁺. The CHEM 1⁺ system (Fig. 18-32) is a continuous flow analyzer that uses extremely small quantities of sample for all of its 35 chemistries. The analyzer has a throughput of 720 tests/hour or up to 1800 tests/hour when an optional electrolyte module is used. This model has many of the same features as its predecessor, the CHEM 1 analyzer, including the formation of Chemistry Capsules. For

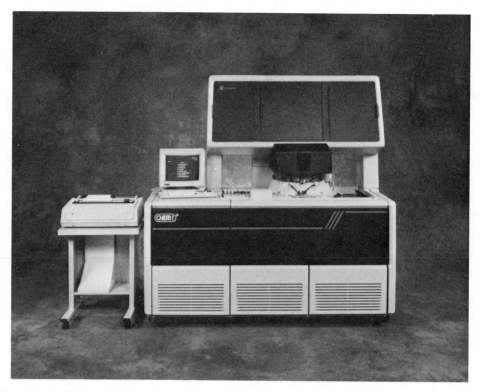

Fig. 18-32 The Technicon CHEM 1$^+$ is capable of performing all of its 35 on-board tests, including ISEs with only 42 μl of sample (courtesy Technicon Instruments Corp.).

each test a "capsule" is generated: first reagent, then specimen, followed by a second reagent separated by small air bubbles. Air bubbles also separate each individual capsule of specimen and reagents; the air bubbles help to minimize carryover.

Programming is optimally performed with the assistance of a bidirectional interface and the use of specimen bar codes. PID, demographic data, and tests requested are downloaded into the CHEM 1$^+$ from a host computer. Either primary collection tubes or specimen aliquot cups are accommodated by the linear sample carrier that continuously loads and unloads samples. Optionally, an operator may manually program assays through the system's keyboard and color CRT.

The reagents of the CHEM 1$^+$ are prepackaged into cassettes. Most reagents have an onboard stability of 30 days. Two reagents are used for each assay, with only seven μl of each reagent required/test. The specimen and reagents flow through an individual tubing path forming a chemistry capsule for a specific test. The capsule is transported through a Teflon tube that is inter-

nally coated with a special fluorocarbon oil to ensure a smooth flow. The three components are mixed when the capsule passes into an enlarged diameter tube called the "vanish zone." Here, a small air bubble that had separated the specimen plus reagent one from reagent two vanishes into the total mixture. Further mixing is accomplished by a corkscrewlike coil. The mixture then moves through a series of optical stations where absorbance readings are obtained.

The test menu has been expanded to include immunoassays and drugs of abuse testing. Electrolytes, routine chemistries, and enzymes are all included in the menu of available assays.

The software features include on-line diagnostic checks, on-line QC data management, and computer link capabilities with Technicon RA systems. This link acts as a built-in backup and offers expanded test menus with merged, individual patient reports.

The Technicon RA-2000. The Technicon RA-2000 chemistry analyzer (Fig. 18-33) is a discrete, selective, random access analyzer suited for medium-volume laboratories. The system has a maximum throughput of 240 tests/hour, or up to

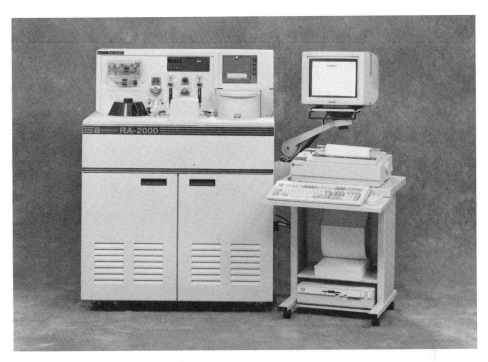

Fig. 18-33 The Technicon RA-2000 offers a 3-hour walk-away capability. This system also has the ability to perform up to 255 different assays, storing both manufacturer and user-defined parameters (courtesy Technicon Instruments Corp.).

720 tests with optional ISEs. The system has an unprecedented capability of performing and storing parameters for 255 manufacturer and user-defined methods and thus is considered an "open" system. The RA-2000 has an on-board refrigerator compartment to improve the stability of the reagents.

Up to 30 samples may be loaded onto the system's carousel; up to 26 tests may be on-board the system. The maximum throughput is achieved when all 30 programmed patient samples have all 26 tests ordered (780 tests/hour).

The optical system uses semidisposable cuvettes that are washed on board the analyzer. The unique feature regarding this wash station is its self-contained nature. No external water hookup is needed nor is a drain. All of the waste is self-contained and is discarded as needed.

A computerized workstation where programming applications appear as symbols is the communication link between instrument and operator. The operator may program tests through the keyboard/computer mouse and the color monitor. The system may be bidirectionally interfaced.

The Technicon DAX Systems. The Technicon DAX is a series of modular, selective, random access analyzers that can be tailored to meet the needs of large, high-volume laboratories. There are four possible configurations of DAX. The DAX 240 has one analyzer module and one reagent module and can perform 26 assays/sample. Its specimen throughput is 100/hour (i.e., 2600 test results are available in 1 hour). The DAX 48 (Fig. 18-34) is composed to two analyzer modules and one reagent module. This system can perform 34 assays/sample and can process 150 samples/hour, giving a maximum throughput of 5100 tests/hour. The DAX 72 has three analyzer modules and two reagent modules. Twenty-six tests may be performed/sample. The specimen throughput is 300/hour, or up to 7800 test results/hour. The DAX 96 system has 4 analyzer modules and 2 reagent modules that permit the analysis of 34 assays on 300 samples/hour, or a maximum throughput of 10,200 test results/hour.

All DAX systems have a walk-away capability of 300 samples, or 60 specimen racks of 5 samples. All systems accommodate 5, 7, and 10 ml evacuated specimen tubes for primary sampling, or a 2 ml sample cup. Sample identification is ob-

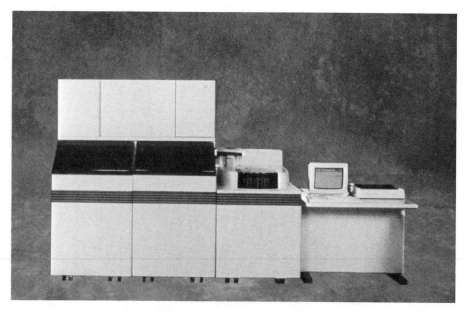

Fig. 18-34 The Technicon DAX 48 System, with a maximum throughput of 5100 results/hour, is suited for large, commercial laboratories (courtesy Technicon Instruments Corp.).

tained through bar codes that are scanned by the system. All patient demographics and requested tests are downloaded directly to the system from a host computer. The bar coded specimen racks are continuously fed into the circular sampler. Operators may also select to manually program tests through a touch-screen CRT or through the on-board computer mouse. The sampler is equipped with a liquid-level sensor that alerts the operator of low sample volume, absence of specimen, and fibrin clots. The analyzer may be programmed to autodilute samples 1:2, 1:4, or 1:8. The required sample volume for colorimetric assays is between 2.5 and 25 μl/test, whereas the electrolytes require 63 μl.

Up to 36 reagents may be stored on-board in each reagent module. One side of each module is refrigerated, whereas the other side is ambient. Most reagents require reconstitution, and once reconstituted they are stable for 14 to 30 days. Calibration is required as new reagents are loaded or as quality control dictates.

The test menu includes electrolytes, routine chemistries, and enzymes. The system is classified as an open-reagent system because user-defined methods may be added to the test repertoire. Sodium and potassium are measured by ISE; the remaining chemistries are measured col-

orimetrically. The colorimetric module uses permanent rectangular glass reaction cuvettes that are washed, dried, and tested for clarity. The cuvette wash system requires 40 L of deionized water/hour. To accommodate the user-defined parameters, 16 different photometer wavelengths between 340 and 804 nm are available.

The DAX systems may be bidirectionally interfaced to most laboratory host computer systems. Software features include review-and-edit options for abnormal test results, on-line QC data management, a complete QC graphics package, specimen status tracking, and workload recording monitoring.

Summary

The instrument that is best suited for a laboratory depends on a number of factors. Listing the strengths and weaknesses of each prospective new analyzer is a good start in the decision-making process. The physical and environmental requirements of an analyzer such as space, reagent storage, electrical, plumbing, and waste disposal are all important issues that need to be addressed, as are the ease of operation and required training. Table 18-1 is a summary of the automated clinical systems discussed in this chapter and some of their salient features.

Table 18-1 Common automated chemistry systems

Analyzer	Category	Maximum throughout	Program mode	Sample volume	Test menu	Reaction/optical design	Unique features
ABBOTT Spectrum EPx	Discrete Selective Random access	225 results/hour	Download through bar code or manual Bidirect Interface	10 μl for most assays	Electrolytes Routines Enzymes	Glass cuvettes washed/reused	Tandem access Bar-coded reagents Teflon probes Primary sampling
BAXTER Paramax 720ZX	Discrete Selective Random access	720 results/hour	Download through bar code Bidirect interface	10 μl for most assays	Electrolytes Routines Enzymes Open-reagent	Disposable plastic cuvettes; heat-sealed	Tabletted dry reagents Closed-container sampling
BECKMAN ASTRA 8	Discrete Selective	480 results/hour	Manual Unidirect interface	150 μl for 8-test profile	Electrolytes Routines	Reaction cup in module	Modular design ORDAC dilutions
BECKMAN Synchron CX7	Discrete Selective Random access	825 results/hour	Download through bar code or manual Bidirect interface	3 μl for most assays 169 μl for ISEs	Open-reagent system, 100 assays available	Pulse xenon lamp Glass cuvettes washed/reused	Concurrent calibration Primary sampling ORDAC Bar-coded reagents
KODAK Ektachem 700 XRC	Discrete Selective Random	750 results/hour	Download through bar code or manual Bidirect interface	10-11 μl for all assays	Electrolytes Routines Enzymes	Reflectance photometry	Dry-reagent slides Sample proboscis Primary sampling Bar-coded reagents
DuPONT ACA Analyzers	Discrete Selective Random	50-76 results/hour	Manual Unidirect interface	20-800 μl	Extensive 80 assays available	Reagent pack acts as cuvette	Binary coded reagent pack
DuPONT Dimension	Discrete Selective Random access	400 results/hour	Manual Bidirect interface	10-12 μl for most assays	Electrolytes Routines Enzymes	Blow-molded Surlyn cuvettes	FLEX Reagent cartridges Ultrasonic probe mixing Bar-coded reagents

Continued.

Table 18-1 Common automated chemistry systems—cont'd

Analyzer	Category	Maximum throughout	Program mode	Sample volume	Test menu	Reaction/optical design	Unique features
IL Phoenix	Selective Sequential	600 results/ hour	Manual Unidirect interface	121 μl for panel	Electrolytes 8-test panel	Coimmobilization	Solid state fluidics Analytic modules
IL Monarch	Centrifugal Random access	600 results/ hour	Download Manual Bidirect interface	2-30 μl for most assays	Extensive Open-reagent system	Rotor/cuvette	Automated change of rotors BoatIL reagent cartridges
OLYMPUS REPLY	Discrete Selective Random access	600 results/ hour	Download through bar codes or manual Bidirect interface	15 μl for most assays	Extensive Open-reagent system	Rectangular, disposable cuvettes	Serpentine chain of samples Color-coded sample holders
OLYMPUS AU5000 Series	Discrete Sample-based Selective	2700-7800 results/ hour	Download through bar codes or manual Bidirect interface	6 μl/test or 200 μl for 27-test panel	Electrolytes Routines Enzymes DAU, TDM	Glass cuvettes washed/reused Test-dedicated cells	Modular design Flame photometer Color-coded racks
ROCHE COBAS-BIO	Discrete Batch centrifugal	400 results/ hour	Manual Unidirect interface	2-80 μl for most assays	Enzymes Esoterics	Disposable cuvettes assembled onto rotors	Air bubble partition eliminates carryover
ROCHE COBAS MIRA S	Discrete Selective Random access	140-204 results/ hour	Download through bar code or manual Bidirect interface	85 μl for ISEs 2-95 μl for other assays	Electrolytes Extensive Open-reagent system	Disposable cuvettes	On-board reagent cooling

Continued.

Table 18-1 Common automated chemistry systems—cont'd

Analyzer	Category	Maximum throughout	Program mode	Sample volume	Test menu	Reaction/optical design	Unique features
ROCHE COBAS FARA II	Discrete Centrifugal	400 results/ hour	Manual Bidirect interface	0.1 to 95 μl in 0.1 μl steps	Extensive Open-reagent system FPIA ability	Disposable rotors Horizontal light path	Microvolume pipetting
COULTER Optichem 180	Discrete Selective Random access	180 results/ hour	Manual Bidirect interface	10 μl for most assays	Electrolytes Extensive Open-reagent system	Disposable multicell cuvettes	Cooled sample and reagent plate
BOEHRINGER MANNHEIM/ Hitachi 717	Discrete Selective Random	750 results/ hour	Download through bar code or manual Bidirect interface	1-20 μl for most assays	Extensive Open-reagent system	Semidisposable cuvettes; washed/reused	Concurrent calibration
BOEHRINGER MANNHEIM/ Hitachi 747 Model 200	Discrete Selective Random access	6600 results/ hour	Download through bar code or manual Bidirect interface	1-20 μl for most assays	Extensive Open-reagent system	Semidisposable cuvettes; washed/reused	Autointegrated maintenance (AIM) Insta-Link reagent tracking
TECHNICON CHEM 1^{+}	Continuous flow Sequential	1800 results/ hour	Download through bar code or manual Bidirect interface	1 μl/assay	Electrolytes Routines Enzymes	Chemistry Capsules	Computer link to RA-2000 Analyzer
TECHNICON DAX Series	Discrete Selective Random access	2600-10200 tests/hour	Download through bar code or manual Bidirect interface	2.5-25 μl/ assay; 63 μl for ISE	Electrolytes Extensive Open-reagent system	Permanent, rectangular cuvettes; washed/reused	Modular design

Review Questions

1. Tandem access, which gives an operator the ability to prioritize the order in which assays are performed, is a unique feature of which analyzer?
   A. The Technicon Dax
   B. The Olympus DEMAND
   C. The Abbott Spectrum EPx
   D. The Coulter Optichem

2. Which feature is found exclusively in the Paramax 720ZX?
   A. Bar-coded reagents
   B. Closed Container Sampling
   C. Flame Photometry
   D. Bichromatic Colorimetric Photometry

3. Modular design, ORDAC, and peristaltic pumps are all features of the:
   A. Beckman Synchron CX7
   B. Boehringer Mannheim/Hitachi 736
   C. Roche COBAS-BIO
   D. Beckman ASTRA 8

4. The Kodak Ektachem Analyzers have many unique features, but the one feature found exclusively in all Kodak Sytems is:
   A. Dry-reagent tablet technology
   B. The employment of reusable slides
   C. Dry-reagent slide technology
   D. Closed container sampling

5. Despite its low throughput time, the DuPont ACA III is still found in many clinical laboratories because of its:
   A. Small sample volume requirements for enzymes
   B. Extensive test menu
   C. Dry-reagent technology
   D. Closed-container sampling

6. Describe the optics of The Instrumentation Laboratory Monarch.
   A. Self-forming cuvettes with reflectance photometry
   B. Reflectance photometry off a shiny surface
   C. Reusable glass cuvettes with bichromatic wavelength
   D. Light passes through a monochromator and disposable rotors.

7. An automatic cuvette loader, refrigerated storage of concentrated reagents, and a continuous chain of interlocking holders are features of the:
   A. Olympus DEMAND and Olympus REPLY
   B. DuPont Dimension and IL Phoenix
   C. Kodak Ektachem 500 and 700XRC
   D. Abbott EPx and Coulter OptiChem.

8. The COBAS MIRA and COBAS FARA differ in that the MIRA is:
   A. A centrifugal analyzer
   B. Capable of performing therapeutic drug assays
   C. In need of manual loading of 72 disposable cuvettes
   D. Able to run only Roche assays

9. Although the Coulter OptiChem is designed for smaller laboratories with low throughput, it is equipped with features found in larger instrument systems including:
   A. On-line QC data management
   B. Workload recording statistics data management
   C. Bidirectional computer interface capability
   D. All of the above
   E. A and B only

10. In 1981, The Boehringer Mannheim/Hitachi 705 was the first automated system in the chemistry laboratory to offer this feature:
    A. Disposable reaction cuvettes
    B. The requirement for large volumes of deionized water
    C. Random access capabilities
    D. Flame photometry

11. The analyzers with the greatest theoretical test throughput are the:
    A. Technicon DAX, Olympus AU5061, and the Boehringer Mannheim/Hitachi 736
    B. IL Monarch, Baxter Paramax 720, and the DuPont Dimension
    C. Coulter Optichem 180, Roche COBAS-BIO, and the Beckman ASTRA 8.
    D. DuPont ACA, Roche Cobas Mira S, and the Abbott Spectrum EPx.

12. Individual sample tips, Teflon-coated probes, wash stations, and Capsule Chemistry are all efforts to eliminate:
    A. Prozone
    B. Downtime
    C. Carryover
    D. Downloading

Answers

1. C   2. B   3. D   4. C   5. B   6. D   7. A   8. C   9. D
10. C   11. A   12. C

Bibliography

Abbott Diagnostics Spectrum EPx Product Brochure, Abbott Laboratories, Abbott Park, Il, 1991.

Alpert NL: Spotlight on the Baxter Paramax 720ZX, Clinical Instrument Systems Newsletter, 10(9), Stamford, Ct, 1989.

Alpert NL: Spotlight on the Olympus Reply, Clinical Instrument Systems Newsletter, 11(6), Stamford, Ct, 1990.

Alpert NL: Spotlight Update on the Hitachi 704 Analyzer, Clinical Instrument Systems Newsletter, 10(5), Stamford, Ct, 1989.

Baxter Paramax 720 Product Brochure, Baxter Healthcare Corporation, Irvine, Ca, 1990.

Beckman Synchron CX3, CX4, CX5, CX7 Clinical Systems Product Brochures, Beckman Instruments Incorporated, Brea, Ca, 1989, 1991.

Boehringer Mannheim Diagnostics Hitachi Series Product Brochures, Boehringer Mannheim Corporation, Indianapolis, In, 1990.

Coulter Optichem 180 Procedure Manual, Coulter Electronics, Incorporated, Hialeah, Fl, 1991.

Davis JE: Automation. In Kaplan LA, Pesce AJ, eds: Clinical chemistry: theory, analysis, and correlation, St Louis, 1984, Mosby–Year Book.

DeCrese R, Lifshitz MS: Profile on the Baxter Paramax Chemistry System, The Instrument Report, Applied Technology Associates, Incorporated, Chicago, Il, 1988.

DeCrese R, Lifshitz MS: Profile on the Instrumentation Laboratory Phoenix, Applied Technology Associates, Incorporated, The Instrument Report, Chicago, Il, 1991.

DeCrese R, Lifshitz MS: Profile on the Olympus AU5000 Chemistry Systems, The Instrument Report, Applied Technology Associates, Incorporated, Chicago, Il, 1988.

DuPont ACA IV Product Brochure, E.I. DuPont de Nemours, and Company, Incorporated, Wilmington, De, 1990.

DuPont Dimension Product Brochure, E.I. DuPont de Nemours, and Company, Incorporated, Wilmington, De, 1990.

Hunter LL: Automated chemistry analyzers. In Bishop ML, Duben-Von Laufen JL, and Fody EP, eds: Clinical chemistry, principles, procedures, correlations, Philadelphia, 1985, JB Lippincott.

Instrumentation Laboratory Phoenix Product Brochure, Instrumentation Laboratory, Lexington, Ma, 1987.

Instrumentation Laboratory Monarch Product Brochure, Instrumentation Laboratory, Lexington, Ma, 1990.

Kodak Ektachem 700 Methodologies Summary, Eastman Kodak Company, Clinical Products Division, Rochester, NY, 1986.

Maclin E, Young DS: Automation in the clinical laboratory. In Tietz NW, ed: Fundamentals of clinical chemistry, ed 3, Philadelphia, 1986, WB Saunders.

Roche Diagnostics FARA Product Brochure, Roche Diagnostic Systems, Incorporated, Montclair, NJ, 1989.

Roche Diagnostics MIRA S Product Brochure, Roche Diagnostic Systems, Incorporated, Montclair, NJ, 1991.

Technicon Dax Product Brochure, Technicon Instruments Corporation, a Subsidiary of Miles, Incorporated, Tarrytown, NY, 1990.

Technicon Chem 1[+] System Product Brochure, Technicon Instruments Corporation, a Subsidiary of Miles, Incorporated, Tarrytown, NY, 1991.

CHAPTER 19

Automation in Immunochemistry

ROBERT H. WILLIAMS
JACK A. MAGGIORE

General Principles of Immunoassay
   Measurement
Basic Modes of Detection and Methods of
   Analysis
Automated Immunoassay Analyzers

In the past most immunoassays were performed using radioisotopes. These **radioimmunoassay (RIA)** methods provided the clinical laboratory with a sensitive technique for detecting compounds that typically occurred at plasma and/or urine concentrations too low to be detected by conventional methods. However, they provided little flexibility in terms of specimen processing.

There are several disadvantages associated with an RIA technique. First, it is a batch technique that is very labor-intensive and difficult to automate. Second, the shelf-life of most assay kits is usually short (i.e., 1 to 2 months) and in laboratories that have small test volumes, the kits tend to expire before they are used. Finally, the use of radioisotopes poses a potential safety hazard to employees and therefore requires licensing and special handling procedures for its disposal.

In the late 1970s there began a major move by manufacturers to develop nonisotopic methods to replace traditional RIA techniques. **Enzyme-linked immunosorbent assay (ELISA)** techniques were among the first to be introduced. These assays were primarily used for serology testing. Although the methods were nonisotopic, they still required batch testing and at that time were not readily automated. One of the first non-isotopic immunoassay systems to become semi-automated was a method called **enzyme multiplied immunoassay technique (EMIT).** However, the detection limit of this methodology was not as sensitive as RIA. It also was used primarily for the analysis of therapeutic drugs. In the early 1980s another technique called **fluorescence polarization immunoassay (FPIA)** was introduced, which demonstrated a level of sensitivity comparable with many isotopic methods. It also was developed initially to measure therapeutic drugs.

With the advent of monoclonal antibody production and the development of new solid phases for separation of bound and free fractions, companies began to revise old technologies and develop new ones that demonstrated greater specificity and sensitivity. These immunoassays have since been processed to be used with analytic instruments that have recently become highly automated. These immunoassay systems, their principles of operation, and their unique characteristics are presented in this chapter. A brief discussion of the fundamental principles of immunoassays will precede this section.

General Principles of Immunoassay Measurement

Immunoassays are primarily used to measure analytes such as therapeutic drugs, drugs of abuse, hormones, polypeptides and proteins, tumor markers, and other compounds, like vitamins, that occur in minute quantities. They are used because other traditional chemical methods are often inadequate in terms of their limit of detection (sensitivity) or too sophisticated to be used routinely. Many of these traditional methods are also nonspecific and are subject to interferences. Immunoassays, on the other hand, involve specific interactions between **antibodies** and **antigens.** The analyte of interest can be either an antigen or antibody. The type of interactions that occur in immunologic assays are not exclusive to antibodies and antigens. Some analytes that react with antibodies in vitro are not antigenic in vivo. Such analytes are then called **haptens.**

Highly specific reactions can also take place between an analyte and a binding protein (i.e., binding of thyroxine by thyroxine binding globulin). These reactions are called **competitive protein binding (CPS)** assays. Although in the strictest sense they are not considered immunoassays, their interactions are similar. Consequently, antibody and competitive protein binding assays are generally grouped together. The preferred term used to represent the analyte being measured by either assay is called the ligand.

To monitor the reaction, an antigen (ligand) or antibody (binding protein) must be chemically bonded (tagged) with a moiety called a **tracer.** The tracer can remain free in solution (free form) or bind to one of the components of the antigen-antibody/binding protein complex (bound form). In the past this tag was usually a radioisotope. However, because of the aforementioned problems associated with its use, many companies have since developed nonisotopic tracers such as enzymes, fluorescent molecules, bioluminescent or chemiluminescent compounds, or micro-latex particles. By monitoring the reaction of the enzyme photometrically, the increase or decrease of fluorescence, the generation of chemiluminescence, or the production of turbidity, a relationship can be established between the analyte of interest and this signal.

Immunoassay techniques can be classified as **homogeneous** or **heterogeneous.** Homogeneous methods do not require an analytic step to physically separate the bound from the free fraction before final measurement. Heterogeneous methods, however, require at least one separation step. This is usually accomplished by a solid support coated with an antigen or antibody that binds one of the fractions. The solid support can be a tube, a bead (glass, polystyrene, or latex), a paramagnetic particle, a glass-fiber filter paper, a dry multifilm layer, or in the case of some ELISA techniques, a microtiter well. By measuring how much free or bound label is present (using the tracer as a means of detection), and comparing it with known standards, the amount of analyte can be determined. Homogeneous methods are often used to measure small, low molecular weight compounds. Hetergeneous assays can be used to measure both large, high molecular weight compounds and small, low molecular weight compounds that occur in low concentrations.

Immunoassay methods can also be classified as being **competitive** or **noncompetitive.** The latter can be further divided into **sequential,** or **sandwich (immunometric)** type immunoassays. With competitive immunoassays, the analyte in the patient sample is first mixed with labeled analyte (Fig. 19-1). Then both unlabeled and labeled analyte compete to bind with an antibody. Either free labeled analyte or bound labeled analyte is then measured (In Fig. 19-1 the label is an

Step 1. Immobilization of Antibody to Solid Surface

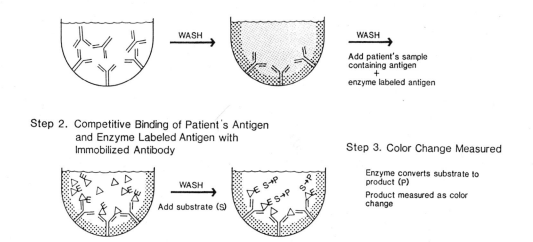

Step 2. Competitive Binding of Patient's Antigen and Enzyme Labeled Antigen with Immobilized Antibody

Step 3. Color Change Measured

Fig. 19-1 Enzyme immunoassay, "competitive binding" technique. (From Kaplan LA, Pesce AJ: Clinical chemistry, ed 1, St Louis, 1984, Mosby–Year Book.)

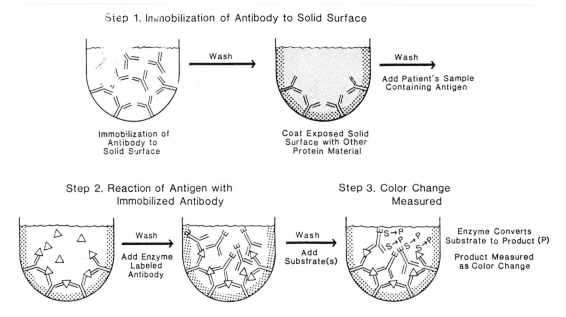

Step 1. Immobilization of Antibody to Solid Surface

Immobilization of
Antibody to
Solid Surface

Coat Exposed Solid
Surface with Other
Protein Material

Add Patient's Sample
Containing Antigen

Step 2. Reaction of Antigen with
Immobilized Antibody

Add Enzyme
Labeled
Antibody

Step 3. Color Change
Measured

Add
Substrate(s)

Enzyme Converts
Substrate to Product (P)

Product Measured
as Color Change

Fig. 19-2 Enzyme immunoassay, "sandwich" technique (antibody-labeled assay). (From Kaplan LA, Pesce AJ: Clinical chemistry: theory, analysis, and correlation, ed 1, St Louis, 1984, Mosby–Year Book.)

enzyme). This technique is commonly used to measure many therapeutic drugs.

During a sequential immunoassay, unlabeled analyte (patient sample) is first mixed with excess antibody and then binding between them is allowed to reach equilibrium. Labeled analyte is added next to bind those antibody sites that are not already occupied by the unlabeled analyte. Either free or bound labeled analyte can be monitored. With this approach a higher fraction of the unlabeled analyte can be bound by the antibody compared with a competitive assay (especially at low analyte concentrations). In general, sequential assays provide a two-fold to four-fold increase in sensitivity compared with competitive assays.

With a sandwich or immunometric immunoassay (also known as an antibody-labeled assay), the analyte in the patient sample binds to an antibody that has been covalently linked to a solid-phase support (Fig. 19-2). A labeled antibody is then added that reacts with a second antigenic site on the analyte, thus forming a complex known as a "sandwich" (the label in Fig. 19-2 is also an enzyme). The advantage of the sandwich technique is that it does not require the use of purified labeled antigens or ligands. This eliminates potential problems often associated with the labeling of these molecules. Antibodies also tend to be more stable during the labeling process.

Basic Modes of Detection and Methods of Analysis

Manufacturers of immunoassay instruments have used several approaches to detect and measure compounds in biologic fluids. Although these methods vary from one manufacturer to the next, all involve direct or indirect measurement of analyte via the use of a tracer in combination with a homogeneous or heterogeneous technique. These methods and their modes of detection are briefly discussed as specific instruments are described in this chapter.

Because many instrument manufacturers have developed novel methods of analysis, they are generally the sole source of reagents/test modules that are needed for their instrument. Such instruments are called **"closed reagent systems,"** meaning that test packs (including calibrators and sometimes controls) are only available from the instrument vendor. Instruments that can use reagents from other vendors are called **"open reagent systems."** The instruments that are reviewed in this chapter are considered closed systems unless otherwise indicated. A summary of these immunoassay systems, their features, and current test menus is given in Table 19-1.

Automated Immunoassay Analyzers

Abbott Diagnostics' TDx, TDxFLx, ADx, IMx, and IMx SELECT Systems

Abbott TDx System. The Abbott TDx is an automated batch analyzer that has the ability to perform a variety of laboratory tests such as therapeutic drugs, immunosuppressants, hormones, clinical chemistries, proteins, and toxic/abused drugs. The TDx uses fluorescent polarization immunoassay (FPIA) technology (Fig. 19-3) and competitive binding immunoassay methodology for many of its assays. The tracer in FPIA is the analyte conjugated to the fluorescent molecule, fluorescein (tracer-antigen complex). Analyte in the patient sample competes with the fluorescein-labeled analyte for binding sites on the antibody. In FPIA the detection of bound vs free tracer is based on the rotation characteristics of molecules in solution and their interaction on excitation with plane polarized light (i.e., light generated in a vertical orientation that excites molecules with subsequent generation of fluorescence). Large molecules such as tracer bound to antibody rotate more slowly than small molecules, like free tracer. When a beam of plane polarized light is passed through a solution containing bound and free tracer, both will absorb light, but only antibody-bound tracer, because of its slow rotation, will emit light in the same vertical orientation ("polarized light"). Antibody-bound tracer thus causes an increase in polarized light being transmitted to the detector (increase in fluorescence polarization).

However, free tracer, because of its rapid rotation, will emit light in a different orientation, causing less polarized light to be transmitted to the detector (decreased fluorescence polarization). The higher the concentration of analyte in the patient sample, the less antibody available for binding to the tracer, and thus the higher the amount of free tracer. Therefore the amount of polarization sensed by the detector decreases. In FPIA the amount of analyte in the sample is inversely proportional to the amount of fluorescence polarization.

FPIA optics have been designed to recognize only polarized light emitted from the fluorophore (Fig. 19-4). The TDx system uses a tungsten halogen lamp as a light source that, in conjunction with an interference filter, produces monochromatic light (blue) at 485 nm. The light is then passed through a liquid-crystal polarizer (that is electrically switched) to produce a single plane of blue light that excites the fluorophore. After excitation the fluorophore emits light (green) at a different energy and wavelength (525 to 550 nm) that is focused onto the phototube. The TDx optical system is completely electronic and thus contains no moving parts.

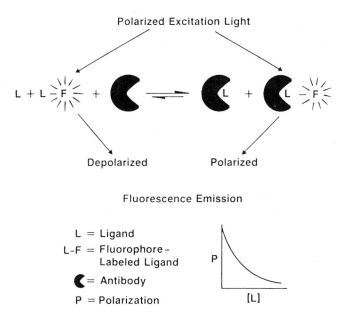

Fig. 19-3 Principle of fluorescence polarization immunoassay (FPIA) and typical dose-response curve. (From Kaplan LA, Pesce AJ: Clinical chemistry: theory, analysis, and correlation, ed 1, St Louis, 1984, Mosby–Year Book.)

Table 19-1 Summary of automated immunoassay systems

Manufacturer (system)	Assays	Mode	Menu	Sample volume dilutions	Samples per tray	Time to 1st result (avg)	Maximum throughput (test/hr)	Primary tube sampling	Calibration stability	Computer interface
ABBOTT TDx	FPIA REA	1,4	A,B,C D,H FLM	50 µl (most)	20	6 min	40-80	No	6-point	Upload only
ABBOTT TDxFLx	FPIA REA NXT	1,2,4,6	A,B,C D,H FLM	On-board 50 µl (most)	20	6 min	40-80	No	2-4 weeks 6-point	Upload only
ABBOTT ADx	FPIA	1,6 Flexible Access	C	On-board 50 µl	20	7 min	40-60	No	2-4 weeks 6-point	Upload only
ABBOTT IMx and IMx SELECT	FPIA MEIA	1,6	B,D,E,F G,H,I,J	250 µl	50-60 FPIA 24-48 MEIA	12-45 min	60-FPIA 24-MEIA	No	2-4 weeks 6-point 2-4 weeks	Upload only
BAXTER STRATUS II and IINTELLECT	RPIA FSF	1,3,5	B,D,E,F G,H,I,J	On-board 200 µl 50 µl On-board (IIntellect)	30	8-10 min	48	No	6-point 2 weeks	II-upload only, Bidirect Iintellect
BECTON DICKINSON AFFINITY	EIA ImmUnits	1,2,3,5	B,E,J	100-350 µl	46	22-60 min	30	No	6-point	Upload only
BIOTROL SYSTEM 7000	EIA paramagnetic micro-bead	1,2,5	B,D,E,F G,H	10-150 µl On-board	36	30-40 min	100	Yes	2 weeks initial 4-point; 2-point/ week (varies)	Bidirect
BOEHRINGER MANNHEIM ES 300	EIA coated tube	1,2	E,F,G H,J	100 µl	160 (10 for controls)	50-210 min	100	No	5-point/ 2 weeks; 1-pt/ run	Bidirect
CIBA CORNING ACS: 180	Chemiluminescence	1,2,3	B,E,F,G H,I,J	10-200 µl	60	15 min	180	Yes	2-point 1 week	Bidirect
CIRRUS IMMULITE	EIA bead, chemiluminescence	1,2,3,5	B,E,F,J	25 µl	42	45 min	120	No	2-point	Upload only

Continued.

Table 19-1 Summary of automated immunoassay systems—cont'd

Manufacturer (system)	Assays	Mode	Menu	Sample volume dilutions	Samples per tray	Time to 1st result (avg)	Maximum throughput (test/hr)	Primary tube sampling	Calibration stability	Computer interface
MILES TECHNICON IMMUNO 1	EIA Paramagnetic and turbidimetric	1,2,3,5	B,E,H,I J	1-50 µl	78	7-35 min	120	No	2 weeks 6-point 4 weeks	Bidirect
PB DIAGNOSTICS OPUS and OPUS PLUS	ELISA, Dry-multi-layer film, Fluorogenic	1,2,3,5	B,E,I,J	10-40 µl On-board (PLUS)	20	6-23 min	75	No	6-point 6 weeks	Upload only
PB DIAGNOSTICS OPUS MAGNUM	Same as OPUS	1,2,3,5	B,E	10-40 µl On-board	30	6 min	190	Yes	6-point 6 weeks	Bidirect
SERONO-BAKER DIAGNOSTICS SR 1	IEMA or EIA	1,2,3,6	B,E,F,J	150-250 µl On-board	80 (1 for calibrator)	60 min	60	No	initial 6-point; 1-pt/4 hr	Upload only
SYVA ETS Plus	EMIT	1,2,6	C	17.5 µl	16	1 min	60	No	2-point daily	Upload only
TOSOH MEDICS AIA-1200 and AIA-600	EIA Paramagnetic and fluorescent IEMA	1,2,3,5	E,F,G H,I,J	110-120 µl	AIA-1200 = 100; AIA-600 = 40	AIA-1200 and 600 50 min	AIA-1200 = 120 AIA-600 = 60	No	2-6 point 4 weeks	Bidirect

KEY: 1 = Batch, 2 = Random access, 3 = Stat interrupt, 4 = Unit dose, 5 = Continuous access, 6 = Panel

A = General chemistries, B = Therapeutic drugs, C = Drugs of abuse/toxicology, D = Infectious disease, E = Endocrinology, F = Fertility, G = Tumor markers, H = Specific proteins, I = Cardiac assessment, J = Anemia, K = Immunosuppressants (cyclosporin)

EIA = Enzyme immunoassay
FLM = Fetal lung maturity testing
FPIA = Fluorescent polarization immunoassay
REA = Radiative energy attenuation
NXT = Immunometrics technology
MEIA = Microparticle enzyme immunoassay
RPIA = Radial partition immunoassay
FSF = Front surface fluorometry
EMIT = Enzyme multiplied immunoassay technique
ELISA = Enzyme-linked immunosorbent assay
IEMA = Immunoenzymetric assays

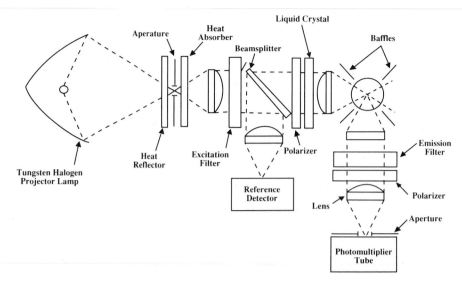

Fig. 19-4 The FPIA optical assembly of the Abbott TDx system (courtesy Abbott Diagnostics, a Division of Abbott Laboratories).

The TDx uses another technology called **radiative energy attenuation (REA)** to measure certain chemistry analytes such as BUN, creatinine, glucose, and cholesterol. It is based on the principle that the measured fluorescence intensity of any solution containing a fluorophore is related to the absorbance of the solution. If an analyte-reagent generates a chromogen that absorbs either the excitation light (primary attenuation), emission radiation (secondary attenuation), or both (total attenuation), attenuation of the fluorescence is observed. The degree of attenuation is directly proportional to the amount of chromogen present in the solution. Thus the final fluorescence intensity is inversely proportional to the concentration of analyte. The amount of final fluorescence intensity is measured by the TDx detector. By using the appropriate calibrators the concentration of an analyte can be determined.

The TDx system can also use a third technology called **turbonephelometry.** It allows for the analysis of certain specific substances (i.e., immune proteins). Nephelometry is based on the measurement of scattered light. Although turbo-nephelometry does not use fluorophores, the TDx optical system is designed to read light within the fluorescence spectrum encountered in nephelometry. To generate the proper radiant energy to measure the light scattering that takes place, a special TDx Turbo Carousel is required. It contains a green light-emitting diode (LED) as the light source. Light scattering is produced

when the patient sample is incubated with a reagent containing antibody specific for the substance to be quantitated. The amount of light scattering is directly proportional to the concentration of the substance.

The TDx system can be operated in one of two modes: batch or unit dose. Each mode has its own special 20-position carousel. The unit dose mode allows the operator to perform up to 20 different assays during a single carousel run. Some assays, such as digoxin, require a pretreatment step. The analyzer automatically takes a sample blank reading when required by the specific assay mode. Even though the TDx can run unit dose assays, it is still considered a batch analyzer meaning that it can only perform one assay at a time. It has no true "stat" interrupt capabilities. Users interact with the analyzer via a touch pad-alphanumeric LED display.

The TDx system calibrators consist of six vials labeled A through F. Controls normally consist of three levels, Low, Medium, and High. A phosphate buffer containing a protein stabilizer is used for all dilutions. Reagents are thermolabile, and thus after sample analysis should not be stored on-board the analyzer but placed immediately in the refrigerator.

The type of TDx system carousel, sample cartridge, and reagent pack that is used depends on the analytic mode that is chosen. Batch testing features a carousel that has a bar coded label position and can accommodate up to 20 cuvettes

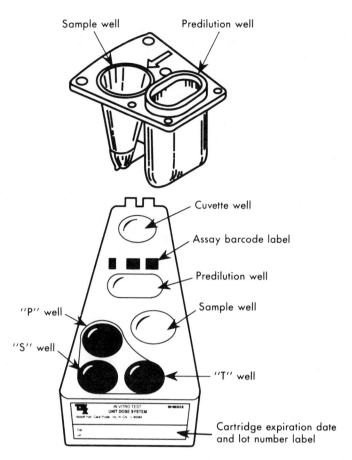

Sample well

Predilution well

Cuvette well

Assay barcode label

Predilution well

Sample well

"P" well

"S" well

"T" well

IN VITRO TEST
UNIT DOSE SYSTEM

Cartridge expiration date
and lot number label

Fig. 19-5 The Abbott TDx "batch" sample cartridge well, **A**, and "unit dose" cartridge, **B** (courtesy Abbott Diagnostics, a Division of Abbott Laboratories).

and sample cartridges for sample analysis. Each sample cartridge contains a sample well and a predilution well (Fig. 19-5, *A*). The reagent packs consist of three vial (3-pot or S, T, P vials) or four vial (4-pot or W, S, T, P vials) reagent packs that are bar coded (W = wash solution, S = serum, T = tracer, P = pretreatment). Unit dose testing uses a special carousel that has a barcoded label position and can accommodate up to 20 individual unit dose cartridges. Each unit dose cartridge consists of an assay barcode label, a cuvette well, a sample well, a predilution well, and three or four wells for reagents (Fig. 19-5, *B*).

The process sequence for both batch and unit dose occurs automatically after the analyzer door is closed, the RUN key is pressed, and the system has passed all initialization checks. After the RUN key is pressed, the Abbott TDx automatically performs 12 initialization checks before its pipetting sequence, including checks on the (1) waste cup volume; (2) door and buffer sensors; (3) sample probe home position; (4) ambient tem-

perature; (5) carousel lock; (6) bar code reader; (7) lamp intensity; (8) LED Turbo carousel (position 21); (9) number of cuvettes; (10) syringe valve movement; (11) reagent pack liquid levels; and (12) cuvette surface temperature. The above checks take approximately 1 minute.

Once the TDx has performed the initialization sequence, the pipetting sequence follows (for most assays this is called Mode 1). During this sequence sample mixed with dilution buffer is added to the predilution well of the sample cartridge. Reagent (P), dilution buffer, and one-half of the prediluted sample volume are then dispensed into the sample cuvette. The remaining samples are diluted and dispensed into their cuvettes in a similar manner. After a blank reading is taken in cuvette, the second half of each diluted sample, additional reagents (T and S), and dilution buffer are added to the cuvette to give the final reaction volume. Depending on the assay, an incubation period may follow. Final intensity readings, corrected for background intensities,

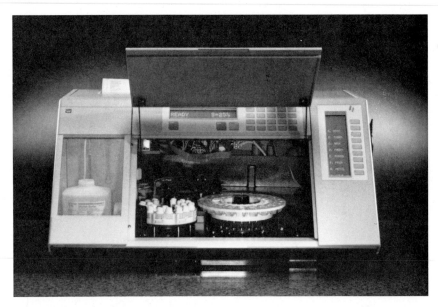

Fig. 19-6 The Abbott TDxFLx system, buffer access door (*far left*), system status display (*top-center*), reagent carousel with wedge-shaped packs for random access testing (*left-center*), sample/cuvette carousel for random access and batch testing (*right-center*), and reagent display panel and key pad (*top-right*) (courtesy Abbott Diagnostics, a Division of Abbott Laboratories).

are then converted to the appropriate concentration. A similar process sequence occurs for unit dose assays.

Abbott TDxFLx System. The TDxFLx is an automated system that is a derivative of the TDx, and thus many of its characteristics and internal components are identical to the TDx (Fig. 19-6). The test menu is also similar to the TDx and depending on the assay can use either FPIA or REA technology. However, unlike the TDx, the TDxFLx has bar code wand/scanner capabilities for entering sample and patient identification numbers.

The TDxFLx also uses **immunometrics (NXT) technology.** NXT technology is based on the principle that the measured fluorescence intensity of a solution is proportional to the concentration of the fluorophore. During the assay the reagents and analyte react to generate an enzyme concentration that is directly proportional to the analyte concentration. This active enzyme subsequently acts on a fluorogenic substrate to generate a fluorescent product. The fluorescence intensity is measured at two points in time. The change in intensity during this time interval is directly proportional to the analyte concentration. By using calibrators and comparing changes in fluorescence intensity, the analyte concentration in the patient sample can be determined.

Unlike the TDx, the TDxFLx can perform one of three modes: Batch, Unit Dose, and Random Access. The pipetting sequence for most batch and unit dose runs is similar to the TDx; the sequence for random access runs has been modified to accommodate the random access function.

The random access mode allows up to 20 patient samples to be tested for any one of 13 different therapeutic drugs during a single carousel run. Eight wedge-shaped reagent packs can be loaded onto the special TDxFLx carousel (see Fig. 19-6) that allows the user to perform, via the random access function, up to 8 different assays on a given sample. A reagent keypad with an LED display is used to select the assays to be run in the random-access mode (see Fig. 19-6). This keypad is activated when the reagent bar code reader scans the loaded carousel. The reagent display shows the assay names and indicates the number of tests used.

Tests that have been incorporated into the random access mode are some of the major therapeutic drugs (antiepileptics, antiarrthymics) and the aminoglycoside antibiotics. Unit dose assays are available for these analytes, as well as ethosuximide and fetal lung maturity testing. Assays for toxicology/abused drugs and clinical chemistries are still limited to testing in the batch mode.

A dilution protocol is available with some assays that are run in the batch mode.

The TDxFLx sample cartridges (X SYSTEM cartridges) that are used for batch and random-access testing are also similar to those used by the TDx. The batch mode requires the use of the TDxFLx 3- or 4-pot reagent packs and the batch-pack adaptor. For the random-access mode, a wedged-shaped, 3-pot pack is used (see Fig. 19-6). The unit-dose cartridge is identical to the one used with the TDx. For immunometric assays, X SYSTEMS Tri-well cartridges are used. They are composed of a sample well, a predilution well, and a tablet well.

Abbott ADx System. The Abbott ADx system (Fig. 19-7) is also a derivative of the Abbott TDx system. However, unlike the TDx system, this tabletop instrument is dedicated solely to screening specimens (serum and/or urine) for the major classes of abused drugs and performing other toxicologic assays. The ADx system uses FPIA technology for drugs of abuse detection and REA technology for ethanol measurements.

The major differences between the ADx and the TDx are the 20-position carousels used by the two instruments and the manner in which the otherwise identical reagents are packaged. The TDx carousel holds only sample cups and cuvettes. A single reagent pack is placed in the an-

alyzer beside the carousel. Thus the TDx when used for screening of drugs of abuse is configured to perform as a batch analyzer. In contrast the ADx offers what is termed **flexible access.** Reagent packs are loaded on the ADx carousel along with the sample cups and cuvettes. Thus the ADx can screen one or more samples for several different tests in a single run. The reagent packs consist of the same type of vials that are used on the TDx (S, P, T and sometimes W). The difference is how the reagent cartridge has been configured to adapt to the ADx carousel.

There are three modes of flexible access with the ADx: paneling, combination testing, and batch testing. Paneling allows the user to perform a series of tests on one or multiple samples without sample splitting. One sample can be analyzed for a maximum of 10 different tests in a given run. In combination testing the operator can run different tests in varied configurations on a series of samples, including simultaneous assays of serum and urine. Any number of configurations are possible, limited only by the space that is available on the carousel. Batch testing can accommodate up to 20 patient samples for a single test.

The ADx determines which assays will be run by reading the bar code on the reagent cartridge labels. It also counts the number of times that

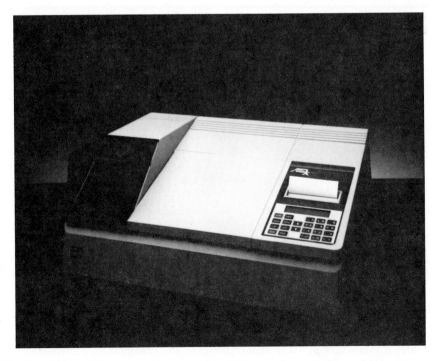

Fig. 19-7 The Abbott ADx system (courtesy Abbott Diagnostics, a Division of Abbott Laboratories).

each pack has been used. In the panel mode the carousel must be configured with the reagent pack followed by the sample cartridges and cuvettes for each patient. The same process is followed for each additional assay. The instrument automatically returns to the correct patient sample to perform each of the assays. In the "run" mode, with combination and batch testing, a sample is required in each of the sample cartridges following a reagent cartridge.

Because the Abbott ADx uses FPIA technology, the inverse relationship that exists between the level of polarization and the concentration means that at low concentrations the system measures a very strong signal. Therefore the ADx, like the TDx or TDxFLx, can detect very low levels of drug, and thus has excellent sensitivity. It also incorporates, as a safeguard, background subtraction that helps to detect the presence of any normal or abnormal fluorescent characteristics of the sample. Blank readings also correct for hemolyzed, icteric or lipemic serum samples, many urine sample adulterations, and reagent integrity.

One of the unique features of the Abbott ADx system is the ability of the operator to adjust the **threshold** to detect lower level of drugs. The threshold is the concentration at which the presence or absence of drug/metabolite is flagged or shown to be greater/less than a **cutoff level** (the level where a significant amount of false positives are likely to occur because of a lack of sensitivity). The manufacturer supplies "suggested thresholds" for each assay that should be followed to prevent a high false positivity rate without sacrificing detection capability. Unlike many other dedicated drug immunoassay systems, the ADx provides the user with numeric, semiquantitative data.

All reagents are fully reconstituted liquids and thus are ready to use. The design of the wash station reduces carryover to less than 0.1%. A number of print options are available that afford the operator the ability to format the printouts to meet specific requirements for identification, chain-of-custody, and qualitative and semiquantitative data interpretation.

Abbott IMx System. The Abbott IMx system (Fig. 19-8) is an automated tabletop batch analyzer that performs a wide variety of immunochemistries on plasma or serum. The test menu is quite extensive and includes assays for hepatitis, endocrinology, fertility, physiologic disorders, cancer/tumor markers, congenital and infectious disease, renal and cardiac assessment, and some therapeutic drug monitoring (theophylline). The instrument performs assays by two established technologies: fluorescence polarization immunoassay (FPIA) (described earlier), and a technology called **microparticle enzyme immunoassay (MEIA).** Homogeneous assays are performed by FPIA, which is generally the method of choice for analytes of low molecular weight. Heterogeneous assays are performed by MEIA, which is generally used for larger molecules of high molecular weight such as protein hormones or antibodies.

The IMx system consists of several integrated

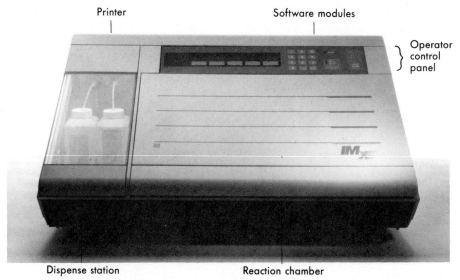

Fig. 19-8 The Abbott IMx system and subsystems (courtesy Abbott Diagnostics, a Division of Abbott Laboratories).

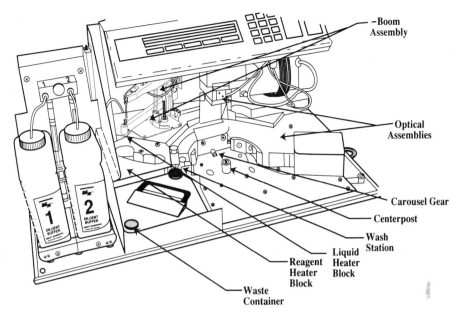

Fig. 19-9 The Abbott IMx reaction chamber/processing area, (courtesy Abbott Diagnostics, a Division of Abbott Laboratories).

subassemblies (see Fig. 19-8); a schematic of the reaction chamber is depicted in Fig. 19-9. Dilutions and calculations are also performed on board so the analyzer can produce a final result. The user interacts with the system via a numeric touch pad and a 40 character per line alphanumeric LED display. The control panel has a numeric pad, five function keys, run and stop buttons, and an assay mode selection key. The system does not permit the operator to enter patient demographics or report comments.

IMx MEIA technology uses submicron (<0.5 μ) microparticles coated with an antibody specific for the analyte that is being tested (capture molecule). The microparticles have an effective surface area that is significantly greater than the traditional ¼-inch polystyrene beads. Also, the diffusion distance between analyte and the solid phase is reduced substantially ($\sim$ 100 times less). Both factors accelerate analyte binding and attainment of equilibrium, thereby decreasing assay incubation times.

The heterogeneous MEIA assays, unlike the FPIA homogeneous assays, require a separation step. This is accomplished by transferring the reaction mixture, consisting of the analyte that has been incubated with the microparticle-antibody complex, to an inert glass fiber matrix where the microparticles bind irreversibly. The immune or microparticle-antibody-analyte complex is re-

tained by the glass fibers while the other components of the reaction mixture (which may contain potentially interfering substances) flow through the large pores of the matrix. Detection of the immune complex is accomplished by adding an alkaline phosphatase-labeled conjugate to the complex, forming an antibody-analyte-conjugate "sandwich." A fluorogenic substrate (4-methylumbelliferyl phosphate) is added, which is hydrolyzed to a fluorescent product (4-methylumbelliferone) by the bound alkaline phosphatase. The amount of fluorescent product formed is directly proportional to the concentration of analyte in the test sample. The MEIA reaction sequence is shown in Fig. 19-10.

The IMx requires two different types of carousels, one for FPIA and one for MEIA assays. The FPIA carousel holds 20 specimens. Each sample cartridge has two wells, one for sample and the other for predilution. Reactions cuvettes must be loaded opposite each sample cartridge. The MEIA carousel holds 24 reaction cells; each cell consists of a sample well and three reaction wells: predilution, incubation, and matrix/blotter (Fig. 19-11). The latter reaction well contains the glass matrix fibers that will bind the microparticle-immune complex and a blotter that will absorb any unbound material that passes through the fibers. The operator may program and load multiple carousels while the instrument runs.

SCHEMATIC REACTION SEQUENCE

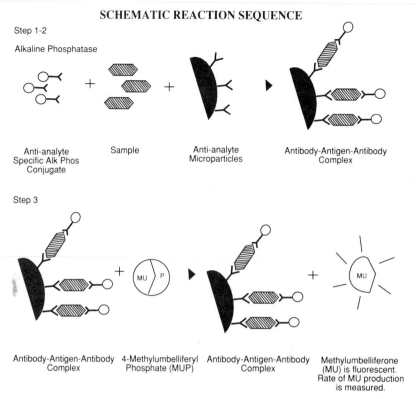

Fig. 19-10 Principle of microparticle enzyme immunoassay (MEIA) (courtesy Abbott Diagnostics, a Division of Abbott Laboratories).

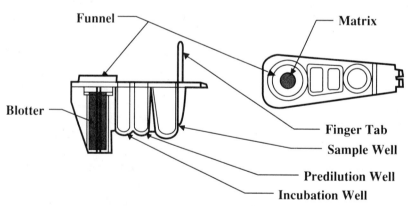

Fig. 19-11 The Abbott IMx MEIA reaction cell (courtesy Abbott Diagnostics, a Division of Abbott Laboratories).

FPIA reagent packs are supplied in bar coded holders and are labeled in the same manner as the TDx reagents. MEIA reagents are also supplied in bar coded reagent packs; however, they contain three or four bottles numerically labeled according to their contents: (1) microparticles, (2) conjugate, (3) substrate, and (4) for specimen dilu-

ent, assay diluent, wash buffer, or assay-specific reagent. The reagent pack/holders are specially designed, so they are placed correctly in the temperature controlled reagent position of the instrument. All buffers and diluents are monitored by a subtraction inventory system.

The IMx has two optical systems that are en-

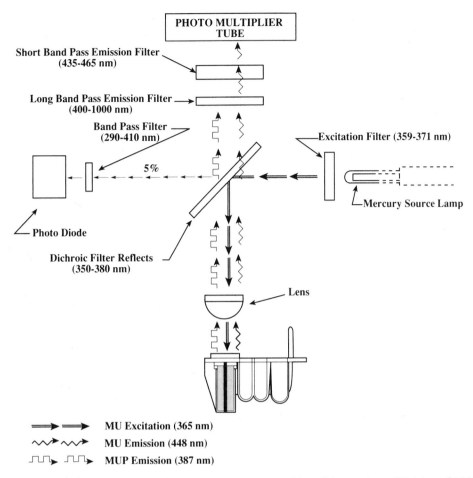

Fig. 19-12 The Abbott IMx MEIA optical assembly (courtesy Abbott Diagnostics, a Division of Abbott Laboratories).

tirely electronic and contain no moving parts. The light source for FPIA is identical to that of the TDx. MEIA tests use a **front-surface fluorometer** and a low pressure mercury arc lamp as its light source (Fig. 19-12). Light emitted from the mercury lamp passes through an excitation filter that selects light with a nominal wavelength of 365 nm. The light is then focused via a dichroic mirror onto the surface of the reaction cell matrix. The MEIA optical assembly measures the intensity of fluorescent light emitted at 448 nm on the reaction cell matrix surface that is produced by 4-methylumbelliferone.

Abbott IMx SELECT. The IMx SELECT enhancement is an upgrade to the Abbott IMx system that provides the user the capability of running up to three different assays on a carousel during a single run, thus enabling the user to run small batch profiles on a single carousel. It consists of a new 24-position carousel that contains a bucket in the center portion where the IMx SELECT reagent packs are placed. The reagent packs contain the same components as the IMx reagent packs except the substrate, 4-methylumbelliferyl phosphate, is supplied in a separate bottle. With an IMx SELECT run the substrate is placed into a reusable holder and positioned in the reagent heater block.

Different assay modules and a different software module are required to run the IMx SELECT and are included with the upgrade kit. This upgrade will allow the user to have the capability of running the MEIA assays, the FPIA assays, and the IMx SELECT assays. The assay modules contain tests that can be run together in any combination on the carousel and are divided into common laboratory profile groups. Rinses have been optimized to eliminate reagent cross-contamination and reduce sample carryover.

A bar code scanner is also part of the IMx SE-

LECT upgrade and is used in the SELECT mode for reading reagent bar coded labels and for scanning patient barcode IDs on sample tubes. The latter provides a mechanism by which patient IDs can be printed on the IMx printout along with the results.

Baxter Diagnostics, Inc., Stratus II and Stratus IIntellect

Baxter Stratus II. The Stratus II is a fully automated, batch immunoassay analyzer (Fig. 19-13). This benchtop instrument has been designed to perform assays for thyroid function, reproductive hormones, cardiac markers, endocrine function, allergy assessment, therapeutic drug monitoring, infectious diseases, and tumor markers. It runs fluorometric immunoassays on small plastic disposable reagent/matrix tabs using the principle of **radial partition immunoassay (RPIA) and front surface fluorometry.**

RPIA is an enzyme immunologic method that uses special antibody-coated tabs that are specific for each assay. The tabs are disks that are composed of a reactive surface of glass-fiber filter paper. The reaction between the analyte (ligand) and enzyme-tracer (analyte or antibody depending on the type of assay) takes place on the tab.

The enzyme tracer is responsible for catalyzing a reaction that generates a fluoroscent product. The amount of fluorescence produced on the front surface of the tab is measured by a detector called a front surface fluorometer. With the Stratus II a low pressure mercury lamp provides the excitation wavelength of 365 nm; the emission wavelength is 450 nm.

In a competitive assay (Fig. 19-14), patient sample that contains the analyte of interest and enzyme-labeled analyte (conjugate) is allowed to react with the antibody bound to the glass-fiber filter paper. If the assay is sequential (Fig. 19-14), a conjugate fluid (containing enzyme-labeled analyte) is added after an initial incubation with patient analyte. After incubation, unbound label is removed with substrate wash fluid. The washing causes unbound analytes (labeled and unlabeled) and proteins to chromatograph to the perimeter of the glass-fiber filter paper. Therefore only labeled analyte remains in the center of the filter paper bound to the immobilized antibody. In a sandwich assay (see Fig. 19-14) a second antibody labeled with enzyme (conjugate) is added to the patient analyte already bound by the immobilized antibody, forming a sandwich. Again,

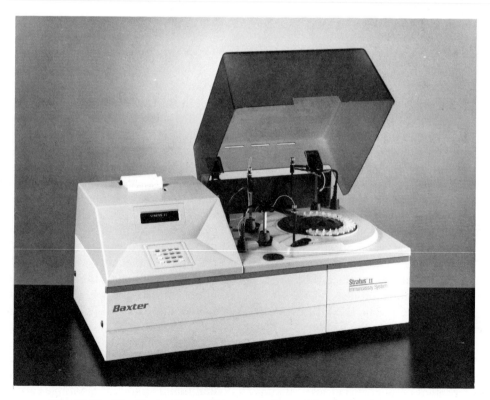

Fig. 19-13 The Baxter Stratus II (courtesy Baxter Diagnostics, Inc.).

Competitive Assays

Patient Sample	Sample/Conjugate	Substrate
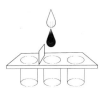	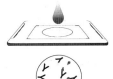 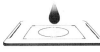	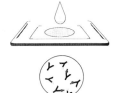
Patient sample and conjugate, an enzyme-labeled analyte, are mixed in a cuvette.	Antigens in the patient sample and conjugate compete to bind with the antibody immobilized in the tab	Excess enzyme-labeled antibody and serum proteins from the patient sample are washed from the reaction zone by substrate.

Sandwich Assays

Patient Sample	Conjugate	Substrate
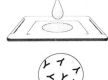 	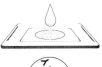 	
The antigen in the patient sample binds to the antibody immobilized in the tab.	In sandwich assays, the conjugate is an enzyme-labeled antibody. This antibody binds to the second antigenic site on the antigen from the patient sample.	Excess enzyme-labeled antibody and serum proteins from the patient sample are washed from the reaction zone by substrate.

Sequential Assays

Patient Sample	Conjugate	Substrate
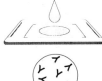	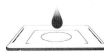 	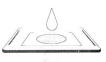
The antigen in the patient sample binds to the antibody immobilized in the tab.	Conjugate is an enzyme-labeled antigen, which binds to the antibody sites that are not already bound by the patient sample.	Excess enzyme-labeled antibody and serum proteins from the patient sample are washed from the reaction zone by substrate.

Fig. 19-14 Principle of radial partition immunoassay (RPIA) using competitive, sandwich, and sequential assays (courtesy Baxter Diagnostics, Inc.).

washing the glass fiber matrix causes diffusion of unbound analytes and proteins to move to the perimeter of the tab. With all assays, as the fluorescence develops in the center of the tab, fluorometric readings are taken sequentially using front surface fluorometry. These readings are compared with a standard curve.

The Stratus II consists of the analyzer and an integrated sampler/dilutor and includes such features as liquid sensing probes, patient identifica-tion number, enhanced data reduction capability, self-diagnostics, and several enhancements to reduce sample carryover. The analyzer requires no special plumbing and can operate over a wide range of temperatures (22° C to 32° C). Daily maintenance requires less than 15 minutes, weekly less than 20 minutes, and monthly about 5 minutes.

The unit is composed of several subsystems: sample carousel/tab magazine, fluid handling system, optical system, and computer. The sample carousel holds 30 sample cups (see Fig. 19-13). Each cup consists of three wells; one for sample, one for mixing of sample and reagents (conjugate, assay buffer, or assay diluent), and the other is reserved for future assays pertaining to infectious disease.

The analyzer has a "stat" add-on feature that allows for the addition of a sample during a run. The "stat" specimen is inserted in the next available position at the end of the batch or can be switched with a routine sample. Using the latter approach, the specimen ID in each position has to be changed. If the "stat" sample requires the same test as the current run, the analytic run does not have to be aborted. However, if the "stat" sample requires a different assay, it cannot be analyzed until the current batch run is complete, or at the option of the operator the routine run is aborted.

Tabs are introduced into the analyzer through a tab loading station (magazine) that is located in the front beneath the carousel. This station can accommodate up to 30 tabs for a particular batch run. The tabs in the magazine are queued within the tab loading station and "peeled off" the stack as the process continues. A cup sensor allows the analyzer to accommodate "stat" samples in a given run. After a run, unused tabs should be removed from the magazine and stored in the refrigerator. Although reagent tabs are stored in the refrigerator, they do not have to be at room temperature before using.

The fluid handling system is composed of three dispensers: sample, conjugate, and wash (see Fig. 19-13). The sampler dispenser tip is washed with distilled water after every patient sample to minimize sample carryover. For some assays a peristaltic pump is activated for additional probe washes. A special decontamination station is provided for those assays (i.e., infectious disease tests that may require additional washing).

A sample that is out of the assay's linear range can be serially diluted on-board. Nine dilution protocols can be programmed and stored. The program allows up to three serial dilutions per sample, thus a second, third, or possibly a fourth sample cup is needed to prepare serial dilutions. The total number of neat samples and dilutions for a given run must be equal to or less than 30. The maximum dilution that can be achieved with three serial dilutions is 1:1000.

Level sensors that are part of the dispensers help to minimize penetration of the probes into sample or reagents and ensure that reagents are available for analysis. Sample carryover is minimized by rinsing the sample dispenser in a specially fitted wash station using Brij/saline solution or distilled water.

The operator interface on the Stratus II is a 16-button numeric keypad. A thermal printer is provided in the analyzer to provide a hard copy of all results, diagnostic readings, calibration curves, and quality control charts. The operator can also select for conventional or SI units. The analyzer's computer can calculate such indices as thyroid binding index (TBI) and free thyroxine index (FTI).

Baxter Stratus IIntellect. The Stratus IIntellect is an upgrade to the Stratus II. It includes an upgraded Intel 386 computer system with increased memory for instrument operations and storage of data. Some of the major features and improvements found with the Stratus IIntellect system compared with the Stratus II are a complete selection to determine patient profiles, calculation of CK-MB index, unlimited storage of QC data, linearity checks, a user-friendly graphic user interface, full-size keyboard, trackball, ability to easily upgrade and backup software, and full bidirectional interface capabilities.

Becton Dickinson Affinity. The Affinity is a compact, random access, immunoassay analyzer (Fig. 19-15). This fully automated benchtop instrument requires no daily maintenance and features individual test units that are bar coded. The Affinity operates by use of a scheduling algorithm. This means that the entire menu of tests that have been requested are viewed, and then individual tests are prioritized to achieve maximum productivity. Throughput is thus determined by the test mix.

The most important feature of the system and central to its design is the self-contained reagent cartridge called the ImmUnit. Each ImmUnit is assay-specific and contains all necessary reagents for an individual test. It consists of six sealed wells: (1) first well or sample well designed to reduce evaporation; (2) wells 2 through 5 for reagents (i.e., substrate solution, chromogen solution, stop solution, conjugate); and (3) well six or reaction/cuvette tube often coated with antibody. This well is star-shaped to increase the reaction surface area. The well contents, which are assay-specific, are opened by the analyzer. Each ImmUnit is bar coded for the test name, lot number, and a unique sequence number that is part of

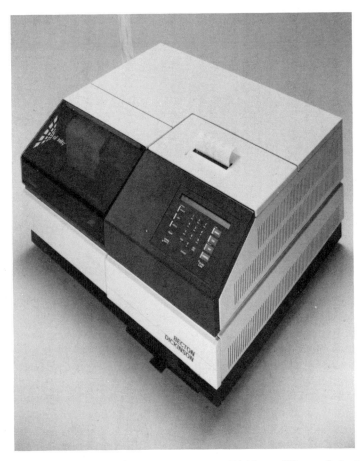

Fig. 19-15 The Becton Dickinson Affinity (courtesy Becton Dickinson Diagnostic Instrument Systems).

the positive patient identification system of the Affinity. The label is divided into two parts: one part is read by the system's bar code reader; the other part (which has an adhesive backing) can be removed and placed on a worklist or vacutainer.

The ImmUnit cartridge has a block marked "CAL" printed at one end. A specific calibrator is added to each cartridge; a special pen is then used to fill in the "CAL" block. The ImmUnits are then loaded onto the tray in ascending order based on concentration. The instrument can be calibrated for two lot numbers of cartridges for each assay.

The Affinity provides the operator with two methods for designating quality control (QC) samples. One approach takes advantage of the analyzer's software and is designed to be used with a three-level QC scheme; the other approach processes individual QC samples like any other test.

The analyzer consists of four functional units:

sample loading/unloading tray, carousel, work station, and detector. The sample loading tray is used to place the ImmUnits' cartridges into the system; it can hold 16 cartridges. The tray also serves as a work station. Once the tray is loaded it is placed into the Affinity. As it moves along a track, the ImmUnits pass under a bar code reader and then move to the Affinity carousel. This process takes less than 1 minute.

The Affinity carousel is a rotating circular rack that has 32 position for ImmUnits (Fig. 19-16). It serves two functions: (1) it acts as a transport device between the work station and detector and (2) it serves as a 37° C incubator. Of the 32 available slots on the carousel, only 31 are available for specimens; the remaining slot is reserved for a special ImmUnit called the Resident ValUnit (RVU). This cartridge contains no reagents and is used as a primer for the system's fluidics and as a reference for the detection system. It is recommended that the RVU be replaced every 2 weeks.

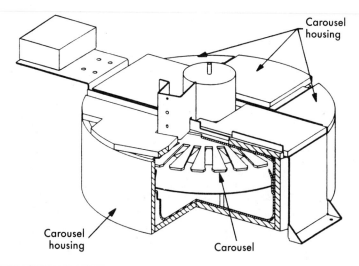

Fig. 19-16 The Becton Dickinson Affinity carousel (courtesy Becton Dickinson Diagnostic Instrument Systems).

The Affinity work station performs all pipetting, mixing, and rinsing operations (Fig. 19-17). The work station has a shuttle mechanism that transports the ImmUnit from the loading tray to the carousel. The work station is composed of three elements: (1) a punch that opens the ImmUnit seals, (2) a transfer pipette that performs all sample/reagent measurements, and (3) a rinse/waste pipette that removes waste from the ImmUnit and washes the reaction cuvette.

The instrument has both fluorometric and photometric detection with the former being detected by a photomultiplier tube and the latter by a photodiode. Therefore its basic design does limit the type of assays that can be run. Different wavelengths can be selected by the use of a filter wheel assembly.

The Affinity can perform enzymatic competitive and noncompetitive (immunometric) assays that use the chromophore, 3,3′,5,5′-tetramethylbenzidine (TMB), hydrogen peroxide as the substrate, and an enzymatic tracer, horseradish peroxidase (HRP). Depending on the type of assay, HRP is either labeled with the analyte of interest (competitive) or bound to a secondary antibody that is directed toward the analyte that is being measured (noncompetitive). After an incubation period and wash cycle the HRP that remains in the reaction mixture catalyzes the formation of oxygen and water from the hydrogen peroxide. The oxygen then oxidizes the TMB (blue) to an oxidized product (yellow) and is read at 450 nm. The oxidation process is stopped by the addition of citric acid. A reference reading is taken at 630

nm that also helps account for variation in the optical surface of the tubes.

The user interacts with the instrument via a membrane keyboard and an alphanumeric 40-character liquid crystal display (LCD). A thermal printer produces results, calibrations curves, Levey-Jennings quality control charts, and other reporting formats.

Biotrol Diagnostics' System 7000. The Biotrol System 7000 is a fully automated, random access immunoassay analyzer that incorporates the principles of ELISA technology using as a solid phase magnetic micropolystyrene beads that have a core of ferrous oxide (Fig. 19-18). This

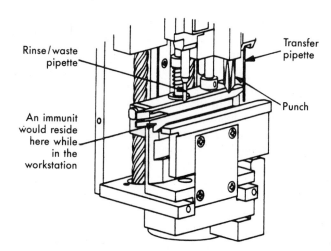

Fig. 19-17 The Becton Dickinson Affinity work station (courtesy Becton Dickinson Diagnostic Instrument Systems).

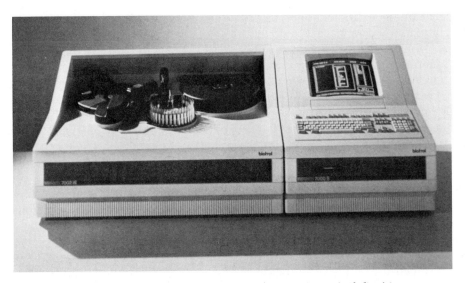

Fig. 19-18 The Biotrol System 7000, control unit (*right*) and processing unit (*left*) with reagent carousel on the right, sample carousel in the center, and reaction carousel on the left (courtesy Biotrol USA, Inc.).

solid phase results in (1) reduced incubation time because of an increase in surface area where the reaction takes place, (2) totally automated dispensing, incubation, separation, and washing steps within each reaction cuvette, (3) a large available test menu that uses ELISA techniques that do not restrict the size of the analyte being measured, and (4) the ability to perform various immunocapture techniques that are used in various serology assays to separate immunoglobulins.

The Biotrol System 7000 is a benchtop analyzer that consists of two main units: the process unit and the control unit. The process unit contains the following subassemblies: (1) reaction carousel, (2) wash station, (3) photometer, (4) reaction carousel, (5) pipetting station, (6) sample carousel, and (7) reagent carousel. The control unit consists of (1) computer-data processing unit with 3.5-inch disk drive, (2) color monitor, (3) alphanumeric keyboard, (4) on-board thermal printer (40 columns), and (5) an RS-232 bidirectional interface.

The reaction carousel (see Fig. 19-18) is refrigerated and can accommodate 100 cuvettes. The pipetting station has separate probes for dispensing sample and reagent. Each probe is equipped with a liquid level detector. Two separate wash solutions are used: one to clean and decontaminate the probes, the other to perform the separation and washing steps in the reaction carousel.

Patient samples can be dispensed from both primary tubes and sample cups. Sample carry-over is prevented by use of a wash station. The system has a 36-position sample carousel that is both removable and interchangeable, thus permitting the operator to preload samples on one carousel while tests are being performed on another (see Fig. 19-18). Sample dilutions can be performed on-board the analyzer.

Depending on the assay, the Biotrol 7000 performs tests using either single or two-vial liquid reagents. The on-board reagent carousel has a capacity for up to 20 single vial or two-vial tests (see Fig. 19-18). Prepared substrate has an on-board stability of 3 days. A positive ID bar code reader is available that provides the instrument with an integrated reagent inventory system. The total number of tests that be accommodated on-board the analyzer is 2000.

The Biotrol System 7000 processes tests at either 2 or 3 fixed cycles. The cuvettes make one complete revolution in approximately 15 minutes. Thus the results from the first patient are available in either 30 or 40 minutes. All results that follow are available 10 seconds after the previous result. The system also has a 24 hour standby mode that results in a "no wait" start-up time.

The maintenance requirements of the Biotrol System 7000 are minimal. It has a software-driven automated maintenance program designated as a "shutdown" procedure that lasts for 5 minutes. There is also a 10-minute weekly maintenance program that has to be performed. The computer capabilities of the system include several features that are important for quality assurance and quality control data management.

Boehringer Mannheim ES 300 System. The Boehringer Mannheim ES 300 System is a fully automated, random access immunoassay analyzer that can perform a wide variety of patient testing for thyroid, fertility, anemia, cancer, and infectious diseases (Fig. 19-19). The assays are based on enzyme immunoassay (EIA) technology using coated tubes as the solid-phase.

This benchtop analyzer consists of two main components: the analyzer and the computer system, which includes a monitor, keyboard, and printer (see Fig. 19-19). The analyzer can be further classified into several subassemblies: (1) sample rotor, (2) reagent rotor, (3) multifunction arm (MFA), (4) incubator rotor, (5) dispensing (pipette) assembly, and (6) photometer.

The sample rotor has 150 positions available for patient sample and standards; 10 additional positions can be used for multiconstituent controls (see Fig. 19-19). The sample rotor is composed of a ring with 6 detachable rotor segments that can be removed from the sample rotor for loading and unloading. Each segment is coded with a geometric marking that prevents them from being accidentally mounted on the sample rotor in the wrong position. The sample rotor also rotates bidirectionally, thus providing for random sample pipetting during an analytic run. The reagent rotor (inner ring) has 12 variable reagent positions and 3 designated positions, two for the universal substrate and one for cleaning solution that is used by the system (see Fig. 19-19). The reagent rotor also moves bidirectionally. The incubation rotor can hold 160 coated tubes; it also rotates in a clockwise or counterclockwise fashion, thus positioning the appropriate tube for loading and processing.

The multifunction arm (MFA) is located in the middle of the analyzer between the sample rotor and the incubation rotor (Fig. 19-20). The MFA is composed of two arms: (1) the sample/reagent needle and the reagent/substrate needle are on opposite ends of one arm; (2) the photometer/mixer needle and the coated tube needle are on opposite ends of the other arm (see Fig. 19-20). These arms move in a scissorlike fashion to perform the pipetting, mixing, and aspiration of sample, reagents, and reaction fluid. To increase the precision and accuracy of pipetting, the ES 300 immunoassay system uses a dispensing or pipetting assembly that is driven by two Hamilton syringes: 250 µL and 500 µL.

The optics of the ES 300 system have a temperature-controlled photometer. It contains a

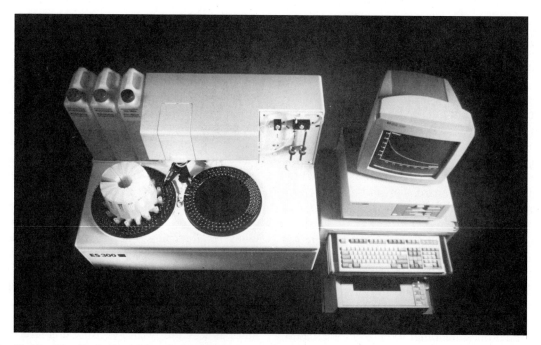

Fig. 19-19 The Boehringer Mannheim ES 300 immunoassay system, sample rotor (outer ring on the left), reagent rotor (*inner ring on the left*), and incubation rotor (*right center*) (courtesy Boehringer Mannheim Corporation).

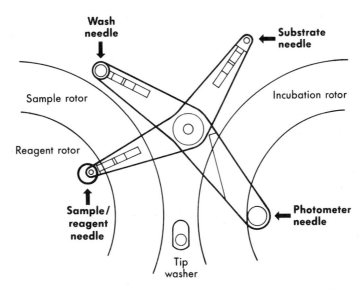

Fig. 19-20 The Boehringer Mannheim ES 300 multifunctional arm (courtesy Boehringer Mannheim Corporation).

halogen lamp, a 422 nm interference filter, and a flow-through cuvette. The 422 nm filter is mounted on a filter wheel that has 3 additional filter positions reserved for future tests.

All assays on the ES 300 immunoassay system use heterogeneous enzyme immunoassay (EIA) techniques that are either competitive, modified-competitive, or sandwich type. The instrument uses a reagent system of specially coated tubes called Enzymun-Test reagents. Because all the assays are heterogeneous, a separation step is required. This is made possible by the specially coated tubes. A typical competitive assay on the ES 300 system involves (1) run initialization, (2) pipetting of sample and reagent, (3) incubation, (4) coated tube washing, (5) pipetting of substrate, (6) second incubation, (7) mixing and photometric measurement, and (8) curve and sample calculations.

In addition to the 3 existing coated-tube methods, new assays for the ES 300 will use the new streptavidin tube technology (Fig. 19-21). The reaction tubes are coated with streptavidin via an anchor protein. The advantages of coating the with streptavidin are (1) more binding sites are available than are needed for the reaction and (2) the excess binding sites compensate for any minute imprecisions that may occur during the tube molding process. This technology is based on the strong binding affinity between streptavidin and biotin; such strong bonding results in greater assay temperature range and faster reaction times. Initially, the analyte in the patient sample

binds to the biotinylated-antibody that is directed against that analyte (see Fig. 19-21). The biotinylated-end of the antibody then binds to the streptavidin on the tube wall. The remaining steps of the assay are similar to the typical EIA methodologies for competitive or sandwich assays.

The computer system controls all necessary functions of the system including daily maintenance and weekly checks using an initialization and end of run process.

Ciba Corning Diagnostics' ACS: 180. The ACS: 180 is a completely automated immunoassay analyzer, capable of operating in a random access or batch mode (Fig. 19-22). The benchtop instrument is capable of performing a variety of assays including tests for thyroid function, reproductive hormones, anemia, cardiac assessment, endocrine function, allergy assessment, therapeutic drug monitoring, and cancer. The ACS: 180 uses a unique chemiluminescent tracer and paramagnetic particles as solid-phase reagents. The use of **chemiluminescence** allows the instrument to detect small quantities of analyte regardless of their molecular size. The micron-sized paramagnetic particles offer maximum surface area (up to 50 times that of coated tubes or microwells), a rapid means of separation without centrifugation, and minimal nonspecific binding.

The ACS: 180 system can be divided into 6 subsystems (Fig. 19-23): (1) cuvette loader/process track, (2) sample handling system, (3) reagent handling system, (4) separation/wash sys-

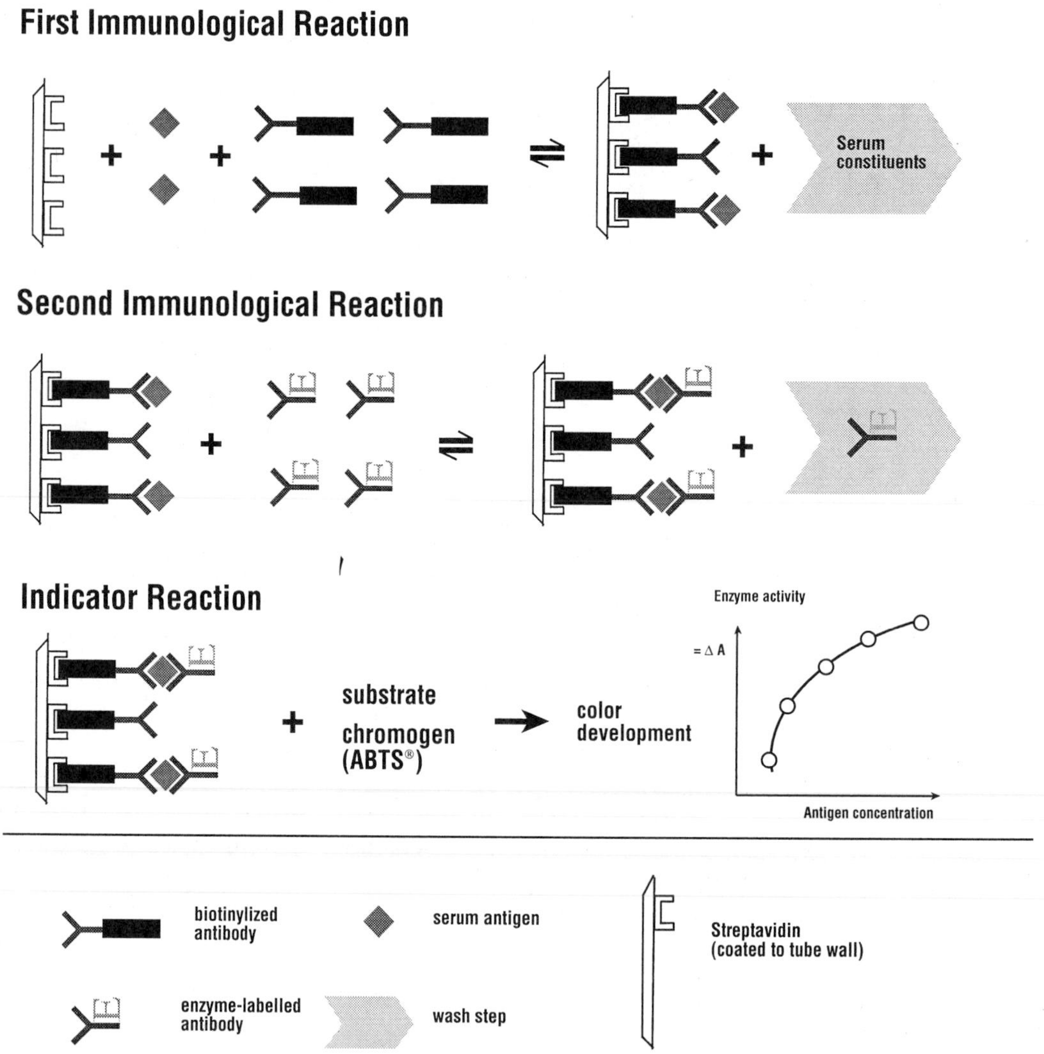

First Immunological Reaction

Second Immunological Reaction

Indicator Reaction

Fig. 19-21 Principle of the streptavidin sandwich technology (courtesy Boehringer Manneheim Corporation).

tem, (5) luminometer, and (6) data reduction system. Reactions between sample and reagents take place in disposable plastic cuvettes. Cuvettes, in quantities of 200, can be loaded into the bin by the operator. These cuvettes are then automatically and sequentially dispensed from the cuvette loader onto a linear process track. This track moves from left to right in increments of 20 seconds. Samples are dispensed into cuvettes by a dedicated probe; reagents are added at select intervals (software-controlled) by means of 3 dedicated probes.

The sample handling system consists of a laser bar code reader, a digital dilutor, and a 60-position tray for loading patient samples, calibrators, controls, and diluents (see Fig. 19-23). The sam-

ple tray consists of 2 concentric rings, each capable of holding primary tubes or sample cups. The outer ring holds 34 samples; the inner ring holds 26.

The ACS: 180 can be programmed to repeat any sample that exceeds a selected range, and for most assays will dilute and re-assay any sample that is above the linear range of the assay. Several dilution ratios can be selected based on sample size. To minimize carryover, the inner/outer surfaces of the probe are thoroughly washed with deionized water.

The reagent handling system has a reagent tray that can hold up to 26 reagent bottles to accommodate up to 13 different assays (see Fig. 19-23). The inner portion of the tray agitates and thus has

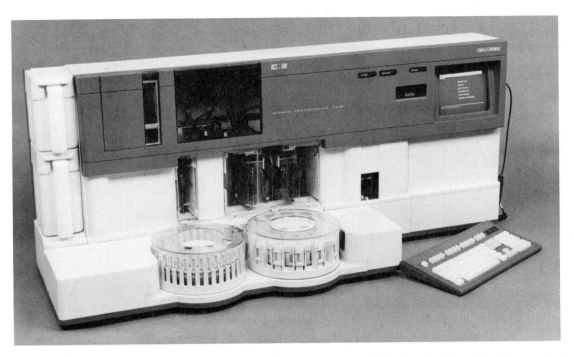

Fig. 19-22   The Ciba Corning ACS: 180 immunoassay system (courtesy Ciba Corning Diagnostics Corporation).

been specifically designed to maintain the solid-phase reagents in suspension. The stability of the reagents is 40 hours on-board the instrument if they are refrigerated when not in use.

The separation/wash station is designed to recover the paramagnetic particles and remove unbound tracer. Particles are rapidly pulled to the back wall of the cuvette by stationary magnets mounted on the process track followed by aspiration of liquid using a spring-loaded probe. After completion of the wash cycle, the particles are resuspended in a hydrogen peroxide/nitric acid solution (flash reagent No. 1).

The luminometer chamber is a rotary housing with 6 wells that contain a photomultiplier tube (PMT) detector (see Fig. 19-23). When the cuvette is positioned in front of the PMT, a solution of sodium hydroxide (flash reagent No. 2) is added to the cuvette. The addition of alkali in the presence of hydrogen peroxide causes the acridinium ester to become oxidized to a product that emits light photons at 430 nm. The flash of light that lasts for about 3 to 4 seconds is detected by the PMT. So-called dark counts are taken before light emission occurs and then subtracted.

The ACS: 180 assays are of the competitive or sandwich type using an acridinium ester as a chemiluminescent tracer. Competititve assays are

used for smaller molecules like digoxin and thyroxine. Competition takes place between the analyte in the patient's serum and analyte tagged with acridinium ester. Sandwich assays are used for larger molecules or when a broader range of measurement response is required (i.e. ferritin, peptide hormones, or CK-MB). In the sandwich assay a second antibody tagged with the acridinium ester binds the analyte in the patient's serum at another site.

The instrument stores a master curve for calibration that is determined by the manufacturer using multiple runs on multiple instruments. Each lot of reagents is supplied with data for a lot-specific dose-response curve. The calibration curve data is entered into the instrument via the keyboard or a bar code wand. The ACS: 180 computer software is designed to calculate and plot quality control data. It also has an extensive diagnostic program to aid in troubleshooting.

Cirrus Diagnostics' IMMULITE. The Cirrus IMMULITE is a fully automated, random access immunoassay system (Fig. 19-24). Central to the operation of this benchtop analyzer is a proprietary assay tube that provides for rapid and efficient washing of a ¼-inch polystyrene bead solid phase. The polystyrene bead within the assay tube is coated with antibody against the analyte

System Operation

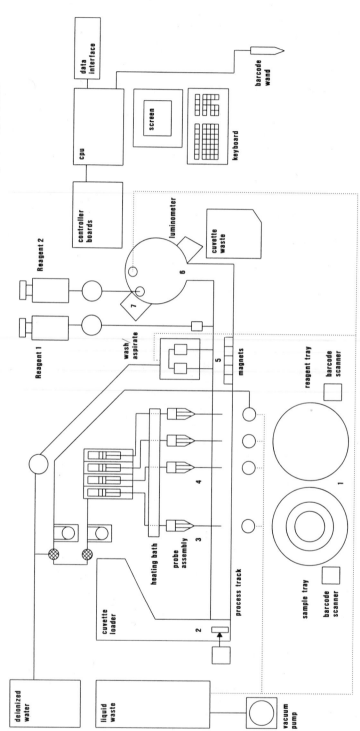

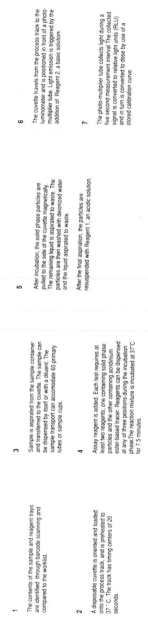

1

The contents of the sample and reagent trays are identified through barcode scanning and compared to the worklist.

2

A disposable cuvette is oriented and loaded onto the process track, and is preheated to 37° C. The track has timing centers of 20 seconds.

3

Sample is aspirated from the sample container and transferred to the cuvette. The sample can be dispensed by itself or with a diluent. The sample transport can accomodate 60 primary tubes or sample cups.

4

Assay reagent is added. Each test requires at least two reagents; one containing solid phase particles and the other containing acridinium ester-based tracer. Reagents can be dispensed at any of three positions during the incubation phase.The reaction mixture is incubated at 37°C for 7.5 minutes.

5

After incubation, the solid phase particles are pulled to the side of the cuvette magnetically. The remaining liquid is aspirated to waste. The particles are then washed with deionized water and the liquid aspirated to waste.

After the final aspiration, the particles are resuspended with Reagent 1, an acidic solution.

6

The cuvette travels from the process track to the luminometer and is positioned in front of a photo-multiplier tube. Light emission is triggered by the addition of Reagent 2, a basic solution.

7

The photo-multiplier tube collects light during a five second measurement interval. The collected signal is converted to relative light units (RLU) and in turn is converted to dose by use of a stored calibration curve.

Fig. 19-23 Schematic of the Ciba Corning ACS: 180 subsystems (courtesy Ciba Corning Diagnostics Corporation).

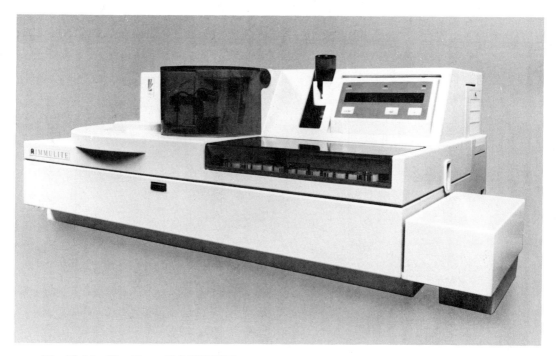

Fig. 19-24 The Cirrus IMMULITE immunoassay system (courtesy Cirrus Diagnostics, Inc.).

of interest and is held captive in the assay tube; this tube serves as the reaction vessel for all incubations, subsequent washes, and signal development (Fig. 19-25).

The system achieves a high degree of sensitivity by using heterogeneous enzyme immunoassay assays coupled with a chemiluminescent detection system. Competitive assays use enzyme-labeled analyte; sandwich assays use enzyme-labeled antibody. The label for both types of assays is alkaline phosphatase, which forms a chemiluminescent product when it hydrolyzes a luminogenic dioxetane substrate.

The major subsystems of the Cirrus IMMULITE are shown in Fig. 19-26. Samples in barcode carriers are loaded onto a continuous conveyor belt (chain loading station) followed by as many as 5 different assay tubes in any order for each patient sample. Additional samples can be loaded at any time, and "stat" samples can be inserted as the next sample to be processed with no loss of throughput. The loading chain has 85 locations for processing sample and assay tubes; new positions are continuously made available every 30 seconds as the chain indexes.

The sample volume is assay dependent. Assays that exceed the linear range of the standard curve are flagged. From the raw signal the IMMULITE can estimate the value of the sample by extrapolation of the standard curve and print out a recommended dilution factor. Samples, however, must be diluted off-line.

The reagent carousel holds as many as 12 resident assays and is thermoelectrically cooled (see Fig. 19-26). There is sufficient reagent for 50 to 100 tests each. All assay tubes are barcoded. After passing a barcode reader, the assay tubes are transferred every 30 seconds to the incubation carousel where the pipettor simultaneously adds sample and labeled reagent (see Fig. 19-26). Tubes in the carousel are agitated every 10 seconds to maximize the reaction. For most assays the incubation time is 30 minutes; tests requiring longer incubation times to enhance their sensitivity have an incubation time of 1 hour. Menu changes can be made during operation by pressing the "Pause" button, which stops the load chain and pipettor.

After incubation of the sample with the alkaline phosphatase labeled reagent, rapid separation and efficient washing of the bead occur by spinning the tube at high speed about its longitudinal axis (see Fig. 19-25). This process causes the unbounded contents to be expelled into a coaxial sump chamber that is an integral part of the tube (see Fig. 19-25). The overall process allows for 4 or more washes to take place within seconds, thus completely removing the unbound

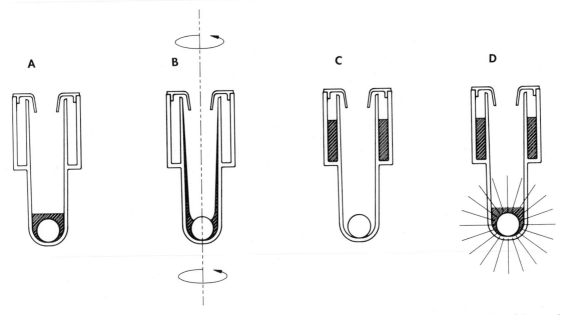

Fig. 19-25 Cross-sections of an IMMULITE assay tube during different operational phases. **A,** tube with sample and label reagent; **B,** tube spinning on its longitudinal axis to transfer sample and reagents to sump; **C,** tube with sample, reagents, and wash in sump; and **D,** tube with luminescent reaction producing light signal (courtesy Cirrus Diagnostics, Inc.).

label from the tubes; it also allows them to be processed sequentially within seconds. The chemiluminescent substrate is then added, and the tube is transferred to the luminometer.

After a 10-minute incubation period at 37° C within the luminometer to develop and maximize the luminescent signal, the light output is measured with a photomultiplier tube. Automatic attenuation of the light signal increases the dynamic range of the measuring system 100-fold. Counts are converted to analyte concentration by use of stored standard curves.

The computer of the Cirrus IMMULITE stores all master standard curves, monthly cali-

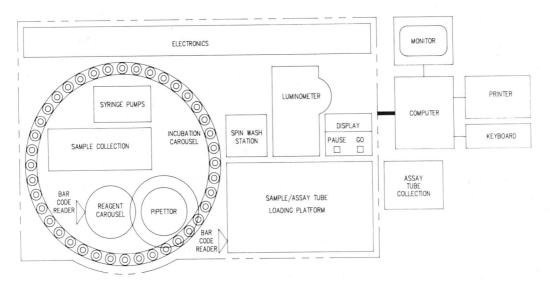

Fig. 19-26 Schematic representation of the major subsystems of the Cirrus IMMULITE (courtesy Cirrus Diagnostics, Inc.).

bration adjustments, and patient and quality control results. This information can be archived, searched, and displayed in a variety of ways or sent to a laboratory information system.

Miles Inc., Diagnostics Division, Technicon Immuno 1. The Technicon Immuno 1 is a fully automated, freestanding immunoassay system that can perform a wide range of tests for thyroid function, therapeutic drug monitoring, anemia, adrenal hormones, and other tests of physiologic importance (Fig. 19-27). The system has been designed to perform testing by patient-orientated random access, batch, or "stat" testing. The system provides for an immunochemistry workstation with throughput and organizational characteristics similar to Technicon's clinical chemistry systems (i.e. Technicon Chem 1).

The Technicon Immuno 1 can perform both homogeneous and heterogeneous assays in any sequence. The separation step for the heterogeneous assays use a universal magnetic particle-antibody conjugate; separation is achieved in less than 1 second. The substrate for all current heterogeneous tests makes use of alkaline phosphatase labels. There is sufficient space on board the instrument to accommodate up to 50 different substrates if future tests require other enzymatic labels. Tests are measured kinetically either by turbidimetry or colorimetry. No pretreatment is required for any assay.

The Technicon Immuno 1 follows 5 basic steps during sample analysis: (1) sample and reagent delivery, (2) incubation and separation, (3) automated detection and signal process, (4) data reduction and calibration, and (5) data reporting. The system is composed of two main modules (see Fig. 19-27). The larger module is the analytic portion of the system. The smaller module is the user interface, which is a full-sized keyboard, printer, and video display terminal (VDT).

A top view of the analytic module is shown in Fig. 19-28. To the left is the sample tray that contains holders for up to 78 samples, including "stats." Samples can be loaded continuously onto the analyzer, generating an expandable worklist. Next to the sample tray (see Fig. 19-28, *top*) is the magnetic particle area where the assays requiring a magnetic particle separation are maintained in 2000 test containers. The large circle in the center is the reaction area that contains reusable reaction cuvettes. All the pipettes required for washing, adding reagent, and substrate are located in this area. Wash solution is used to decontaminate pipettes and reaction cuvettes between tests. To the far right in Fig. 19-28 is the refrigerated reagent storage housing that can

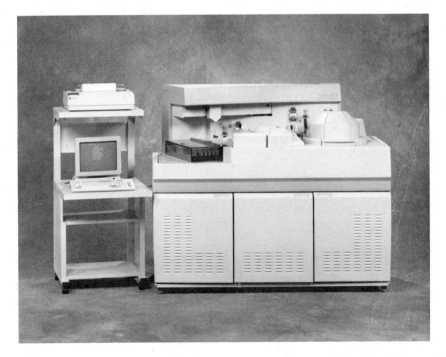

Fig. 19-27   The Technicon Immuno 1 immunoassay system (courtesy Miles, Inc., Diagnostic Division).

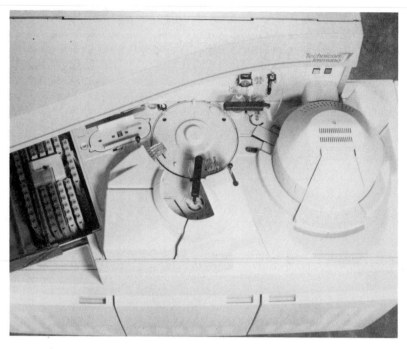

Fig. 19-28   Top view of the Technicon Immuno 1 immunoassay system depicting analytic module (courtesy Miles, Inc., Diagnostic Division).

store up to 22 different reagent (assay) packs. This feature provides extended stability and continuous test flexibility. Reagents are monitored by a reagent inventory system.

Both homogeneous and heterogeneous testing can occur simultaneously in adjacent cuvettes. The incubation time is dictated by the assay. Unlike most immunoassay systems, the Technicon Immuno 1 can alter the incubation times when there is a need for ultrasensitive assays (i.e., thyroid stimulating hormone [TSH]). It does so by taking a reading after the initial incubation and then determining if the assay requires additional incubation to obtain the appropriate test result.

The system's computer has a large storage capacity for samples and test results. It can also generate full page reports for patient, calibration, and quality control data, and produce Levey-Jennings charts.

PB Diagnostics' OPUS, OPUS PLUS, and OPUS MAGNUM

PB Diagnostics' OPUS. The OPUS is a fully automated, continuous-access immunoassay system that has been designed to perform tests for thyroid function, reproductive/fertility hormones, therapeutic drug monitoring, tumor markers, and infectious disease. This benchtop analyzer operates in random-access and "stat"

modes and has the additional capabilities of performing preset panels and batches. For most assays, external pretreatment of specimens is unnecessary (except for Total T_3, where a single dilution step is performed).

Assays are performed using **dry multilayer film** and **fluorogenic enzyme-linked immunosorbent assay (ELISA)** technologies using test modules that are assay specific. There are two types of modules: one for multilayer film assays and the other for fluorogenic ELISA assays.

The multilayer film test module is shown in Fig. 19-29, *A*. This 1½-inch plastic module contains "dry" reagents and is used for analysis of low molecular weight analytes. It consists of a polyester film base coated with an antibody bound to fluorescent-labeled analyte (immune complex) immobilized in an agarose matrix. This layer is called the "signal layer." Above this layer is a second layer composed of agarose containing iron oxide that serves as an "optical screen" preventing the passage of light to the top layers. The topcoat layer contains buffers, surfactants, and additional reagents. This layer also acts as a "molecular sieve," preventing the passage of large molecules and allowing only the smaller analyte molecules to pass on to the signal layer. The topcoat layer is in contact with a grooved surface that promotes uniform spreading and metering of the

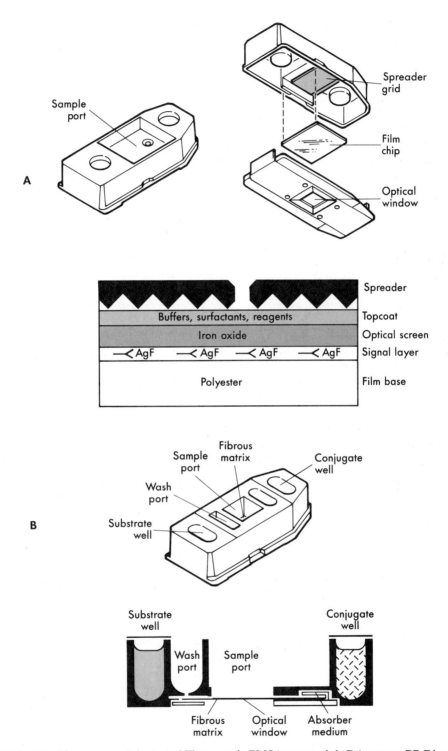

Fig. 19-29 Multifilm test module **A**, and Fluorogenic ELISA test module **B** (courtesy PB Diagnostics, Inc.).

sample. The fluorescent signal is read from below through an opening in the base of the plastic module.

In the multilayer film assay, patient sample containing the analyte of interest is dispensed into the test module via a sample port. The sample then spreads through the top layer and the iron oxide screen layer before it comes into contact with an immune complex in the signal layer. In the signal layer competition occurs between the analyte in the patient sample and the fluorescent-labeled analyte for a limited number of antibody binding sites. Free fluorescent-labeled analyte diffuses into the layers above where it cannot be detected by the optical system. As with other competitive assays, the more analyte in the patient sample, the less fluorescent-labeled analyte that is bound to the antibody of the immune complex. Thus the fluorescence measured is inversely related to the concentration of analyte in the patient sample.

The fluorogenic ELISA test modules use a sandwich immunoassay for large analytes or a sequential-binding immunoassay for smaller analytes (Fig. 19-29, *B*). The ELISA test module is composed of a 1½-inch plastic housing that has individual foil-covered wells for reagents. In the center of the module is the sample port that also contains a fibrous glass matrix coated with an antibody. This area is known as the "reaction zone." The front end well of the module contains the enzyme-antibody conjugate. At the opposite end of the module is a substrate well and a wash port; the latter serves for dispensing substrate.

During a fluorogenic assay, patient sample is applied to the sample port containing the fibrous glass matrix and allowed to incubate for a few minutes with the immobilized antibody (antibody No. 1). After incubation enzyme-antibody conjugate (antibody No. 2) is pipetted into this reaction zone whereby a "sandwich"-immune complex is formed (antibody No. 1-patient analyte-antibody No. 2/enzyme). Substrate is applied to the wash port and migrates to the reaction zone by capillary action. At the same time unbound conjugate is picked up by an absorber medium. The substrate (4-methylumbelliferyl phosphate) is converted into a fluorescent product (4-methylumbelliferone) by the enzyme (alkaline phosphatase) that is conjugated to the antibody. With the sandwich-type assays the amount of fluorescence is directly proportional to the concentration of the analyte in the patient sample; with the sequential-type assays the amount of fluorescence is inversely proportional to the concentration of the analyte in the patient sample.

The OPUS consists of several subassemblies: (1) operator interface (touch screen/display and thermal printer), (2) tray assembly, (3) internal barcode reader, (4) loader/ejector, (5) incubator rotor, (6) pipetting station, (7) optics module/fluorimeter, and (8) computer/data reduction system (Fig. 19-30).

All functions are initiated through the interactive touch screen/display. The operator simply selects the tests by touching the screen. The OPUS also has an optional bar code wand that can be used to enter alpha-numeric patient information directly from the sample tube. Results of calibrations, raw instrument readings, and calculated results are printed by a built-in 40 column thermal printer with alpha-numeric and graphic capabilities.

The operator inserts assay-specific, bar coded test modules one at a time into the loading port of the analyzer. The OPUS accepts 20 modules in about 2 minutes. The operator then loads the sample and pipette trays onto the tray assembly. The tray assembly holds a single tray of up to 20 patient samples and two trays of pipette tips. Once the modules, samples, and pipettes have been loaded onto the tray assembly, the load/ejector transports the test modules to a 20-position incubated rotor. The incubated rotor has several functions: (1) it rotates the test modules to the pipetting station, (2) it rotates test modules to the reading station, and (3) it brings test modules back to the loader/ejector where they are ejected into the waste drawer.

Between the tray assembly and the incubator is the pipettor assembly that automatically dispenses the sample/reagent onto the test module (see Fig. 19-30). The pipettor assembly consists of an automatic pipettor mounted on a motor-driven arm that has both vertical and horizontal movement. The arm moves the pipettor over the tray assembly for access to pipette tips and sample cups. The arm then moves the pipettor to the pipettor port of the incubator where it transfers patient samples and reagent (conjugate, substrate) to the sample port of the test module. After the pipette tip has been used it is discarded. Because the analyzer changes pipette tips before each pipetting step there is no sample carryover between measurements. After the appropriate incubation time, the test module is rotated via the incubator rotor to the "reading" station where a

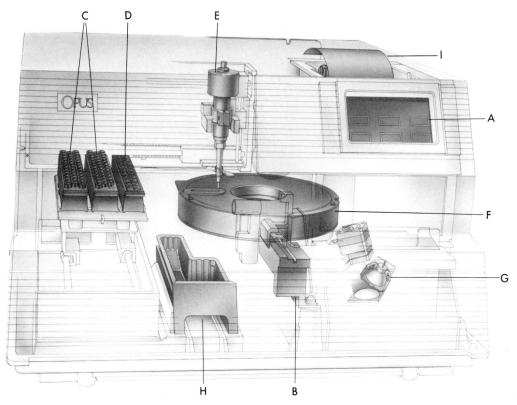

Fig. 19-30 Subassemblies of the PB Diagnostics OPUS. *A*, touchscreen; *B*, loader; *C*, pipette tip tray; *D*, sample tray; *E*, pipettor; *F*, rotor; *G*, optics; *H*, waste drawer; and *I*, printer (courtesy PB Diagnostics, Inc.).

fluorescent signal is detected by the fluorimeter and subsequently converted into a test result by the data reduction system and printed using the thermal printer. Dilutions are performed off-line if the patient test result exceeds the upper range of the instrument.

The optics module/fluorimeter consists of a tungsten halogen light source, excitation and emission filters, and two photodiodes (Fig. 19-31). The optics module (fluorimeter) reads diffuse fluorescence from the test module surface. Light from the lamp passes through a 3-position filter wheel that has 1 blocking filter and 2 pairs of matched excitation/emission narrow band filters, 360 nm/450 nm (for ELISA-based assays) and 550 nm/580 nm (for multilayer film assays). The light passing through the excitation filters excites the fluorescent tag and thus illuminates the surface of the module. This light excites the fluorophore molecules in the test module to fluoresce. The emitted light passes through the 450 nm or 580 nm emission filter before it is focused onto a silicon photodiode. This photodiode produces a current proportional to the intensity of the incident light. The second photodiode converts light from the excitation filter to provide a reference reading. For multilayer assays two fluorometric readings are taken; multiple readings are taken for ELISA-based assays. After the test module has been read, the rotor then moves it to the loader/ejector where it is ejected into the waste drawer.

The OPUS computer controls and monitors all instrument functions. It also provides on-screen help messages and monitors an internal inventory system for pipette tips, waste drawer capacity, and used test modules. The operator responds to instrument prompts to empty the waste drawer and to refill pipette tips. Maintenance requirements with the OPUS are minimal.

PB Diagnostics' OPUS PLUS. The OPUS PLUS is a recent derivative of the OPUS Immunoassay system. It is based on the same multilayer dry film and fluorogenic ELISA technology and has many of the same features as the OPUS. The subassemblies that are unique to the OPUS Plus are those required for making dilutions. Two dilution trays hold on-board diluent packs

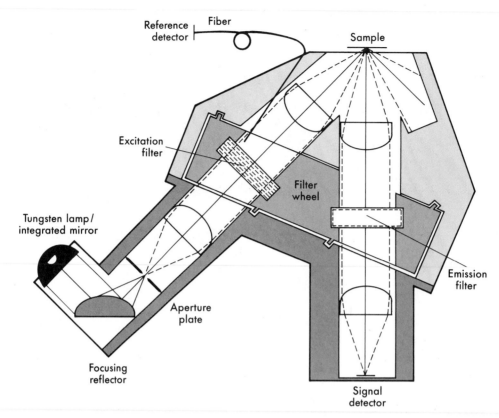

Fig. 19-31 Optics module of the PB Diagnostics OPUS (courtesy PB Diagnostics, Inc.).

and cups for serial dilutions and pretreatment solutions; each holds up to 7 different solutions. The OPUS Plus also inventories these supplies and prompts the operator if more dilution cups are needed.

The pipettor assembly consists of a microprocessor-controlled pipette that not only delivers all samples and reagents, but also performs onboard dilutions (for such assays as hCG) and pretreatment steps (for analysis of T_3). The automatic dilution sequence allows selection of up to 3 dilutions along with the neat sample (i.e., with hCG, a dilution sequence could be 1:10, 1:100, and 1:1000), and calculates values in terms of concentration in the undiluted specimen. In the stat mode all 3 dilutions are performed. The bar code reader has the capability of identifying appropriate diluents and pretreatment solutions.

In addition to the key features mentioned previously, the OPUS Plus has an increased storage capacity for pipette tips and provides for immediate "stat" access. The stat interrupt feature allows the operator to load stat samples in 1 minute; the maximum wait time is only 4 minutes. Two separate tray drives allow for faster access for processing of stat samples.

PB Diagnostics' OPUS MAGNUM. The OPUS MAGNUM is PB Diagnostics' newest and most sophisticated immunoassay system (Fig. 19-32). This fully automated benchtop model is a high throughput, random and continuous access analyzer; stats are processed in 6 minutes. Like the OPUS and OPUS Plus, all tests employ their own sample tips that are changed with each sample/pipetting step, ensuring no carryover between samples.

The OPUS MAGNUM can use sample cups or primary tubes for loading samples. The instrument has an internal barcode reader that can read the barcoding of the primary tube and thus ensures positive sample ID and patient demographics. Specimens can be added via the sample handling port by the addition of several sample trays. The operator simply loads the samples into the trays, selects the proper test, and presses a "run" button. Samples are then automatically entered

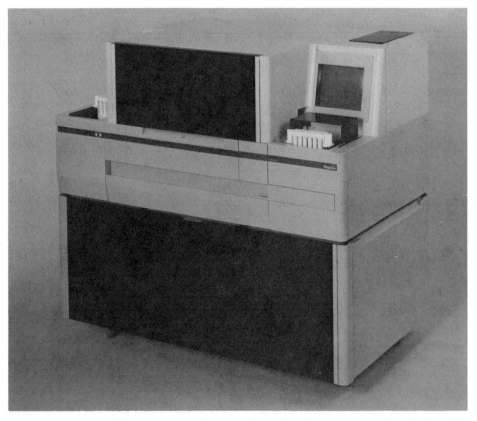

Fig. 19-32   PB Diagnostics OPUS MAGNUM (courtesy PB Diagnostics, Inc.).

into the instrument for processing. After the sample is aspirated the sample tray moves to the exit port.

The test modules are identical to those used on the OPUS and the OPUS PLUS. The difference is in the magazine configuration that holds these modules. With the OPUS MAGNUM reagents are stored on board the instrument in test-specific magazines, each capable of holding 10 modules. Each magazine is self-contained with test module, desiccant, and a foil protective cover. The operator simply loads the magazines onto the specially designed crescent-shaped rack. A total of 36 test-specific magazines can be loaded and stored on board at one time, thus the on-board capacity is 360 tests. Bar coding at the base of each magazine tells the OPUS MAGNUM the test lot number and date of the assay that has been loaded. The multi-tasking software of OPUS MAGNUM also allows the operator to reload magazines during instrument processing. Depending on the test mix and volume, single or

multiple assays can be placed on the reagent carousel, allowing the operator to batch one assay or randomly select up to 36 different assays.

The operator interfaces with the OPUS MAGNUM via the alpha-numeric keyboard or with the special operations provided by the interactive touch screen. The touch screen also displays a status update of the current inventories of each assay that is on board, providing such information as the test name, lot number, and quantity per one third of the carousel. The analyzer has a unique way of displaying and prompting operator functions for routine processing, stat processing, calibration, quality control assessment, and selection of the test menu. A color coded/highlighted system is used to prompt the operator with additional information. For example, tests that are highlighted can be processed; tests colored in green are on board and calibrated; tests highlighted in amber are on board, but not calibrated; and tests highlighted in red are not on board the analyzer; however, they may be calibrated if in current use. The OPUS MAGNUM can also calibrate different lots of the same assay; calibration curves are displayed on the same plot in different colors. Multiple lots can be stored on board at one time providing for immediate use of a new lot number of reagents.

Serono-Baker Diagnostics' SR1. The Serono-Baker SR1 is a fully automated immunoassay system with the ability to perform a variety of laboratory tests such as thyroid and reproductive hormones, cardiac markers, tumor markers, therapeutic drugs (i.e., digoxin) and tests related to nutritional assessment and infectious disease. This compact benchtop analyzer is designed to perform in a discrete, random access mode or in single or multiple batch modes; any combination of analytes can be processed in batch mode.

Central to the operation of the Serono-Baker SR1 are its self-contained, reagent cartridges that are bar coded for each specific assay. The polystyrene cartridges contain several wells (Fig. 19-33). All reactions occur in the 2 long reaction chambers with absorbance readings being taken via the optical windows. Each reaction chamber contains a 2-mm steel ball that enhances the mixing of reagents. Next to the reaction chamber are 3 narrow wells that contain predispensed reagent specific for a given assay. The top of the cartridge, composed of the reaction and reagent wells, is foil-sealed. The 2 circular wells are used to hold sample (patient specimen, controls, and/or calibrators); the 2 square wells are for sample dilutions.

The SR1 uses a unique approach to standardization. Every cartridge houses a well that contains a prepackaged standard (see Fig. 19-33). Using this standard a one-point calibration is performed every 4 hours with a sample run. A 6-point calibration is recommended on receipt of a new shipment of reagents, every 2 weeks thereafter, or as quality control dictates.

The SR1 system uses monoclonal and polyclonal antibodies, magnetic solid phase separation technology, and enzyme/substrate color development to carry out either direct immunoenzymetric assays (IEMA) or competitive enzyme immunoassays (EIA). The direct configuration is used for large molecules such as protein hormones (Fig. 19-34). In this method hormone in the patient sample is first incubated along with two antibodies directed toward different sites of the hormone; one is labeled with fluorescein (FITC), the other with the enzyme alkaline phosphatase (E). The reaction forms a sandwich that

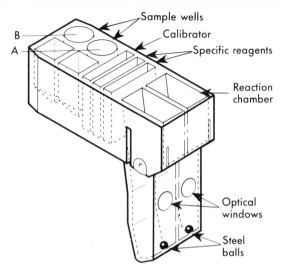

Fig. 19-33 The Serono-Baker SR1 sample/reagent cartridge (courtesy Serono-Baker Diagnostics).

is directly proportional to the amount of hormone present.

The competitive assay is used for small molecules such as T_4 and T_3. A conjugate of the same hormone labeled with FITC is added to compete with the hormone in the patient sample for an enzyme-labeled antibody (i.e., with alkaline phosphatase). Thus at equilibrium the amount of FITC-labeled hormone bound to the antibody is inversely proportional to the amount of hormone in the patient sample.

To separate the bound fraction from the free fraction, magnetic particles conjugated to a fluorescein antibody (separation reagent) are added (see Fig. 19-34). In the IEMA-type assays the magnetic particles combine with the FITC-antibody/hormone/antibody-enzyme complexes, as well as nonreacted FITC-antibody. With the EIA assays the magnetic particles combine with the FITC-labeled hormone/enzyme-labeled antibody and the free FITC-labeled hormone. In both types of assays, only FITC-labeled antibody that is part of the hormone-antibody-complex bound to enzyme will be measured photometrically after the addition of a chromogenic substrate.

Before the substrate is added the magnetic particles are separated from the liquid containing nonreacted constituents by use of a powerful magnet. After removing this liquid the magnetic particle complex is incubated with the chromogenic substrate, phenolphthalein monophosphate. The enzymatic reaction produces free phe-

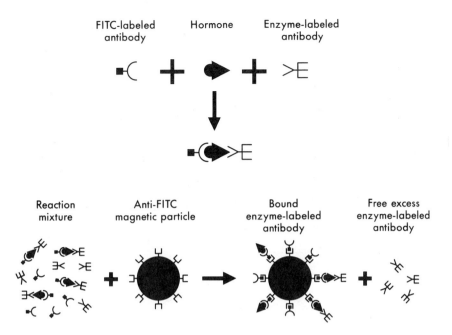

Fig. 19-34 Principle of the SR1 direct immunoenzymetric assay (IEMA) (courtesy Serono-Baker Diagnostics).

nolphthalein. The reaction is stopped by the addition of a highly alkaline solution that also causes the indicator, phenolphthalein, to produce a pink color. The amount of pink color is proportional to the amount of hormone. In an IEMA, the color development is directly related to the concentration of hormone; with an EIA the color development is inversely proportional.

The SR1 system is composed of the following subsystems: (1) computer console (keypad covered with a sealed membrane, display screen, and disk drive), (2) cartridge loading ramp, (3) cartridge extractor, (4) syringe/valve assembly for dispensing sample/reagent, (5) common reagent compartment, (6) carousel, (7) photometer assembly, and (8) thermal printer (Fig. 19-35). The display screen provides the SR1 operator with menu-driven on-screen instructions that tell the operator of the system's status and any instructions required before and during analysis. The instrument has a barcode wand for automatic entry of all calibration parameters, assay types, and specimen IDs. The SR1 also has on-line dilution capabilities.

Before the cartridge is processed an aliquot of the patient's sample is pipetted into the appropriate sample well of the cartridge. The manner in which the sample is added to the reagent cartridge depends on the mode of testing: random access, batch, or profile. For random access mode

the patient sample is placed in the first sample well **A**, and calibrator in the second well **B**; for a batch mode the sample is placed in the first well, **A**, and calibrator in the second well, **B**, of the first cartridge only; for profile testing the sample is placed into the first well, **A**, only (see Fig. 19-33).

After the sample has been added to the cartridge, it is placed onto a conveyor belt that has an 11-cartridge capacity (see Fig. 19-35). A stat sample can be placed on the belt before other unscheduled cartridges by reversing the conveyor belt. This belt advances cartridges onto a continuous-loading platform, the incubation carousel. In the center of the carousel is a holder for the separation reagent. As an empty position opens on the carousel, the cartridge is loaded via the cartridge extractor to the pipetting and separating stations. As the extractor moves the cartridge onto the carousel, it passes a barcode reader that scans the bar code label on the side of the cartridge.

The syringe/valve assembly controls liquid aspiration and delivery via the sample probe. Once the cartridge is on the carousel a pipetting sequence takes place whereby the probe aspirates a measured volume of sample and then dispenses it into the reaction well. The sample probe picks up a measured quantity of reagent from the first reagent compartment and transfers the reagent to the reaction chamber containing the sample.

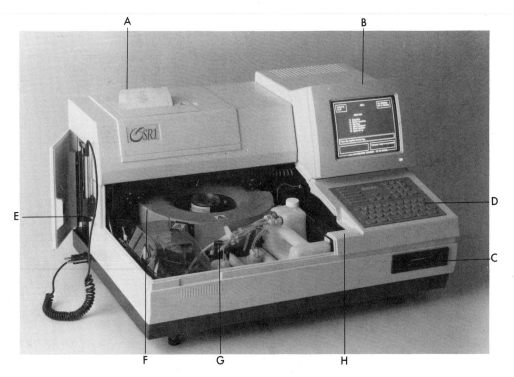

Fig. 19-35 The subsystems of the Serono-Baker Diagnostics SR1. *A*, printer; *B*, display panel; *C*, 3.5″ floppy drive (software updates); *D*, sealed keypad; *E*, barcode wand; *F*, temperature-controlled carousel; *G*, common reagents; and *H*, cartridge-loading ramp (courtesy Serono-Baker Diagnostics).

This sequence is repeated for the second reagent. However, depending on the assay, it may take place immediately after a predetermined incubation period or after the separation reagent is added and incubated. Mixing is accomplished by stainless steel beads located in the reaction cells. To minimize sample carryover, the outside of the probe is washed during the pipetting sequence. The common reagents (wash solution, enzyme substrate, and stop solution) are supplied in bottles and are delivered via specific needles positioned over the right-hand end of the cartridge extractor.

After incubation the cartridges are transported via the carousel to the right-hand end of the extractor and into contact with the SR1 permanent magnet. The magnetic housing is used to separate the magnetic solid phase. While the magnetic particles are drawn to the side of the tube, the reaction mixture is aspirated to waste followed by resuspension of the particles in wash solution. After the cartridge is replaced on the carousel for a brief incubation period, this process is repeated with no incubation phase. Substrate solution is added to the washed beads, followed by incubation, and then addition of stop reagent to develop

the pink color of phenolphthalein. Toward the front of the carousel shield is an eject mechanism to remove cartridges that have been completely processed.

The optical system is also located on the same housing as the permanent magnet. It consists of two tungsten halogen lamps, a filter wheel assembly that contains 3 interference filters (490 nm, 554 nm, 650 nm), and the photocell detectors. These detectors are the broad-band gallium arsenide type with a range of 400 to 760 nm. During color measurement the filter wheel turns to send light of all 3 wavelengths through the reaction chambers to the detectors where absorption is measured. Depending on the concentration the absorbance at 554 nm (peak absorbance for low concentration of analyte) or 490 nm (low absorbance for high concentration of analyte) is used. The 650 nm reading is taken to reduce any interferences because of variations in the optical surfaces of the cartridges and turbidity of solutions.

The SR1 computer monitors all system parameters including temperature, pressures, diluent inventory, and the status of the disposable waste container. The waste container can be emptied without shutting down the system via the maintenance menu program. From the applications program the instrument can perform daily or weekly cleaning. The Catalyst software provides the instrument with several new enhancements related to storage of calibration curves and patient data and the ability to run batch samples in a continuous access mode.

SYVA ETS and ETS Plus Systems. The Syva ETS is a fully automated analyzer for qualitative screening of drugs of abuse in urine. The Syva ETS Plus system is an upgrade to the ETS system that allows it to perform quantitative analysis of ethyl alcohol in serum/plasma and urine and qualitative analysis of barbiturates, benzodiazepines, and tricyclic antidepressants in serum. The upgrade also includes an enhanced software package with troubleshooting features that provide error detection, a new pump design, and sample tray cover. Because both analyzers are similar in design only the Syva ETS Plus system will be discussed.

The drugs of abuse assays are based on Syva's enzyme multiplied immunoassay technique (EMIT) technology (Fig. 19-36). It involves competitive binding technology using the enzyme, glucose-6-phosphate dehydrogenase, bound to a drug as a conjugate tracer. Competition for an antibody specific for a particular drug occurs between drug in the patient sample and the drug bound to enzyme. If the enzyme-bound drug is not bound by antibody it will remain active. Active enzyme will catalyze the substrate, glucose-6-phosphate, converting the coenzyme NAD to NADH. This reaction produces a photometric change that can be detected at 340 nm by the analyzer. The higher the concentration of unlabeled drug in the patient sample, the less antibody available to bind to the enzyme-labeled drug. More of the enzyme-labeled drug remains free and thus becomes available to catalyze the aforementioned reaction. The amount of NADH generated, and thus absorbance change, is directly proportional to the amount of analyte present in the serum/plasma or urine sample.

The drugs of abuse assays are not quantitative. Photometric absorbance readings are taken on assay reactions over timed intervals. By comparing the absorbance change for a sample with that

Emit Drug Assay Principle

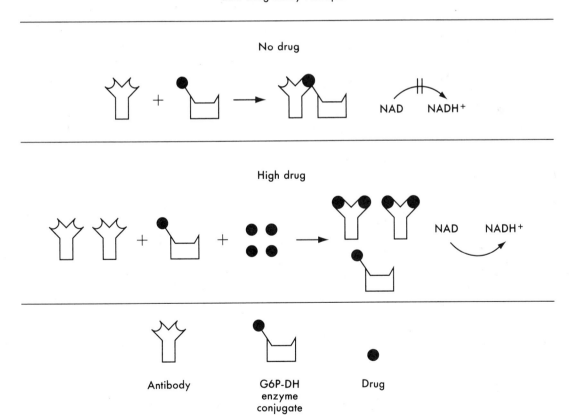

Fig. 19-36 Principle of homogeneous enzyme-multiplied immunoassay technique, EMIT (courtesy SYVA Company).

of a low calibrator containing a known quantity of drug or drug metabolite, the presence of drug in the sample can be determined. Three calibrators are supplied: negative (containing no drug), low (representing the cutoff level), and medium (representing a positive). The reaction rate of the low calibrator serves as the "cutoff" or reference point for determining sample results. A sample is considered positive if its reaction rate is equal to or greater than that of the low calibrator. The negative and medium calibrators serve as controls to monitor and validate reagent and instrument performance.

Unlike drugs of abuse assays the assay for ethyl alcohol is a quantitative assay. It uses alcohol dehydrogenase to catalyze the oxidation of ethyl alcohol and the reduction of the co-enzyme NAD to acetaldehyde and NADH, respectively. The formation of NADH causes a photometric change that is directly proportional to the amount of alcohol present in the sample. The change in absorbance of a calibrator that contains a known amount of ethyl alcohol is compared with the sample to determine the concentration of ethyl alcohol.

The Syva ETS Plus system automatically measures and mixes samples, reagents, and buffer. The system computer interprets operator input, processes assay data, and interprets results. The operator can select up to 6 assays for each sample to be run in batch panel screening or random access mode. Identification numbers can be preassigned for up to 96 samples.

The operator interacts with several major components either during operation of the system or for maintenance. A schematic of these components is presented in Fig. 19-37. The keypad/display unit is composed of 7 lights that indicate whether the instrument is in one of the following modes: standby, processing, assay selection, sample identification, or calibration. These keys are used for assay entry, sample identification, and control of system functions. The display shows the assays selected for each sample and the tray, cup, and ID number. It also prompts the operator and provides error or status messages. The carousel consists of (1) a 16-position sample tray for calibrators, controls, or samples, (2) a reagent rack that holds up to 6 reagent vial cassettes, and (3) a carousel cover that protects samples, calibrators, and reagents.

The Syva ETS Plus system has two fluid reservoirs, one for assay buffer and one for distilled or deionized water. A syringe (pipettor/dilutor) assembly dispenses the appropriate volume of sample, reagent, and buffer. A liquid-sensing probe assembly transfers samples, reagents, and buffer to cuvettes. An internal heater serves to regulate buffer temperature. The cuvette compartment accommodates a 24-well cuvette; it is kept in a thermally controlled block that moves into the photometer unit for reaction rate measurement. The operator is prompted to replace cuvettes when there are no usable wells remaining before or during an analytic run. The photometer takes readings of the reaction mixture through the cuvette over a 30-second period. The amount of transmitted light is measured by the detector.

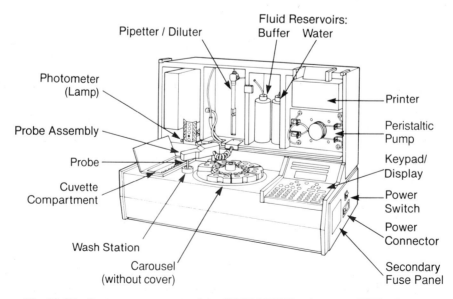

Fig. 19-37 System components of the SYVA ETS Plus (courtesy SYVA Company).

Test results and stored parameters are generated in a 20-character-per-line format using a dot-matrix printer. An RS-232 port is also provided that can be used to interface the instrument with the Syva EDMS, a PC-based data management and reporting system that automates data collection and storage of calibration and test results.

Unlike most of the immunoassay instrument manufacturers, Syva's EMIT reagents do not have to be used exclusively with the Syva ETS instrument line. They can be and are often used on other "open" systems where a high volume of drug screens are being performed. However, for laboratories that have low to medium volumes, the Syva ETS and/or ETS Plus systems are quick, easy to use automated analyzers that will simplify the task of screening for drugs of abuse. With higher volumes, linking several ETS Plus analyzers (up to 5) to the Syva EDMS data management system will facilitate the workflow and will in result faster processing.

Tosoh Medics AIA-1200 and AIA-600. The Tosoh Medics AIA-1200 and AIA-600 are fully automated, continuous random-access immunoassay analyzers that use fluorescent rate enzyme immunoassay methods. The AIA-1200 is a floor model (Fig. 19-38), whereas the AIA-600 is designed to be a benchtop model (Fig. 19-39). Both instruments are capable of running all analytes in a "true" random access mode. The test menu includes assays for thyroid assessment, fertility hormones, insulin, human growth hormone, tumor markers, cardiac assessment, and anemia.

Both instruments are also based on the same enzyme immunoassay technology. They can perform heterogeneous immunoenzymometric (sandwich) and competitive binding assays. Alkaline phosphatase is used as the label and catalyzes the conversion of 4-methylumbelliferyl phosphate to the fluorescent compound, 4-methylumbelliferone. All reactions require an incubation time of 40 minutes at 37° C.

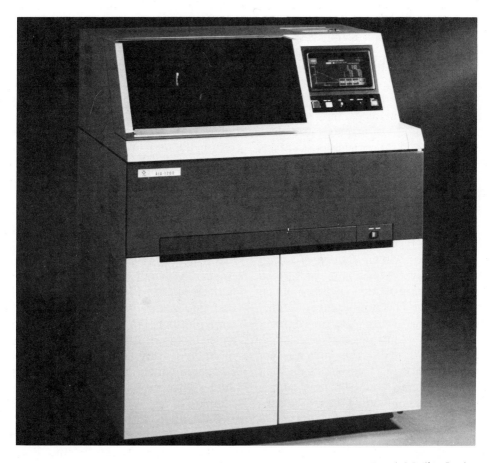

Fig. 19-38 Tosoh Medics AIA-1200 immunoassay system (courtesy Tosoh Medics, Inc.).

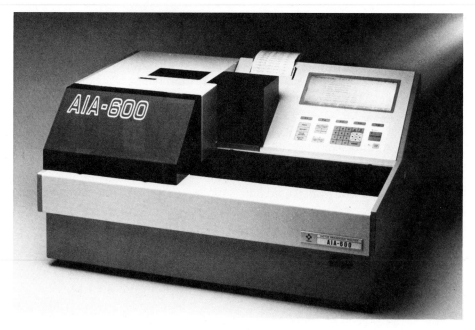

Fig. 19-39   Tosoh Medics AIA-600 immunoassay system (courtesy Tosoh Medics, Inc.).

Central to the operation of the AIA-1200 and AIA-600 is the AIA-PACK reagent system (Fig. 19-40). The AIA-PACK is a readily disposable plastic test cup that contains all the necessary reagents to perform an assay procedure using either a sandwich assay or competitive assay. All reactions and final measurements occur within this reagent pack. The reagents are lyophilized to permit long-term storage. The capture antibody is immobilized on a solid support composed of ferrite-coated microbeads (paramagnetic particles) that are used to separate the free labeled conjugate from that of the bound. The AIA-PACK reagents are stored in plastic bar coded trays (20 cups/tray).

In the sandwich-type assays (used for larger molecules), two monoclonal antibodies are directed at different sites of the analyte of interest. One antibody is immobilized on the paramagnetic particles; the other is conjugated to alkaline phosphatase (see Fig. 19-40). With the competitive assays (used for smaller molecules), alkaline phosphatase is conjugated to the antigen rather than a second antibody. This conjugate then competes with the analyte in the patient sample for a limited number of binding sites on the antibody-coated paramagnetic particle (see Fig. 19-40).

In both assays, after incubation and a series of washes, fluorogenic substrate is added to the re-

agent test cups to produce a fluorescent signal that is either directly proportional (sandwich assays) or inversely proportional (competitive assays) to the analyte concentration. The overall process is illustrated in Fig. 19-40. Both the AIA-1200 and the AIA-600 have a positive reagent identification system. The AIA-1200 uses the bar code on the reagent trays to identify the analyte and provide an automated mechanism for assessing the reagent inventory. The AIA-600 contains a video camera that reads the pattern recognition code that is found on the top of each test cup.

The optical system of the analyzers uses **top-to-top fluorescence detection** with a discrete excitation wavelength of 365 nm and an emission wavelength of 440 to 500 nm. Light of the appropriate wavelength is directed to the upper surface of the reagent test cup. Fluorescence produced in each cup by the conversion of 4-methylumbelliferyll phosphate to 4-methylumbelliferone is detected by the optical system. This fluorescence is monitored every second for 100 seconds and compared with a reference channel. The rate of fluorescence production is calculated for each sample.

Calibration can be performed at any time during a patient run and can be analyzed in any number of replicates up to nine. Both systems recognize a new lot number of reagents and

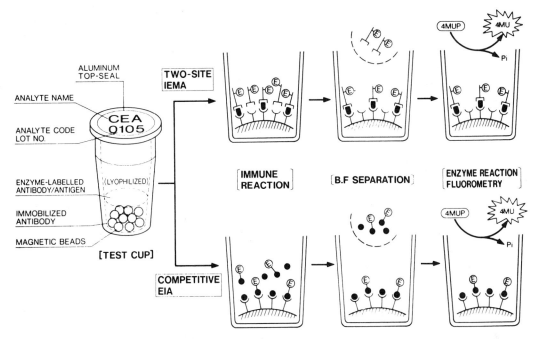

Fig. 19-40 Reaction schematic of the Tosoh Medics AIA-PACK test cup technology (courtesy Tosoh Medics, Inc.).

prompt the operator that a calibration is warranted. The software also keeps track of the time since the last calibration and alerts the operator of the need for recalibration. The recalibration interval can be set by the operator.

Tosoh Medics AIA-1200. The AIA-1200 measures samples with a positive displacement syringe using disposable pipette tips. The pipette tip is rinsed between tests on the same sample and changed between samples, thus eliminating any possibility of carryover. If a dilution is required it must be performed "off" line. The AIA-1200 has an optical, noncontact type of infrared sample level sensor. Up to 100 patient samples can be initially loaded into the sample racks (10 racks with 10 samples/rack); samples can be added at any time during the operation of the instrument. Twenty-one different analytes can be kept on board simultaneously; the on-board assay capacity is 420 AIA-PACKs.

With the AIA-1200 immunoassay system, there are three approaches to entering sample and test request information: (1) direct operator interaction via a touch screen, (2) downloading from a diskette, or (3) by downloading from a host computer. After generating a worklist, sample cups and pipette tips for each specimen are loaded into the racks that are placed on the top left of the instrument.

After the assay process begins, the instrument selects the AIA-PACK test cups from the reagent inventory drawer and transfers them to the transport blocks using a bar code reader and cup sensor (Fig. 19-41). The test cups are then transported to the sampling station via an elevator where, after a 10-minute preincubation period, the cup's foil seals are broken. The instrument attaches a pipette tip to the sampling arm and dispenses sample and diluent into the test cups to annotate the immune reaction; the pipette tip is then discarded. The test cups are then incubated for 40 minutes at 37° C during which they are agitated over the course of the reaction. After the 40-minute incubation period the contents of the test cups are washed twice under magnetic agitation using preheated wash solution. Substrate is then added and the incubation is continued. The AIA-1200 completes the analysis by reading the fluorescence rate of five test cups simultaneously, using top-to-top fluorescence detection. A schematic of the functional components involved with this overall process is shown in Fig. 19-41.

A stat sample can be placed in the analyzer at any time. The analyzer will interrupt its loading process and process the stat sample in the next available position. There is one stat position on the analyzer that can be used repeatedly.

The instrument has the capabilities of per-

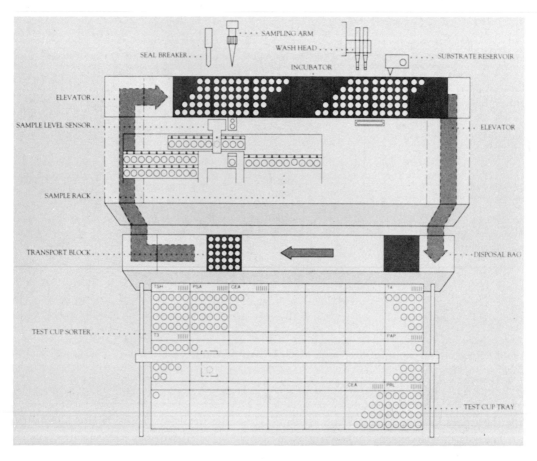

Fig. 19-41   Schematic of the functional components of the Tosoh Medics AIA-1200 immunoassay system (courtesy Tosoh Medics, Inc.).

forming automatic workload recording, generating patient histograms, and providing a wide selection of reporting formats for patient results. One of the most unique features of the instrument is its capability for remote diagnostics through a telephone modem.

Tosoh Medics AIA-600. The AIA-600 uses two independent continuous chains, one for samples and one for the AIA-PACK test cups (Fig. 19-42). Up to 40 specimens and 40 test cups can be initially loaded, providing about 50 minutes of walk-away time. As soon as the assay process is initiated additional sample cups and/or test cups can be added at any time. The design of the AIA-600 is such that there is no need for a dedicated "stat" position. A stat sample can be placed on the sample line at any time in the first available position.

The operator can request tests via a membrane keypad or by downloading from a host computer.

Tests can also be automatically generated by the on board video camera once the assay process has begun. After the patient sample has been placed on the sample cup chain (line) and the AIA-PACK test cup in the corresponding position on the test cup chain (line), the instrument is ready for sample processing.

The AIA-600 moves test cups past a video camera that scans for a pattern recognition code. The analyzer then generates a worklist if one has not been entered. If one has been entered via the keypad or by downloading from a host computer, the instrument verifies proper placement of the test cups. The AIA-600 then breaks the test cup seal and dispenses the required amount of sample and diluent to annotate the immune reaction. The sample probe is then washed internally and externally before it is used again for another sample. The sequence of events that follow (i.e., incubation time, washing, and measurement of flu-

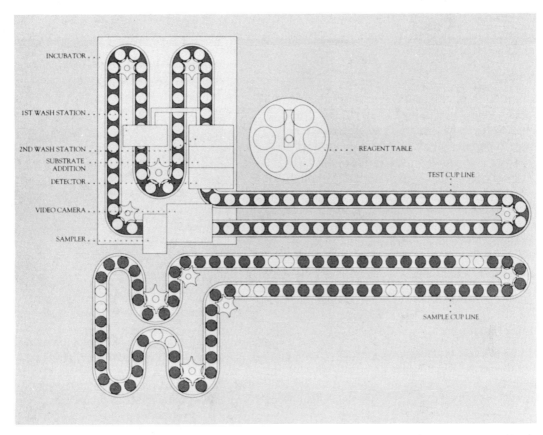

Fig. 19-42 Schematic of the functional components of the Tosoh Medics AIA-600 immunoassay system (courtesy Tosoh Medics, Inc.).

Automated Immunoassay Systems: Benefits and Drawbacks

Benefits

Accuracy
  Computer-defined (robotic) pipetting
  Calibration-curve storage
Cost
  Fewer repeat analyses
  Fewer disposables
  Smaller sample size
Labor
  No dedicated operator
  Ease of training
  Ease of use
Safety
  Nonisotopic reagents
  Reduction in hazardous waste

Versatility
  Extensive menu of specialized tests
  Reagents packaged in different sizes
Workstation consolidation
  Bench space
  Reagent storage

Drawbacks

Analyzer downtime
Cost
  Acquisition
  Maintenance contract
Closed-reagent systems
Limited test menu

orescence) is similar to the AIA-1200. A schematic of the functional components pertaining to these events is depicted in Fig. 19-42.

Summary

Automation of nonisotopic immunochemistries has had a major impact in all clinical laboratories. Many tests that traditionally had to be performed by reference or specialty laboratories can now be performed on-site in hospitals, clinics, and physician office laboratories. Although there are many benefits in performing such assays in-house, there are some drawbacks. Both have been summarized in the box on p. 357. In general the benefits outweigh the drawbacks. These instruments have provided a mechanism to produce accurate, reliable test results with a reduction in turn-around-time, thus improving overall patient care.

Review Questions

1. The drawbacks of performing analyses by radioimmunoassay (RIA) include all of the following except:
   A. Poor sensitivity
   B. Very labor-intensive
   C. Short shelf-life of reagents
   D. Handling of radioactive waste
   E. Difficult to automate

2. Which one of the following statements is false regarding the general principles of immunoassay measurement?
   A. The analyte of interest may be either an antigen or antibody
   B. Haptens are highly antigenic in vivo and therefore are often incorporated into in vitro analyses
   C. The term "ligand" refers to the analyte being measured
   D. A tracer is chemically bonded to a ligand to help monitor the reaction
   E. Isotopes are examples of early tracers

3. Regarding homogeneous and heterogeneous techniques, which one of the following statements is false?
   A. A separation step is required for heterogeneous assays
   B. Low molecular weight analytes are often measured by homogeneous techniques
   C. ELISA techniques are classified as homogeneous
   D. Heterogeneous assays often incorporate a means of solid support
   E. The final mixture that is analyzed in a homogeneous system contains both free and bound analyte

4. Regarding competitive and sequential immunoassays, which one of the following statements is false?
   A. Sequential (noncompetitive) methods are more sensitive than competitive methods
   B. Therapeutic drugs are often monitored by competitive methods
   C. The analyte competes with a labeled analyte for binding sites in a competitive assay
   D. Only the free labeled analyte may be quantitated when using competitive methods
   E. The component in excess in sequential immunoassays is the antibody to the analyte

5. Features of the Abbott TDx include all of the following except:
   A. True random access capabilities
   B. Use of fluorescein as a tracer
   C. Extensive test menu
   D. A 6-point calibration curve
   E. Ability to perform nephelometric assays

6. Which statement is false regarding the Abbott IMx?
   A. Microparticle enzyme immunoassay (MEIA) is a heterogeneous assay used for larger molecules
   B. The reaction cell cuvettes serve as the separation medium in MEIA procedures
   C. The fluorescent polarization immunoassay (FPIA) methodology is identical to the TDx
   D. Two optical systems are contained within the analyzer
   E. All FPIA procedures from the TDx may be run on the IMx

7. The analyzer that employs the principle of radial partition immunoassay (RPIA) is the:
   A. Abbott TDxFLx
   B. Cirrus IMMULITE
   C. Serono Baker SR1
   D. Baxter Stratus II
   E. Ciba Corning ACS:180

8. Analyzers with a "stat" interrupt capability include all of the following EXCEPT the:
   A. Becton Dickinson Affinity
   B. Boehringer Mannheim ES 300
   C. Tosoh Medics AIA-600
   D. Baxter Stratus II
   E. PB Diagnostics OPUS

9. Which statement is false regarding ImmUnits, the self-contained reagent cartridge of the Becton Dickinson Affinity?
   A. Each cartridge is bar coded to contain the test name and lot number
   B. The cartridges are used for running calibrations, controls, and patient samples
   C. The cartridges act as the solid (separation) phase in the heterogeneous EIA techniques employed by the system

D. Each cartridge may be used to analyze 50 to 100 samples

E. Reagent stability approaches 6 months when properly stored

10. The Syva ETS exceeds the capabilities of the Abbott ADx in terms of:
   A. Sample carousel capacity
   B. Test menu selection
   C. Throughput time
   D. Sample volume requirements
   E. Panel testing

11. Immunoassay analyzers currently employing chemiluminescence technology include:
   A. The Cirrus IMMULITE and the PB Diagnostics OPUS
   B. The Ciba Corning ACS:180 and the Cirrus IMMULITE
   C. The Abbott IMx and the Abbott TDxFLx
   D. The Serono Baker SR1 and the Boehringer Mannheim ES 300
   E. The Tosoh Medics AIA-1200 and the Baxter STRATUS IIntellect

12. Dry, multilayer film reagent technology is unique to the:
   A. Becton Dickinson Affinity
   B. PB Diagnostics OPUS
   C. Boehringer Mannheim ES 300
   D. Syva ETS Plus
   E. Cirrus IMMULITE

13. Paramagnetic EIA technology is employed by which systems?
   A. The Biotrol System 7000 and the PB OPUS
   B. The Technicon Immuno 1 and the Biotrol System 7000
   C. The Tosoh AIA-600 and the PB OPUS MAGNUM
   D. The Becton Dickinson Affinity and the Boehringer Mannheim ES 300
   E. Only the Baxter Stratus II

14. What features do the Cirrus IMMULITE and Ciba Corning ACS:180 have in common?
   A. Chemiluminescence technology and "stat" interrupt
   B. Heterogeneous principles and dry-reagent film technology
   C. Continuous feed capabilities and automatic dilutions
   D. Drugs of abuse testing and nephelometric techniques
   E. None of the above

15. Refrigerated on-analyzer reagent storage is a feature of the:
   A. PB Diagnostics OPUS PLUS
   B. Abbott ADx
   C. Becton Dickinson Affinity
   D. Abbott IMx
   E. Technicon Immuno 1

16. Which of the following techniques are homogeneous assays?

A. EMIT
B. RPIA
C. ELISA
D. FPIA
   1. A and C
   2. B and D
   3. A and D
   4. B and C
   5. All of the above

17. Which of the following immunoassay analyzers features continuous random access?
   A. Tosoh Medics AIA-1200
   B. Biotrol System 7000
   C. Boehringer Mannheim ES 300
   D. Becton Dickinson Affinity
   E. Cirrus IMMULITE

Answers

1. A 2. B 3. C 4. D 5. A 6. E 7. D 8. B 9. D 10. C 11. B 12. B 13. B 14. A 15. E 16. 3 17. C

Bibliography

ADx System Operator's Guide, Abbott Laboratories, Diagnostics Division, Abbott Park, Il, 1988.

Alpert N: AIA-1200 Automated Immunoassay Analyzer, Clinical Instrument Systems, 11(9), Stamford, Ct, 1991.

Babson AL: The Cirrus IMMULITE Automated Immunoassay System, J Clin Immunoassay, 14(2), 83-88, 1991.

Bassion S: Immunological reactions, In Kaplan LA, Pesce AJ, eds: Clinical chemistry: theory, analysis, and correlation, St Louis, 1984, Mosby–Year Book.

Buffone GJ: Principles of immunochemical techniques. In Tietz NW, ed: Fundamentals of clinical chemistry, ed 3, Philadelphia, 1987, WB Saunders.

Dudley RF: The Ciba Corning ACS:180 Automated Immunoassay System, J Clin Immunoassay, 14(2), 77-82, 1991.

Duncan T, Engelberth L, and LaBrash B: The Boehringer Mannheim ES 300 Immunoassay System, J Clin Immunoassay, 14(2), 105-110, 1991.

Freier C, Kan B, and Cicquel T: Biotrol System 7000: Automated Immunoassay Analyzer, J Clin Immunoassay, 14(2), 111-114, 1991.

Hurtubise PE, Bassion S, Gauldie J, and Horsewood P: Immunochemical techniques. In Kaplan LA, Pesce AJ, eds: Clinical chemistry: theory, analysis, and correlation, St Louis, 1984, Mosby–Year Book.

IMx System Operation Manual, Abbott Laboratories, Diagnostics Division, Abbott Park, Il, 1988.

Jefferson R: The Becton Dickinson Affinity Immunoassay System, J Clin Immunoassay, 14(2), 89-93, 1991.

Keller CH, Fitzgerald KL, Barnes A: The Abbott IMx and IMx Select Systems, J Clin Immunoassay, 14(2), 115-119, 1991.

Lifshitz, M, DeCresce R: Abbott IMx Immunoassay System, The Instrument Report, 2(6), 1990. Applied Technology Associates, Inc., Chicago, Il.

Lifshitz M, DeCresce R: BD Affinity Immunoassay System, The Instrument Report, 3(2), 1991. Applied Technology Associates, Inc., Chicago, Il.

Lifshitz M, DeCresce R: Baxter Stratus II Immunoassay System, The Instrument Report, 2(8), 1990. Applied Technology Associates, Inc., Chicago, Il. 1990.

Loebel, JE: Tosoh AIA-1200/AIA-600 Automated Immunoassay System, J Clin Immunoassay, 14(2), 94-102, 1991.

Olive C: PB Diagnostics' OPUS Immunoassay System, J Clin Immunoassay, 14(2), 126-132, 1991.

OPUS Immunoassay Operator's Manual, PB Diagnostics Systems, Inc., Westwood, Ma, 1990.

Plaut DS, McLellan WN: The Baxter Diagnostics Inc., Dade Stratus II Automated Fluorometric Immunoassay System, J Clin Immunoassay, 14(2), 120-125, 1991.

Schneider NE: Technicon Immuno 1 Automated Immunoassay System, J Clin Immunoassay, 14(2), 103-104, 1991.

SR1 Instrument Manual, Serono Baker Diagnostics, Allentown, Pa, 1991.

Syva ETS Plus System Operator's Manual, Syva Company, Palo Alto, Ca, 1990.

TDxFLx Operation Manual, Abbott Laboratories, Diagnostics Division, Abbott Park, Il, 1990.

TDx System Operator's Guide, Abbott Laboratories, Diagnostics Division, Abbott Park, Il, 1985.

Thompson SG: Competitive binding assays. In Kaplan LA, Pesce AJ, eds: Clinical chemistry: theory, analysis, and correlation, St Louis, 1984, Mosby–Year Book.

CHAPTER **20**

Automation in Hematology

MARY ANN DOTSON

Particle Counting
Histogram Analysis
Automated Differential Counting
Reticulocyte Automation SYSMEX R-1000
Quality Control

In the early 1960s, medical technologists spent an appreciable amount of time at the microscope manually counting red and white blood cells using a counting chamber. This method provided an estimate of the average number of red and white cells in a patient's blood sample. In most laboratories, a total of 30 counts a day for one technologist was considered a heavy load. In performing a manual red cell count, the technologist would count about 500 cells out of a total of nearly 5,000,000 cells/cubic mm. Random sampling, dilution and preparation, glassware-calibration, and human judgment and fatigue often produced inherent error.

One of the most significant changes in laboratory equipment has been the introduction of clinical instruments that perform quick and precise counting of peripheral blood cells. These instruments have progressed from simple discrete counters to highly sophisticated multiple parameter counters with computers capable of bivariate data analysis; many of their electronic function checks are now performed by on-board computers at the touch of a button. Modern instruments are also programmed to perform start-up and shut-down procedures. Some units are so automated that the technologist may "walk away" once the samples are loaded and analysis has begun.

Technologists operating these sophisticated analyzers may not be aware of the finer details of analyzer performance if "key" operators are assigned to perform maintenance and troubleshooting duties.

Before the advent of today's instruments, attempts were made at estimating cell populations by indirect methods. Measuring the total absorbance of diluted red cells was one such attempt. Another method used a "nephelometric principle" of light dispersion. Both of these approaches failed to measure red cell populations satisfactorily.

In addition to devices for counting peripheral blood cells, electronic technology has made it possible to determine red cell volume and hemoglobin and to calculate from these parameters the various indices that describe the red cell. Platelet counting has been added to selected automated counters, thus generating eight parameters for each sample tested. Recently, advances in instrumental technology have brought white blood cell classification into the realm of automation.

Automated hematology instruments are now manufactured with 20 to 30 plus parameters for each processed sample together with the power to flag samples with populations beyond expected limits. They can generate interpretive comments for leukocyte, erythrocyte, and platelet population morphology and provide quality control (QC) statistics and generate charts on demand. They may be interfaced with laboratory or hospital computer systems for automatic reporting and record storage.

Particle Counting

The particle counters found in clinical laboratories today are based on one of two principles. One type uses an optical principle to identify cell characteristics by the physical scattering of light. Simultaneously the cells are counted by monitoring the number of times the focused light beam is interrupted. The second type uses the Coulter principle in which a flow of electrical current between two electrodes is interrupted by cell passage and the number of interruptions is counted to enumerate the cells. Several variations of these two general methods have evolved, generating a great deal of research into the physics and mechanics of cell counting, sizing, and identification. Research in this field continues to refine and expand the functions of cell counting and classification by size and type.

Coulter Cell-Counting Devices. In 1958 Joseph and Wallace Coulter designed and marketed the first cell counters using this Coulter principle, which is still basically employed in today's state-of-the-art in instrumentation. The basic components of this system are shown in Figure 20-1 and are briefly presented to illustrate the basic Coulter principle.

The system consists of a simple arrangement for holding the sample, establishing sample flow, and "metering" the flow so that an electronic counter can be activated as a selected sample volume is drawn through and scanned by the orifice. A dilute suspension of cells, *E*, is contained in a sample beaker. The tube, *B*, contains the aperture, *A*, through which the sample is drawn. The electrodes are designated by *C* and *D*. When the stopcock, *F*, is opened, an external vacuum source, *P*, initiates flow through the orifice and causes the mercury, *J*, in the manometer to assume the position shown with the mercury in the open leg of the manometer drawn slightly below the horizontal branch. When the stopcock, *F*, is

closed, the unbalanced manometer functions as a syphon to continue the sample flow through the orifice.

As the mercury in the open leg rises into the horizontal branch, it makes contact with a wire electrode, *L*, sealed in the manometer wall and energizes a high-speed decade counter that begins counting all pulses that reach or exceed the threshold level. A few seconds later the mercury column makes contact with a second wire electrode, *M*, which stops the counter. The syphoning action continues until the mercury column comes to rest at a level near that of the mercury in the reservoir. Contact, *K*, provides a ground return path for the start and stop electrodes. The contacts, *L* and *M*, are very carefully located so that the volume contained in the tube between the contact is ½ ml. As a consequence of the arrangement the counter is actuated as ½ ml is drawn into the system. In practice the horizontal section is a U tube in the horizontal plane so that contacts are nearer together. By this means the vacuum in the system at the start and stop contacts is kept substantially equal so that any elasticity in the system because of bubbles will introduce less than 0.01% error in the syphoned volume under the worst conditions.

The function of inlet, *O*, and stopcock, *G*, which is normally left in the closed portion, is to allow rapid filling of the system when setting it up instead of depending on the relatively slow flow through the orifice.

Fig. 20-2 is a block diagram of the electrical functions of an early Coulter Counter. The pulses produced at the orifice are amplified and displayed on the oscilloscope screen and appear as vertical lines or spikes (Fig. 20-3). The height of an individual pulse spike from the baseline is a measure of relative size of the cell producing the pulse, and because the rate at which they are produced is several thousand/second, the viewer obtains an immediate impression of the average cell size and cell size distribution. The threshold control dial located below the oscillosope screen enables the operator to select the height or level above the baseline, which if reached or exceeded by a pulse, will result in the pulse being counted. The height or level corresponds to a particular cell size.

The original Coulter Counter Model A was introduced and used in laboratories in the early 1960s. It was hand wired and used a total of 30 vacuum tubes. Blood cells were diluted in a medium that was a good conductor of electricity.

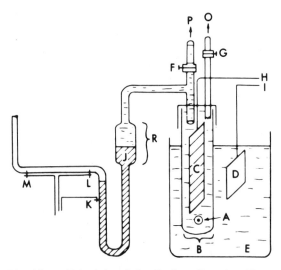

Fig. 20-1   Principle of the Coulter Counter. (From Coulter W: High speed automatic blood cell counter and cell size analyzer, Chicago, 1956, Coulter Electronics, Inc.)

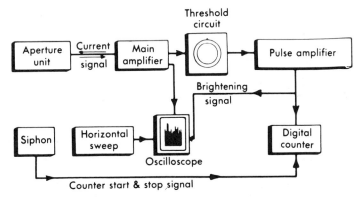

Fig. 20-2 Electronic circuitry of the Coulter Counter (courtesy Coulter Electronics, Inc.).

Large dilutions were necessary to space out the particles (cells) in solution thereby facilitating individual cell measurement. Blood cells, being poor conductors of electricity, displace conductive (diluting) fluid during passage through the aperture and interrupt the flow of current as they are pulled through the counting device. The volume of fluid that a cell displaces is proportionate

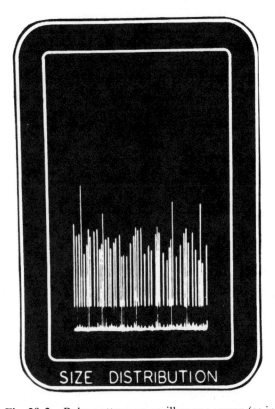

Fig. 20-3 Pulse pattern on oscilloscope screen (as in Fig. 20-1). Horizontal axis represents time (passage of cells through the aperture orifice); vertical axis represents cell size (courtesy Coulter Electronics, Inc.).

to the accompanying drop in current and thus is a measure of the cell's volume. The number of cells, as well as the volume of each cell, is measured as they pass through the sensing zone of the instrument.

The Model A was soon replaced by Models FN, ZBI, and others that used solid-state circuitry, printed circuit boards, and digital electronic displays. The digital and mechanical registers of the Model A were replaced, first by glow tubes in the Model F and then by numeric readout tubes in Models FN and ZBI. The aperture viewing lens was replaced by a viewing screen. Major electronic advances were made by replacing all tubes with transistors and by using printed circuit boards. However, these early models with their improvements still used a single aperture, required manual dilutions, and counted one type of cell at a time. Although Coulter Models F, FN, and ZBI have been reliable instruments, the single channel counter in use today is the Coulter ZM (Fig. 20-4).

Coulter Counter, Model S (Coulter Electronics, Inc.). The first multiparameter hematology counter was the Coulter Model S; it is the prototype of all modern hematology counters. The basic principles of operation of this instrument serve as a foundation for the newer models. The single aperture for counting has been replaced by two sets of apertures, making it possible to count white cells and red cells at the same time. The apertures are immersed in glassware called "baths." Each triplicate set of apertures contains three internal electrodes (one within each aperture tube) and one associated single external electrode immersed in the bath of conductive fluid surrounding the apertures. Fluid and cells are drawn at a constant rate through the three apertures, where

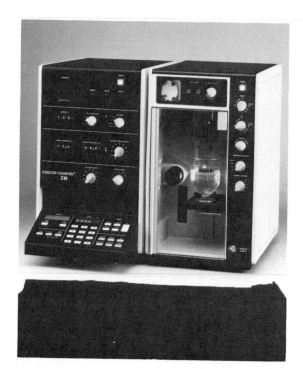

Fig. 20-4 Coulter Counter ZM (courtesy Coulter Electronics, Inc.).

each cell's passage interrupts the electric current, producing a "blip" or signal that can be counted. Three separate white blood cell counts (WBC) and three separate red blood cell counts (RBC) are obtained during each cycle of this instrument. These triplicate counts are compared, and, if results are within reasonable limits, they are averaged. If one count is out of limits, the other two are used. If the three are widely separated (no two agree), no result is reported. Dilution of the whole blood sample for white cell and red cell counting will be described in a later section.

Dilution of whole blood for the white cell count and addition of a red cell hemolyzing agent are simultaneously accomplished. The bath from which the white count is drawn becomes optically clear and forms a "cuvette" of about 1 cm from front to back. A small exciter lamp at the front of the WBC bath beams through the WBC solution to a photocell behind the bath. The absorbance of the hemolyzed blood dilution is measured. From this reading a hemoglobin (Hb) value is generated.

As each cell crosses the electrical field for counting it produces an electrical signal that is actually the instantaneous decrease of the current through the aperture. The size of this signal mea-

sures the electrical resistance created by the cell, which is a function of the cell's volume. Measuring the total of these electrical signals and dividing the total by the number of impulses (cells) produces an average signal that corresponds to average cell volume. Applied to the red cell-counting sequence, this technique reveals the mean red cell volume (MCV).

Methods for obtaining four parameters (RBC, WBC, Hb, and MCV) have been discussed. Three other parameters are calculated from these four measured values. To derive the mean corpuscular hemoglobin (MCH), the hemoglobin value is divided by the number of red cells/unit volume. This is done electronically using the electrical signals produced by the sample.

The hematocrit is defined as the packed cell volume or the percentage of blood sample that is red cells. This value is usually obtained by centrifuging a blood sample until cells are "packed" followed by measurement of the volume of the red cell layer as a percentage of the total. If the average volume and number of red cells in a sample are known, the product of these values will indicate the total red cell volume in a given volume of whole blood. Because red cells do not pack without leaving interstices between the cells (even under ideal centrifugation conditions), the electronic hematocrit value is not identical to the manual method. The manual microhematocrit is considered the reference method. This value is assigned to the electrical signal to calibrate the instrument to a known hematocrit value.

The mean corpuscular hemoglobin concentration (MCHC) represents the average hemoglobin in a given volume of red cells. This can be determined from the electrical information corresponding to the mean corpuscular volume and the hemoglobin.

A whole blood sample arrives at the appropriate point of measurement within the instrument by the fluid-handling system of the Model S, which is fully automated; the number of operations involve a complex fluid-moving, pneumatic system. Movement of fluid is propelled either by pressure or by vacuum with many valves placed in a continuous line that, on signal, open or close to move the diluted sample in the right direction. The command center for all valves is a bank of small induction motors accessible from the back center of the counting module. Vacuum is provided by a pump in a separate module.

Measurement of each sample is by segmentation. The sample fills a tube that has a very con-

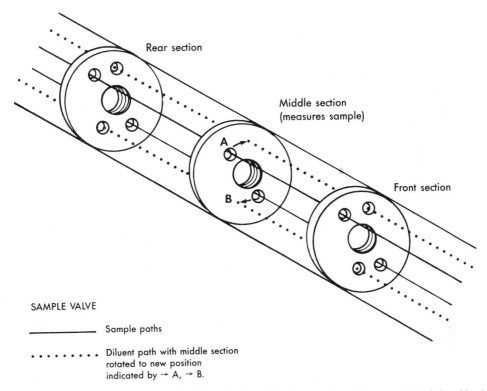

Rear section

Middle section
(measures sample)

Front section

A

B

SAMPLE VALVE

——————— Sample paths

· · · · · · · · · Diluent path with middle section
rotated to new position
indicated by → A, → B.

Fig. 20-5 Blood sampling valve diagram. Fluid paths through valve are shown for sample (*solid and broken lines*) and for diluent (*dotted line*). The middle section rotates on its central axis to segment (measure) a sample for its initial dilution. **A** and **B** mark the spots where the sample segment is located following rotation of the middle section of the sampling valve. The sample is now aligned with the diluent stream pathway.

sistent and accurate internal diameter. This tube is "cut" into a precise length thus accurately segmenting a portion of the sample. The mechanism used to segment each sample into precise lengths is called the blood sampling valve (Fig. 20-5). This valve is made of three ceramic cylinders through which accurate lengthwise channels have been bored. Holes in each cylinder match up to provide channels for fluids and samples to be transported from the front section through the middle and back sections of the ceramic valve. The front and rear sections of the valve are stationary. The center sections, which segments the sample, is designed to rotate on its center axis. When it rotates to a new position, precisely measured amounts of fluid contained in the channel(s) are isolated (segmented).

Blood is drawn into the sampling valve by vacuum. The valve is turned, segmenting a precisely measured blood sample. The repositioned valve is aligned with a new set of channels present in the front and back ceramic sections. A measured stream of diluent washes the blood out of the sampling channel and performs the necessary di-

lution at the same time. This primary white cell dilution of the blood sample proceeds to a chamber where a secondary aliquot of it is aspirated, measured, and rediluted for the red count. This secondary dilution is delivered to a bath on the left side of the instrument. Both the primary white cell dilution and the secondary rediluted red count sample are swirled in their respective mixing chambers. A few drops of a hemolyzing agent are added to the white cell dilution in the mixing chamber to destroy the red cells, thereby releasing their hemoglobin contents. The red cell and white cell dilutions then proceed to their respective counting baths where the aperture tubes will draw off ½ ml portions at a controlled rate for counting and sizing. Between successive counting cycles the counting baths and aperture tubes are well rinsed with diluent.

The Coulter Model S was the first seven-parameter automated hematology counter widely used in the United States. Fig. 20-6 is a block diagram of the fluidic and electrical pathways of the Coulter Model S. It proved to be a workhorse in the laboratory; many systems were used for 10 to

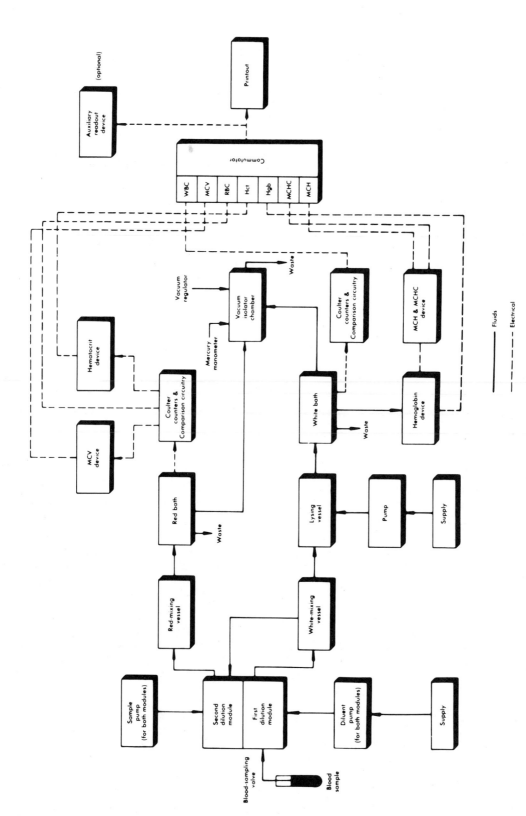

Fig. 20-6   Block diagram of the Coulter Model S blood-counting system (courtesy Coulter Electronics, Inc.).

15 years, processing hundreds of samples/day with relatively little down time. This type of performance was virtually impossible with clinical laboratory equipment 30 years ago.

Beyond the Model S. Coulter counters that were manufactured after the Model S continued to employ the same counting technology while implementing changes and improvements including the addition of new parameters, a decrease in sample and reagent volume, improved electronics, refinements in computer programming, and the addition of QC programs. The name of the models changed as improvements were incorporated. Following the Model S came the Model S Sr and then the third generation "Plus Series": S Plus II, S Plus III, S Plus IV, S Plus V, S Plus VI, and the STKR (Stacker). Several of these major additions will be explained in detail later in this chapter.

The first new parameter to be added to the original seven on the Model S Coulter Counter was the platelet count. The small size of the platelet presented a difficulty in separating it from background noises (electronic, dust, debris, bubbles) and other blood cells. Two changes made it possible to separate and count red cells and platelets together. First, the red cell apertures were reduced in diameter and length from $100 \times 75\ \mu m$ to $50 \times 60\ \mu m$. The white cell aperture diameter and length remained at $100 \times 75\ \mu m$. The change in the red cell apertures increased the instrument's sensitivity such that platelet-sized particles could be identified and counted.

Samples exiting each aperture must be carried away immediately because the sensing zone (electrical field) of each aperture extends beyond its edges (Fig. 20-7). A stream of fluid is directed past the rear of the red cell apertures during the count period that carries the sample away from this area of the sensing zone. This fluid stream, called "sweep flow," prevents the red blood cells from swirling back to the edge of the sensing zone (where a partial interruption in the current would be mistaken for a platelet). Reducing the size of the apertures and adding sweep flow allowed the addition of platelet counts to the Coulter Counter menu. An electrical "burn" circuit was also added to automatically clean protein buildup from the aperture orifices thus reducing the need for repeated manual cleaning.

The platelet count is derived from the raw count obtained from counting all particles between the sizes of 2 and 20 fl. This raw count data is analyzed and a mathematic formula is applied to extrapolate a reported platelet count representing platelets from 0 to 70 fl in size. This procedure will be discussed in more detail in the section on histograms.

The Coulter STKR (Stacker) is the last model in the S Plus series; it incorporated a three-part leukocyte differential displayed as a histogram with interpretation of eosinophil and basophil populations. This fully automated instrument could accommodate 12 sample racks (each holding 12 sample tubes). Each rack automatically dropped to a conveyor belt to mix the samples by

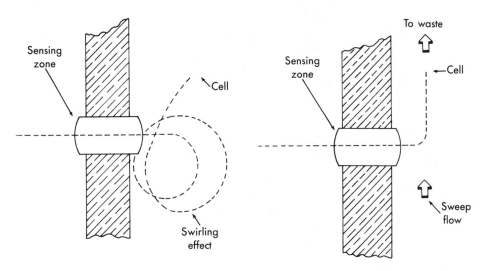

Fig. 20-7 The path of a red cell through apertures (cross-sectional view) is shown without sweep flow, **A,** and with sweep flow, **B.** As red cells exit the aperture orifice, sweep flow prevents them from recirculating into the sensing zone. Sheath fluid is not part of this design (courtesy Coulter Electronics, Inc.).

a rocking motion while laterally carrying the rack toward a bar code reader and aspirating needle to identify each sample before aspiration into the system. The double lumen aspiration needle pierced the tube stopper and aspirated the sample while venting the tube. The STKR system claims a maximum throughput of 114 (200 μl) samples/hour; it measures 16 parameters and generates 2 interpretive reports. Dilution ratios for cell counting are 1:251 for WBCs and 1:6250 for RBCs and platelets.

The fully automated (new generation) model developed by Coulter Electronics, Inc. is the Coulter STKS (Stack S) (Fig. 20-8). It incorporates the previously described Coulter technology (for all red cell parameters, platelet parameters, and the total white count) with new technology to differentiate the white cells into five subpopulations. The new technology was first developed as a "stand alone" differential counter that Coulter named "VCS." The V stands for volume, which is the original technology used by Coulter to size and count cells using direct current. C represents conductivity that uses radio frequency (RF) to gather information about cell nuclear size and density. S indicates scatter of laser light. Forward angle light scatter provides information about cell shape and refractability. These three simul-

taneous analyses evaluate each cell measured. The VCS has now been combined with the STKR to become the STKS, which will be discussed later in this chapter.

LASER Hematology Counters. The technology of **hydrodynamic focusing** was first described by Crosland-Taylor in 1953. In 1965 Kamentsky measured multiple cell characteristics with laser-based spectrophotometry. In the late 1970s Ortho Diagnostics Instruments revolutionized cell counting by incorporating a helium/neon laser and principles of flow cytometry into their instruments. Their original "Hemac" instrument was replaced by the ELT (erythrocyte, leukocyte, thrombocyte) series incorporating improvements in stability and speed. The ELT-8 will be discussed here; discussion of the ELT-15 will be in the Histogram section. The photograph of the ELT-8 (Fig. 20-9) is representative of the ELT-15 also. The units housing the ELT-8 and ELT-15 are the same; only internal changes and additions to the ELT-8 resulted in the production of the ELT-15.

Laser (Light Amplification by Stimulated Emission of Radiation) light is of a single wavelength (monochromatic), travels great distances with very little spread (coherent), and its parallel waves travel in one direction (in phase). The tech-

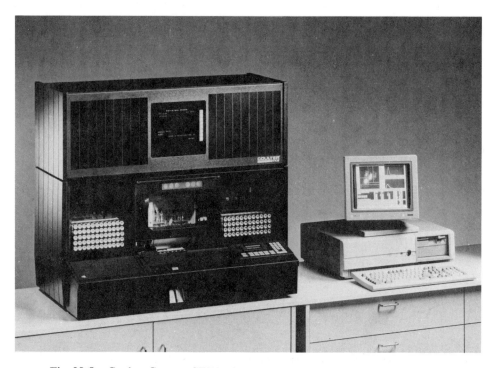

Fig. 20-8 Coulter Counter STKR (Stacker). (Courtesy Coulter Electronics, Inc.)

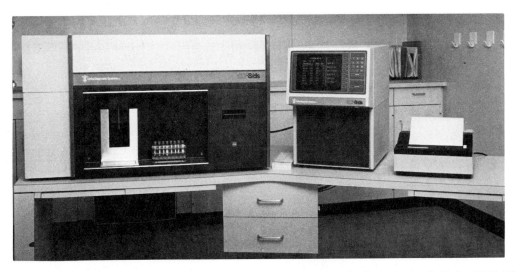

Fig. 20-9 Ortho ELT-8 Hematology System (courtesy Ortho Diagnostics Systems, Inc.). Ortho ELT-15's appearance is identical; all differences are internal.

nical advantage of a laser beam is its extremely sharp focus of discrete, monochromatic light. Focused to about 20 μl, laser light is ideal for cell counting because the beam approaches the total diameter of the sample stream.

Flow cytometer principles were incorporated into Ortho hematology instruments, making it possible to count thousands of cells in a matter of seconds. The "fluidic aperture" concept incorporates a unique idea. The sample stream column, bearing the cells to be counted, is centered in a high-speed stream of liquid passing through the laser beam. This method of presenting a very narrow stream of diluted sample to the counting area is one of the unique features of the instrument. A diluted sample is injected into the center of a stream of isotonic fluid (sheath stream) at the base of a funnel-shaped flowcell (Fig. 20-10).

Hydrodynamic focusing of the sample stream is produced by the configuration of the flowcell. Its cone shape produces a symmetric decrease of its cross-sectional area. This shape, together with the precise regulation of flow pressures, is such that the sample stream evolves into an 18 μm column in the center of the larger stream of isotonic fluid. The condition of two different liquids traveling together without mixing is known as laminar flow. The larger stream (the sheath stream) completely surrounds the sample stream. Laminar flow conditions are created in the absence of turbulence. The sheath stream and sample stream travel at different velocities. The particles in these two streams of liquid travel in parallel

lines to one another. Under conditions of laminar flow the cells in the sample stream are hydrodynamically focused in an effective "fluid aperture" at precisely the center of the laser beam (Fig. 20-10). The flowcell is made of quartz because quartz does not alter the laser beam as it enters or exits the flowcell. Laser light is scattered in all directions by the presence of a particle in the sensing zone of the flowcell. Because of the unique properties of laser light very small particles (e.g., platelets) can be easily identified and precisely counted.

Blood is drawn into a sampling valve and split into two streams. One of the streams is diluted with a lysing solution and then sent to a flow cell where white cells are counted as they interrupt the laser beam.

The other stream (used for red cell, platelet, and hemoglobin measurements) is first diluted with isotonic solution and then further split into two secondary streams. Each of these secondary streams is diluted a second time. Isotonic solution is used for one of the dilutions, which then passes through the laser beam. As red cells and platelets in the dilution pass through the beam, they are counted and their size is determined by the degree to which they scatter the laser beam. This red cell sizing information is totaled to report the hematocrit.

The other secondary stream dilution is further diluted with a hemoglobin diluent that converts hemoglobin to cyanmethemoglobin. It is directed to the special colorimeter where Hgb is

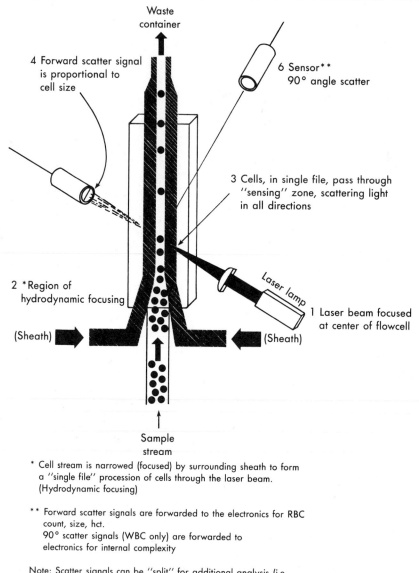

Waste
container

4 Forward scatter signal
is proportional to
cell size

6 Sensor**
90° angle scatter

3 Cells, in single file, pass through
"sensing" zone, scattering light
in all directions

2 *Region of
hydrodynamic focusing

Laser lamp

1 Laser beam focused
at center of flowcell

(Sheath)

(Sheath)

Sample
stream

* Cell stream is narrowed (focused) by surrounding sheath to form
a "single file" procession of cells through the laser beam.
(Hydrodynamic focusing)

** Forward scatter signals are forwarded to the electronics for RBC
count, size, hct.
90° scatter signals (WBC only) are forwarded to
electronics for internal complexity

Note: Scatter signals can be "split" for additional analysis (i.e.,
hgb content, fluorescence)

Fig. 20-10   Flowcell and optics bench design of the Ortho ELT-15 (courtesy Ortho Diagnostics, Inc.).

measured. A light emitting diode (LED) providing light at 539 nm is used as the radiation source in this colorimeter, and a photomultiplier is used as a detector.

Red blood cells and platelets are counted simultaneously. Three cell characteristics influence the light scattering signals that are used to separate red cells and platelets. Light scatter signals represent the cell volume, time of flight, and refractive index. Forward light scatter represents the overall volume of each cell. Time of flight represents the diameter of each cell. Time of flight is measured in nanoseconds (ns). It measures the

time it takes a cell to traverse the laser beam (sensing zone). Hemoglobin (found in red cells) has a constant refractive index that helps in separating platelets, which lack hemoglobin, from red blood cells.

The electronic system calculates MCV, MCH, and MCHC. Eight parameters are reported from a sample size of less than 100 μl of blood. Hydrodynamic focusing and laminar flow allows a more concentrated cell suspension to be used than when employed with earlier impedance (Coulter) counters. ELT dilutions used are white cells 1:19 and red cell/platelet 1:600. On average about 25,000 red cells and 7000 white cells are counted. The amount of diluent used is also very low. All solutions for one sample total less than 14 ml.

Ortho Diagnostic Systems introduced newer ELT versions that allow a speed of over 100 samples/hour using 100 μl of sample. The on-board computer stores patient data and automates the QC data handling. It can tabulate and display patient data or selectively recall and print out patient information including histograms; abnormal results are flagged. The current versions of the ELT-8 and ELT-15 include a platelet count. The ELT-15 also provides a red cell morphology index (RCMI) and a three part histogram differential in both percent and absolute numbers. Unfortunately these instruments are no longer marketed.

Hematology Systems. Over the past two decades Technicon has introduced a considerable number of blood-counting instruments including the SMA-4 and SMA-7, the modified 4-A and 7-A, the Hemalog and Hemalog-D, and the HS-90 System. These instruments employed the light scatter principle of detecting cells in a flowcell using hydrodynamic focusing and laminar flow technology. The Hemalog-D introduced in 1975 was the first automated differential counter that used cytochemical staining and cell size to classify white cells into five basic types. The Hemalog D and the faster D-90 were ultimately replaced by the H-6000, which combined CBC analysis and differential counting into one system. The H-6000 was followed by the H-1, which is smaller in size and uses smaller volumes of sample and reagents. Recent improvements to the H-1 have produced the H-2. Because the basic technology of both of these instruments has changed very little, the H-2 will be described (Fig. 20-11).

The H-2 has four modules: (1) analytic module, (2) electronic module (power, vacuum, pressure supplies, disk drives), (3) CRT/keypad/ticket printer module, and (4) screen printer module.

The analytic module houses a four channel (A to D) system using light scatter and fluidic principles of hydrodynamic focusing and laminar flow with quartz flowcells. Computer technology has made it possible to analyze the data extensively with the development of special algo-

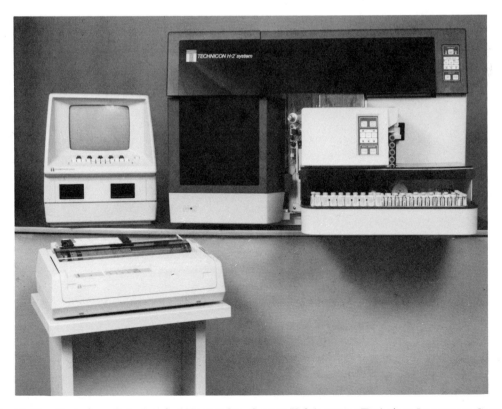

Fig. 20-11 Technicon Cytochemical Hematology System H-2 (courtesy Technicon Instrument Corp.).

rithms. Several new parameters are derived from this system: large unstained cells (LUC), cellular hemoglobin concentration mean (CHCM), lobularity index (LI), and mean peroxidase activity index (MPXI). These parameters will be described later along with the flagging system for suspected abnormals.

The hemoglobin channel, *A,* uses a modified cyanmethemoglobin procedure to measure hemoglobin colorimetrically at 546 nm. The dilution ratio is 1:25.

The RBC/platelet channel, *B,* uses laser optics along with the principles of hydrodynamic focusing and laminar flow for its analysis of red cells and platelets. The red cells are isovolumetrically sphered and then fixed by the diluting fluid using a 1:625 dilution ratio. The light scattered by the red cells at low and high forward angles is simultaneously collected. Low angle forward scatter signals (0 to 5 degrees) provide cell size measurements for each red cell, whereas high angle scatter analysis (5 to 15 degrees) provides absorbance measurements for each red cell. The red cell absorbance is due to the hemoglobin concentration in the cell. Red cell absorbance measurement is compared with that obtained from the hemoglobin channel's measurement of cyanmethemoglobin. When a preset difference between these measurements occurs, all red cell parameters are flagged.

The peroxidase channel, *C,* performs the total white cell count and differential analysis using the same fluidic principles with a tungsten light source rather than a laser. Red cells are lysed, and

Table 20-1 Hematology systems with reported parameters

	STKR	STKS	ELT-15	H-1 H-2	E 5000	NE 8000	CD 1600	CD 3000
WBC	X	X	X	X	X	X	X	X
RBC	X	X	X	X	X	X	X	X
HGB	X	X	X	X	X	X	X	X
HCT	X	X	X	X	X	X	X	X
MCV	X	X	X	X	X	X	X	X
MCH	X	X	X	X	X	X	X	X
MCHC	X	X	X	X	X	X	X	X
PLT	X	X	X	X	X	X	X	X
RDW-CV	X	X		X	X*	X	X	X
RDW-SD					X*	X		
RCMI			X					
HDW				X				
CHCM				X				
MPV	X	X	X	X	X	X	X	X
P-LCR					X	X		
PDW		X**		X**	X	X	X**	X**
PCT		X**		X**			X**	X**
NEUT #	X	X	X	X	X	X	X	X
NEUT%	X	X	X	X	X	X	X	X
LYM #	X	X	X	X	X	X	X	X
LYM%	X	X	X	X	X	X	X	X
MONO #	X	X	X	X	X	X	X	X
MONO%	X	X	X	X	X	X	X	X
EOS #	I	X		X		X		X
EOS%		X		X		X		X
BASO #	I	X		X		X		X
BASO%		X		X		X		X
LUC #				X				
LUC%				X				
LI				X				
MPXI				X				

I = Interpretive report only.

* = One is selected by user.

** = International only.

the white cells are fixed and stained for peroxidase in a 1:41.6 dilution ratio. All leukocytes containing peroxidase stain with an intensity relative to their peroxidase content. Eosinophils stain intensely, neutrophils stain moderately, and monocytes stain weakly. Lymphocytes do not stain, and other cells that are larger and do not stain are classified as LUCs.

There are two detectors in this leg of the optics bench. One is a dark field detector that gathers scattered light that represents the size of each cell. The other detector is for the bright field and detects the amount of staining in each cell. These measurements are made simultaneously to indicate both size and staining characteristics of thousands of cells/second. The total white cell count and differential are determined in this channel. A new parameter representing an index of the mean peroxidase activity of the neutrophils, the mean perioxidase activity index (MPXI), is determined in this channel.

The last channel, D, in the system is the basophil/lobularity (nuclear) channel. This channel provides a basophil count and analyzes the different nuclear shapes. The basophil is the only cell that retains its cytoplasm in this channel because it is resistant to lysis by the low pH reagent in combination with a surfactant. All other cells including neutrophils, eosinophils, lymphocytes, and monocytes are stripped of their cytoplasm leaving only a nucleus to be counted in this 1:41.6 dilution. The previously described fluidic technologies are combined with laser technology for analysis of the cells at two different forward scatter angles. Low forward angle scatter is related to the size of the cell, whereas the high forward angle scatter is related to nuclear lobularity.

The test results include an eight-parameter CBC and six leukocyte subpopulations in percent and absolute numbers. Table 20-1 lists the various models discussed in this chapter along with their respective reported parameters.

The automated closed tube sampler on the H-2 requires 145 μl of whole blood/aspiration at a rate of 102 samples/hour. Only 125 μl of sample is needed for open vial aspiration. The H-2 may be equipped with a direct cytometry port that can be used for research purposes in performing lymphocyte subset analysis for Pan T, Helper T, Suppressor T, and B cells.

TOA Medical Electronics. The Sysmex E-Series instruments combine automated sample mixing and bar code reader identification with CBC analysis and a three-part histogram differential. Electronic impedance technology is combined with fluidic principles of hydrodynamic focusing and laminar flow. The E-5000 uses 200 μl of whole blood to determine results of 18 parameters and 3 histograms in the automated mode. Automated sampling options include open vial mixing and sampling using the rack sampler or closed tube (cap piercing) sampling with the CP-1000 unit.

The E 5000 system (Fig. 20-12) consists of a main analyzer unit, a computer/data analysis unit, a power supply unit, and an optional ticket printer or graphics printer. Blood is drawn into a ceramic blood sampling valve that rotates and isolates segments of the sample for appropriate dilution and direction to the analysis area. Details of this type of sampling valve have been described earlier (see Fig. 20-5). Analysis includes hemoglobin determination, RBC/platelet separation, and WBC analysis. Hemoglobin is determined using a modified cyanmethemoglobin method and is read colorimetrically at 540 nm.

The unit housing the apertures for cell counting and sizing is called a "transducer" in instruments made by TOA. The RBC/PLT transducer has a single aperture with a diameter of 50 μm. Red cells and platelets are counted and sized as they traverse the electrical field (of the aperture) produced by internal and external electrodes. The unit is designed with hydrodynamic focusing and laminar flow that directs cells to pass through the center of the aperture in single file formation. Front sheath fluid surrounds and hydrodynamically focuses the sample stream, and back sheath fluid carries the sample away from the back of the aperture preventing red cell recirculation. The count time is divided into increments, and the counts from these increments are compared to ensure uniformity of cell passage through the aperture. Disruptions in the flow of cells result in uneven distribution of counts among these time intervals and generate an analysis error message. A dilution ratio of 1:750 is used in the E-5000, whereas a 1:500 dilution is used in the NE-8000 for red cell and platelet analysis. These low dilution ratios are possible because of the use of hydrodynamic focusing and laminar flow technologies.

The electronic thresholds that separate debris from cells and separate cells by type are called discriminators. Discriminators are controlled by the computer program and adjust from sample to sample to accommodate for cell size variations from patient to patient. These adjusting elec-

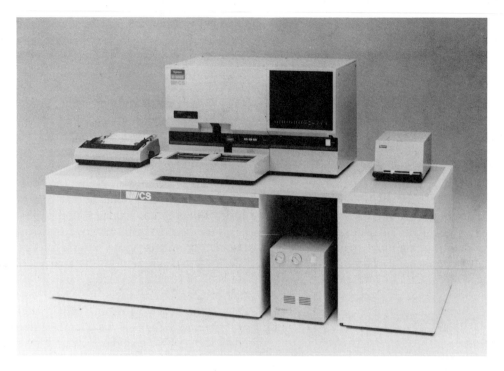

Fig. 20-12 Sysmex E-5000 system (courtesy TOA Medical Electronics, Inc.).

tronic thresholds are called floating discriminators. The lower discriminator for red cell counting adjusts between 25 and 75 fl and the upper one adjusts between 200 and 250 fl. Red cell counts and platelet counts are directly measured. The height of each red cell pulse is totaled to produce a hematocrit value.

The white cell transducer also contains a single aperture through which a 250 μl volume of diluted sample is drawn. A volumetric, nonmercury, ball float type of manometer controls the volume of sample passing through the aperture. The WBC dilution is 1:250. The lysing reagent performs two functions. It lyses the red cells and produces controlled shrinkage of the white cells for analysis into three subpopulations. The total white cell count is determined following placement of the lower discriminator that floats between 30 and 60 fl. The upper white cell discriminator is the only fixed discriminator and is set at 300 fl.

The E-5000 computers process data, store sample results and histograms, provide QC files, and incorporate a moving average indices program using patient data to monitor instrument performance.

Histogram Analysis

Histograms are distributional plots. The histograms of interest are those for red cells, white cells, and platelets. Technicon also produces a hemoglobin histogram. The Y axis of the three common histograms is concentration or relative number (of cells), and the X axis is measurement of cell size in fl (Fig. 20-13, *A*).

RBC Histograms. There are no major differences among the red cell histograms generated by the different manufacturers of hematology analyzers. The normal red cell population produces a histogram with gaussian distribution (see Fig. 20-13, *A-2*). As the MCV gets smaller or larger the histogram pattern will shift along the X axis to the left or right, respectively. The histogram pattern will widen as there is more variation in red cell size and this is reflected in the red blood cell distribution width index (RDW) parameter that is a measure of anisocytosis. The small population of cells to the right of the single cell population represents doublets. Correction for coincidence is automatic in all instruments because coincidence is mathematically predictable, based on the cell concentration. Red cell fragments or very small red cells appear on the left side of the

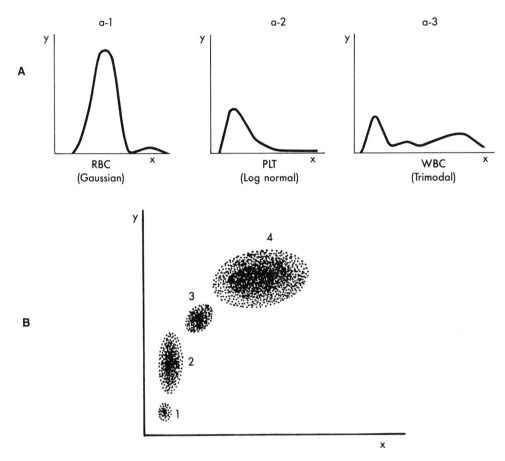

Fig. 20-13 **A**, Histogram displays: X axis represents cell size, Y axis represents relative number; A-1 Gaussian distribution (RBC), A-2 Log normal distribution (PLT), A-3 Trimodal distribution (WBC from three part differential analysis instruments). **B**, Scattergram (cytogram, dot plot): Y axis represents cell size, X axis represents a second cell characteristic measurement such as internal complexity (nuclear size or staining intensity). The density of the dots represents cell concentration. Cell concentration is represented by different colors on instruments with color monitors. Cluster 1 = debris, 2 = lymphocytes, 3 = monocytes, 4 = granulocytes.

histogram. If either type of red cell form crosses the lower threshold, the red count will be falsely lowered. In addition the hematocrit and other red cell parameters will be affected. Red cell agglutination interferes with counting, and the histogram pattern may reflect these cell groups by an increase in the "doublet" population.

Platelet Histograms. All multiparameter instruments that count platelets do so from the red cell dilution while the red cells are being counted and sized. Platelet size distribution is log normal (see Fig. 20-13, *A-2*).

Automated Differential Counting

Geometric Data Corporation, Coulter Biomedical Research Corporation, and Abbott Laboratories each made pattern recognition differ-

ential counters during the 1970s and early 1980s. Automated counting of white cell differentials by computer-directed pattern recognition was based on information concerning size, shape, color, and density that was acquired by electronic analysis of microscopic images. Each stained, blood film was scanned until a cell was located, then the image was broken down into a large number of data points. Each point was analyzed for information, which was fed to a computer where the cell was classified on the basis of the characteristics mentioned previously. These systems performed reliably on normal blood films, greatly reducing the tedium of manual differential counting, but had at least four major drawbacks. First, 100 cells were routinely identified and this did not enhance the precision of the manual differential (it only relieved the technologist fatigue factor). Second, if more cells were counted (i.e., 200 or 500 total cells [for statistical purposes]) much more time was required to find the additional cells. Third, a clean, monolayer film of cells was required with consistent staining characteristics. Fourth, review of "other" cells was required and "other" could be debris, stain precipitate, atypical, or abnormal white cells. The pattern recognition differential counters are no longer being manufactured.

WBC Histogram (Screening) Differentials. The more popular routine cell counters have been enhanced by addition of the histogram differential. The first attempt was to identify only two cell populations: lymphocyte and all other white cells. Next, three-part histogram differentials were introduced, lymphocyte, mononuclear (monocytes), and granulocyte (see Fig. 20-13, *A-3*). Most manufacturers of multiparameter hematology counters now have models that perform a three-part screening differential.

The histogram differential is based on analysis of subpopulations of white cells. The population distribution is displayed on the data terminal screen of these instruments or a hard copy may be printed. The two-part histogram differential was introduced by Coulter Electronics in their S Plus II. The red cell lysing reagent lysed the RBCs and stripped away the white cell cytoplasm, leaving the nucleus to be counted. The lymphocyte nucleus was separated from all other white cells by its size difference giving rise to a two-part differential that was introduced as part of the routine report generated by the Coulter S Plus II. The three-part differential was introduced by Coulter Electronics, Inc. and by Ortho Diagnostics Systems in 1983.

The five-part cytochemical differential provided by the Technicon instruments (since 1975) is usually found in more sophisticated laboratories with special interests in hematology/oncology patients and in larger hospitals with research interests.

In 1990 four companies manufactured instruments with five-part white cell differential analysis. Technicon Instrument Corporation continues to use light scatter analysis and cytochemical staining in its system. The three other manufacturers do not use stain to separate white cells into subpopulations. Coulter Electronics, TOA Medical Electronics, and Unipath (Sequoia-Turner) each make multiparameter cell counters that include five-part white cell differential absolute

counts and percentages. They use electrical resistance technology, light scatter technology, or a combination of both to analyze thousands of white cells in a matter of seconds.

Scattergrams (Dot Plots) or Cytograms. Scattergrams are two-dimensional displays of cell analysis data. Each axis represents measurement of a cell characteristic. Cells with similar characteristics form clusters, and the density of a cluster represents cell concentration (see Fig. 20-13, *B*). All instruments performing five-part screening differentials evaluate cell size and at least one other measurement (characteristic) of each cell. Cell size is measured by either electrical resistance or light scatter. The second cell measurement employed and the technology behind it form the basis of how the instruments differ.

Reticulocyte Automation: Sysmex R-1000

Flow cytometers can be configured to count reticulocytes but they require manual sample preparation before analysis by these instruments. A flow cytometer that is dedicated to reticulocyte counting is manufactured by TOA Medical Electronics. The Sysmex R-1000 shown in Fig. 20-14 is a fully automated reticulocyte counter. It uses an argon laser with sheath flow, hydrodynamic focusing, and laminar flow principles that have been described. This system consists of an analyzer unit, a pneumatic unit, and a laser power supply unit. The analyzer unit includes the fluidic system, the optical system, the electrical system, and a CRT with a control panel to operate the instrument. The pneumatic unit provides a regulated vacuum source and pressures to propel a sample through the analyzer. The electrical system changes the scattered light signals into electrical signals from which cell numbers and reticulocyte identification are obtained.

One hundred μl of whole blood are aspirated into a sample valve for precise measurement before dilution and staining with a fluorescent dye (Auramine-O). The staining reaction is controlled at a constant temperature to ensure reproducible results. Auramine-O is taken up by ribonucleic acid (RNA) in the immature red cells. The intensity of the staining is proportional to the amount of RNA in the cell. Approximately 30,000 cells pass through the flowcell to be analyzed for size and staining intensity. The laser light scattered by the passage of a single cell through the beam contains information characteristic of the cell. The forward light scatter signal

CHAPTER 21

Automation in Hemostasis

JEANINE M. WALENGA

Development of Hemostasis Instrumentation
Instrumentation for Clot-Based and Chromo-
   genic-Based Assays
Instrumentation for Platelet Evaluation
Instrumentation for Immunologic Based Assays
Future Trends in Coagulation Instrumentation

Development of Hemostasis Instrumentation

Laboratory assessment of coagulation disorders is no longer limited to monitoring clot formation and/or its dissolution employing such
basic tests as the bleeding, whole blood clotting,
prothrombin time (PT), activated partial thromboplastin time (APTT), and thrombin time. New
diagnostic tests based on biochemical, physiologic, radiochemical, pharmacologic, chemical,
physical, and immunologic principles have
emerged to identify the site and nature of a hemostatic defect. Along with the new tests numerous instruments have been developed. Table 21-
1 summarizes the types of instruments that can
be found in a modern hemostasis laboratory. The
detection system for each class of instruments
and the technique for which they are used in the
laboratory are also listed.

The development of coagulation methods on
automated instrumentation opens a new era in
the diagnosis and management of hemostatic disorders that will provide not only better information in terms of reliability of data, time, and cost
effectiveness but also more specific and sensitive
data on diagnostically decisive parameters.

Clotting Assays. Clinical coagulation testing
began in the early 1900s with physicians measuring simple bleeding times. In the early 1920s the
whole blood clotting time was introduced in
which venipuncture blood added to a glass tube
was timed for clot formation. A few other whole

blood assays were developed at this time. The
thrombelastograph can still be found in laboratories. This instrument gives a recorded tracing of
the kinetics and physical nature of whole blood
(or plasma) clot formation, its strength, time to
begin clotting and end complete clot formation,
and fibrinolysis if present.

During the next 30 years many of the basic
concepts of the mechanisms of blood coagulation
were learned, including the introduction of the
one-stage PT assay by Quick in 1935, the discovery of factor V in 1947, and the discovery of factor VII in 1951. The APTT was formulated during the following years and was associated with
the study of hemophilia.

In the late 1950s the first coagulation instrument was introduced to the laboratory. The Fibrometer (BBL, a division of Becton Dickinson,
Cockeysville, Md), a semi-automated clot detection device, uses a mechanical system attached to
electrodes to measure the clot endpoint. The fibrometer provided an objective approach to coagulation testing and the possibility of comparing
data from lab to lab or technician to technician.
Throughout the 1960s coagulation laboratories
relied on either the fibrometer or the tilt-tube
technique. Today fibrometers, proven to be a
workhorse and a highly versatile instrument, can
still be found in most coagulation laboratories.

The move toward complete automation took
place in the 1970s. This was fueled by the increasing number of assays being requested, which was
probably because of an increasing incidence of
venous thrombosis, introduction of more sensitive tests for the diagnosis of thrombosis, increased use of warfarin and heparin as anticoag-
ulants, the use of invasive diagnostic tests
requiring anticoagulation, and more sophisticated surgeries (e.g., use of extracorporeal circu-
lation).

Table 21-1 Instrumentation for today's hemostasis laboratory

Instrument class	Detector	Assay technique
Clot detectors	Electromechanical, viscoelastic, electromagnetic, light transmission	Clotting
Spectrophotometers	Light transmission	Synthetic substrate
Cell counters	Impedance	Platelet count
Aggregometers	Visible light transmission or impedance	Platelet function
Microtiter plate washer/reader	Light transmission	ELISA
β or τ counters	Radiation	RIA

For automated instrumentation, optical endpoint detectors evolved. As in a spectrophotometer where a change in light transmission is used to record a biochemical reaction, the new generation of coagulation instruments incorporated the use of recording light transmission to monitor a **clot endpoint.** The mechanics of these instruments are based on the principle that a change in light transmission occurs when plasma is converted from a fluid phase to a gel phase. Although this principle works under almost all conditions, lipemia, hemolysis, as well as some abnormal clotting reactions, can cause false readings. The electromechanical, principle of the fibrometer is usually the method of choice to confirm a suspicious test result.

Other detectors of clot endpoints were considered. Electromagnetic, ultraviolet light, fluorescence, laser, radioactivity, and electrical current detectors were developed. However, measurement of visible light transmission, or light scatter in some instances, seemed to be the most practical and economic method.

Chromogenic Assays. The developments in the knowledge of the hemostatic system led to the need for different types of laboratory instruments. To measure individual enzymes, inhibitors, or isolated reactions the clot based assays proved to have too many variables (sensitivity of detecting a clot; activators and inhibitors present in plasma that could cause interferences in the assay interpretation). By developing **chromogenic** based assays, specific isolated biochemical reactions could be monitored without the need for an intact coagulation system to produce the clot endpoint.

The principle of **synthetic substrate assays** is based on a specific enzyme-substrate reaction. The substrate is a synthetically prepared sequence of three or four amino acids that mimics the enzymatic active site of the natural substrate. These reactions are specific for the enzyme-substrate combination and do not rely on the multiple reaction steps of the coagulation cascade for an endpoint as clotting assays do.

$$Tos - Gly - Pro - Arg - pNa \xrightarrow{\text{thrombin}}$$
$$\text{(colorless)}$$
$$Tos - Gly - Pro - Arg + pNa$$
$$\text{(yellow)}$$

Synthetic substrates have been made for many of the coagulation and fibrinolytic factors including activators, inhibitors, and cofactors. Using these substrates, assays have also been developed to measure plasma levels of drugs such as heparin, streptokinase, and tissue plasminogen activator (TPA) based on their activation or inhibition of specific enzymes. These assays can be made for direct analysis of an enzyme (as shown previously in an assay for thrombin). If a substrate is not available for a particular enzyme, an indirect measurement of the enzyme can be made. In these assays the enzyme in question acts as the limiting factor in a reaction, and another enzyme in the reaction is quantitated.

Step 1: Plasmin $+ \alpha_2 -$ antiplasmin $\rightarrow$ plasmin $-$
    (reagent)   (plasma)

    antiplasmin complex $+$ excess plasmin

Step 2: H $-$ D $-$ Val $-$ Leu $-$ Lys $-$ pNa
    excess plasmin
    $\rightarrow$ H $-$ D $-$ Val $-$ Leu $-$ Lys $+$ pNa

For the chromogenic assays, color development is quantitated and enzymatic activity of the unknown analyte is determined through extrapolation of activity from a previously constructed standard curve.

For chromogenic assays, sometimes referred to as **amidolytic assays,** spectrophotometers are required. These can be simple one-cell manual instruments or elaborate fully automated systems. Synthetic substrate assays are easily adaptable to any spectrophotometer and they are easily automatable.

Platelet Function Assays. Laboratory assays for platelets include several techniques that have remained in routine practice over the years. The platelet count using a microscope is standard in all labs. However, a count cannot give any indication of functionality. The bleeding time assay is considered one of the better assays to assess overall platelet and coagulation function.

Platelet aggregation is at this time one of the better assays to evaluate platelet function. This method, developed by Born in 1963, is based on the concept that light transmission through platelet rich plasma (PRP) will increase when platelet clumps because platelet aggregation has occurred. Activated platelets will adhere to one another (adhesion) and then undergo further shape change, releasing their granular content to form an irreversible platelet clump (**aggregation**). This response is easily followed by a change in light transmission.

Other platelet assays that have been devised to quantitate platelet adhesion, platelet factor 3 (thromboplastin) availability, and clot retraction do not require special instrumentation. They can be performed with microscopes, fibrometers, or visualization of blood clot formation.

Immunologic Assays. The most recent development in hemostatic testing has been the immunologic-based assays and instrumentation. In addition to the well-known hemostatic enzymes and inhibitors there are substances released during activation of the hemostatic processes. These substances, termed **molecular markers,** are well-defined chemical entities of low molecular weight found in minute quantities in the blood and are derived from specific enzymatic reactions or released from activated cells. Some have functional activities, whereas others are only byproducts of a reaction. The evaluation of molecular markers has greatly enhanced the diagnostic ability of the hemostasis laboratory. These markers provide a site-specific indication of where an activation is occurring or a specific deficit that is leading to a bleeding or thrombotic disorder. Moreover, because of their origin, molecular markers indicate the initial stage of an activation process.

Finding elevated levels of markers related to thrombin generation, platelet activation, or decreased fibrinolytic activity would indicate a hypercoagulable state in a patient. This patient could then be treated prophylactically with low doses of an antithrombotic agent, and a clotting episode (stroke, heart attack) can be avoided. The molecular markers can indicate these changes, whereas the routine PT, APTT, fibrinogen, and platelet count assays would not show any abnormalities. In addition to the molecular markers, several newly identified enzymes are currently measured by the enzyme-linked immunosorbent assay (ELISA) technique because reliable functional assays (e.g., chromogenic assays) have not yet been developed.

The clotting and chromogenic assays do not have the level of sensitivity required to measure these parameters (10^{-6} gm/ml limit of sensitivity). ELISA and radioimmunoassays (RIA) that can measure 10^{-12} g/ml are commonly adapted to these measurements. Be aware, however, that immunologic assays do not measure the function of a protein, they only measure the presence of a protein. A normal ELISA result can be accompanied by an abnormal clotting or chromogenic activity. Thus immunologic assays only quantitate protein; they do not measure the activity of a protein.

For larger proteins (e.g., fibrinogen, antithrombin III) the older immunologic techniques such as radial immunodiffusion (RID) or the Laurell rocket technique can be employed. A modification of the Laurell technique is two-dimensional electrophoresis that provides a higher degree of separation of the antigens.

Several manual and automated systems are available for these assay techniques. Combinations of pipettors, dilutors, washers, and readers can be made.

Instruments for Clot-Based and Chromogenic-Based Assays

The primary instrument used in the clinical coagulation laboratory is one that is used to determine the capacity of blood to clot. This can be done globally by measuring clotting time. In association with clotting assays, specific quantitation of the individual enzymes, inhibitors, and activators that compose the coagulation (also fibrinolytic and platelet) system, it is also important to determine the exact source of a disorder. These specific parameters can be measured with chromogenic, biochemically defined assays.

Several companies have developed instruments that are capable of measuring both clotting assays, such as the PT and APTT, as well as the

Table 21-2   Coagulation instrumentation

Manufacturer	Model	Probe
MLA	Electra 700, 750, 800, 900	Clot
	Electra 900C, 1000C	Clot/chromogenic
Organon Teknika	Coag-A-Mate XM, RA4, X2	Clot
	MDA	Clot/chromogenic
Ortho	Koagulab 16-S, 32-S, 40-A, 60-S	Clot
	Koagulab CTS	Clot/chromogenic
Biodata	MCA 110P, 110WP	Clot
Helena	Dataclot 2	Clot
	Cascade 480	Clot/chromogenic
IL	ACL 100, 200	Clot
	ACL 300, 300 Plus	Clot/chromogenic
DuPont	Aca	Clot/chromogenic
	Coumatrak	Clot
Ciba Corning	512	Clot
International Technidyne	Hemochron	Clot
HemoTec	Hepcon/HMS	Clot
Miscellaneous	Spectrophotometers (manual and automated)	Chromogenic

chromogenic substrate assays. These **multiprobe** instruments have the feature of performing the classical global coagulation assays plus specific chromogenic assays on one machine rather than two, a potential advantage for the expanding coagulation laboratory. Table 21-2 lists the various manufacturers of coagulation instrumentation, the different models they carry, and whether the systems are single or multiprobe.

Medical Laboratory Automation Instrumentation. Medical Laboratory Automation, Inc. (MLA, Pleasantville, NY) offers a wide range of automated coagulation instrumentation including the MLA Electra 700, 750, 800, 900, 900C, and 1000C, which measure clot formation by the photometric clot detection principle. The photo-optical system consists of two photolamps and photodetectors with logarithmic amplifiers. This technique is used to compute the mathematic second derivative of the optical density signal. If a sample is too transparent or too opaque, an off-scale warning will be printed. Each of the instruments allows for continuous loading of patient samples. All of the MLA instruments are capable of performing the PT, APTT, thrombin time, fibrinogen, and factor assays. They will also prepare dilutions of plasma in saline for the factor and fibrinogen assays.

The Electra 700 (Fig. 21-1) has a turntable with 30 cuvette positions (60 samples). The turntable locks after indexing to prevent disturbing the sample in the test station. Color-coded cuvettes are used for PT/APTT user identification,

and used cuvettes are automatically discarded into a disposal catch bin. The reagent pump system consists of three independent peristaltic pumps. Reagents are primed directly into the reagent reservoir to eliminate waste. In addition to the basic test menu the 700 will perform a two-stage PT, factor substitution tests, and other special tests. This instrument also has a selectable incubation time switch for either 200 or 300 seconds that allows for the variable incubation requirements of different reagents. In the PT mode the throughput of the instrument is 180 tests/hour. The APTT mode will run 68 tests/hour. The 700 has a built-in instrument QC and the confidence test, which assesses the clot detection system by simulating a clot and printing the verification times. As with most newer instrumentation these instruments can be interfaced with the hospital mainframe computer. The 700 is suitable for the needs of a laboratory requiring an automated instrument with the ability to intersperse PTs and APTTs with single-patient and batch-processing capabilities.

The newest series of MLA Electra instruments are the 900, 900C, and 1000C systems. The Electra 900 is a random access photo-optical clot detection system capable of performing all clotting assays including the PT (with derived fibrinogen), APTT, actual fibrinogen (Clauss method), thrombin time, and up to 99 user-defined special clotting assays. The operator can program the number of channels to be used, reagent volumes (25 to 500 μl), incubation time, activation time,

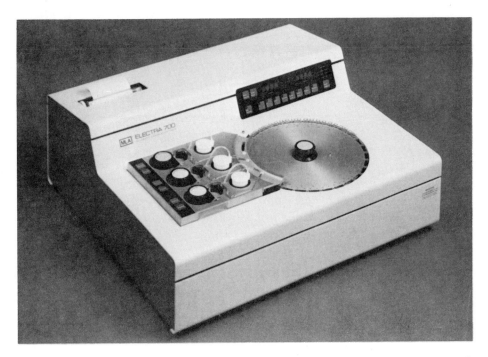

Fig. 21-1 The Electra 700 automated coagulation instrument (courtesy Medical Laboratory Automation, Pleasantville, NY).

and step time (interval between feed belt movements). This allows for easy adaptation of new tests and reagents from different manufacturers. An on-board CRT allows the user to review and edit standard curve data before printing.

The 900C and 1000C offer the capability of performing the chromogenic assays in addition to the routine clot-based assays. The programmed chromogenic assays include antithrombin III, protein C, plasminogen, antiplasmin, heparin (high and low levels), factor VIII, factor IX, factor X, PT chromogenic, and APTT chromogenic. These assays can be performed in batches or mixed modes. Each assay channel is standardized by a reference channel that automatically balances the filter optic system and calibrates the photo-optical cell.

The Electra 1000C (Fig. 21-2) is an Electra 900C with the addition of an MLA automatic **primary tube sampler.** This system has the capacity to hold 100 blood collection tubes of varying sizes. The sample probe determines the size of the tube, and, based on a normal hematocrit, the instrument calculates the amount of plasma available for aspiration. The different MLA systems are compared in Table 21-3.

Organon Teknika. Organon Teknika (Durham, NC) has developed a wide range of coagu-

lation instruments that are suited to meet the needs of individual laboratories. The principle of operation is similar in all of the Coag-A-Mate instruments in that clot formation is detected from the rate of change in light intensity. The photo-optical clot sensing system consists of detector cells, each with its own red light emitting diode (LED) light source, which is driven by a constant current regulator to give each a noise-free light beam. This light beam passes through the cuvette to a diffuser and then to a sensor that converts the light into an electrical signal. This signal is converted into a digital value that is displayed by the printer.

The smaller of the Organon Teknika instruments is the Coag-A-Mate XM (Fig. 21-3), which is designed for use in a small laboratory or as a backup unit in a larger hospital. The Coag-A-Mate XM is capable of performing PT, APTT, thrombin time, quantitative and semiquantitative fibrinogen, and factor assays. The double photo-optical system reads four samples simultaneously; however, this instrument requires an operator to be present at all times to add plasma and reagents at specified intervals. Therefore it is only suitable for low volume needs.

The newest instrument of Organon Teknika is the MDA (Multi-Channel Discrete Analyzer)

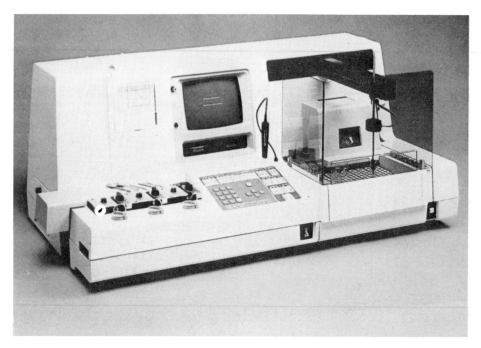

Fig. 21-2 The Electra 1000C automated coagulation and chromogenic substrate assay instrument (courtesy Medical Laboratory Automation, Pleasantville, NY).

Table 21-3   Features of the MLA Electra coagulation instrument series

	MLA 700	*MLA 800*	*MLA 900/900C*	*MLA 1000C*
Throughput (number/hour)	PT: 180/hr	360/hr	360/hr	360/hr
	APTT: 68/hr	136/hr	136/hr	136/hr
Random access	Yes	No	Yes	Yes
Reagent pumps	3	2	3	3
Sample ID	No	No	Yes	Yes
Bar code	No	No	Yes	Yes
INR	No	No	No	No
Quality control	No	No	Yes	Yes
PT with derived fibrinogen	No	No	Yes	Yes
Printed standard curves	No	Yes	Yes	Yes
Factor assay dilutions	No	No	No	Yes
Chromogenics	No	No	No/Yes	Yes

Table 21-4   Features of the Organon Teknika Coag-A-Mate coagulation instrument series

	XM	*RA4*	*X2*	*MDA*
	Manual	PT: 108/hr	320/hr	180 test/hr
Throughput (number/hour)		APTT: 60/hr	96/hr	
Random access	No	Yes	Yes/No	Yes
Reagent pumps	0	4	2	4
Bar code	No	No	No	Yes
INR	Yes	Yes	Yes	Yes
QC	No	Yes	Yes	Yes
PT with derived Fibrinogen	Yes	Yes	No	Yes
Printed standard curves	No	No	Yes	Yes

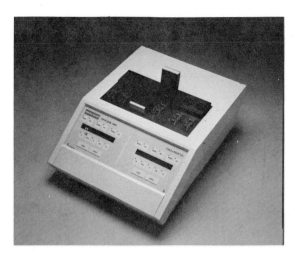

Fig. 21-3 The Coag-A-Mate XM automated coagulation instrument (courtesy Organon Teknika, Durham, NC).

(Fig. 21-4). It is a random access analyzer that can perform clotting, chromogenics, and immunoassays. It features a closed, primary tube sampling system that automatically pipets plasma sample from a closed-blood collection tube.

Identification of samples is done by bar coding. The instrument is driven by four syringe pumps that have access to over 30 reagents or controls on-line at one time. With a throughput of 180 tests/hour, the MDA is a fully automated instrument with microsampling capabilities. Up to 120 samples can be loaded in a single run. The MDA is useful for research laboratories and routine laboratories because of its ability to run 12 separate tests on a single sample. This instrument is still under development and will be released in 1992. The different systems from Organon Teknika are compared in Table 21-4.

Ortho Diagnostic Systems. Ortho's (Raritan, NJ) line of coagulation instrumentation includes the Koagulab 16-S, 32-S, 40-A, and 60-S. These instruments are capable of performing the PT, APTT, thrombin time, quantitative fibrinogen, and factor assays.

A unique feature to the Koagulab clotting instruments is the clot detection system. By an automatic light modulation the variability in the opacity of each patient plasma is compensated by adjusting the intensity of the light source for each specimen. This is done by providing a blank time at the beginning of each assay during the time reagent is dispensed into the cuvette. A photodetec-

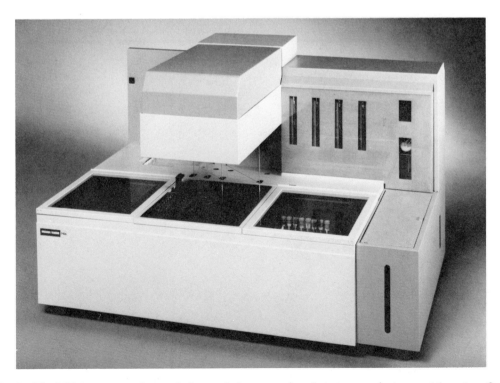

Fig. 21-4 The MDA automated coagulation and chromogenic substrate assay instrument (courtesy Organon Teknika, Durham, NC).

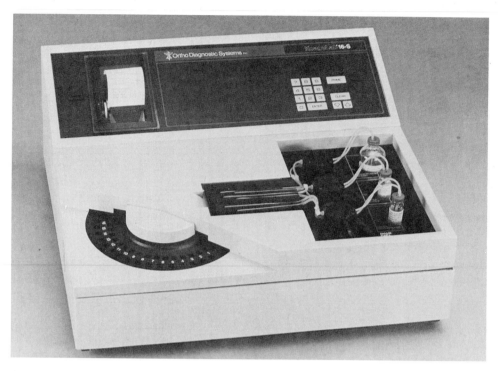

Fig. 21-5   The Koagulab 16-S automated coagulation instrument (courtesy Ortho Laboratories, Raritan, NJ).

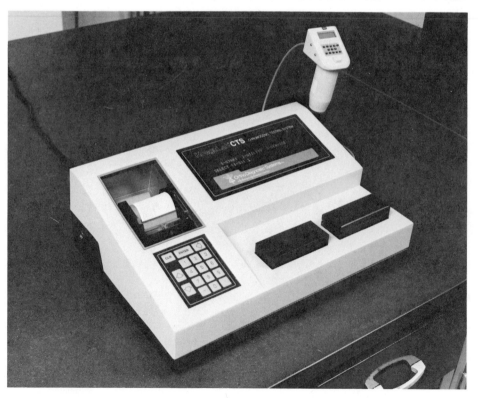

Fig. 21-6   The Koagulab CTS automated coagulation instrument and chromogenic substrate assay instrument (courtesy Ortho Laboratories, Raritan, NJ).

tor records the LED signal. To avoid interferences (e.g., electronic noise) during the clotting process, clot formation is monitored over its entire time course. A graph of the clot formation in which turbidity vs reaction time is plotted (i.e., the **clot signature**) can be printed on request. The Koagulab systems are equipped with a QC data management program, computerized pump calibration, bar code reading, incubation time flexibility, and computer interfacing.

The Koagulab 16-S is the most widely used of the Koagulab models (Fig. 21-5). It has built-in data management software that will automatically enter QC data into the appropriate population. Other features include sample identification, Coefficient of Variation (CV) flag, adjustment of incubation times, maximum endpoints, and International Normalized Ratio (INR). The cuvette trays are composed of 16 wells. Four trays can be loaded/run. Up to 202 PTs and 101 APTTs/hour can be run.

The latest instrument introduced by Ortho is the Koagulab CTS (Fig. 21-6). This system was designed to perform chromogenic substrate assays. The system's test menu includes antithrombin III, antiplasmin, protein C, plasminogen, heparin, and factor VIII. This chromogenic system is capable of analyzing eight samples simultaneously in 5 minutes. The CTS is equipped with a computer-controlled pipettor to add reagents. Standard curves can be stored for future use. This instrument is not walk-away (semiautomated) and requires hands-on attention. A comparison of the different Ortho instruments is given in Table 21-5.

Helena Laboratories. The Dataclot 2 (Fig. 21-7) from Helena Laboratories (Beaumont, Tx) is an updated model of the original BBL Fibrometer. As with the fibrometers, the clot is detected by an electromechanical probe (Fig. 21-8, *A*) which has two electrodes. One electrode remains stationary in the plasma while the other moves in and out of the plasma (Fig. 21-8, *B*). When a clot forms, the electrical circuit is completed by the fibrin strands when the moving electrode would otherwise be out of the plasma. This stops the timing mechanism.

The Dataclot 2 has built-in stopwatches to monitor incubation times and a digital display of the temperature and clotting time. This is a semiautomated instrument that lends itself to a small laboratory because of the low throughput and the hands-on time required to run an assay; however, it has the versatility to do any type of clotting assay using any reagents.

Recently Helena has introduced a new hemostasis analyzer, the Cascade 480, with the capability of performing PT, APTT, fibrinogen, and thrombin time in any order with rapid throughput. Four samples are read simultaneously for a throughput time of up to 360 PTs/hour or 144 APTTs/hour. The Cascade is equipped with five reagent pumps so there is no requirement for changing reagents between runs. Special features include computer memory storage of reference curves, INR calculations, options for derived fibrinogens, and a half-volume mode that will run an assay at reduced reagent and plasma volumes. A comprehensive data management system allows the operator to print all patient-related he-

Table 21-5 A comparison of the Ortho Koagulab coagulation instrument series

	16-S	*32-S*	*40-A*	*60-S*
Throughput (number/hour)	PT: 202/hr APTT: 101/hr	202/hr 101/hr	166/hr 114/hr	360/hr 180/hr
Random access	Yes	Yes	Yes	Yes
Reagent pumps	3	3	3	4
Sample delivery	Manual	Manual	Automatic from sample tube	Manual
Bar code	Yes*	Yes*	No	Yes*
INR	Yes	Yes	Yes	Yes
Printed standard curves	Yes	Yes	No	Yes
Clot signature	Yes	Yes	No	Yes
Display	Dot matrix	Dot matrix	LED	VFD (vacuum fluorescent display)
Auto pump calibration	Yes	Yes	Yes	Yes

*Option available but must be purchased separately.

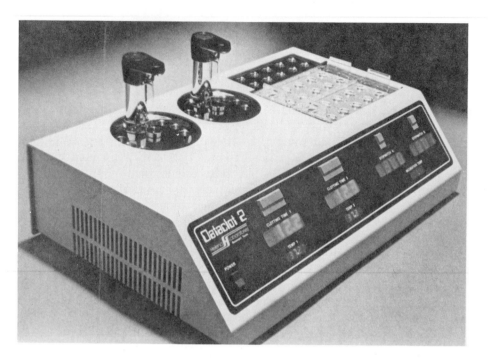

Fig. 21-7   The Dataclot 2 coagulation timer (courtesy Helena Laboratories, Beaumont, Tx).

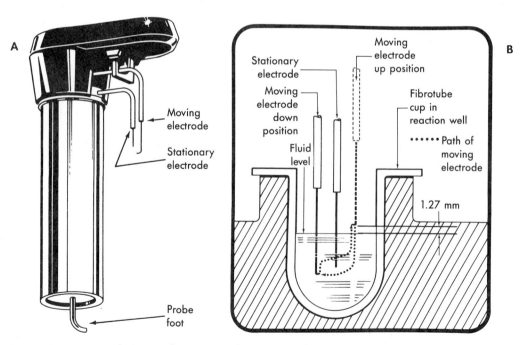

Fig. 21-8   **A**, Electromechanical probe for clot detection by the Fibrometer (courtesy BBL, Cockeysville, Md). **B**, Mechanics of the operation of the fibrometer probe.

mostasis information on report sheets. QC data can be easily archived and evaluated against a pool of peer laboratories. In addition a stand-alone chromogenic analyzer included with the Cascade allows 17 different chromogenic assays to be performed without interrupting the routine clot testing.

Troubleshooting. Each of the coagulation instruments has a troubleshooting guide in its accompanying manual for problems specific to that instrument. Furthermore, many of the clotting analyzers have diagnostic modes that can take the technologist through a program to diagnose and correct the malfunction.

In general there are some important things to be aware of for all clotting instruments. Inaccurate clotting times can be obtained because of temperatures being too cold or too warm. Temperature is controlled automatically and can be monitored at all times on most instruments to ensure that the clotting assays are being performed at 37° C. Equally important is that the reagents are kept at 4° C to avoid deterioration. Peristaltic pumps accurately deliver the amount of plasma and reagent needed; however, these pumps should be calibrated and checked according to each manufacturers' specifications to ensure that they are working properly. It is also very important to keep the tubing clean and to change it as required. Also, tubing should be designated for each reagent so that cross-contamination does not occur. Normal and abnormal controls should be run on each shift to check that the instrument and the reagents are working properly.

Similarly, for chromogenic assay instrumentation temperature, timing, and pipet calibration are critical. Particularly when microsample/reagent volumes are used, pipetting errors can result in extremely erroneous results. Although proper reagent handling is important for both clotting and chromogenic assays, the chromogenics are probably more sensitive to changes in reagent conditions and the reagents are more susceptible to degradation. The purified enzymes are not as stable as the common PT/APTT reagents, making it important to run proper controls during the testing period. As with the coagulation instruments, cross-contamination of reagents/samples should be avoided and cleanliness of the instrument should be maintained.

For both coagulation and chromogenic assays probably the most critical factor in achieving accurate results is the manner in which the sample is collected and processed. Special precautions should be followed to avoid activation or degradation of the sample. In addition lipemia and hemolysis can cause false readings on optical based clotting and chromogenic instruments.

Instrumentation for Platelet Evaluation

Platelets, the first line of defense against bleeding, play a key role in the balance of hemostatic mechanisms. They react to a wide range of stimuli responding by shape change, adhesion, aggregation, and degranulation. Platelets can be either hyperactive, causing thrombosis, or inhibited, causing bleeding. Each of these responses are quantitated by laboratory techniques. Several new technologies make it possible to measure platelet functions and to some extent monitor antiplatelet treatment. See p. 391 for a list of instrumentation used for platelet testing.

Bleeding Time Devices. The **bleeding time test** has been widely used for the screening of platelet dysfunction and general hemostatic defects. Quite simply, an incision is made on the forearm and the time to stop bleeding is measured. Today several companies, such as International Technidyne and Organon Teknika, manufacture spring-loaded lancets that produce a more standardized incision than the original scalpel-type blades.

Platelet Aggregometers. The functionality of platelets is studied by platelet aggregometry, a technique in which platelets are isolated in platelet-rich plasma, stimulated by various agents, and monitored for their ability to aggregate (i.e., undergo shape change, release granular contents, and aggregate to one another). Several different types of platelet aggregometers are available.

Biodata Corp. (Hatboro, Pennsylvania) has the Platelet Aggregation Profiler (PAP) 4 (Fig. 21-9). This instrument has four independently operated aggregation channels. Aggregation is measured by optical means. LEDs transmit light through test tubes containing PRP. The light passes to detectors, becomes amplified, and is then sent to a multiplexer. When platelets are in a nonactivated state, the PRP is translucent. After aggregation, the PRP becomes clear (platelet clumps can be visually observed).

The PAP 4 offers the capability of performing a von Willebrand's test. For this assay the data is printed on a log-log chart and reported as percent activity. The standard curve is made by pipetting dilutions of plasma into a platelet suspension

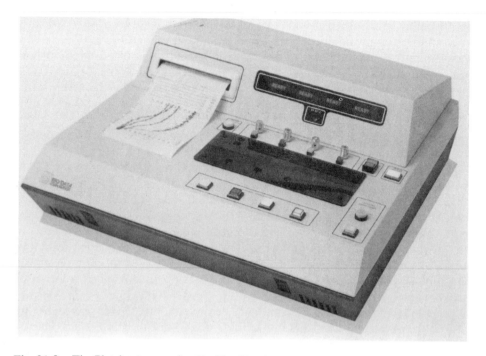

Fig. 21-9 The Platelet Aggregation Profiler (PAP) 4 aggregometer (Biodata; Hatboro, Pa).

mixed with ristocetin. The standard curve is then plotted and stored for future use in the instrument's memory.

Additional features of the PAP 4 include automatic 0% and 100% baseline settings, microsample volume capabilities, and the ability to perform leukocyte aggregations. With the special function keys individual aggregation curves can be reprinted. The chart reader is built into the PAP 4.

Chronolog Corporation (Havertown, Pennsylvania) makes four types of platelet aggregometers. The Model 430 is a single channel automatic aggregometer and the Model 440 is a dual channel automatic aggregometer. The principle of operation is based on quantitation of infrared light that is simultaneously passed through platelet-poor plasma and PRP. By depressing a button, the baselines are automatically set. Light transmission is compared digitally, and a difference in voltage is generated, amplified, and recorded on an auxillary linear strip chart recorder. A front panel range error lamp signals if the platelet count is too low (<30,000 platelets/mm³). A constant stir speed of 1200 rpm controls the stirring action. Although it is recommended to use the Chronolog recorders, most strip-chart recorders can be attached to the aggregometer.

Chronolog also has a Lumi-aggregometer Model 400, 450, or 460 that is used to simultaneously measure platelet aggregation and secretion of ATP from the granules of the activated platelets. The general operation of the lumi-aggregometer is identical to the 430 and 440 models. In addition, however, at a right angle to the aggregation channel is a sensitive photomultiplier tube that simultaneously measures the luminescence created by luciferin-luciferase in the presence of ATP. The simultaneous recording of both platelet aggregation and secretion of ATP is a powerful tool in the investigation of platelet function disorders. It also represents an advance over studies of serotonin release from activated platelets that requires radioactive labeling and cannot be performed simultaneously with aggregation studies.

Chronolog makes a whole blood aggregometer (Model 500, 530, or 540) that measures platelet aggregation in whole blood by impedance changes. Whole blood is opaque, and therefore aggregation cannot be measured photometrically. Electrical impedance between two fine elec-

---

Instrumentation for Platelet Evaluation

Cell counters/microscopes
Bleeding time devices
Aggregometers
    Platelet rich plasma
    Whole blood
    Luminescence
    Platelet ionized calcium
Miscellaneous (for evaluation of clot retraction, PF3 availability, platelet adhesion, and flow cytometry)

---

trodes is used. When the electrodes are immersed in blood, a monolayer of platelets coats the electrodes. On aggregation additional platelets adhere to the monolayer, increasing the impedance between the electrodes. This change in resistance is converted to a DC voltage that is recorded on a linear chart recorder.

Another platelet aggregometer available from Chronolog is the Platelet Ionized Calcium Aggregometer (PICA), which can simultaneously measure cytoplasmic ionized calcium and platelet aggregation. Aequorin luminescence is the marker used to measure ionized calcium concentration. This system has been useful to study the dependence of calcium on platelet shape change, aggregation, and the effect of inhibitors on platelet function.

Troubleshooting. General troubleshooting guidelines for platelet function testing are as follows: care should be taken to ensure the wells of the aggregometer are at 37° C because platelets will not aggregate optimally at other temperatures. The stir speed of the reaction wells should be periodically checked. Proper stir bars should be used with all tests. Also, cuvettes should be handled at the top to avoid fingerprints on the area where light transmission is measured. Most problems stem from the preparation and handling of the blood sample and PRP.

Instrumentation for Immunologic-Based Assays

Immunologic assays provide highly sensitive tools to determine minute amounts of substances in serum, plasma, and other biologic fluids. Older techniques such as latex agglutination, radial immunodiffusion, and nephelometry are used to measure the larger proteins (e.g., antithrombin III, protein C). These techniques are not recommended because these assays only measure the presence of proteins; they do not measure their functionality. More sophisticated techniques such as rocket (Laurell) immunoelectrophoresis, enzyme linked immunoassays (ELISA), and radioimmunoassays (RIA) of higher sensitivity are needed to measure the smaller sized molecular markers that circulate in minute quantities. The ELISA technique seems to be the most widely accepted because of its ease of operation, no need for isotopes, and quantitative precision. Newer instrumentation has been developed for these new test methodologies to be performed quickly, accurately, and in a batch processing manner.

ELISA Instruments. Several companies have developed instrumentation for performing ELISA-based assays. The technique for performing these assays incorporates multiple fill/aspiration steps in which the reaction chambers (usually a 96-well 8 × 12 configuration microtiter plate) are filled with antigens, antibodies, or reagents followed by a washing procedure to remove the unbound material. Instrumentation includes washers to perform washing procedures and microtiter plate readers to quantitate the reactions. Commonly a multichannel pipet (8 or 12 tip) is used to add reagents, although samples are still pipetted manually one at a time. Several manufacturers have undertaken the development of automated walk-away 96 tip multichannel pipettors; however, these are not in common use.

Bio-Tek Instruments (Winooski, Vermont) offers a complete line of manual and automated ELISA microtiter plate washers and readers. The features of these instruments are compared in Table 21-6. The EL 401 Manual Washer allows for 8 or 12 channel washings of a plate/strip (Fig. 21-10).

The EL 403 Autowasher is an automated system designed for high volume ELISA work. It can be programmed for five different wash cycles, dispense volumes, soak times, plate shaking, QC on the aspiration and dispense function, and automated maintenance programs. Aspiration is performed from the top down, minimizing fluid contact with the probes and thus minimizing high background resulting from cross-contamination of samples. The EL 403 can also be interfaced to a robotic arm for less hands-on operation.

Bio-Tek also has several ELISA readers with varying capabilities. The EL 301 and EL 307 are manual readers with single/dual wavelength photometers. The EL 301 Microwell Strip Reader is a portable reader (Fig. 21-11) with filters at 405

Table 21-6 Features of the Bio-Tek ELISA instrument series

	EL 301	*EL 307*	*EL 311*	*EL 312*	*EL 340*	*EL 320*
Wavelength range	400-700 nm	380-750 nm	380-750 nm	380-750 nm	340-750 nm	340-750 nm
Absorbance range	0-2.500	0-2.000	0-3.000	0-4.000	0-4.000	0-3.000
Linearity	0-2.000	0-2.000	0-2.000	0-3.000	0-3.000	0-2.000
Manual or auto/	Manual	Manual	Auto	Auto	Auto	Auto
speed			30 secs/plate	9 secs/plate	9 secs/plate	45 secs/plate
Kinetics capabilities	No	No	Yes	Yes	Yes	Yes
Agglutination	No	No	Yes	Yes	Yes	Yes
Temperature control	No	No	No	No	Yes	?
Bar code	No	No	No	No	Yes	Yes
Plate agitation	No	No	No	No	Yes	Yes
Stacking capabilities	No	No	No	No	No	Yes

All models have a tungsten halogen light source and a silicon photodiode detector.

and 490 nm. The EL 307 Manual Reader has filters that range from 380 to 750 nm. The photodetectors of the EL 301 and EL 307 consist of a silicon diode with a tungsten-halogen lamp. The EL 301 is useful when only a few strips of a microtiter plate are used, whereas the EL 307 can read a full 96-well microtiter plate.

The EL 320 Stacking Autoreader is an auto-mated instrument with capabilities that include 20 programmable protocols and stacking flexibility for up to 25 microtiter plates (Fig. 21-12). It can read up to 80 plates/hour in an endpoint or kinetic mode. The EL 320 has the basic capabilities of the other Bio-Tek auto readers. It is best adapted to a laboratory that performs large batches of ELISA assays.

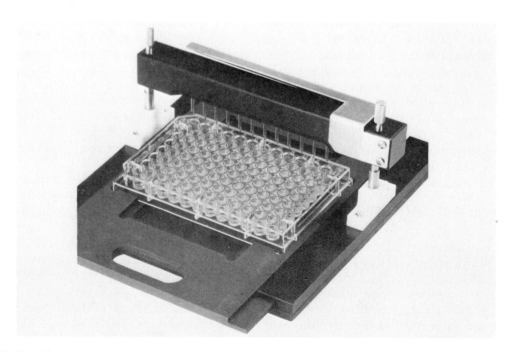

Fig. 21-10 Bio-Tek's EL 401 manual microplate washer assembly (courtesy Bio-Tek, Winooski, Vt) and example of a 96-well plate for ELISA testing.

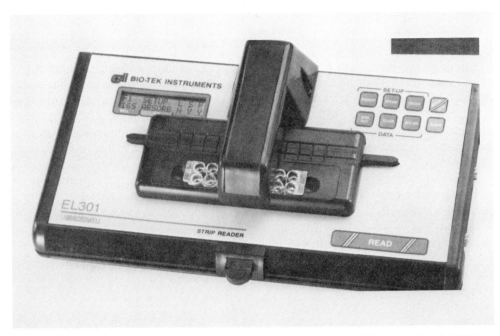

Fig. 21-11 Bio-Tek's EL 301 (courtesy Bio-Tek, Winooski, Vt). Microwell Strip Reader for ELISA testing.

Dynatech (Chantilly, Virginia) offers several models of both microtiter plate washers and readers for ELISA testing that range from manual to fully automated systems. The Handi-Wash and Miniwash are manual washers that will fill/aspirate from 12 or 8 rows at once. The Minireader is a manual photometer for measuring absorbance values from a microtiter plate.

The Ultrawash II and the MR 700 Reader are the most automated systems available from Dynatech. The Ultrawash II will dispense and aspirate washing buffer from a 96-well microtiter plate. An entire 5-cycle run can be completed in less than 3 minutes, a process that could take up to 15 minutes manually. The wash volume, soak time, and number of wash/aspirate cycles are adjustable and fully automated through a built-in program. One disadvantage of this instrument is that it can only wash a 96-well plate. The heads, however, can be manually changed to accommodate strips of reaction wells or partial plates.

The MR 700 is a photometer designed to measure the light absorbance of samples in a 96-well microtiter plate. The instrument can be operated in either a single wavelength or dual wavelength mode that includes five different wavelength settings in the range of 340 to 700 nm. The dual wavelength mode measures the absorbance of a sample at two preselected wavelengths. The peak wavelength is set near the absorption maximum,

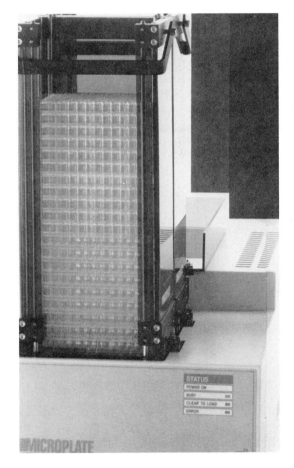

Fig. 21-12 Bio-Tek's EL 320 (courtesy Bio-Tek, Winooski, Vt) automated stacking microplate reader.

and the reference wavelength is chosen outside this area to correct for variations because of scratches, dirt, and imperfections. A tungsten halogen lamp projects a light beam horizontally through two lenses into a 90 degree prism from which the light is projected vertically down through the sample well and onto a rotating filter disc. A silicon photodetector measures the energy of the light beam.

Troubleshooting. The ELISA washers should be kept clean to avoid mechanical problems. Tubing should be rinsed with distilled water followed by air to avoid precipitation or crystallization of buffers in the tubing or in the aspiration and dispensing probes. If this occurs, inaccurate and inefficient washing will occur. All 96 wells of a microtiter plate should be filled/aspirated with equal volumes. It is important to visually inspect a plate after aspiration to be sure no buffer remains because this will cause a dilution error when reagents are added. Most problems with ELISA washers require a service person.

Common problems with ELISA assay results stem from improper collection and handling of the specimen. Particularly when working with molecular markers, the sample can be easily activated or degraded if not collected by the accepted technique in the proper anticoagulant/preservative and processed appropriately. In addition certain precautions in reagent handling (e.g., keeping the substrate in the dark) are very important to follow. Users should try to avoid spillage from overfilled microtiter plate wells. In particular the acid used to stop the reaction will ruin the optics and decrease the life of the instruments.

Future Trends in Coagulation Instrumentation

Technologic advances in methodology and instrumentation have changed the scope of almost all coagulation laboratories. The dramatic growth and development have resulted from the influences of clinical chemistry, clinical immunology, pharmacology, biochemistry, and biotechnology. Analytic instruments for use in hemostatic testing go beyond the clot-based readers and platelet aggregometers to a range of automated discrete chemistry analyzers, batch processors, microtiter systems, and the newest multiprobe instruments designed to simultaneously measure different assay endpoints. Moreover, automation has the distinct advantages of operational simplicity, microsampling, low reagent consumption, cost-effectiveness, and computer compatibility for fast and accurate data reduction. Instruments are designed for batch processing of single tests on multiple samples or multiple test panels on a single sample. Versatility ranges from instruments that only measure the final reaction solution by endpoint or kinetic analysis to instruments that automatically pipet reagents and sample, incubate, and analyze the reaction.

These advances in methodology and instrumentation and other developments such as dry chemistry, dip-stick screening, flow cytometry, physician's office testing, and disease panel profiling are providing the clinical hemostasis laboratory with tools to provide needed patient care against the risks associated with thrombosis and for monitoring of the new drug therapies.

Review Questions

1. What are the components of hemostasis that should be considered in a thorough diagnosis?
   A. Coagulation factors
   B. The cardiovascular system
   C. Coagulation enzymes and inhibitors, fibrinolytic enzymes and inhibitors, cellular elements including platelets, leukocytes, and endothelium.
   D. The liver and cardiovascular system
2. Pathologic events associated with abnormalities of the hemostatic system include:
   A. Thrombosis (clotting) and bleeding
   B. Heart attack, stroke, deep venous thrombosis
   C. Heparin induced thrombocytopenia
   D. All of the above
3. The difference between a fibrometer and an optical detection coagulation instrument is that:
   A. Different assay systems have to be used on the two kinds of instruments
   B. The optical systems can be more easily automated and therefore have better versatility to new assays and reagents than the fibrometer
   C. The fibrometer shows strong interference to lipemic samples resulting in falsely shortened clotting times
   D. The fibrometer uses an electromechanical detector, which is a more physical way of detecting a clot than a change in light transmission
4. A synthetic substrate assay is based on the following principle:
   A. A peptide sequence is made that mimics the active site of the natural enzyme
   B. A substrate with specificity for one enzyme is used to quantitate the activity of that enzyme
   C. An intact coagulation system is required for accurate activity measurements
   D. Enzymatic activity releases pNA, a photo-op-

tical tag, from the synthetic substrate that can be quantitated at 305 nm

5. Platelet evaluation:
   A. By platelet count is usually adequate to assess overall platelet function
   B. Using the bleeding time test is a very accurate and objective method
   C. By platelet aggregation measures the functionality of platelets
   D. Is limited to platelet aggregation in plasma without available techniques to quantitate the release response

6. Molecular markers are best measured by the ELISA or RIA technique because:
   A. They are found in minute quantities in plasma
   B. They are of very small size
   C. Many are byproducts of a reaction and do not have a functional activity
   D. All of the above

7. The primary difference between ELISA and synthetic substrate testing is:
   A. Synthetic substrate assays have higher sensitivity and lower specificity than ELISA assays
   B. The higher sensitivity and lower specificity of the ELISA test over the synthetic substrate test
   C. The ability of the synthetic substrate assay to measure functionality of an enzyme that an immunologic assay cannot do
   D. Synthetic substrate assays are difficult to automate, whereas ELISA methods are easy to automate

8. A multiprobe instrument is defined as an instrument:
   A. That is capable of performing both manual and automated functions
   B. That can handle a multiple number of samples
   C. That has multiple reagent reservoirs
   D. That has the ability to perform both clotting and chromogenic assays in the same system

9. The unique advantage of centrifugal analysis over other instrumentation techniques is:
   A. Immediate and numerous absorbance readings can be taken on multiple samples in a kinetic assay
   B. Fast turnaround time
   C. Small sample and reagent volumes are used
   D. Increased precision over manual techniques

10. Common problems associated with ELISA techniques include:
    A. Available sample amount is often too little
    B. Excess wash buffer; reagent remaining in microtiter plate wells after aspiration
    C. Specificity is too low, leading to frequent interfering substances in the assay
    D. Sensitivity is not high enough to detect the low sample concentration

Answers

1. C   2. D   3. D   4. B   5. C   6. D   7. C   8. A   9. A   10. B

Bibliography

Bick L: Disorders of hemostasis and thrombosis, New York, 1985, Thieme Stratton.

Colman RW, Hirsh J, Marder VJ et al, eds: Hemostasis and thrombosis: basic principles and clinical practice, ed 2, Philadelphia, 1987, JB Lippincott.

Corriveau DM, Fritsma GA, eds: Hemostasis and thrombosis in the clinical laboratory, Philadelphia, 1988, JB Lippincott.

Fareed J: Perspectives in hemostasis, New York, 1981, Pergamon Press.

Fareed J, ed: Automation in coagulation testing: parts I and II, Semin Thromb Hemost 9(3, 4): 139–400, 1983.

Fareed J, ed: Molecular markers of hemostatic disorders, Semin Thromb Hemost 10(4): 215–340, 1984.

Hemker HC: Handbook of synthetic substrates for the coagulation and fibrinolytic system, The Hague, 1983, Martinus Nijhoff.

Hirsh J, Brain EA: Hemostasis and thrombosis. A conceptual approach, ed 2, New York, 1983, Churchill Livingstone.

Murano G, Bick RL: Basic concepts of hemostasis and thrombosis, Boca Raton, Fla, 1980, CRC Press.

Ogston D: The physiology of hemostasis, Cambridge, Mass, 1983, Harvard University Press.

Parvez Z: Immunoassays in coagulation testing, New York, 1984, Springer-Verlag.

Ratnoff OD, Forbes CD: Disorders of hemostasis, Orlando, Fla, 1984, Grune & Stratton.

Thompson AR, Harker LA: Manual of hemostasis and thrombosis, ed 3, Philadelphia, 1983, FA Davis.

Thomson JM: Blood coagulation and haemostasis, New York, 1980, Churchill Livingstone.

Triplett DA: Hemostasis. A case oriented approach, New York, 1985, Igaku-Shoin.

Verstraete M, Vermylen J: Thrombosis, Elmsford, NY, 1984, Pergamon Press.

CHAPTER 22

Automation in Microbiology

BARBARA LEWIS
KATHY RISTOW

Automated Blood Culture Instruments
Urine Screen Instruments
Identification and Susceptibility Instruments

The clinical microbiology laboratory has been one of the last laboratory disciplines to incorporate automated instrumentation into routine laboratory procedures. The need to streamline procedures and increase productivity finally provided the incentive to develop automated testing in microbiology laboratories. Conventional testing methods for the detection, identification, and susceptibility testing of organisms in the clinical microbiology laboratory were traditionally growth dependent. However, overnight incubation was not compatible with rapid testing. Automation also had to overcome such obstacles as the addition of reagents and interpretation of test results.

During the past decade automation in clinical microbiology has overcome these obstacles and experienced extensive growth and development. The first semiautomated instruments developed for the detection, identification, and antimicrobial susceptibility testing of bacteria required manual preparation with overnight off-line incubation and manual reading. Eventually computer assistance was included in the instrumentation through personal computers. These instrument-assisted systems proved to be reliable, reduced lab costs, and subsequently became widely used in both small and large laboratories during the 1980s.

Meanwhile, totally automated instruments for detection, identification, and antimicrobial susceptibility testing of aerobic bacteria with more rapid, same-day results became more widely

available and used. The automated models first introduced during the last half of the seventies were improved and developed, thereby decreasing equipment downtime. Companies learned they needed to provide adequate service and support for their instruments in the field, and they did just that. In addition the excellent correlation obtained in numerous studies comparing automated equipment with conventional testing supported the ever-growing acceptance and use of automated instrumentation in both clinical and industrial microbiology laboratories.

Most recently the use of methods that are not growth-dependent has contributed to a new generation of automated instrumentation that produces results during a given shift. Some manufacturers have upgraded existing automated instruments, whereas other systems represent entirely new designs. Video image processing, colorimetric sensors, fluorogenic substrates, infrared spectroscopy, and bioluminescence are just a few of the technologies that have been incorporated into instruments that continuously monitor samples with computer assistance. These totally automated instruments are capable of processing large test volumes and require minimal technologist time for sample preparation and equipment operation. Troubleshooting is well-constructed and user-friendly. Enhanced data management programs reduce the amount of time required to retrieve results and increase the reporting capabilities of these instruments. The 1990s have been ushered in by the need for rapid, reliable results that are readily available to the laboratorian, physician, and pharmacist. Consequently the instrumentation of the 1990s is being developed to anticipate and meet those needs.

396

Automated Blood Culture Instruments

For many years blood cultures were performed using large bottles that were visually inspected daily for signs of microbial growth. In addition each bottle had a small aliquot of fluid removed at specified intervals for a stain (to detect organisms present) and "blind subculture" (to culture any bacteria present on solid media for further identification and susceptibility testing). Blood cultures were time-consuming to process for a small percentage of bottles with microbial growth, and positive cultures were not detected very rapidly.

Automation was developed to reduce the handling time and shorten the time required to detect the presence of microorganisms. The Bactec System was a pioneer analyzer in clinical microbiology and became the first automated instrument in many clinical laboratories. With the wide acceptance of this method, advances have been made that further decrease labor time and reduce the time needed to detect microbial growth. The newest blood culture instruments feature walk-away automation.

Bactec System. The Bactec System consists of a group of instruments designed to detect the presence of microorganisms in blood specimens. Originally manufactured by Johnston Laboratories, Bactec instruments are currently manufactured and marketed by Becton Dickinson Diagnostic Instruments. The Bactec 460 was the first widely used automated blood culture system. The next generation of instruments is more automated and computerized, although the detection principle has remained the same: analysis of the air space in blood culture vials for the presence of CO_2 elaborated as a microbial metabolic byproduct.

The Bactec 460 system uses bottles that are filled with measured amounts of media containing ^{14}C. Because the weak beta radiation in the media cannot penetrate the glass, the bottles are safe to handle. However, the use of radioactive materials does require adherence to safety guidelines for handling and disposal that may require additional training. Several media types are available for the growth of aerobic and anaerobic organisms, including optional resins for antimicrobial inactivation, hypertonic (10% sucrose) media, high volume, and pediatric volume vials. The blood culture vials are inoculated with 3 to 5 ml of blood, placed in 4-vial racks, and incubated at 35° C on a shaker in a standard microbiology incubator for the first 24 hours. Agitation during this primary incubation period results in more rapid organism growth, hence faster detection. The detection of organisms is based on use of ^{14}C-labeled glucose and other substrates with subsequent release of $^{14}CO_2$ in a vial.

Once the vial tops are wiped with alcohol, up to 15 racks are placed on the sample changer and the instrument automatically tests all vials present. Each vial requires 60 seconds test time; therefore 60 vials will be tested in 1 hour. The instrument begins its test operation by producing a partial vacuum in the ion chamber, at the same time heating two 18-gauge needles. The head valve then closes, lowering the movable head down onto the vials, and driving the needles through the rubber septum on top of the test vial. The atmosphere above the broth level is flushed into the ion chamber by closing the outlet valve and opening the inlet valve, drawing gas from a reserve tank through a filter and the culture vial. The radioactive gas passes through the chamber and changes the impedance between the two poles. The impedance is converted into a numeric value, or **growth index** (GI), which is printed on tape or datalog card. If this value exceeds a preset threshold, the vial is determined positive for bacterial growth and a red light corresponding to the location of the vial will be seen. The test head rises, the valve head closes, and the pump draws room air through the dust filter, flush valve, and the ion chamber, transferring all the $^{14}CO_2$ into a soda-lime trap where it is retained. This cleanses the measurement system before the next reading cycle while the sample changer moves the next vial into position.

The Bactec 460 can also be employed for the detection, identification, and susceptibility testing of mycobacteria. The system requires a different instrument hood and uses special Bactec vials, with 7H12 broth containing ^{14}C palmitic-1 acid. The labeled CO_2 released by metabolism of palmitic acid is used to detect growth. Specimens are decontaminated, concentrated, and injected into culture vials. The vials are read on the instrument with positive cultures detected in 7 to 12 days.

The Bactec 460 system has been superseded by the NR-660, NR-730, and the recently released NR-860 systems. All of these models use **infrared detection** of microbial metabolic CO_2 byproduct, thus eliminating the problems of working with radioactive material. These newer models complete each vial test cycle in about half the time of the original 460.

The smallest of the nonradiometric instruments is the NR-730. It is a single unit that includes an LCD panel, tape printer, and automatic test chamber (Fig. 22-1). The NR-730 can test up to 30 vials on each tray. Tabs encoded on each tray assure selection of proper gas mixture (aerobic or anaerobic) for each tray run. The NR-730 has a 2 to 8K memory chip with 16K nonvolatile ram, a 6502 microprocessor chip, and battery backup. The user loads the tray onto the tray carrier and initiates the testing. The instrument retains test results in memory until the next testing cycle is initiated.

The NR-660 consists of an automatic test module, monitor, printer, and an incubator/shaker (Fig. 22-2). The incubator/shaker module contains 2 orbital shakers and 10 vial trays: 5 aerobic and 5 anaerobic. Each tray holds up to 60 vials, giving the NR-660 a total capacity of 600 vials. Vials are logged on the system via the keyboard and given a designated position on a tray. All trays are equipped with identification tabs that ensure proper sequencing in the daily test cycles and trigger selection of the proper culture gas. When prompted by the computer, the user removes the tray from the incubator module and loads it onto the tray carrier. The instrument begins testing when prompted by the user. The NR-660 also has a 2 to 8K memory chip with 16K nonvolatile ram, a 6502 microprocessor chip, and battery backup.

The recently introduced NR-860 (Fig. 22-3) is fully automated. This instrument is a single unit that contains a tray transport mechanism designed to move trays between the test area and storage drawers. Separate doors between the test area and storage drawers allow the instrument to perform testing while the user is loading or unloading vials. Bar-coded labels, including a unique sequence number and media type, mark each test vial. There are 8 storage drawers containing trays of 60 vials, and a double decker shaking unit that holds a maximum of 120 vials. A pressure sensitive sensor has been incorporated into the test head to detect the excessive pressure that may be produced in positive vials. Because tray testing is automatic, there is no handling of vials until a positive is flagged or a negative is discarded. Hardware includes a 20 megabyte hard drive with a 3.5-inch floppy disk port. Floppy disks are used for data backup and/or installation of software updates. The NR-860 does not have continuous monitoring capability, although it may be programmed to read each vial up to 4 user-designated times within a 24-hour period.

The test and detector systems on all three instruments are the same. Infrared light is used to measure the amount of CO_2 present in the bottle headspace. Vials are automatically disinfected with ultraviolet light. Bottles are brought into the test chamber by the tray carrier and positioned under the test head. The analysis loop is flushed with room air and then culture gas. Previously heated needles enter the vials. These needles are heated over their full length by a clam-shell heater thus preventing any cross-contamination. A pump mixes the vial head space gas with culture gas present in the analysis loop. The needles are removed from the vial and reheated. The test sample and a reference vial are alternately exposed to infrared light. Each reading is zeroed

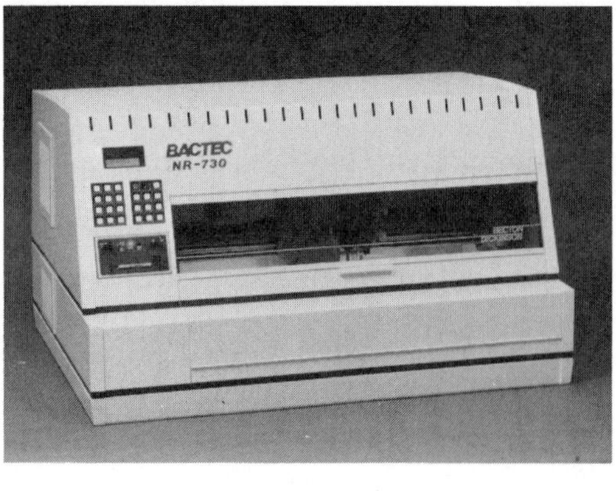

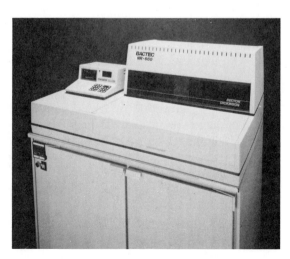

Fig. 22-1 Bactec NR-730 Blood Culture System (courtesy Becton Dickinson Diagnostic Instruments).

Fig. 22-2 Bactec NR-660 Blood Culture System (courtesy Becton Dickinson Diagnostic Instruments).

against culture gas from the external tanks. The detector registers the amount of light that was not absorbed by CO_2, and the amplifier converts this into voltage. Voltage is converted into a numeric or growth value (GV) calculated by the computer and is displayed on the terminal or sent to the printer. The amount of CO_2 generated by microbial metabolism is inversely related to the amount of infrared light detected and measured. Increased CO_2 present in the test sample results in more light being absorbed and less light registered by the detector. Thresholds for the GV have been determined by the manufacturer but can be adjusted by the user. Positive vials may also be detected by using a Δ growth value. Because the NR-660 and NR-860 retain the GV of each test vial, they are able to compare each new test result of a vial with its prior GV. If the difference between the values exceeds a Δ value, the bottle is flagged as positive. This value can be user-defined or the manufacturer recommended values can be used.

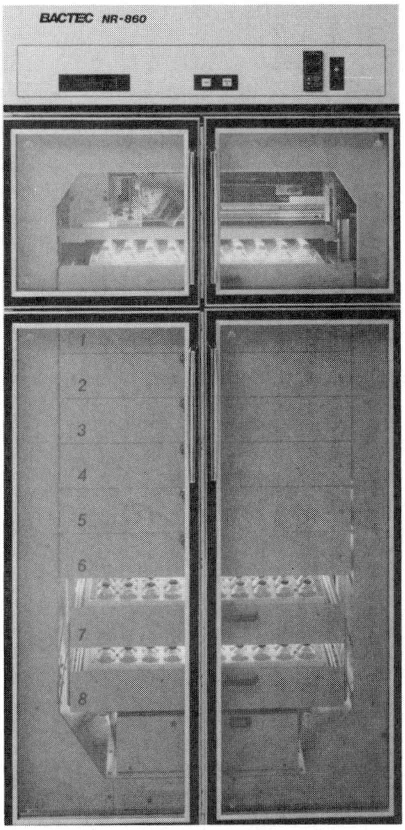

All instrument parameters are electronically monitored, and an audible alarm sounds to alert operators. Malfunctions are displayed visually or are printed to facilitate corrective action. Both the NR-660 and NR-860 have a self-check program that is used to troubleshoot electronic malfunctions. In the event a problem has been diagnosed as component related, the Bactec has been designed in modular units that allow for quick replacement. The user receives the modular unit that contains the replacement component and installs the new unit on the instrument.

Organon Teknika BacT/Alert. The BacT/Alert (Organon Teknika) is a self-contained instrument with total walk-away automation that continually agitates and monitors blood cultures (Fig. 22-4). Microbial growth is detected through noninvasive monitoring of the level of CO_2 within each sample bottle by a **colorimetric sensor** attached to the bottom of the bottle.

Each BacT/Alert instrument contains 10 horizontal rows stacked vertically. Each row consists of 24 adjacent cells, providing an overall testing capacity of 240 bottles or 120 blood culture sets. The cell blocks provide both continuous agitation and incubation, eliminating the need for such daily activities as visual inspection or manual loading and unloading of bottles. Each bottle

Fig. 22-3 Bactec NR-860 Blood Culture System (courtesy Becton Dickinson Diagnostic Instruments).

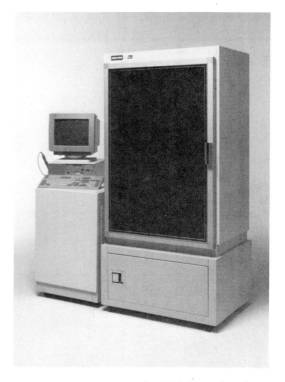

Fig. 22-4 BacT/Alert Microbial Detection System (courtesy Organon Teknika Corp.).

cell is scanned at 10-minute intervals or 144 times/day.

Aerobic and anaerobic bottles are each inoculated with 10 ml of patient blood. A bar-code label displaying media type and a unique identification number is used to track test bottles. This labeling system reduces data entry and clerical errors. The instrument guides the user to the correct placement of the bottles inside the unit with a series of light-emitting diodes (LEDs) placed next to each cell. When the test cycle is complete, the bottles are discarded.

The culture bottles contain an internal colorimetric sensor to detect microbial growth. Production of CO_2 causes the sensor to change color from green to yellow. The BacT/Alert uses solid-state **reflectometers** to monitor the sensors. Excited light is directed toward the sensor, which is reflected back to a light-absorbing photodiode. The instrument measures the amount of light returned and compares this with an initial threshold or the sample's own past performance (rather than a common threshold). A sample is determined positive when one of three criteria is met: (1) a sustained increase in the rate of change, (2) an acceleration of CO_2 production (how the rate has changed from baseline), or (3) amplitude of signal (the threshold that is applied on initial entry). Background CO_2 produced by blood components is differentiated from microbial CO_2 production. Blood components produce CO_2 in gradually increasing amounts, but have a decreased rate of production whereby microbial growth results in an increase in the amount and rate of CO_2 production. The system will alert the user of positive cultures by LEDs, monitor display, hardcopy printout, and/or audible alarm.

The system is driven by a Compaq Deskpro 286e computer that has 1 megabyte of RAM, a 40 megabyte hard disk drive, a floppy disk drive, an internal tape backup system, and an internal modem. Up to four data units can be interfaced to one computer system for a total of 960 tests. Also available are data management capabilities such as comprehensive data handling, reporting, and graphing.

Urine Screen Instruments

A variety of instruments using different methodologies have been developed to screen for **bacteriuria** (the presence of microorganisms in urine). The value of these instruments rests in the ability to send out negative results as a final report on completion of testing without waiting 24 to 48 hours for a negative culture result. A positive urine screen is not diagnostic; it reflects the presence of microorganisms. Routine cultures must be performed to assess the clinical relevance.

Los Alamos UTIscreen. The Los Alamos UTIscreen (LAD) 633 (Los Alamos Diagnostics) is a fully automated instrument that uses the UTIscreen bacterial test kit to estimate the quantity of bacteria and yeast present in a urine specimen (Fig. 22-5). This rapid screening test uses **luciferin/luciferase** to detect bacterial or yeast adenosine triphosphate (ATP). The assay involves three steps: an initial incubation step for the release and destruction of urinary somatic cellular ATP; a second step for the release of ATP from living microbial cells; and a final step for the

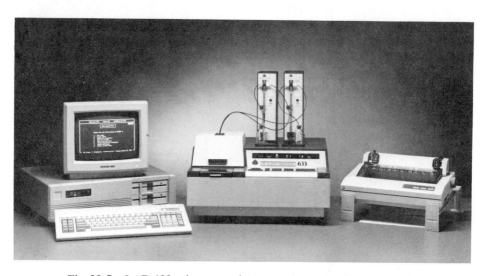

Fig. 22-5 LAD 633 urine screen instrument (courtesy Los Alamos).

detection of light emitted as a by-product on the addition of luciferin/luciferase to any microbial ATP present.

The LAD 633 will process up to 25 samples in a single run that takes less than 10 minutes to complete. This instrument is fully automatic and programmable, features walk-away automation, contains a full-function computer that can interface with other lab computer systems, and prints results for a permanent record. The instrument dimensions are width, 20 inches; depth, 20.5 inches; and height, 12 inches. The LAD 633 weighs 77 pounds and has standard electrical requirements.

Minimal technician time is required to operate the instrument. Twenty-five μl of urine are dispensed into tubes in a carousel and loaded into the instrument that automatically injects reagents, performs calibrations, incubates, interprets, and displays results on the monitor screen. Test results are automatically printed at the end of the test run.

Results obtained with the LAD 633 luminometer and UTIscreen test kit are comparable with other rapid bacteriuria screens, including microscopic, enzymatic, and filtration methods. The advantages offered by the fully automated urine screening instrument over other screening methods and standard culture include ease of performance and more rapid and objective results.

Vitek Bac-T-Screen. The Bac-T-Screen (Vitek Systems, Inc.) instrument is used to screen urine specimens for the presence of bacteriuria and **pyuria** (Fig. 22-6). This simple, rapid, nongrowth-dependent test uses a colorimetric technique to detect the presence of bacteria and/or white cells in urine.

The BAC-T-SCREEN instrument has 2 sample-testing barrels to enable continual processing of specimens; one barrel is testing while setting up the other. The testing process begins with the insertion of a Dynadepth filter card into one of the two slots on the front of the instrument. One ml of urine is poured into the active barrel, and the start button is pushed to activate automatic dispensing. The specimen is diluted with 3 ml of diluent, allowed to mix, and vacuumed through the filter card. Bacteria or white cells are attracted to and subsequently adhere to the filter. This step is followed by addition of 3 ml of safranin dye, which, after a 30-second period, is vacuumed through the filter. Bacterial cells, white cells, and background fibers are stained by the safranin. The filter is then decolorized twice by vacuuming 3 ml of solution through the filter. The decolor-

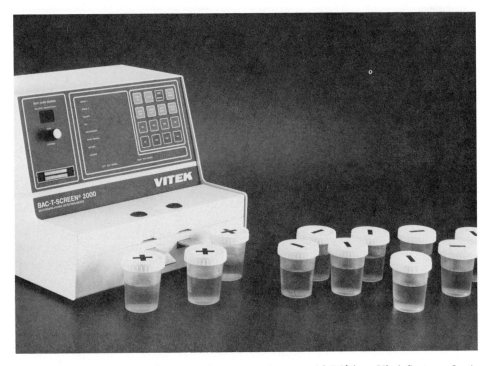

Fig. 22-6 Bac-T-Screen urine screen instrument (courtesy bioMérieux Vitek Systems, Inc.).

ization step provides selective removal of the dye from the filter but not from the bacteria and white cells. Stained bacterial and white cells produce a pink to red pigmentation of varying intensity on the filter.

The filter card may be read visually or with a test card reader. The test card reader provides a more objective interpretation and may simplify interpretation of questionable results. The LED printout reports results in relative absorbance units. Positive values may either be user-defined or follow the manufacturer's recommended values.

The Bac-T-Screen is simple to use and processes each specimen in less than 2 minutes. Indicator lights show which barrel is ready for use. Clogs in the barrel are detected and aspirated by a probe in the dispenser cap. The instrument requires minimal maintenance.

Identification and Susceptibility Instruments

Conventional microbial identifications and susceptibility testing methods have been replaced by a variety of instruments offering same day, even same-shift, results. A variety of principles are employed by commercial manufacturers. All systems described here have been tested extensively and show excellent correlation with conventional standard test methods.

Vitek AMS. The Automicrobic System (AMS) (Vitek Systems, Inc.) consists of a monitor, a printer, and 3 modular components: the filler/sealer, the reader/incubator, and a computer (Fig. 22-7). The system is fully automated from sample loading to results printout and provides same-day identification and susceptibility testing of most aerobic gram-negative and gram-positive bacterial isolates. In addition the AMS offers enteric pathogen and urine screen capabilities, overnight identification of yeast isolates, and rapid (enzymatic) identification of anaerobic and fastidious gram-negative isolates.

Test inoculum is prepared from primary isolation plates. Several isolated colonies are picked and suspended in 0.45% sterile saline in an uncapped tube. A **nephelometer,** available from Vitek, is used to adjust the density of the test inoculum to a McFarland standard specified for the type of test card.

Disposable test kits consist of clear plastic cards about the size of a playing card (Fig. 22-8). Each test card contains 30 test wells connected by a series of capillaries and is sealed on both sides with clear tape. The wells contain lyophilized biochemicals or specific dilution of antimicrobial solutions. Filling stands are configured to hold up to 10 test cards and corresponding inoculum tubes. The prepared inoculum is placed adjacent to the test card desired and connected with a transfer tube. The filling stand is placed in the chamber of the filling module, the door is closed, and air is evacuated from the chamber. During this process air is forced out of the card wells via the transfer tube. When the vacuum is subsequently released, the pressure difference between the interior and exterior of the card forces specimen through the capillary channels into the wells

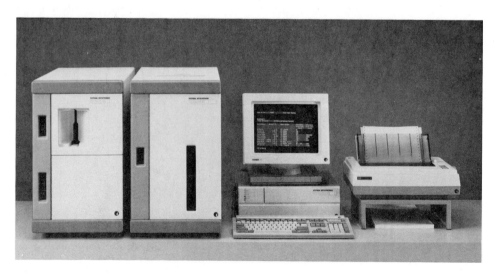

Fig. 22-7 Vitek AMS 120 (from left, filler/sealer module, reader/incubator, monitor, computer module, and printer) (courtesy bioMérieux Vitek Systems, Inc.).

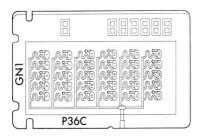

Fig. 22-8 Outline of a typical test card used by the Vitek AutoMicrobic System. Note that 30 media are inoculated by injecting the inoculum through 1 port (courtesy bioMérieux Vitek, Inc.).

containing media. The tray stand is removed from the chamber, each transfer tube is cut, and the card is sealed using the sealing unit.

Filled and sealed test cards are loaded into the reader/incubator module. The interior of this module contains a revolving carousel that holds 4 trays. Each tray contains up to 30 test cards stacked vertically. During the test period each card is scanned hourly by the reader head; reading time is 12 seconds/card or 7 minutes/tray of 30 cards. Vertical drive mechanisms move the reader head down the tray as it is read. An electrooptical detection system aligns the reader with each card. The reader extracts the card with a horizontal drive mechanism, moves it through the optical system, and returns the card to the tray. The optical system consists of 12 LEDs that emit light of 660 nm through the test card. Any attenuation of light is measured by phototransistor detectors. Card type and specimen number are also read by the optical detectors. Incubation time required for identifications and/or susceptibilities ranges from 4 to 18 hours.

Data readings are stored in the reader module and the computer module. The computer features a Motorola MC68010 16 bit microprocessor, hard drive (up to 85 megabyte, depending on model), large data base, and unidirectional and bidirectional laboratory computer interface options. It directs the reader/module functions and data analysis and automatically sends final reports to the printer. The AMS can provide support for multiple components (e.g., several terminals, printers, and up to 2 reader/incubator modules).

The growth rate in the presence of specified dilutions of antimicrobial agents in susceptibility cards is monitored and compared with the growth rate in the positive control well to determine the **minimal inhibitory concentration (MIC)** of each antimicrobial. The MIC value of an antimicrobial agent is calculated from the composite slope and the coefficients for that particular organism/drug combination.

Biochemical reactions in test wells of identification cards are compared with known reactions and probabilities. The two closest patterns are compared, the identification probabilities are computed, and subsequent identifications are reported as normalized percent probabilities. The yeast identification card requires off-line incubation.

Vitek also offers an information management software package (IMS). The IMS provides user-defined epidemiology and susceptibility data, selective antimicrobial reporting, and chartable patient reports as configured by the user.

Sensititre Microbiology System: ARIS. Same-day (5-hour) or overnight (18-hour) bacterial identification and susceptibility testing may be performed with an automated instrument manufactured by Radiometer America Inc. The Sensititre Microbiology System has two separate modules, the Automatic Inoculator and the AutoReader, which are interfaced with a Digital Professional 380 computer with P/OS operating system that drives the readers, collects and stores data, and a software package for complete analysis and epidemiologic evaluations of the data.

The Sensititre system uses fluorogenic technology to detect and correlate bacterial enzyme activity to antibiotic susceptibility testing. Specifically defined fluorescent probes for detection of carbohydrate metabolism, deamination of tryptophan, presence of four bacterial enzymes, use of four carbon sources, decarboxylase reactions, and other tests for urea and esculin hydrolysis are used for identification of bacterial organisms.

The test inoculum is prepared by emulsifying several well-isolated colonies directly from the primary isolation plate and emulsifying them in sterile, demineralized water to achieve a turbidity equivalent to a 0.5 McFarland standard. The Automatic Inoculator includes a built in nephelometer to achieve this final concentration. A strip containing fluorescent product from a **fluorogenic** (nonfluorescent) **substrate** is then added for 5-hour testing. Enzymatic action of the test organism surface enzymes on the fluorescent label releases the fluorescent product, which is detected by the autoreader. The amount of fluorescence is directly related to bacterial growth. In some cases incubation must be extended overnight. The addition of the fluorogenic marker to the inoculum does not interfere with overnight, nonfluorogenic reading.

The Sensititre Automatic Inoculator is a rapid, microprocessor-controlled dispensing instrument that automatically delivers inoculum to a 96-well microtiter tray. Each prepared inoculum tube is fitted with a disposable dosehead to dispense the preprogrammed volume of inoculum into each microtiter plate well and clamped into place on the bridge of the automatic inoculator. The labeled microtiter plate is placed into the plate holder, and the technologist selects the desired dosing pattern desired with the keypad. Inoculum is dispensed into the microtiter tray wells through positive displacement action occurring in the dosehead. After inoculation, the plate is removed and undergoes **off-line incubation** in a standard 35° to 37° C incubator for 5 hours or overnight.

After the off-line incubation, plates are loaded onto the Sensititre AutoReader for reading and interpretation. The reader contains a single excitation/detection wavelength fluorometer to measure the intensity levels of fluorescence emitted by the test well. As the plate is transported over the reading optics, raw fluorescence values are counted and transmitted to a microcomputer. For susceptibility testing, the presence or absence of bacterial growth is determined by the amount of fluorescence in each well. Optics consist of interference filters and a beamsplitting cube with wavelength selective coatings in conjunction with lenses to focus the light onto the sample and the detector. The light source is a boardband xenon flash lamp that generates microsecond pulses of high intensity light. The detector is a photomultiplier tube that provides the means for measuring low levels of fluorescence. The autoreader transports the microtiter plate over the excitation/detection optics while infrared LEDs and phototransistors relay binary signals to the microprocessor for exact well-positioning information.

Susceptibility panels are available for determination of full-range minimum inhibitory or breakpoint concentrations of antimicrobials for testing gram-positive, gram-negative, and urinary isolates. A variety of standard plate formats and custom formats using any standard antimicrobics are available in 2000 plate lots. Dry form plates are individually foil wrapped in lots of 10. Inclusion of a desiccant in each pack permits room temperature storage for 1 to 2 years from the date of manufacture.

Auto identification panels provide organism identification for aerobic gram-negative bacilli. Each plate is designed to test 3 organisms by repeating 32 biochemical tests 3 times across the 96-well plate. Stabilized, dried plates are sealed with foil seals and wrapped individually in foil pouches containing a desiccant. Plates are stored at room temperature and have a minimum shelf life of 6 months from the date of manufacture. The automatic inoculator automatically adds oil to overlay specified wells. The 5-hour fluorogenic substrates do not routinely require addition of reagents to any test wells, although additional biochemical tests for the production of oxidase, indole, motility, and pigment may be required to confirm an identification.

After auto identification panels are read by the autoreader, the raw fluorescence data is transferred to the DEC PRO 380 computer where the final identification is determined by two methods. Initially a biocode match is sought in the biocode library. If there is not a match in the library, the final identification is calculated by the computer, using probability and data matching routines. The auto identification system will identify over 140 taxa comprising Enterobacteriaceae, oxidase-positive fermenters, pseudomonads, and other nonfermenters.

Final patient reports may be printed in selected formats displaying desired patient and specimen information, isolate identification, and susceptiblity results with interpretations.

The Sensititre Aris automated reading and incubation system is a module that can be retrofitted to the Sensititre AutoReader module. This system features on-line incubation, bar-coding technology, and automatic reading on completion of the required incubation period. The Aris holds up to 64 panels and is a strictly fluorogenic system. Currently there is a one-way interface from the Aris to laboratory information systems. Also, the Aris and the autoreader use the same identification and susceptibility panels.

Microscan autoSCAN-W/A. The autoSCAN-W/A (Baxter Diagnostics Inc., Micro-Scan Division) is a fully automated instrument capable of providing identifications within 2 hours and susceptibilities within 3.5 to 7 hours with rapid panels or performing overnight testing with traditional panels. The autoSCAN-W/A system consists of an incubator/processor and a data management system (DMS) (Fig. 22-9). In addi-

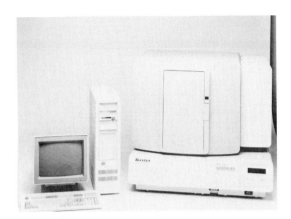

Fig. 22-9 MicroScan autoSCAN-W/A fully automated microbial system (courtesy Baxter Diagnostics Inc.).

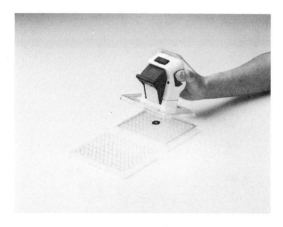

Fig. 22-10 The RENOK Rehydator/Inoculator used to inoculate the dried identification and susceptibility panels (courtesy Baxter Diagnostics Inc.).

tion the RENOK Rehydrator/Inoculator (Fig. 22-10) is used to inoculate the dried identification and susceptibility panels.

The autoSCAN-W/A uses rapid fluorescence technologies (fluorogenic and fluorometric) for rapid panels and turbidity and/or color development in standard identification and susceptibility panels.

Rapid bacterial identification is based on bacterial enzymatic activity detected using synthetic fluorogenic substrates and fluorescent pH indicators. Rapid susceptibility testing measures growth or inhibition of growth in the presence of fluorogenic substrates and antimicrobials. The autoSCAN-W/A contains a fluorometer optics module that consists of a section for excitation of the fluorophore and a section for detection of the subsequent fluorescence.

The rapid chromogenic identification panels use colorimetric optics to read each well at six different wavelengths during each read cycle. Subsequently the computer selects the wavelength reading that best discriminates the reaction for each well. Antimicrobial susceptibility wells are read at two different wavelengths.

The preparation of test inoculum begins by picking several morphologically similar colonies from primary isolation plates and emulsifying this growth in a specified inoculation liquid to achieve a 0.5 McFarland turbidity. The fluid is poured into the ID section of the inoculator set transfer seed trough. This is followed by the addition of either inoculated MIC broth (for combo panels) or 25 ml of uninoculated inoculum water with Pluronic-D. The transfer lid is replaced, the

RENOK rehydrator/inoculator is attached, and incubation is completed.

Before loading panels into the autoSCAN-W/A, patient demographics are entered in the computer. Bar codes are then printed and affixed to the panels (either before or after panel inoculation). Panels are loaded (and subsequently removed) through the operator's door at the center top of the instrument.

Inside the instrument is a carousel holding 8 towers, each of which has 12 shelves to hold test trays. A bar-code reader, the spectrophotometer, the fluorometer, reagent dispenser, and panel-accessing apparatus surround the carousel. The reagent compartment contains reagents that are automatically added after an appropriate incubation period.

After loading labeled panels into the instrument and initiating the autoSCAN-W/A, the operator's hands-on work is completed. The bar-code reader scans all trays to create an internal map of each panel, and the computer schedules the processing and reading of all panels and begins operation independent from the computer. On completion of each panel of any type, results are automatically uploaded to the data management system where a variety of report printing options are available to the user (e.g., automatic or batch).

Rapid fluorogenic panels provide 2-hour identification of aerobic gram-negative and gram-positive bacteria. Rapid chromogenic panels are available for 4-hour identification of fastidious gram-negative bacteria, yeasts, and anaerobes. Rapid fluorogenic susceptibility panels are avail-

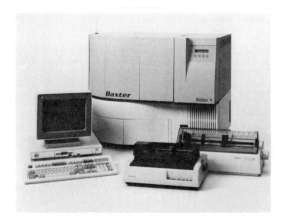

Fig. 22-11 MicroScan WalkAway-40 Microbial System (courtesy Baxter Diagnostic Inc.).

able to determine minimal inhibitory concentrations for gram-negative and gram-positive bacteria and also to determine breakpoint susceptibilities of gram-negative and gram-positive isolates.

The data management system features both unidirectional and bidirectional laboratory interface options that allow for cost-effective and rapid reporting of patient test results. Reporting algorithms may be used to selectively report the most cost-effective and/or formulary antibiotics. The epidemiology program provides capability for multiple-parameter searching as specified by the user. Repeat isolates are automatically excluded from epidemiology reports to prevent skewing of the data.

The autoSCAN-W/A can incubate and process up to 96 test panels simultaneously. Rapid and conventional panels may be tested during the same run. A smaller version of the autoSCAN-W/A, the WalkAway-40 Microbiology System (Fig. 22-11), has a maximum capacity of 40 rapid or conventional panels. The WalkAway-40's data management system can also be linked to a pharmacy computer to enable the pharmacist to review antibiotic use. Additional software is available that allows the pharmacist to interact with the report information generated in the data management system by the analyzer. The MicroScan pharmLINK software enhances the ongoing, concurrent drug usage evaluation process required of hospitals by accreditation organizations.

Review Questions

1. The Bactec NR 660 blood culture system is based on:

A. Bioluminescence
B. Internal colorimetric sensor
C. Infrared spectrophotometer
D. Radiometry

2. Bioluminescence detects the presence of bacteria in urine by detecting the presence of:
A. Bacterial ATP
B. Somatic ATP
C. Growth in a test card
D. Kinetic analysis

3. The Bac-T-Screen is able to detect the presence of:
A. Pyuria
B. Bacteriuria
C. Dysuria
D. A and B
E. B and C

4. Which of the following system(s) produce same day results:
A. Sensititre ARIS
B. Micro Scan Walk-Away
C. Vitek AMS
D. A and B
E. A, B, and C

5. The BacT/Alert blood culture system is based on:
A. An internal colorimetric sensor
B. Kinetic analysis
C. Bioluminescence
D. Infrared analysis

6. Which of the following is (are) important parameter(s) in the selection of automated methods?
A. Easy to use
B. Cost effective
C. Accuracy
D. A and C
E. All of the above

7. The AMS Vitek test cards are filled:
A. Using inoculation trays
B. By ion exchange
C. By transfer of log phase growth into lower chamber
D. Using a vacuum chamber

Review Answers

1. C   2. A   3. D   4. C   5. A   6. E   7. D

References

Becton Dickinson Diagnostic Instrument Systems, 660 Operator Manual. Document MA-0018. June, 1990. Sparks, Md.

Becton Dickinson Diagnostic Instrument Systems, 860 Operator Manual. Document MA-0070. May, 1991. Sparks, Md.

bioMerieux Vitek, Inc. Bac-T-Screen Test Package Insert, Cat. No. 26-20-10. Jan, 1987. Hazelwood, Mo.

bioMerieux Vitek, Inc. Reference Manual Part No. 510578-1, 1991. Hazelwood, Mo.

bioMerieux Vitek, Inc. Technical Bulletin 007167-5, rev, June, 1991. Hazelwood, Mo.

Clayland BG, Clayland C, Tomforde KM, and Wallace S: Full spectrum automation for the clinical microbiology laboratory, American Clinical Laboratory. May, 1989.

Instrument Application Note Model 633 UTIscreen Bacterial ATP Test, Document P-036, August, 1988.

MicroScan Division, Baxter. MicroScan Rapid Identification Procedural Manual. Document 3250-03050. October, 1988. West Sacramento, Ca.

Organon Teknika Corporation, Product Information: BacT/Alert Microbial Detection System. Document M1-101-90. Durham, NC.

Pezzlo M, Ige V, Woolard AP, Peterson E, and DeLa Maza LM: Rapid bioluminescence method for bacteriuria screening, J Clin Microbiol 27: 7160629, 1989.

Sensititre Gram Negative Auto Identification System Product Information, Sensititre LTD, The Manor, Manor Royal, Crawley, West Sussex RH10 2PY, England.

Sensititre Instrumentation Product Information, Sensititre LTD, The Manor, Manor Royal, Crawley, West Sussex RH10 2PY, England.

Shedding New Light on Microbiology, Sensititre LTD, The Manor, Manor Royal, Crawley, West Sussex RH10 2PY, England.

UTIscreen Bacterial ATP Test Package Insert, Document P-009. August, 1988.

Thorpe TC, Wilson ML, Turner JE, DiGuiseppi JL, Willert M, Mirrett S, and Reller RB: BacT/Alert: an automated colorimetric microbial detection system, J Clin Microbiol 28: 1608, 1990.

CHAPTER 23

Automation in Physician Office Laboratories

LARRY E. SCHOEFF

Evolution of Physician Office Laboratories
Instrument Systems for Physician Office Laboratories

Evolution of Physician Office Laboratories

Physician office laboratory testing is the fastest growing area in laboratory medicine. These laboratories currently account for at least 50% of all diagnostic testing performed in the United States. It is estimated that there are currently about 80,000 physicians' office laboratories operating in this country. The test volume generated by these laboratories is estimated to be at least ten billion tests annually, with a potential revenue source of approximately a half billion dollars.

Laboratory testing in the physician's office is not a new phenomenon. Dipstick urinalysis, occult blood screening, hematocrits, throat cultures, and glucose testing have been performed in doctors' offices for years. In recent years technologic advances and miniaturization of computerized instruments, new and improved technology in diagnostic reagents/kits, changes in federal health care reimbursement policies, and a more competitive health care delivery market have all contributed to a tremendous growth in physician office laboratory testing.

New federal laws enacted to reduce healthcare spending have had a major impact on clinical laboratory diagnostic testing moving to new settings. More and more tests are being performed in laboratories that are outside the boundaries of the present regulatory structure, such as physicians' offices. The shift of testing to physician offices and the patient's right to quality test results offers both a challenge and an opportunity to the clinical laboratory profession. The

most essential guideline for development of physician office laboratories (POL) is that minimum quality assurance standards must apply to these laboratory settings as they do other clinical laboratory environments (i.e., hospital and reference labs).

The primary challenge will be effective, realistic, and fiscally viable approaches to quality management in physician office laboratories. The clinical laboratory profession must prepare new professionals for appropriate liaison roles to an industry involved in manufacturing and marketing new technologies and instrumentation for these new laboratories.

While there are problems, the opportunities offered by POL testing include more than just a welcome potential for easier patient access to health care and speedier test results. They also include broadened employment opportunities for the laboratory profession that is ready to meet the challenge of change. It must be emphasized again that the prompt development and maintenance of appropriate quality assurance standards in POLs, as well as in other laboratory settings, is the key to everyone's intended goal—improved patient care. This will occur in an orderly fashion as clinical laboratory professionals are educated to the unique circumstances and needs of POLs and become actively and directly involved in communicating with, consulting for, and operating these increasing popular laboratories.

With the advent of DRGs and related prospective payment mechanisms, ambulatory care clinics are seeing a tremendous influx of patients formerly cared for as in-patients. More and more patients are now examined and diagnosed before hospital admission. Acute illnesses of patients are now being managed in an out-patient clinic in lieu of lengthier hospital stays. This shift in patient care is having a significant impact on the scope and volume of POL testing, especially for the primary care physician.

Diagnoses are made in the physician's office assisted and confirmed by that office's laboratory testing; this type of medical practice is increasing rapidly. Office-based diagnostic testing will continue to increase in volume and complexity for a variety of reasons: rapid advances in, and proliferation of, technology; convenience to both the patient and the physician; faster turnaround time of lab results; and the need to supplement medical practice income in the current reimbursement framework. The shift in patient health care and diagnostic testing from the hospital to the ambulatory setting is creating a demand for educational and technical assistance for those individuals performing laboratory procedures in physicians' offices. Planning the educational training and consultation services for these individuals is difficult because of their varied job roles, educational backgrounds and lack of laboratory experience.

In the last decade much attention has been focused on the quality of small office laboratories; however this attention to quality has generally come from outside the primary care physician group. Currently, small laboratories in physicians' offices are practically the only laboratories that have no standards or regulations imposed on them by governmental agencies, which promotes little incentive for implementing any system of quality control. As a result, speculation about the quality of service provided in office-based laboratories persists compared with the present-day standards of hospital-based laboratories.

Current reimbursement mechanisms encourage the expansion of small office laboratories that cannot afford to employ highly educated and trained personnel. The average number of individuals performing tests in physicians' offices is approximately 2 per office. The level and type of formal training of these personnel varies widely. Up to half of these personnel have no formal laboratory training or certification. These "laboratorians" may vary from doctors to nurses to office assistants to receptionists. Because patient care has largely shifted to the outpatient setting, an ever-increasing number of medical offices are now performing laboratory testing, often by these nonlaboratory personnel. The clinical laboratory profession has a strong obligation to provide consultation and education toward quality assurance

and appropriate instrumentation to meet the needs of these laboratories at a level commensurate with the background of their personnel.

Instrument Systems for Physician Office Laboratories

POLs have become one of the markets most pursued by chemistry and hematology instrument manufacturers. The new instrumentation and reagent packages allow many more physicians to set up laboratories in their offices. The rapid growth of office-based physician laboratories has been made possible by advances in medical technology; the use of microprocessors, dry chemistry reagents, ion-specific electrodes, and other advanced instrument and reagent systems has brought the newest technology from the hospital and research laboratories into the POL.

The specific instrumentation used in a physician's office laboratory depends on many factors: the physician's medical specialty; the size of the practice; the degree of automation required; the test menu needed; the physician's degree of need for ease of operation; the necessary turnaround time; the reagent, instrument, and supply budget; and particular requirements for quality control programs and result-reporting systems.

The analyzers that are being marketed for POLs can be automated, semiautomated, or manual. The advantages of automated instrumentation include the level of training needed to operate the instrument is minimal; turnaround times for test results are short; and a hard copy of the test results can be obtained while the patient is still in the office. The major disadvantage of using automated instruments is the cost of the analyzer itself. Manual and semiautomated instruments are not as expensive as their automated counterparts, but they usually have longer turnaround times and a considerable amount of time may be required to train office personnel to operate them.

Other factors that should be considered before obtaining an instrument are its ability to perform test profiles, the ease of converting from one test to another, and reagent preparation requirements. Calibration curves should be stable for at least 1 month, and a quality control program and 24-hour service should be available from the instrument manufacturer. Many instrument manufacturers provide ready-to-use reagents, controls, and standards for each assay, which decreases the likelihood of errors in reagent preparation. Dry chemistry reagents can usually be stored in a small area, which is a significant advantage in an office laboratory.

Chemistry Analyzers. Clinical chemistry analyzers can be automated, semiautomated, or manual and can use serum, plasma, or preferably, whole blood for analysis. "Dry" chemistry reagent systems and "wet" reagent systems are available. Most chemistry analyzers use sample volumes of less than 50 μl, with turnaround times of less than 10 minutes. Many of the systems have ready-to-use, unitized reagents, controls and calibrators with a shelf life of 12 months or more. Almost all of the systems can be purchased for under $15,000.

Dry Reagent Systems. The Seralyzer III Blood Chemistry Analyzer from Miles Inc., Diagnostic Division (Fig. 23-1) uses test strips consisting of cellulose fibers impregnated with reagents. The reagent strips are stored in vials and are stable for 1 to 4 months after the container is opened. The reaction parameters for each assay are programmed by a dedicated module that is inserted into the analyzer. The sample, which usually requires predilution, is pipetted into the strip, and the strip is moved into the analyzer. Light from a xenon lamp strikes the strip, and the vertically re-

flected light is passed through a collimator to the interference filter and is sensed by the sample photodetector. Reflected light is also passed through the reference photodetector. The ratio of the sample to reference reflectance is used to compensate for the drift in electronics and variations in the intensity of the lamp. Profile testing is difficult because each test requires a separate plug-in module.

The Kodak DT System (Fig. 23-2) uses a multilayered film technology similar to that of the Ektachem 700 analyzer. Each test slide is bar coded to identify the assay and the lost number of the reagent. The reagents are stable for about 1 year. With a specially designed battery-driven pipet, the sample is placed on the slide and incubated for 5 minutes at 37° C. Light illuminates the slide, and the amount of reflected light is related to the concentration of analyte in the sample. The incubator can hold up to 5 slides thus allowing for batch or profile testing of up to 5 assays. The DT-60 can perform only colorimetric assays. The DT-SC Analyzer, which uses a xenon lamp as a light source with UV or visible wavelength detection, is available to perform enzyme assays and some therapeutic drug testing. The

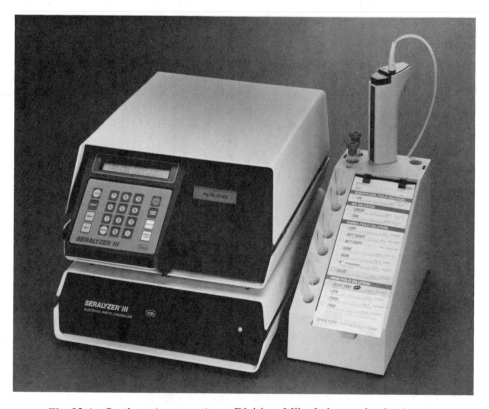

Fig. 23-1 Seralyzer (courtesy Ames Division, Miles Laboratories, Inc.).

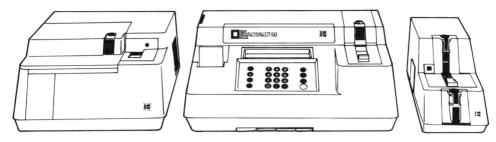

Fig. 23-2 DT-60 (courtesy Eastman Kodak Co.).

DT-E module can be obtained for measuring electrolytes.

The Reflotron system from Boehringer Mannheim Diagnostics uses solid phase reagent tabs containing a magnetic code to identify the tests, reaction parameters, and the calibration curve for each assay. With each reagent lot, the calibration curve is established by the manufacturer. Therefore the laboratory does not have to calibrate the system. The shelf life of each test tab is from 1.5 to 2 years. Blood is placed on a glass fiber pad, and the plasma is separated from the erythrocytes. Plasma is transported away from the erythrocytes by capillary action, and the required sample volume is added to the reagent at a temperature of 37° C. Excess plasma is removed from the reaction area. The concentration of analytes is determined by reflectance photometry. With this system blood obtained by finger or heel stick can be used for analysis. Because this is a single test system, profile testing is not practical.

The ChemPro system uses individually barcoded test cards that contain liquid calibrators and an ISE system. Each card contains two compartments: one for an aqueous calibrator and one for the sample. After the sample is pipetted onto the card, the calibrators and the sample are transferred by capillary action to ISEs where the measurements are made. With this system, the analytic measurements are determined directly on whole blood and some profile testing is possible.

The Analyst from DuPont is a desktop system that consists of specially designed disposable plastic rotors. The rotors contain the bar-coded reagents and are stable for 1 year stored in a refrigerator. Rotors are available for profile or discrete analysis. Sample, which must be prediluted with pipettes supplied by DuPont, is automatically pipetted into the rotor. By centrifugal force the sample is transferred through capillaries into the reaction cuvettes along the rotor's perimeter. These cuvettes contain the reagent tablets. The chemical reactions are monitored at 37° C using bichromatic spectrophotometry. After each test profile the rotor must be discarded whether a complete or partial chemistry profile is formed. With the Analyst, rotors are available for performing a 7- or 12-test general chemistry profile, a lipid profile, or a discrete analysis of a single analyte. An ISE system for measuring sodium and potassium is also available from DuPont.

Dry reagent technology is well suited to the office-based physician laboratory because the space required for storage of reagents is small, the reagents are ready-to-use, and the calibration curves are stable for long periods of time. An adequate supply of reagents for several months of work can usually be stored in a small refrigerator. Because of the ease of operation of these instrument systems they may not require the services of highly trained laboratory personnel.

Wet Reagent Systems. The Vision system from Abbott (Fig. 23-3) uses two-dimensional centrifugation with specially designed disposable reagent packs for analysis. The reagent pack is a self-contained unit with cuvette, liquid reagents,

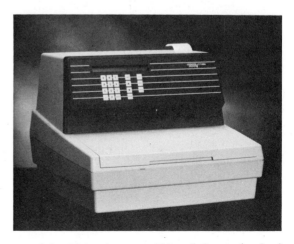

Fig. 23-3 Vision (courtesy Abbott Laboratories, Inc.).

and bar codes to identify the assay. Two drops of sample, either blood, serum, or plasma, are placed into the multichambered reagent pack, and the packs are placed into a 10-position rotor in the analyzer. By centrifugal force the plasma is separated from the erythrocytes. The packs are rotated at a 90-degree angle, which results in a premeasured amount of sample and reagent being transferred into the cuvette. The reactions are monitored at 37° C, and the absorbances are measured bichromatically. Blood can be obtained by finger or heel stick in a special tube provided by Abbott. The tub is inserted directly into the reagent pack, eliminating the pipetting of blood from the capillary tube into the analyzer. The reagents are stable for several months, and with this system 1 to 10 analytes can be measured. The Vision system is suitable for batch, profile, or stat assays.

The Gemstar from Electro-Nucleonics (Fig. 23-4) is a random-access analyzer that can be used either for batch or profile analysis. Most reagents are supplied in lyophilized form. Reconstituted reagents are usually stable for 5 to 12 days. The Gemstar can operate in three modes: the profile, batch, or mix-match mode. In the

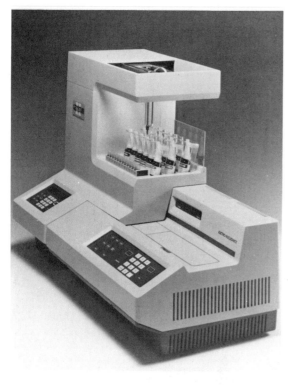

Fig. 23-4 Gemstar (courtesy Electro-nucleonics, Inc.).

profile mode, it is possible to run as many as 12 different tests on a single sample. In the batch mode the same test can be determined on 11 different samples, and in mix-match mode a profile can be determined on a small batch of samples. The reagents are manually pipetted into disposable cuvettes, and the samples are dispensed into these cuvettes with a special 12-position pipettor system from Electro-Nucleonics. The cuvettes are placed in the analyzer and maintained at 37° C, and the absorbance is measured.

The ASSIST is a benchtop random-access analyzer. A disk that contains the chemistry programs is loaded into the disk drive. Reagents must be reconstituted and placed in the reagent tray. From 1 to 16 samples are loaded on the sample tray, and the disposable cuvettes are placed into the analyzer. Samples and reagents are automatically pipetted into the cuvettes and mixed and the absorbances monitored bichromatically. The reagents are stable for 5 days after being reconstituted. The ASSIST analyzer can perform either batch, profile, or stat assays.

The Uni-Fast system uses unitized, lyophilized reagent vials. The reagent is reconstituted with sample and diluent by a pipettor-dilutor system that is supplied with the analyzer. The operator aspirates the reaction mixture directly from the vial into a flow-through cuvette where absorbance is measured. For tests that require preincubation, the vial is placed in a separate compartment before the contents are aspirated into the cuvette. Because the Uni-Fast uses a single reagent vial for each test, it is suitable for stat testing.

The following box lists test menus for some of the commonly used POL chemistry analyzers. A more extensive listing of POL chemistry systems, including glucose and electrolyte analyzers is summarized in Table 23-1.

Hematology Analyzers. The hematology systems designed for the physician's office are semiautomated to automated and use less than 50 µl of blood to measure red blood cells, hematocrit, hemoglobin, and white blood cells. Some of the more sophisticated hematology systems can also determine platelet counts and RBC indices. An extensive list of POL hematology analyzers is summarized in Table 23-1. They all have similar principles of analysis and measure the electrical conductivity differences between the cells and the diluted solution. With all these systems blood must be placed in the cups, diluted, and aspirated into the analyzer. The results are usually ob-

Test Menus of POL Chemistry Instruments

GEMSTAR	VISION	ANALYST	SERALYZER	DT-60	REFLOTORN
Albumin	Albumin	Alk phos	ALT	Colorimetric	ALT
Acid phos	Alk phos	ALT	AST	Ammonia	AST
Alk phos	ALT	AST	T. bili	Amylase	BUN
ALT	AST	T. bile	BUN	BUN	Chol
Amylase	BUN	BUN	Chol	Chol	GGT
AST	Chol	Ca	Creat	HDL Chol	Glucose
D. Bili	Creat	Chol	CPK	Creat	Hb
T. Bili	Glucose	Creat	Glucose	Glucose	Trig
BUN	T. protein	GGT	Hb	Hb	Uric acid
Ca chol	Trig	Glucose	LDH	T. protein	
MDL-chol	Uric acid	Trig	K	Trig	
Chloride	K	Uric acid	Trig	Uric acid	
CO$_2$	Theophylline		Uric acid	RATE	
CPK	Creatine		Phenobarbital	Alk phos	
Creat	kinase		Phenytoin	ALT	
GGT	Amylase		Theophylline	AST	
Glucose	Hemoglobin		Digoxin	CK	
Hb	Calcium		Carbamazepine	GGT	
Iron	Serum HDL-		HDL	LDH	
LDH	cholesterol			Theophylline	
Phos	Total			ELECTROLYTE	
T. protein	billirubin			Na	
Trig	GGTP			K	
Na	Prothrombin			Chloride	
K	time			CO$_2$	
Digoxin	CRP				
Phenytoin	LHD				
Theophylline	Thyroxine				
T4	(T-4)				
TU	Phenytoin				
	Glycated				
	hemoglobin				
	Sodium				

tained in less than 1 minute on most cell counters. A few of the analyzers have CRT displays that help identify abnormal cellular patterns by giving the operator visual interpretation of histograms.

Summary. The number of POLs is rapidly increasing because test results can be obtained while the patient is in the office, allowing the physician to provide prompt patient care and affording the patient greater convenience and decreased anxiety; and the revenue generated by these laboratories will provide the added incentive for many physicians to remain in practice.

Many reliable, accurate, and user-friendly instruments are available for the physician to choose from when starting or expanding a POL. Many manufacturers have complete departments devoted to the POL market. Before purchasing an instrument several should be evaluated and the advantages and limitations of each compared. Most local hospital and reference laboratories are willing to help with this evaluation.

The ideal instrument for the office laboratory should use whole blood for clinical chemistry analyzers thus eliminating the time-consuming step of centrifugation and separation of serum from cells. Ideally, reagents should be available already prepared; the reaction parameters and pipetting of samples and reagents should be automatically performed. Test results should be available in under 5 minutes. The price of the analyzer should be less than $15,000 with a cost/test of less than $1. Leasing an instrument should be optional by the manufacturer. In addition to the routine chemistry tests, special tests (e.g., theapeutic drugs and hormone levels) should be possible with the analyzer. Careful logistic information should be documented on the analyzer's test re-

Table 23-1 Summary of POL chemistry systems

Company	Product	Notes
Glucose systems		
Ames Div. Miles Labs	Glucometer	Dry chemistry whole blood analyzer uses DEXTROSTIX test strips and a reflectance photometer
Boehringer Mannheim	Accu-Chek II	Blood glucose monitor uses Chemstrip bG
Diatron Biomedical	Diatron Easytest	Meter for blood glucose strip tests
Home Diagnostics	Diascan Blood Glucose	Personal bedside blood glucose system using reagent strips. QC program available
Larken Industries	Glucochek II	Meter for blood glucose strip tests
Lifescan	Glucoscan 2000 and 3000	A personal Blood Glucose monitoring system with a dual-beam optics system that includes test strips, control, and meter. Model 3000 contains memory chip for last 29 readings
Orange Medical	Betascan	Meters for blood glucose strip tests
Ulster Scientific	Glucokey	Meter for blood glucose strip tests
Dry chemistry systems		
Miles Inc., Diagnostics Division	Seralyzer III Blood Chemistry Analyzer	Dry chemistry system based on cellulose strips. Many tests available (see box)
	Clinimate TDA Blood Chemistry Analyzer	Dry chemistry system performing theophylline and digoxin tests
	Clinistat Dry Chemistry Analyzer	Dry chemistry using advanced film technology. Processes up to 19 tests/run
Boehringer Mannheim	Reflotron	Whole blood dry chemistry system uses a reflectance photometer and performs a variety of chemical tests (see box)
DuPont	Analyist	Reagents unitized in disposable rotors; profile or discrete analysis; ISE available (see box)
Eastman Kodak	Ektachem DT-60	Chemistry analyzer using dry film technology. Many tests available (see box)
ILEX	Prompt	Automated system uses whole blood systems. Unitized test cards with test, control, and calibrator
Electrolyte systems		
AMDEV	Lytening	ISE Na/K analyzer with prompting and tape print
AVL Scientific	Blood gas analyzer	Whole blood analyzer for blood gases
AVL Scientific	Electrolyte Analyzer	Uses whole blood to determine sodium and potassium by ISE
Baker Diagnostics	ANA-LYTE+1 +2	Direct measurement of sodium and potassium by ISE using whole blood. +2 also measures pH and ionized calcium.
Wet chemistry systems		
Abbott Laboratories	Vision	Highly automated whole blood chemical analyzer. Many tests available (see box)
Arden Medical	Chempro 1000	A novel, fully automated system for variety of common chemistry tests and electrolytes; uses a disposable cartridge
Baker Diagnostics	1-2-3	Blood cell and capillary blood glucose materials for quality control
Bio-Analytics	Smart Alex II	Semiautomated instrument for wide range of chemistry and immunoassay tests
Boehringer Mannheim	Chem 400	Test tube chemistry system including instruments, reagents, standards and control. Tests available: 16 chemistry tests and 5 enzyme reactions
Boehringer Mannheim	Unitest	A test tube and dry chemistry system including instrument, reagents, standards and controls. Tests available: 28 chemistry tests

Continued.

Table 23-1   Summary of POL chemistry systems—cont'd

Company	Product	Notes
Boehringer Mannheim	Unimeter 330 K	Test tube and dry chemistry instruments, reagents, standards, and controls. Tests available: 23 chemistry tests including Potassium by ISE
Chemtronics Labs	Chemistry test systems	Wet chemistry systems for glucose, hemoglobin, cholesterol, HDL chol. Systems are self-contained, marketed for nonlab screening settings
Cooper Biomedical	Request	A random sample access chemistry analyzer with a small computer for 28 tests. Test reagent kits, standards, and controls are also available
Cooper Biomedical	Analyzer II Plus	A semiautomated system programmed for 40 tests and includes reagents and controls
Cooper Biomedical	Assist	A fully automated system programmed for 40 tests and includes reagents and controls
EM Diagnostics	Unipack 500	Wet chemistry system for bilirubin, glucose, cholesterol, HDL cholesterol, and hemoglobin
EM Diagnostics	Unipack 100	A single-beam mini-chemistry analyzer for glucose, hemoglobin, and erythrocytes
EM Diagnostics	Easy-ST	Chemical analyzer uses bar-code cuvettes filled with reagents in powder form
Electro-Nucleonics	Gemstar	Includes 21 chemistry tests with reagent kits. See box
Electro-Nucleonics	Gemini	A fast centrifugal analyzer with reagent kits capable of doing 40 chemistry tests
Phytec	Versamate A	Semiautomated system for a variety of chemistry tests
Sclavo	Unifast	Semiautomated chemical analyzer and reagent systems for a variety of common chemistry tests
Seragen Diagnostics	StaEase	Programmable analyzer can be set up for 25 tests
Seragen Diagnostics	Quick-Chem	Test-tube chemistry system including reagent kits, standards, controls, incubator and calculating colorimeter for 19 common chemistry tests
SmithKline Beckman	Eskalab-CCS	A test tube system with kits for albumin, alkaline phosphatase, amylase, BUN, bilirubin, calcium
Technicon	Assist	Automated random access system for general chemistries and enzymes

Hematology systems

Company	Product	Notes
TOA Medical Electronics (American Scientific Products)	Sysmex: CC-130, CC-150, PL-110	Blood cell counters that range from 3 to 8 parameters
Baker Instruments	Series 130	3-parameter cell counter (RBC, WBC, Hgb) that uses 40 μl of blood
Baker Instruments	Series 150, System 8000	5-parameter cell counter (RBC, WBC, MCV, Hgb, Hct). 8000 also has MCH, MCHC, and Plt
Boehringer Mannheim	Hemo-W	Small system for WBC and Hct
Boehringer Mannheim	M430	System for WBC, RBC, Hgb, and Hct
Clay-Adams	QBC, QBC Plus	Novel blood cell instrument that uses Hct and fluorescent stained buffy coat to RBC, WBC and Plt. QBC Plus includes 7 chemistry tests
Coulter Electronics	CBC-4, CBC-5, T540, S550, S770	Systems range from RBC-WBC counters to those with many parameters
Diagnostic Technology	Picoscale	4-parameter system (WBC, RBC, Hgb, Plt)
Mallinckrodt	390, S670, Profile 700	Broad range of cell counters
Phytec	Versacount	3-parameter analyzer (RBC, WBC, Hct)
Sequoia-Turner	Cell-Dyn Systems	Range from simple to complex cell counters
Seragen Diagnostics	Quick Count, QC/ Plus 2, Pronto 5	2- and 4-parameter counters (WBC, Hgb plus RBC, Hct)

port to enable the laboratory to keep a record of which tests are being ordered by each physician in a group practice.

The lack of quality control protocols for POLs can result in poor performance and questionable accuracy of the test results. For each analyzer a quality control program should be written that will prevent the operator from starting a test unless control material is measured. In addition proficiency testing for the POL should be established by the appropriate organizations to provide some assurances of quality control.

"Doc-in-the-box" analyzers that are advertised as "fool-proof" are emerging as the predominant systems in POLs. They can be operated by personnel without laboratory training, (i.e., nurses or office assistants). Such instruments would likely be cost effective because the intense competition between manufacturers will keep costs down. However, in large group practices a laboratory technician or technologist may be required because of the increased volume of work and the many different types of laboratory procedures likely to be requested.

Review Questions

1. Discuss how federal legislation has impacted the evolution of POLs.
2. What is the single greatest challenge and potential problem that POLs face?
3. List five criteria to consider before acquisition of specific instrumentation for a POL.
4. Name two specific chemistry analyzers that use dry reagents and describe the principle of operation of each.
5. Name two examples of "wet" chemistry analyzers and describe how they operate.
6. Why is dry reagent technology advantageous to POLs?
7. Name four POL hematology analyzers and their testing capabilities.
8. Give two reasons why POLs will survive and most likely increase in the future.

Bibliography

Aziz K: Assuring quality in the physician's office laboratory, Amer Clin Lab, July, 1989, 8.

Bills J et al: Comparison of four chemistry analyzers for physician office and clinic laboratories, Clin Lab Sci 2:11, 1989.

Clinical chemistry devices for physicians' office laboratories: premarket notification, Am Clin Prod Rev, August 1987, 19.

Etnyre-Zacher P, Miller S: An educational program for physicians' office laboratory personnel, Am Clin Lab, Jan/Feb 1990, 10.

Ferron D: Guidelines for POL instrument selection, Medical Laboratory Observer, Jan 1990, 53.

Jackson J, Campbell J: State regulation of physicians' in-office laboratories, Am Clin Prod Rev, Feb, 1988, 38.

Jackson J, Conrad M: Diagnostic instruments for the physician's in-office laboratory, Am Clin Prod Rev, August 1987, 10.

Ng R: Instrumentation for physician's office testing, Am Clin Prod Rev, November 1987, 48.

Pesce M: Instrument systems for the physician's office laboratory, J Med Tech 2-9:566, 1985.

Shaikh A: Laboratory instrument evaluation and selection procedure designed for physician office laboratories, Clin Lab Sci 2:118, 1989.

Simon V, Mobley R: Physicians' office laboratories and clinical laboratory improvement amendments of 1988, Diag Clin Test 27:24, 1989.

Stevens R et al: Training and educational needs in small office laboratories, J Med Tech 2(9):577, 1985.

CHAPTER 24

Maintenance and Repair

LARRY E. SCHOEFF

Equipment Maintenance
Equipment Repair

Medical laboratories exist to provide analyses that can be used in patient diagnosis or treatment. The only product the laboratory provides is a report that is quantitative, descriptive, or both. If the report is inaccurate or unreliable, the purpose for the laboratory's existence is defeated; when the report is sufficiently misleading, it may do considerable harm. Errors are much more common than generally realized or admitted and are almost certain to occur routinely unless a well-organized program of error avoidance is put in place. This program is generally referred to as quality control or quality assurance. In this chapter various aspects of quality control measures involving maintenance and repair of instrumentation are examined.

With medical laboratory reports only a few quality judgments can be made by looking at the report, and the information is most often used before there is a chance to evaluate its quality. An error in any step in the production of the report can cause a serious error in its validity that may not be apparent.

The ultimate reason for quality control of laboratory work is to ensure the best care of the patient. The laboratory's responsibility is to ensure that each report reflects the patient's condition accurately, reliably, and promptly so that diagnosis and treatment can be carried out in the most effective and expedient manner.

Effective quality control needs to anticipate all possible variables that might affect the test report. The following list is representative of the potential sources of error that may affect the laboratory tests:

Patient identification
Specimen labeling

Specimen collection technique
Specimen preservation and storage
Mixing or sampling
Reagent quality (including water)
Instrument performance
Instrument calibration
Electrical supply
Transposition of data
Standard and reference quality
Calculation
Choice of test method
Pipetting or weighing
Timing and timer accuracy
Temperature

No simple program of quality control can anticipate all possible errors. The need is not so much for a rigid system as for an attitude and state of mind that compels each analyst to question everything about personal performance and the instrument's performance. Because this attitude is not universal and because even the best workers have lapses, rules that help avoid the more common errors are needed. These rules must be followed.

Equipment Maintenance

It is not unusual for an analytic instrument to be blamed for one of the errors previously mentioned. When poor instrument performance is suspected, it is wise to consider all of the elements that might affect results before instrument problems are considered.

Instruments and analytic systems used in the laboratory vary greatly in their principles of operation and complexity. There are many different pieces of equipment, and new ones are frequently introduced. Adaptation to these may be time consuming and troublesome. A number of general rules may be applied that can make the process simpler and more problem free. These general rules also contribute considerably to quality control.

Understanding the Equipment. No new piece of equipment should be operated before the operator understands what it does and how it functions. It is impossible to make reasonable judgments about such factors as temperature, timing, carry-over, and contamination without a clear understanding of the principle of operation of the equipment.

Operator manuals generally provide most of the necessary information, and they should be studied carefully before tests are run. Obviously, more complex equipment requires more detailed study and training.

Regular Performance Checks. Before an instrument is used each day, the necessary steps should be taken to ensure that it will perform properly. The nature of the equipment will determine what these steps might be. Certainly it should be clean and in good condition. If there are reagents or expendable supplies used, these should be checked. Often the checking of some electrical function is required. Temperature may be critical. If it is, the operating temperature should be observed and made a matter of record.

Often the instrument must be zeroed or blanked or checked for background to ensure that no value is indicated in the absence of a sample. Many devices require operation through a cycle to ensure that all systems are functional and to prime pumps and fill lines and chambers. Others may require changing of membranes or charging with reagents. With computer-associated systems, certain programs or information may need to be furnished. All such requirements should be combined into a start-up procedure, and the appropriate steps followed and checked off or recorded each day. Simple, small equipment naturally does not require involved start-up procedure, but even centrifuges and baths should be conscientiously checked for proper function.

Calibration. Calibration is important. This simply means ensuring that the measuring device is accurately reporting what it was meant to measure. Thermometers should be checked periodically against a certified thermometer or one of guaranteed accuracy. Timers should be compared with some accurate timepiece. Spectrophotometers should be checked against a standard calibrating filter, and gamma counters should be calibrated with a standard energy source. Calibrating standards must be analyzed and their values "locked in" on automated instruments. All calibrating procedures should be recorded.

Preventive Maintenance. Preventive maintenance refers to all those functions that may be regularly done to avoid downtime for repairs, adjustments, or restocking. This may include lubrication, retubing, changing membranes, and replacing small parts. For each instrument there should be a description of these activities, and their frequency should be defined. A record should be kept that explains what was done on each date. Even very simple devices should be observed for proper condition and function. Frayed cords, defective switches, and worn parts should receive prompt attention.

Correct calibration or function of instruments should not be assumed just because test results seem to be right. Each element that can be checked should be tested independently of the test to be done.

Reference Controls. Reference controls are assayed sera that chemically resemble patient samples. It is recommended that at least three levels be used to establish the linearity of the procedure through the expected range of patient values. These should be run with each test run.

These reference, or control sera, are used to provide data of precision, which can indicate any unusual problem with the testing procedure or instrument. For them to serve a purpose, limits of acceptability must be established and observed. Whenever these limits are exceeded, the procedure must be considered to be out of control and no results should be reported until the problem is resolved. It is useful to prepare a list of steps that might be taken to evaluate and correct the problem so that time is not lost in guessing and in aimless activity. As soon as the problem seems to be corrected, the controls should be repeated.

The test sequence should not be considered to be in control until reference control values fall within the established limits of acceptability. When limits are exceeded, some record should be made of the problem and of the steps that were necessary for its correction. A review of the record of problems and their corrections at the end of the month may prove instructive and helpful.

Method Correlation. The quality control policy of the laboratory should also recognize the need to correlate the results of different testing methods on different instruments. It is not uncommon for laboratories to use two or more methods or instruments for testing a single substance.

Both instruments may be giving appropriate quality control data, but because of different methods and reference material, the two may not agree with each other. In studying the correlation of various methods, it is important to check for agreement at extremely high and low levels because these are the results that would be significant when sick patients are tested. If reasonable correlation cannot be achieved, it may be necessary to quote different normal ranges and to alert the medical staff to the differences found.

Equipment Repair

Laboratory equipment has changed a great deal over the last 10 to 15 years. At that time it was not only possible but also advisable for laboratory workers to thoroughly understand their equipment and to perform many simple repairs. Electronics has been revolutionized by semiconductor devices. Transistors have been adapted to perform a large range of functions, and solid-state crystals have been fashioned into fantastically small integrated circuits that can be designed to perform complex calculations using algorithms. Sensitive and sophisticated transducers are able to detect nearly any type of physical change and convert it to an electrical force that can be quantitated.

Ion-selective electrodes have been developed to the point where they can accurately measure many elements. Solid-state devices have been engineered into microprocessors and computers that can sort, count, calculate, and perform quantitive judgments with great speed. All of these devices have been miniaturized and engineered into instruments that are extremely fast, accurate, convenient, and remarkably small. Thanks in large part to solid state electronics, these devices are, for the most part, trouble free and easy to maintain.

It has become difficult to diagnose problems that pertain to the technical detail of these instruments, and the temptation is to plug them in and accept the fact that they work until the time when they obviously do not.

Specific diagnoses of problems are presented in the next section, following a general review of troubleshooting including problem recognition, identification, and correction.

Steps in Problem Solving

Problem Recognition. An instrument malfunction cannot be identified or corrected until it is apparent to the instrument operator that there is a problem. As basic and self-evident as this may seem, many malfunctioning instruments continue to produce inaccurate results because the instrument operators are not aware that a prob-

lem exists. Instrument malfunctions manifest themselves in many ways. Symptoms of instrument problems are sometimes apparent and sometimes subtle. The accuracy of laboratory test results is jeopardized more by subtle problems than by the readily apparent instrumental problems. Readily apparent problems include malfunctions that make a required analytic determination impossible (i.e., a burned out light source in a spectrophotometer, a blown fuse, a ruined photodetector in any photometric instrument, depletion of fuels and/or reagents required for instrument function, or an unplugged power cord). Examples of subtle malfunctions include slight misalignment of the optical system in spectrophotometric instruments, dirty or damaged optical surfaces in optical analytic instruments, contamination of required fuels and/or solutions for instrument operation, damaged or worn electrical potentiometers, and alteration of reference voltages in potentiometric analytic instruments.

Subtle problems require the alert, keen perception of an operator who is able to make fine distinctions between normal and abnormal instrument response characteristics. When these indistinctly expressed malfunctions are not detected, test result inaccuracies unfortunately may be accepted as valid.

Problem/Cause Identification. Once the effect of a problem is perceived, the cause or causes of that problem must be identified. Problem identification is therefore the matching of cause and effect. Experienced instrument operators may readily relate a specific faulty response to its cause because of the frequency with which they have previously observed that malfunction. The continued exposure of the operator to characteristic instrument responses and their identification produces a mental index of cause-effect relationship. However, not all practicing technical laboratory personnel have this index of experience on which to rely. Therefore each malfunction may be a new problem to solve.

The apprehension of facing a new problem can be replaced gradually with the self-assurance that comes from being able to apply knowledge to problem solving in a logical, stepwise fashion. The familiarity of the problem solving approach diminishes or eliminates the uneasiness produced by the unknown.

The logical steps to be followed in troubleshooting are: state the perceived problem, list its possible causes, and then proceed to prove or disprove each cause. Stating the problem caused by readily apparent malfunction is easy (i.e., the light bulb went out in the spectrophotometer). More difficult are the subtle problems. These subtle problems present a constant challenge to the conscientious instrument operator. Persistent monitoring and vigilance are required for identification of these malfunctions. Calibration and quality control checks are the monitoring devices used for detection of subtle malfunctions or for forewarning of possible instrument problems. Preventive maintenance is a means of avoiding problems. Preventive maintenance procedures are well worth the time and effort invested because the direct result is the avoidance of instrument problems that are detrimental to the speed and accuracy with which clinical laboratory analyses are performed. Calibration, quality control, and preventive maintenance are all too frequently approached with a casual attitude. However, these procedures are extremely important in indicating the presence of a subtle problem.

Possible causes of a problem should be listed in order of most to least probable. In the example of the spectrophotometer light bulb going out, the most probable cause would be a burned out bulb followed by no current available to the bulb.

The second possibility has a number of probable explanations: the power switch is off or the plug is not plugged into the power outlet (both of which are frequently responsible for inoperative instruments), a fuse is blown, the light bulb leads are not securely connected to the circuit connections, or no current is available from the power outlet. Additional causes of symptoms manifested by malfunctioning instruments are listed in most instrument operation manuals. If the most probable causes are proved not to be responsible for a problem, then these more comprehensive lists are very useful.

The procedure followed in proving or disproving hypothesized causes of a problem depends heavily on common sense. In the example of the light bulb in the spectrophotometer, a quick visual check of the bulb will determine whether it is burned out. If the bulb is not burned out, further investigation is required. By observing whether other electrically operated parts of the circuit are functioning, the operator can determine whether the problem is limited to the bulb or has affected the entire circuitry of the instrument. If all electronic functions of the instrument are inoperative, then the following checks should be made: "on-off" switch in "on" position, power line plugged into power outlet, fuse not blown, and current available at the power outlet

(check with a simple indicator light or a voltmeter or ask an electrician). Frequently, one of these obvious, easily checked, probable causes is found to be responsible for the malfunction.

If all the obvious causes are eliminated as the responsible problem, additional circuit analysis procedures may be required. Even the electronics novice can visually check a circuit for melted, scorched, or damaged components. The odor of overheated components is also a good indicator of a problem within a circuit. Voltage and signal waveform checks require the use of an oscilloscope; voltage checks require only a voltmeter. Competence in the use of these test instruments and experience in obtaining electrical readings from circuits provide the needed expertise to follow the simple test point measurements given in many instrument manuals.

Problem Correction. Problem correction also should be the responsibility of the instrument operator. Two options are available. First, the operator may decide that the minor repair and/or replacement needed for correction of a malfunction is within his or her capabilities. Second, the operator may conclude that additional troubleshooting or malfunction correction requires additional expertise. With this conclusion, expert assistance should be obtained. Of utmost importance is the expedient, effective repair of malfunctioning clinical laboratory instruments. The malfunction must be recognized and identified promptly.

Diagnosis of Problems. Many of the devices in the laboratory are small, simple instruments such as pumps, heaters, dilutors, and simple spectrophotometers. These should be understood by qualified laboratory personnel, and their failure or malfunction should be diagnosable and in many cases repairable. Often solutions to problems with simple equipment involve common sense more than profound knowledge. When confronted with an instrument that does not work, consider the following:

1. Is it plugged in? Maybe the janitor pulled the plug.
2. Is the overload breaker in the breaker panel not thrown out? Try a desk lamp or a test light in the receptacle to be sure there is electricity available.
3. If there is no electricity at the plug, find the breaker box that furnishes that area of the building. It is probably a small metal door in the hallway close by. Rocker-type

circuit breakers in the box have a small element that heats and expands when overloaded, throwing out the breaker and thus cutting off electricity to that circuit.

4. In older buildings there may be screw-in fuses in the box. They are rated as to the number of amps they will carry. Look at the mica front window to check if the fuse is blown. If it is smoked up and the little metal band under it is melted, the fuse is blown and must be replaced. More than likely the rocker-type circuit breakers will be in the panel instead of the older, screw-in type of fuses.

5. Do not replace the fuse or reset the breaker until the cause of the blown fuse is found. It may have been a direct short from a broken wire or some obvious defect. It could also be from too much load on the line (e.g., too many heating devices). If no immediate cause is found, unplug as many items as possible, replace the fuse, and reconnect the devices one at a time until the new fuse blows. This will indicate which item is responsible for the overload. By taking everything else off the line and trying again, the operator can tell if the total load was too much for the fuse or if there was an electrical problem in the device previously reconnected.

6. When breakers throw out, the operator cannot always easily tell by glancing at them. They may be pushed only slightly up from the "on" position. Run a finger down the line of breakers; the one that is out will be slightly raised. Immediately after a circuit breaker throws out, it may feel warm or even hot. However, other breakers that are heavily loaded may also feel warm.

7. To put the circuit back in use, push down on the off (or out) side and then depress the on (or in) side as far as it will go. If it throws out again and the problem cannot be located, call an electrician.

8. If the instrument is still dead although plugged in and there is electricity in the line, check the instrument's fuse. Usually the fuse holder is a little black or brown knob close to the point where the power cable goes into the instrument. Some fuse holders have a cover with a milled edge that can be easily removed with the fingers. Others are threaded and must be

screwed out, whereas still others have a bayonet lock that requires only a half-turn. Some fuse covers require a screwdriver to turn. The fuse holder is spring loaded so that the fuse will usually spring out, and one end may be clamped to the fuse cover.

9. Look at this small glass minifuse to see whether it is smoked up and whether the metal band or wire inside is melted. If it is a tiny wire, it may burn up completely. If not sure whether it is burned out, check it with a multimeter or replace it with another fuse of the metal band at one end.

10. To check the fuse with a meter, set the meter to ohms and turn the selector knob to the lowest setting, which is usually marked X1 (or 1). Touch the two meter leads together. The needle should move to the right side of the meter. (This indicates the proper meter setting.) Now touch the two meter probes to either end of the fuse. If the needle responds, the fuse is all right.

11. If the fuse is good and the instrument still does not respond, check the lamps. If an exciter lamp is out, a photometer will obviously not respond. Try a new exciter lamp. It is probably best to unplug the instrument while checking and changing lamps to avoid the possibility of shock. Never work with an instrument's wiring while standing on a wet floor or leaning against metal surfaces unless it is disconnected. Do not forget to plug it in again before trying it.

12. If the instrument still does not respond, remove the cover and start hunting for obvious problems such as the following: (A) A blackened spot may indicate a short circuit. (B) A loose wire that goes nowhere may indicate a broken lead. Check to see where it should have been connected. If this is not apparent, do not guess. This could cause damage. (C) Melted resin, smoke deposit, or a strong smell around a transformer or motor may indicate that it is burned out. (D) Look for resistors that are split open. Sometimes excess heat or humidity may destroy a resistor, leaving a circuit open. (E) Check for any rarely used switches on the back or inside the instrument that might cancel the function. (F) With the multimeter on the ohms position, attach a lead to one prong of the

power cable and touch the other lead to the point inside the instrument where the power comes in. Repeat with the other side of the cable. A little searching will show where terminals connect inside the instrument. One side of the power cord will almost certainly go to the fuse holder. If continuity cannot be demonstrated (if the needle will not move), there may be a break in the cable. While checking, it is a good idea to bend or flex the cable to be sure that the wires inside the insulation are not broken and only occasionally making contact. Also check between the two wires for shorts. (G) If a three-strand power cable is used, the round peg of the plug-in is the ground and it is probably attached to the frame of the instrument. Check this for continuity with the ohmmeter also. (H) Attach the meter leads (still on ohms) to the two sides of the main power switch and throw the switch. The meter should deflect in the on position and return to the peg in the off position. (I) Switch the meter to AC volts and set it on 110 V or higher to see whether, with the instrument plugged in and turned on, 110 V (more or less) can be measured at the point where the power cord enters the instrument. If so, follow the two lines along to see how far the current can be traced. The defective element may be found in this way after a little experience with the instrument. Be careful not to shock yourself or produce a short by touching two hot points with the same probe. Handle the probes on the insulated portion only. If the problem has not been solved by this time, turn the instrument over to a qualified repair technician.

13. When a meter responds erratically and the controls do not produce a smooth response, the problem may be in a faulty potentiometer. Try turning the control, as evenly as possible, from one end of its travel to the other. If the meter needle does not respond smoothly, the pot may be defective. Try tapping the control knob with a finger and notice whether the meter needle remains relatively steady. If not, this is an additional indication of a defective pot. Try this latter test in several positions of the control knob. The defect of the pot may be at only one point. A pot is not difficult to change after a little practice with a soldering iron. Be sure to replace with the proper type of pot. The size indicates the wattage, whereas the ohms and the percent accuracy are usually stamped on the back. Be sure to note which lead goes to which contact of the pot. If wired backward, the meter will move in the wrong direction when the knob is turned. Also, be sure that all contacts are tightly soldered and that no loose drops of solder have fallen where they can cause shorts.

14. Soldering is not difficult but requires some practice. For instrument work a small pencil-type is preferred over a solder gun. The latter heats more quickly but produces more heat than is needed and is harder to get into small places without causing damage to delicate parts. Remove as much of the old solder as possible. Hook the wires to be soldered into the solder holes or otherwise secure them.

    Place the tip of the iron on the point to be soldered so that both the wire and the contact are heated. Touch the solder to the iron at the point of contact and let the solder fuse completely before withdrawing the iron. If the contact is not hot enough the solder will not bond to it and a "cold-solder joint" may be made: this could result in a poor electrical connection. Avoid using excess solder and dripping hot drops of the metal onto other parts. A resin-cord solder (no. 20 G or 22 G) is right for this type of work. The soldering iron should not be left plugged in for extended periods of time. Occasionally retinning the tip of the iron helps to keep it in good shape. This is done by melting a drop of solder on the point and quickly wiping it over the hot surface with a piece of waste material.

15. When electric motors will not function, the following checks may be made: (A) Is electricity getting to the motor? Check whether the motor is plugged in, check the line circuit breaker, the instrument fuse, etc., as noted earlier. (B) Check whether the motor can be turned freely by hand. (C) If it can, unplug the device and check the brushes. They are accessible through small plastic caps on either side of the motor. Be sure that plenty of carbon is left on the brushes, that the brushes are actu-

ally touching the armature (is the lower edge worn shiny?), and that the spring or wire making electric contact in the brush holder is not broken. The brush should fit snugly in the brush holder. If it is so loose that the brush is worn off at an angle, it is probably the wrong size brush. If the brush does not slide easily into the holder, it may fail to feed down against the commutator as the carbon is worn away.

This may be due to the brush being too large or to a deposit of carbon building up in the brush holder. Carbon may be cleaned out with a cotton-tipped applicator soaked in carbon tetrachloride or some similar solvent. Dry out any excess solvent. Special solvents for cleaning motors are available. (D) If the motor turns but not easily, there is a good chance that a bearing has become so dry that it is impeding the motor and could result in burning the motor out. Work light oil into the bearings, and turn the motor back and forth on its bearings until the bearings are completely free and the motor will turn easily by hand. Try it under power to see whether the problem has been solved. Next time, oil the bearings before they get dry. (E) If the motor cannot be turned by hand, a bearing is probably "frozen" from lack of lubrication and possibly too much heat. An attempt can be made to work the bearing loose with lubricants and carefully exercised force. If this does not work, the motor must be torn down and the bearings replaced. If the bearing has been frozen and under power for very long, it is possible that the motor is badly burned and will require extensive repair or replacement. (F) If the motor turns freely and the brushes are in good shape, it is possible that there is a break in either the field coil or armature winding and the motor will need to be sent to a shop for rewinding. (G) If the motor hums but does not move or moves only slightly, there may be a short, which will also require rewinding. (H) If the motor runs noisily and occasionally hangs up, the bearing may be badly worn. To check end play, with the motor in a vertical position (as in a centrifuge), lift the shaft as much as possible and let it drop a few times. A little play with just a faint click can be heard as the shaft falls back into place. A barely perceptible end play is necessary for the motor to run smoothly. If considerable play exists or if a definite metallic clank can be heard, the bearing is probably worn.

Some motors are mounted on rubber grommets, and the whole motor may move when moving the shaft in its bearings.

16. Laboratory power lines are often overloaded, because planners often do not realize the considerable amount of electricity used by the dozens of laboratory devices. One danger signal is excessive heat at the circuit breaker panel. If a circuit is heavily loaded, that particular breaker will be hot, and, if the circuit is overloaded, the breaker will throw out occasionally. Sometimes it is possible to physically move some high-consumption devices to other circuits, or the electrician may move some circuits from one breaker to put them on a less-used position in the breaker box. When the entire lab load begins to be too heavy for the system supplied, voltage may drop.

    This may cause many serious problems with laboratory equipment. Voltage can be checked at the wall plug with a voltmeter. For current to be adequate, the voltage difference between the two should be 117 V or close to it and fluctuation should not occur. Recording voltmeters are available to monitor voltage over a period of time if this seems desirable. Most laboratory instruments will compensate fairly well for drops to about 100 V, but some will not. A lower drop may cause motors to stall and burn. Surges of very high voltage, occasionally associated with overloading, can be very damaging to some components.

17. The person responsible for the care and maintenance of laboratory equipment is seldom able to keep up with all the potential problems. If an awareness of equipment is developed, many breakdown situations may be avoided. The tools should be closely available, loose screws should be tightened, dry bearings lubricated, and dirty contacts cleaned.

18. As experience is gained, comprehension of diagrams can be picked up that will en-

able the technician to follow wiring plans and better understand their function and their potential problems. There are no instant electronics or instrument experts. Only experience, observation, and interest can develop the abilities necessary to cope with instrument failure. It is hoped that the information contained herein will help students acquire some understanding and interest.

19. The following tools and supplies are suggested for any reasonably active laboratory:

Tools
Pliers: needle-nosed and ordinary
Wire cutter and stripper
Vise-grip wrenches
Files: crosscut, rattails, and triangular
Set of small end wrenches
Set of screwdrivers: small to large, and offset screwdriver
Philips screwdrivers
Set of Allen wrenches
Small vise
Small soldering iron
Flashlight
VOM multimeter
Test lamp
Small knife
Hemostats
Small hammer
Supplies
Solder
Spool of 18- or 20-gauge hook-up wire
Electrician's tape
Emery paper
Epoxy cement
Spade terminals or other types
Fuses for all instruments
Brushes for all motors
Replacement lamps for all instruments on hand
3-in-one oil and centrifuge lubricant
Instruction manuals for all instruments
Any repair or replacement parts recommended by manufacturer
Collection of miscellaneous hardware—nuts and bolts

Maintenance/Repair Records and Service. As equipment becomes more sophisticated and automated, it becomes less possible for medical laboratory personnel to perform adequate repairs.

One of the simplest laboratory policies intended to avoid serious repair problems with down time is to insist that all personnel who use equipment carefully read the operating and maintenance instructions. All steps in care and maintenance should be posted and should be followed in all cases. Deviations from normal instrument performance should be noted and investigated. A record should be kept of repairs, calibrations, and maintenance procedures.

It is now mandated, by accrediting agencies and third-party payers, that detailed records be kept of instrument performance, including dates of calibration and repair. Each year the records required become more specific and detailed. At least two types of records should be kept on all equipment. First, the record of performance must be kept by the person responsible for its use. This record would provide temperature checks of heating and cooling devices, calibration corrections and dates of such devices as colorimeters, calibration checks of measuring equipment such as pipettors, and verification of function of mechanical devices such as rotators and shakers. Second, a property record should record the date and price of purchase, name of manufacturer, and the dates and details of repair or maintenance procedures. Most devices should be placed on some type of schedule for periodic cleaning, repair, and calibration. Laboratories with any considerable quantity of equipment may elect to use a computer schedule and record of repair.

It is absolutely essential for laboratories to have access to maintenance and repair capability. Most hospitals now have electronic repair sections with some level of competence with certain types of laboratory devices. The most sophisticated equipment will probably require the services of factory trained service personnel from the manufacturer or vendor. Such services are usually available under warranty or service contract.

Environment. As equipment becomes larger and more complex, the environment becomes increasingly important.

1. Most solid-state circuits are sensitive to extreme change in temperature. Adequate temperature control is imperative.
2. Dust and dirt around mechanical and electrical equipment is both dangerous and apt to cause malfunctions.
3. Corrosion and shorts are caused by mois-

ture and spillage of acids, alkalies, and other corrosive chemicals.

4. All equipment should be plugged into a wall receptacle. Do not use extension cords, multiple (octopus) plugs, or other temporary wiring.

5. All circuits must be grounded. Wall receptacles should provide for a three-pronged receptacle. The ground terminal should be checked to be certain that it is indeed connected to an adequate ground and that it has no electric potential.

6. Circuits should be checked at the instrument site to determine whether adequate voltage is maintained when a full working load is imposed on the line. If there is any indication for it, the sine wave pattern of the AC supply should be checked to be sure there is no distortion.

7. There should be no exposed wiring in work areas, and covers should be kept on equipment to protect it and the operator unless repair or maintenance is actually being performed.

8. Work areas around equipment should be kept clear and free of trash, debris, and stored supplies. Floors should be clean and dry. Traffic should be kept to a minimum.

All these precautions are necessary for the optimal performance of the equipment and the safety of the operator. The medical laboratory represents a huge investment in equipment and its overhead expense. A thorough appreciation of this equipment, its application, maintenance, repair, and replacement is crucial.

WHEN ALL ELSE FAILS

READ THE DIRECTIONS

Review Questions

1. Why is preventive maintenance of equipment so essential in a clinical laboratory?
2. Describe the logical steps to be followed in troubleshooting equipment malfunction.
3. Make a checklist of potential problems that could cause equipment malfunction.
4. Make a list of tools and supplies that should be available for equipment repairs in a clinical laboratory.

CHAPTER 25

Selection of Laboratory Instruments

LEMUEL J. BOWIE

Performance Considerations
Design-Associated Considerations
Economic Considerations
Performance Verification

The selection of any piece of laboratory instrumentation requires a thorough understanding of the needs of the laboratory and some appreciation for how the instrument may be able to satisfy those needs. This understanding may require a complete analysis of such factors as laboratory workflow, staffing on all affected shifts, test mix and turn-around-time requirements, physical limitations imposed by the site of the instruments, fiscal limitations on mode of acquisition or on capital outlay, and instrument performance capabilities. Some of this data may be readily available (e.g., laboratory workload data), whereas other information may be more difficult to acquire. In this chapter a systematic approach toward getting all of this information, making the actual selection of the instrument, justifying its acquisition to the administrator, and documenting its performance on site will be presented.

Performance Considerations

Workload. Two workload recording methods are widely used in the United States. The College of American Pathologists workload recording method is probably the primary system in use in nongovernment institutions. The Automated Management Information System (AMIS) method is the system widely used in government laboratories. Although both systems assign unit values/test (in minutes) based on time-motion studies, some preanalytic and postanalytic steps are difficult to incorporate (e.g., specimen processing, phoning of emergency results). Moreover, it is difficult to keep unit values current with the rapid introduction of new analytic systems or

significant performance enhancements on current analytic instruments. Therefore for the purpose of instrument selection it is best to use individual test volumes for the tests to be performed on the analytic instrument to be considered and calculate instrument-specific and test-mix-specific analysis times and actual operator-instrument required times. The overall analysis time will depend on three major factors: (1) the type of sample, (2) the processing mode, and (3) the analytic characteristics of the instrument.

Sample Type. Although serum is the type of specimen predominantly used for most automated analytic instruments today, the use of serum has a number of disadvantages. First, it must be produced by allowing the blood to clot. This process can take 30 minutes or more for certain specimens. The serum must be physically separated from the blood, usually by centrifugation, and then moved into a separate tube by pipetting or pouring. These processes can easily add 45 minutes to the overall analysis time. Some specialized analytic devices (e.g., Abbott VISION) can use whole blood directly for measurements of a variety of analytes. This has obvious advantages in saving time. However, it must be remembered that whole blood values may be slightly lower than serum values because plasma contains 12% more water than whole blood. If the whole blood is obtained from a finger stick, other biases may be present.

Fortunately, **"primary tube" sampling** devices on newer analytic instruments may lessen the time lost in the pipetting or aliquotting of specimens. Note that there are two types of primary tube sampling devices. Both devices require that the sample be allowed to clot and that it be centrifuged. The most useful type, frequently called **"closed tube" sampling** is accomplished by actually puncturing the stopper and withdrawing an aliquot of serum from the supernatant. The second type requires the operator to remove the stopper, but the sample can be aspirated directly from the original tube. An advantage of primary tube sampling is that it eliminates one potential source of specimen mix-up by eliminating the manual transfer of sample to another tube. A major benefit of the closed-tube sampling device is that it eliminates the hazard for the operator of being exposed to potential infectious aerosols produced when the original tube is opened to transfer a sample aliquot.

Analysis of fluids other than blood is a frequent requirement for most laboratories. Urine specimens often require dilution before analysis (e.g., potassium), and many instruments incorporate automatic dilution and calculation protocols if the sample is identified as a urine. Different methods may be required for urine and other fluids than would be required for the same constituent in blood (e.g., protein). The system should also be able to detect potential chemical or physical interferences to the analytic procedure such as those resulting from hemolyzed, icteric, or lipemic samples.

Sample volume is also an important consideration. If the analyzer is to be used for pediatric samples, it should require minimum amounts (e.g., 1 to 5 μl) per test and there should be adequate protection to prevent concentration by evaporation while the sample is on the analyzer waiting to be tested. Obviously the ability to perform analyses on small amounts of fluid can be very useful when there is a limited amount of specimen available initially or after some testing has been performed. This makes it possible to perform repeat testing or additional testing that might not be possible if larger sample volumes were required.

Processing Mode. Although analyzers can be classified in a number of ways based on how they actually perform the analysis (e.g., continuous flow, discrete, centrifugal, random access), the most meaningful classification from the standpoint of workload handling capability is based on batch vs STAT analysis capabilities.

STAT analyzers are systems designed to provide a limited number of results on a sample with very little time between the time the sample is placed on the analyzer and the time the complete set of results is available or printed. This "lag time" can be as short as 1 minute for 8 results (e.g., Beckman Sychron CX-3). On the other hand, **batch analyzers** are designed to provide

one or multiple tests on a large number of specimens at the maximum analytic rate. Although the analytic rate may be 1000 to 3000 tests/hour, the systems generally have a significant lag time before the first result is available. This lag time may be 5 to 20 minutes. In addition even more time is required to get these more complex devices set up, primed, and running before any samples can be introduced. This start-up time can be 1 hour or more.

The term **throughput** has been used to describe the actual performance of an instrument in analyzing a fixed number of specimens with a specific mix of tests. This overall analytic throughput expressed in sample/hour or tests/hour is generally higher for batch analyzers, particularly when analyzing large numbers of samples with multiple tests continuously over an extended period of time. However, it is easy to see that throughput on these analyzers (when analyzing only a few tests on a sporadic basis) can be significantly lower than a STAT analyzer, which is designed to handle this type of task. Because most laboratories have a need to perform both types of analyses, instruments have been designed to try to accomplish both tasks on a single analytic system. These analyzers are called random access analyzers and are particularly popular for small to moderately large laboratories. These analyzers are capable of performing any number of tests available on the system on any or all of the samples to be analyzed. For example, a glucose test can be performed on each sample or a 20-test profile on all samples or a different mixture of tests on each sample. The advantage of this general approach is that a single analyzer can perform as a STAT or batch analyzer. The disadvantage of this approach is that such random access systems are not as good as the best STAT or batch analyzers for their respective tasks. If the laboratory can only purchase a single instrument, however, this may be an acceptable approach. If the primary concern is either maximum analytic throughput or minimum lag time, then a dedicated batch or STAT analyzer is appropriate.

A word of caution is appropriate, however, when comparing analyzer throughputs particularly for random access analyzers. Throughputs are test-mix specific. A good example is the throughput obtained with an instrument that can perform electrolytes and nonelectrolyte chemistries. Because these methods use different analytic techniques that may be run simultaneously with inherently different throughputs, the overall

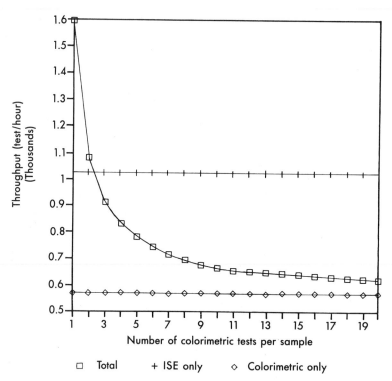

Fig. 25-1 Analytic throughput. Throughput when specimens are only analyzed for sodium, potassium, and carbon dioxide by a separate electrolyte channel, $+$; throughput when specimens are only analyzed for colorimetric constituents, $\Diamond$; throughput when increasing numbers of colorimetrics tests are ordered on each sample, $\square$.

analytic throughput can differ depending on the percentage of electrolyte tests performed. Because three to four electrolytes can be analyzed in the same period as one to two nonelectrolyte chemistries, the higher the number of nonelectrolyte tests/sample the lower the throughput (Fig. 25-1).

No discussion of mode of operation would be complete without a discussion of the importance of backup capability during scheduled or unscheduled downtime. If a new piece of equipment is being purchased to replace a functional but not as efficient system, the easiest solution to the backup problem would be to retain the old instrument and keep it operational as a backup. Another option is to purchase two less capable systems whose combined analytic capabilities would meet the laboratory's requirements and whose cost might be comparable with a more expensive and complex instrument. This approach ensures that exactly the same methods, normal ranges, and specimen limitations apply to the primary system and the backup system. It also ensures that in case one analyzer is completely down, the maximum drop in throughput should

be 50%. If, however, only one method or group of methods is affected, the effect on the laboratory would be much less. It should be remembered that although high throughput analyzers operating at near capacity are very efficient and cost effective, they may be difficult or impossible to back up if the entire instrument is out of service for more than a few hours. Therefore careful planning toward providing adequate backup is essential, if such high speed systems are used.

A concern related to the subject of backup is method comparability. Obviously, the result that the laboratory reports should be independent of the mode in which the sample was analyzed, or on which instrument the sample was analyzed. From a practical point of view there will be slight differences in the calibration of different instruments that will result in different reported values if no adjustments are made. These differences can result from instrument-specific biases, matrix effects of calibration materials, method-specific biases, and differences in target value assignments. It is therefore necessary that both instruments give the same numbers by adjusting one instrument's calibration parameters. This should be done by analyzing approximately 40 fresh samples and determining the reproducibility of each system and the constant and proportional biases that exist between them. The technique for analyzing the data will be described later in this chapter.

Analytic Capabilities. One of the major practical concerns for new instrumentation is that they be accurate and relatively free from interferences. Fortunately the problem of method accuracy and susceptibility to interferences is not as great as it was 10 years ago. Manufacturers have been able to incorporate new analytic technologies into their instruments. More specific enzymatic methods have replaced most of the simple chemical methods that were prone to chemical interferences. Immunoassays, which in the past used polyclonal antibodies of lesser specificity, now use well-characterized monoclonal antibodies of known specificity or even mixtures of monoclonals if multiple specificities are desired. In some instruments (e.g., DuPont ACA) column chromatography is incorporated to eliminate interferences, whereas others use membrane technology to accomplish this (e.g., Kodak Ektachem). Nevertheless it is incumbent on the user to verify accuracy by comparison with a reference method and/or by comparison of fresh samples with an instrument whose accuracy or susceptibility to interferences is known. This comparison should include any known or suspected physical or chemical interferences (e.g., lipemia or icterus) and disease or therapy related interferences (e.g., uremia or salicylate therapy).

No matter how theoretically accurate an instrument or method may be, the achievable accuracy will depend on accurate calibration. Each analytic instrument will therefore have to be calibrated on a periodic basis. The frequency may be as often as once/hour or as infrequent as once every 6 months. When calibration is required on a relatively frequent basis, it can be very expensive because special calibration materials must be used and significant amounts of reagent may be consumed. The process itself may be time consuming, thereby lowering analytic throughput and using valuable technologist time. It is therefore important to ascertain the calibration stability of the various methods that will be used on the instruments under consideration.

A second major practical concern for any analytic instrument is the precision exhibited over a range of concentrations expected in the population of samples to be measured. One of the major strengths of automated devices is that they can perform a given task or set of tasks reproducibly. For most laboratory instruments the analytic reproducibility meets or exceeds the minimum required for clinical use. This is dictated by the range of concentrations seen in normal patient samples and is usually acceptable if the variability of the method is 25% to 50% of the physiologic variability seen in patient samples. The most useful parameter to describe the imprecision of an instrument is the relative standard deviation, or coefficient of variation (cv), inasmuch as it takes into account the concentration at which the imprecision is measured. For constituents that are tightly regulated (e.g., serum sodium), the analytic method may require a maximum cv as low as 2% to be useful to follow changes in patients. For constituents for which the physiologic variability is much greater and the analytic methods are more complex (e.g., hormone receptor assays), the acceptable imprecision may be as high as 10% (cv). Table 25-1 lists some target cvs that may be used as "rules of thumb" to judge how well a particular instrument can perform. Verification of reproducibility can be accomplished by any of the methods described at the end of this chapter.

Reagent stability is another important concern to be addressed when comparing instruments. Stability should be considered in two categories: (a) shelf stability and (b) on-instrument or reconstituted stability. Shelf stability may be as long as 1 year or more when stored under the proper conditions. However, it is important to clarify whether the longest stability stated requires storage at refrigerator temperatures. This could be a hidden cost. The reconstituted stability or on-instrument stability should be judged against the volume of testing anticipated to ensure that the reagent does not expire before being used for some low volume tests. If such stability is a problem, smaller package sizes may be available to prevent outdating.

Table 25-1 Precision guidelines

	cv(%) *
Electrolytes	2
Metabolites (e.g., glucose, cholesterol)	3
Enyzmes	5-7
Immunoassays	7-10

*Numbers represent the upper limit of the cv for multiple analyses in the same analytic run.

The linearity of each method on the instrument must be known to assess the useful range of concentrations outside of which results should not be reported without dilution or other correction to allow values to be quantitated accurately. The Clinical Laboratory Improvement Amendments of 1988 (CLIA '88) has stipulated specific criteria for reporting of results by linear and non-linear methods. From a practical point of view, the wider the analytic range, the higher the effective throughput because fewer samples will have to be diluted. On some analytic instruments this dilution process is fully or partially automated and makes the problem less onerous. There can be large differences in the analytic range for a specific analyte on different instruments such that evaluation of these ranges is important.

Design-Associated Considerations

One of the most important decisions related to the design of automated equipment is whether or not the system can incorporate reagents or methods supplied by the user. If the instrument is not capable of incorporating user reagents it is called a **closed-reagent system.** This is generally the result of the instrument requiring special reagent packaging (e.g., DuPont ACA, Kodak Ektachem). This special packaging frequently results in extended reagent stability and extended calibrated stability for the methods. The manufacturer is completely responsible for the performance of the reagents if there is a problem because the user has no control over its quality. This is also a disadvantage if the manufacturer is not responsive to the user complaints. Another major disadvantage of these closed systems is that they are generally more expensive on a per test basis than **open-reagent systems** with user-prepared reagents. Open systems have the theoretic advantage of being less expensive because the reagents themselves are much less expensive. The true cost of user methods, however, must include the cost of preparing the reagents, the cost of verifying equivalence of materials, the cost of increased calibration frequency (if applicable), and the cost of troubleshooting problems when they arise. User methods may be the most appropriate or the only choice under certain circumstances (e.g., unacceptable accuracy/precision of closed system methods, no commercial method available) and could warrant the selection of an open system if these concerns are sufficiently important.

Another factor in the selection of a particular instrument is the available test menu. This can be as large as 80 or more tests. Obviously the more tests available on the system the more flexibility the system will provide for the laboratory. All instruments have a finite limitation on the number of methods (reagents) that can be on-line on the instrument at one time. This is the number that determines the maximum size of the profile available on the instrument assuming no computer or related limitations in result reporting. Frequently, even though there may be a relatively large menu of tests available, the test in which the user is most interested is not present. It is therefore important to make sure that the tests that the user needs are available. With regard to availability, manufacturers like to announce methods as available at some future date. It is important to consider a method as truly available only if it is released and available for purchase. Future release dates are often unreliable because even if the minor problems with a method have been resolved the final documentation and processing may have to go through the FDA for approval, a process over which the manufacturer has no control. These same general concerns regarding availability also apply to the instrument itself and modifications, upgrades and add-on modules. If the instrument or the additional capabilities are not currently available they should be regarded as absent in the selection process.

Walk-away capability is another feature that manufacturers like to use in describing their instruments. The implication is that, once loaded, the instrument will function on its own without the need for monitoring or intervention. Unfortunately, because no analyzer is immune to breakdown and no operator is so perfect that he or she never sets up or programs the instrument incorrectly, all instruments should be monitored. Although this type of monitoring can be accomplished while the operator is performing other tasks, it does require that the operator be in the vicinity of the instrument. Another aspect of the walk-away capability has to do with the maximum number of samples that can be loaded onto the instrument at one time. In other instances it may be due to a limitation in the maximum number of tests that can be performed in one batch by certain methods or the maximum number of disposable reaction vessels or cuvettes that the system will accommodate. For example, if a sample tray can only hold 50 samples and the instrument is capable of processing 200 samples/hour, the operator will have to return 3 times to process a batch of 200 samples. For these reasons walk-away capability is frequently overstated, and such claims must be interpreted correctly.

In most laboratories space is at a premium, and space needed for storage of reagents and consumables is a major consideration. Instruments that use dry reagents or that require small amounts of reagent/test generally require much less space than instruments that use large volumes of wet reagents. Storage of consumables can also use large amounts of space. For example, some random access systems use large irregular disposable cuvettes that occupy significant amounts of space because the cuvette packages must be individually wrapped to ensure freedom from contamination and cannot easily be packaged to eliminate dead space. As stated previously, the requirement for refrigerated storage is also a significant factor to consider. The actual total amount of storage space required may differ by more than twofold between one instrument and another. The actual amount of space occupied by the instrument (sometimes called its footprint) is perhaps the easiest parameter to note when comparing instruments. However, even here there is a caveat. Most instruments require additional free space for adequate ventilation and service access. This can actually double the amount of floor space that must be allocated to the instrument.

An additional cost to the acquisition of any instrument is the cost of renovation or modification of existing space to accommodate the instrument. This cost should be included as part of the total cost picture presented at the time of justification. Although this cost will exist no matter which instrument is selected, there may be significant differences related to instrument space or utility requirements. Many instruments require a dedicated line for electrical power to the instrument. In addition some instruments require 220 V lines. Others require a conditioned line in some geographic areas because of the poor quality of the electrical power in those areas. Some instruments use a significant amount of water for washing cuvettes and flushing lines. Systems that use large amounts of wet reagents require close drain access if frequent manual disposal of waste is to be avoided. The amount of heat generated and humidity tolerated by different instruments varies significantly and therefore will require different amounts of air conditioning to ensure stable operation, as well as a comfortable environment for the operator. The amount of noise generated by various analyzers is a factor that is frequently overlooked particularly if the instrument is observed in a noisy environment such as a large instrument exhibit at a convention. Unfortunately the solution to the noise problem could be a very costly one if a new room or enclosure must be built. All of these factors must be completely assessed if an accurate determination of the utility-related costs is to be achieved. Moreover, the limitations of the physical plant or available space may determine whether or not a certain instrument is feasible or not. If a 220 V line is not available and a particular instrument requires it, obviously it should not be selected.

Because of the increasing use of laboratory information systems in the laboratory and the advantages of direct communications with laboratory instruments, the capability to interface or connect these two systems has become increasingly important. Although most devices manufactured today have serial ports that can provide a direct cable connection to laboratory computers or other devices, these ports alone do not constitute an interface. For data to be transferred between the instrument and the laboratory computer, a serial port with the ability to interface to a laboratory computer can be a very costly error because the software is the expensive part of the interface. Even if both the instrument manufacturer and computer company indicate that they have software interfaces for all devices currently in widespread use, it is imperative to clarify that these interfaces work with the specific model of the instrument selected and the specific version of the software being used in the laboratory. If either party does not have the software, this will be impossible to accomplish. Even if both parties are interested in modifying their software to accomplish this, it may result in significant expense and time delays. However, once accomplished, test requests can be "downloaded" from the laboratory computer to the instrument computer. This not only results in labor and time savings but also eliminates two major sources of laboratory errors.

There are two types of laboratory interfaces, unidirectional and bidirectional. **Unidirectional interfaces** allow data to be sent to an external device from the instrument, but the instrument cannot receive data or commands from the external device or computer. This interface is the least complex but requires that the computer always be able to receive data because there is no way to control the flow of data. **Bidirectional interfaces** are more complex and expensive but allow for the instrument and computer to "talk" to each other by exchanging messages regarding the status of each device, and data is only sent from one to the other when the one receiving it is ready for it. Downloading of test requests and uploading of patient results generally require a bidirectional interface.

The availability of prompt, competent, and reliable service is of prime importance for all laboratories. Unfortunately the ability to provide this service may differ between geographic locations even for the same manufacturer and instrument model. Nevertheless, it is important to investigate the service availability by manufacturer and instrument model in the local area. This is accomplished best by talking to users of the same or similar instruments from the same manufacturer in the area. Finding out the number of instruments already available and the number of personnel assigned to service these instruments from the manufacturer may also give some feel for the expected level of service support. The frequency of on-site service calls has been diminished by some manufacturers by offering programs that include more extensive training of selected laboratory personnel coupled with the provision of complete replacement modules on-site for the most troublesome or complex instrument subsystems. Although these programs are offered at additional cost, they can benefit both the manufacturer and the laboratory and may be more cost effective because downtime, lost revenue, and dissatisfaction may be reduced for the laboratory. Moreover, the number of service personnel required to cover a certain area may be reduced for the manufacturer.

A frequently overlooked property of laboratory instruments is their "user-friendliness." This is an important concern particularly for instruments that are highly flexible and can provide a variety of functions. This flexibility often leads to complicated instructions or many manipulations for even the simplest procedures. Not only does this make it less efficient and more difficult to operate but it can lead to more errors. For systems operated from computer keyboards, the fewer the number of keystrokes the better. A very useful property of some systems is the ability to use a simple, self-explanatory but less-efficient system for novices and a very efficient, more complex system once the operator becomes more experienced. Other "human engineering" concerns should also be addressed (e.g., room for writing on the instrument, height of sample trays and reagent compartments, height of displays). Appropriate types of message systems and alarms can also be a significant help.

Economic Considerations

One of the most critical activities with regard to instrument selection is the financial justification and the economic effect upon the laboratory. Because this process is intimately connected to the performance capabilities of the various instruments that have been discussed, it is important to understand the relationships. Because professional financial managers in the hospital or institution administration will be evaluating the instruments based on information that the laboratory technologist provides, it is important that it be presented in the most effective manner.

One of the ways in which to accomplish this is to become familiar with some basic financial concepts and associated vocabulary. A list of the most important terms and concepts related to instrument acquisition is given below for reference purposes.

Break-even analysis: Analytic technique for studying the relation between fixed costs, variable costs, and profits. A break-even chart graphically depicts the nature of break-even analysis.

Break-even point: Volume of revenue where revenues and expenses are exactly equal (i.e., the level of activity where there is neither a gain nor a loss from operations).

Budget: Financial plan for future operations.

Capital expenditure: Expenditure chargeable to an asset account where the asset acquired has an estimated life in excess of 1 year and is not intended for sale in the ordinary course of operations. The opposite of revenue expenditure.

Capitalization rate: Discount rate used to find the present value of a series of future cash receipts; sometimes called discount rate.

Cash-flow statement: Statement of actual or projected cash receipts and disbursements for a given period of time.

Cash inflows: Revenues actually received by the hospital.

Cost-based reimbursement: Reimbursement approach generally used by third-party payers. Under this approach, the third party pays the hospital for the care received by covered patients at cost with the expense elements included and from cost determined by the third party.

Depreciation: Annual estimated cost of expired services of fixed assets.

Direct cost: Cost that can be easily identified with a specific process or area.

Expected return: Rate of return a firm expects to realize from an investment. The expected return is the mean value of the probability distribution of possible returns.

Expenses: Costs that have been used up or consumed in carrying on some activity and from which no measurable benefit will extend beyond the present. Expenses are expired costs and ordinarily are accompanied by the surrendering of an asset or by the incurring of a liability.

Gross revenues: Value, at the hospital's full established rates, of services rendered and goods sold to patients during a given time period.

Hurdle rate: In capital budgeting, the minimum acceptable rate of return on a project; if the expected rate of return is below the hurdle rate, the project is not accepted. The hurdle rate should be the marginal cost of capital.

Incremental cash flow: Net cash flow attributable to an investment project.

Indirect cost: Costs that are not directly attributable to a specific process or area and are allocated on a statistical basis.

Internal rate of return (IRR): Rate of return on an asset investment. The internal rate of return is calculated by finding the discount rate that equates the present value of future cash flows to the cost of the investment.

Investment of tax credit: Business firms can deduct as a credit against their income taxes a specified percentage of the dollar amount of new investments in each of certain cateogories of assets.

Net income: Excess of revenues over expenses for a given period of time as presented in the income statement.

Net present value (NPV) method: Method of ranking investment proposals. The NPV is equal to the present value of future returns, discounted at the marginal cost of capital, and minus the present value of the cost of the investment.

Net revenues: Excess of gross revenues from patient services over revenue deductions. Also called net earnings from patient services.

Opportunity cost: Measurable advantage foregone in the past or that may be sacrificed as a result of a decision involving alternatives.

Payback period: Period of time it will take a new line of equipment to produce revenues or result in savings equal to its cost.

Present value: Value today of a future receipt or payment, or successive receipts or payments, discounted at the appropriate discount rate.

Prime rate: Rate of interest commercial banks charge large, strong, corporations.

Pro forma: Projection. A pro forma financial statement is one that shows how the actual statement will look if certain specified assumptions are realized. Pro forma statements may be either future or past projections. An example of a backward pro forma statement occurs when two firms are planning to merge and shows what their consolidated financial statements would have looked like if they have been merged in preceding years.

Revenue: Revenue results from the sale of goods and the rendering of services and is measured by the charge made to patients, clients, or tenants for goods and services furnished to them. It also includes gains from the sale or exchange of assets, interest, and dividends earned on investments and unrestricted donations of resources to the hospital.

Salvage value: Estimated amount for which a plant asset can be sold at the end of its useful life. Also called scrap value. It is the current market price of an asset being considered for replacement in a capital budgeting problem.

Third-party payers: Agency such as Blue Cross or Medicare program that contracts with hospitals and patients to pay for the care of covered patients.

Useful life: Estimate of the number of years equipment will be used by a hospital.

Unbundling: Separation of expense items included in the purchase price of a capital acquisition such as training, installation, and freight so that these may be expensed the first year. The remaining cost of the asset itself is then capitalized and depreciated.

Working capital: Refers to the hospital's investment in short-term assets, cash, short-term securities, accounts receivable, and inventories.

One of the more important general guidelines for laboratory capital acquisitions is that the depreciable life of an instrument is approximately 5 years. This can be significantly different from the actual useful life of the instrument. For example, a spectrophotometer can have a useful life of more than 10 years, yet it will most likely be depreciated financially over a 5-year period. Another important guideline for administrators is the **payback period.** This time is related to the volume of testing and is generally expected to not exceed half of the useful life of the equipment. Here again, however, there may be circumstances in which the payback period may be expected to be within 1 to 2 years. It is important to distinguish between the payback period and the **break-even point.** Figure 25-2 summarizes the total cost vs anticipated revenue and distinguishes between the payback period and break-even point. As can be seen, the break-even point occurs before the payback period and indicates the point at which the total costs of testing on the new instrument are equal to the revenues generated by the tests performed on the instrument. **Total cost** is com-

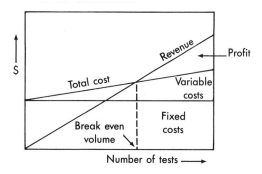

Fig. 25-2 Break-even analysis. The relationship between number of tests or time (if test volume is relatively constant over time) and fixed costs, variable costs, revenue, and profit. (Data redrawn from Gochman W, Bowie LJ: 35th Annual Meeting of the American Association for Clinical Chemistry, New York, July 27, 1983.)

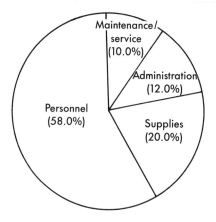

Fig. 25-3 Pie chart of laboratory costs. Each section represents approximate percentage of overall cost for a typical hospital laboratory. Personnel costs include benefits.

posed of both fixed and variable costs. **Fixed costs** are independent of the volume of tests and include such items as lease/depreciation expenses, overhead costs, maintenance contracts, and fixed salaries. **Variable costs** depend on workload and include such items as reagents, standards/calibrators, controls, supplies, and workload-related salaries.

It is exceedingly important to determine total cost/test for each instrument to be considered. It is even better to calculate total cost/reportable result or billable procedure because calibration frequency, disposable costs, and operator time can vary significantly from instrument to instrument. The single most expensive item contributing to total cost is salary expense. Figure 25-3 shows the relative contributions to total cost of the various expense items in a typical laboratory. Note that personnel expenses account for greater than 50% of the total cost of operating a laboratory. If costs are analyzed on a per test basis, a similar conclusion results. DuPont took full advantage of this when it designed and marketed the ACA Clinical Analyzer. Their reagent costs were 3 to 10 times higher than reagents of other available instruments at the time, yet the instrument was an outstanding success in the clinical laboratory market. The reason was simply that operator time and training required were significantly reduced so that the total cost/test was less, even though the reagent cost was clearly higher. It should also be understood that because an instrument may require only one person to perform the work that formerly required two persons, it does not mean one person must be terminated to achieve the

cost savings. The person that is freed up can perform other revenue producing jobs (e.g., run new tests), which can actually result in an increase in net revenue. It is therefore important not to place too much significance on the reagent costs/test quoted by manufacturers because it is the total cost that matters. Fig. 25-4 indicates the danger of this approach by representing the various hidden costs as the invisible portion of an iceberg.

An awareness of the changing legal and political environment also is important in effectively justifying equipment acquisitions. Before the implementation of the prospective payment system using diagnosis related groups (DRGs), laboratories generated revenue that could not be generated by other areas of the hospital. Because they generated large revenues, equipment acquisitions were not as difficult to justify. A new wave of legislation (CLIA '67 and CLIA '88 final rules) will also have an impact on the kinds of analyzers that will be produced and the sites in which analyzers can be operated cost effectively. Although capital costs were initially "passed through" the prospective payment system (they were reimbursed on a reasonable cost basis, independent of case mix or DRGs involved), the reimbursement rate is continuing to drop. The reimbursement rate is currently at 85% for inpatients and outpatients except for those in community hospitals where the rate is 100%. Clearly, the less the hospital or institution is able to reduce instrument costs as a result of legislation, the more difficult will be the justification. However, it is important to be aware of differences in reimbursement rates (e.g., inpatients vs outpatients, urban vs rural) so that

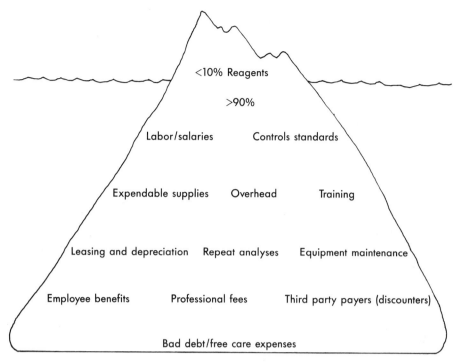

Fig. 25-4 Cost iceberg. A representation of the hidden costs of instrument acquistition.

their impact on the financial justification can be accurately accounted for.

The final consideration with regard to financial justification is the **mode of acquisition**. The most popular modes of acquisition are summarized in the box at right. The simplest acquisition mode is outright purchase by the institution. This assumes that capital is available for purchasing capital items. Even if money is available within an institution, there may be competition with other departments or laboratory sections for the available funds so that effective justification is important. Moreover, even if the institution has funds it may wish to take advantage of other acquisition modes so that the capital funds can be used for other projects where such options are not available. If an institution does not have the capital to purchase equipment outright, rentals, leases, or reagent rentals provide a way to acquire instruments with no capital outlays. A lease is a long-term (3 to 7 year) rental that allows the laboratory to take advantage of potential volume discounts on reagent costs. Leases can be arranged directly with instrument manufacturers or through leasing companies that will purchase the equipment and lease it to the laboratory. The most frequent arrangement for acquisition that does not require a capital outlay is the reagent

---

Modes of Equipment Acquisition

Outright purchase: Full cash payout less appropriate discounts.

FULL SERVICE PRICE/TEST: A renewable short-term agreement (6 or 12 months) whereby the customer agrees to purchase a minimum amount of reagents/day in exchange for use of the full instrument system.

RENTAL: A renewable short-term lease (6 or 12 months) whereby the customer pays a flat rate for use of the instrument system and purchases consumerables (no minimum) from standard price list.

STRAIGHT LEASE: A long-term lease (usually 3, 5, or 7 years) whereby the customer pays a flat rate for use of the instrument system and purchases consumables (no minimum) from standard price list. At end of lease term the customer may buy system at fair-market-value.

CONDITIONAL SALES CONTRACT: A method of financing the acquisition of new equipment by installment payments over a period of months. The seller retains title until all payments have been completed.

REAGENT RENTAL: A long-term agreement (generally 3 to 5 years) whereby the customer agrees to purchase a minimum amount of reagents for the contract period in exchange for use of the full instrument system. It may or may not include maintenance or credits toward a nominal buy-out at the end of the agreement.

rental agreement. With this type of acquisition mode the cost of the instrument and interest expenses are spread out over the agreement period. This cost is then added to the projected cost/test for reagents alone. This sum is then treated in the laboratory expenses budget as an operating expense. This obviously artifically inflates the reagent cost/test, but the laboratory acquires an instrument that it might not have been able to acquire by any other approach. At the end of the contract period the laboratory can purchase the equipment for a nominal amount (e.g., $100). Because manufacturers make the majority of the profit on the reagents themselves and not on the equipment, some manufacturers will allow laboratories to use their equipment if the laboratory contracts to purchase a minimum amount of reagents over a fixed period of time. In this arrangement the laboratory will not own the equipment at the end of the contract. However, maintenance is usually included in the price of the reagent rental contract because it is in the best interest of the manufacturer to keep the instrument running so that the net profits from such a volume-based contract will be realized. This concern on behalf of the manufacturer to keep the instrument running is one of the most attractive aspects of the reagent rental approach. In rentals and leases the cost of maintenance is generally handled separately and should be budgeted for. Because new instrument warranties frequently cover the first 3 to 12 months of the contract after acquisition, the maintenance costs for this period are negligible.

Performance Verification

Because the cost of automated laboratory instrumentation may be $200,000 or more, it is important to see the actual system in operation. Although this can be accomplished at an instrument exhibit associated with a professional meeting or a manufacturer-sponsored demonstration at a local or regional facility, this kind of evaluation only provides a general view of the analytic capabilities. To get at other practical concerns such as reliability, impact on workflow, or workload-specific analytic problems it is better to see the instrument in operation in an environment similar to the one in which it is expected to be used. The best situation is to be able to actually have the instrument brought in on a trial basis before purchasing or signing a contract. Although some large analyzers cannot be installed on a evaluation basis without significant cost to the user and the manufacturer, it should be done

whenever possible. Once installed, the instrument should be thoroughly evaluated regarding the analytic capabilities described earlier in the chapter. In addition, the other concerns discussed under Design-Associated Considerations should be investigated.

The actual evaluation of analytic performance should be accomplished with the use of fresh patient specimens that have been analyzed with a method of known accuracy to provide target values. Fresh patient specimens are preferred because lyophilized materials may display biases that do not exist with actual specimens. If the potential risk of exposure to infectious agents from fresh specimens is perceived to be too great, commercially available products that have been screened for these agents can be used. A simplified protocol for estimating the accuracy, precision, and linearity of analytic instruments has been published by the National Committee for Clinical Laboratory Standards (NCCLS). The procedure requires only the use of 11 specimens, serum pools, or commercial controls in each run at 3 different concentrations. The evaluation should, however, cover at least 5 days. Specific details on how to inspect the data and eliminate outliers are provided, as well as procedures for determining precision, bias, and linearity. Should the instrument be available over a more extended period of time and a more complete evaluation is desired, the NCCLS has also published protocols for more complete evaluation of precision, interferences, method biases, and linearity.

Linear regression using the least-squares method for data reduction has been the accepted tool to analyze data from method comparison experiments. This method assumes that there is no error in the x-data set, which is not the case for even the most precise reference method. As a result the slopes and intercepts used to determine proportional and constant biases may be in error if proper attention is not paid to the handling of outliers and the range of the x-axis data. Although it is clear that the improper inclusion of outliers can lead to erroneous conclusions, the impact of the x-data set range is not as well known. For any constituent whose range of expected values is relatively narrow (e.g., sodium, chloride, calcium), there is a danger that the imprecision of the method used to generate the x-data set (obtained by measuring a single sample multiple times by this method and calculating a standard deviation) is greater than 20% of the spread exhibited by the range of x values (ob-

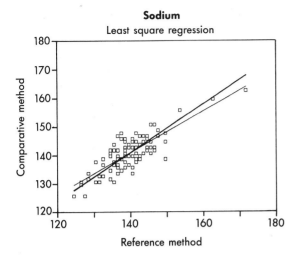

Sodium

Least square regression

Fig. 25-5 Errors in least squares regression analysis. Serum sodium analyses (99 samples) run on two instruments. Least squares regression line (—); Deming regression line (—). See Table 25-3 for value of regression parameters.

Table 25-2 Comparison of regression methods for serum sodium

	Least squares	*Least squares after data reversal*
Slope	0.7358	1.1169
Intercept	37.85	−13.976
Correlation coefficient	0.8117	0.8117
Deming slope	0.8568	0.8569
Deming intercept	20.868	24.35
Sex/Sx	0.1586	0.2036
Sey/Sy	0.2036	0.1586

Number of data points = 99; Sex and Sey = standard deviation of x and y respectively, determined by 10 analyses each on a single sample for x and for y; Sx and Sy = standard deviation of x and y data sets respectively.

tained by calculating the standard deviation from all x values). Under these circumstances the slope and intercept could be significantly in error unless special techniques are used. The method of Deming has been shown to be very useful under these circumstances. Fig. 25-5 shows the difference in calculated slopes and intercepts using the least-squares linear regression approach and the Deming approach. One way of determining whether the least-squares method will give erroneous data for the particular instrument and method is to reverse the data for the x and y axes and recalculate the slope. If the reciprocal of the slope obtained after this reversal is significantly different from the original slope determined before this reversal, the least-squares method is inappropriate and a method such as that of Deming should be used (Table 25-2). Even though the imprecision of y compared with the spread of the y data set (Sey/Sy) is only slightly above 20%, there is a significant difference in slope.

Another way of evaluating instrument analytic performance is to compare results of proficiency testing surveys. These surveys provide a wealth of information on relative instrument biases and user-to-user variability on the same specimen. It is important to understand that there may be biases that are instrument or method specific that result from how the sample was prepared, lyophilized, or stored and that these biases may not be present in fresh patient samples. The surveys also give information on the types of technologies used to measure analytes. For example, data on thyroxine excerpted from the the College of American Pathologists 1990 comprehensive chemistry survey are summarized in Table 25-3 and indicate that radioimmunoassay is no longer the most widely used technique for measuring serum thyroxine. Highly automated, nonisotopic techniques currently account for greater than 80% of results submitted from the 3224 participants in this survey. This data also shows that the precision exhibited by various instruments and methods is highly variable as indicated by the cv. Finally, the data also clearly shows that some methods have significant biases when compared with the mean of all methods reported. Although it is not possible to say which value is the most correct, it is very easy to see how results from a particular instrument would be expected to compare with results from another instrument of interest. These types of proficiency testing surveys are available for the majority of high volume analytes from a variety of professional societies, as well as state and national agencies.

Obtaining Raw Data. To assist prospective buyers in obtaining the maximum amount of useful information from various manufacturers, the questionnaire on p. 438 is provided. It should be used once 3 to 5 instruments of interest have been selected. If it is completed by the manufacturers or by the potential user with information provided by the manufacturers, it will provide data that allow a more objective comparison of the various instruments.

Equipment Acquisition Questionnaire

General

What are the types of chemistry analyzers presently marketed?

Give a brief description of each model.

What is the cost of each model?

What is the warranty period for each analyzer?

Is the analyzer available for reporting results 24 hours a day?

What is the daily start-up time required to prepare the analyzer for operation?

How much time is required to shut down the analyzer after operation?

How much instrument and technologist time are required to process the various batch sizes of one test (e.g., glucose)?

Batch size	Instrument time	Technologist time
1	_____	_____
5	_____	_____
10	_____	_____
20	_____	_____

How much change over time is required to go to a different test?

How long does it take to process a 6-test panel (e.g., 6 enzyme tests)? How much technologist time is required?

How long does it take to process a 20-test panel? How much technologist time is required?

When changing from one method to another, does the analyzer require priming with reagent? If so, how much reagent is needed?

Please supply the names of several hospitals in the area that use the analyzer.

A. Small hospital, less than 100 beds.

B. Medium hospital, 200-300 beds.

C. Large hospital, over 500 beds.

Can the analyzer be interfaced with laboratory computer?

What is the normal delivery time for the analyzer?

Economic

Is a leasing plan available?

Is there a reagent rental program available?

If so, what is the minimum number of tests/month to qualify for the reagent rental program?

What is the minimum dollar outlay/month on this rental program?

Does the analyzer use consumables other than reagents?

What are these consumables, and what is the cost in relationship to batch size?

Batch size	Cost/test
1	_____
5	_____
10	_____
20	_____

What are the fixed start-up costs on a daily basis?

What are the terms and conditions associated with the purchase of the analyzer?

Technical

How many different tests can be performed on the analyzer?

Are the reagents supplied for each of these tests?

Can other companies' reagents be used on the analyzer?

On the average, how frequently must standards and quality controls be run on the analyzer (e.g., with every run, once/hour, once/day)?

Under the following conditions, how many standards, controls, and blanks must be run?

Batch size	Standards	Controls Normal	Controls Abnormal	Blanks
1	____	____	____	____
5	____	____	____	____
10	____	____	____	____
20	____	____	____	____

What are the sample volumes required for each test performed?

How much reagent is required for the tests listed above?

Please submit technical data for the available methodologies.

Training

Does the company offer a training program for the analyzer?

How many people can attend this training program?

Where is the location of the training program?

Does the company provide operator instruction manuals?

What is the cost of this training course when the analyzer is purchased?

Installation

What are the overall dimensions of the analyzer?

What is the total space required for the analyzer and miscellaneous equipment?

What are the electrical requirements?

What are the plumbing requirements?

What are the ventilation requirements?

What other special installation requirements are necessary?

Does the company supply an individual to do the installation of the equipment?

How long does it take to install the analyzer?

Service

What is the yearly cost of a service warranty or maintenance contract?

What is included in the service, warranty, or maintenance contract?

Does the cost of the maintenance contract increase as the equipment gets older?

List the cost of the service, maintenance, or warranty contract for equipment that is new, 1, 2, 3, 4, and 5 years old.

Does the company offer 24-hour service and response?

Where is the location of the closest service representative?

Where is the location of the closest service center?

Table 25-3 Comparison of thyroxine data

Thyroxine (mcg/dl)	No. labs	Mean	SD	CV	No. labs	Mean	SD	CV
Abbott IMX	251	7.15	0.41	5.7	251	16.79	0.86	5.1
Abbott TDX	1343	7.07	0.48	6.8	1336	15.69	0.99	6.3
Abbott Tetrabead	21	7.22	0.63	8.7	22	16.33	1.16	7.1
Baxter Stratus	313	5.73	0.52	9.1	315	13.49	1.20	8.9
Becton Dickinson	28	5.06	0.86	17.1	28	11.67	1.92	16.5
Ciba Corning Magic	114	7.15	0.52	7.3	112	13.20	0.95	7.2
Clinical assays	120	7.09	0.53	7.4	119	15.73	1.49	9.4
Diag Prod/Coat-a-count	85	7.12	0.53	7.5	85	17.23	1.07	6.2
DuPont ACA	340	7.33	0.76	10.4	338	15.49	1.35	8.7
Dupont Dimension	166	8.10	0.62	7.6	163	19.73	1.94	9.8
Kallestad Quanticoat	33	7.17	0.54	7.6	33	15.12	0.80	5.3
Microgenics	43	6.03	0.72	12.0	43	13.23	1.09	8.3
Organon/NML Tetra Tab	28	7.81	0.45	5.8	29	16.40	1.04	6.4
Organon/NML Tetra Tube	39	7.79	0.48	6.1	40	15.46	1.07	7.0
SYVA Ehit	72	5.99	0.62	10.4	72	12.93	1.59	12.3
SYVA Ecp	24	6.16	0.57	9.2	24	13.05	1.80	13.8
Technicon Ra Systems	23	5.59	0.46	8.2	23	13.67	1.14	8.4
All Reagent Manufacturers	3224	6.97	0.83	12.0	3185	15.49	1.85	11.9

From the College of American Pathologists' 1990 Comprehensive Chemistry Survey.

Review Questions

1. What are the disadvantages of using serum as opposed to whole blood or plasma for automated analysis?
2. Describe the main advantages of batch, STAT, and random access analyzers.
3. Discuss the advantages and disadvantages of open vs closed-reagent analytic systems.
4. List at least five major considerations that do not relate to analytic performance but could be critical in the selection process for an analyzer.
5. Describe three modes of instrument acquisition and list the advantages of each.
6. What is the major disadvantage of least squares regression analysis for comparing instruments/methods?

Bibliography

Bachorik PS, Rock R, Cloey T, et al: Cholesterol screening: comparative evaluation of on-site and laboratory-based measurements, Clin Chem 36:255, 1990.

Cotlove E, Harris EK, Williams GZ: Biological and analytical components of variation in long-term studies of serum concentrations in normal subjects, Clin Chem 16:1028, 1970.

Caraway WT, Watts NB: Carbohydrates: In Tietz NW, ed: Fundamentals of clinical chemistry, ed 3, Philadelphia, 1987, WB Saunders.

Deming WE: Statistical adjustment of data, New York, 1943, John Wiley and Sons.

Gochman N, Bowie LJ: Selection factors for automated analytical instrumentation (workshop), 35th Annual Meeting of the American Association for Clinical Chemistry, New York, July 27, 1983.

Cornbleet J, Gochman N: Incorrect least-squares regression coefficients in method-comparisons analysis, Clin Chem 25:432, 1979.

Laboratory Workload Recording Method, Skokie, Ill, College of American Pathologists, 1980.

National Committee for Clinical Laboratory Standards. Interference testing, proposed guideline, NCCLS publication EP7-P, Villanova, Pa, 1985.

National Committee for Clinical Laboratory Standards, Performance claims, proposed guideline, NCCLS publication EP6-P, Villanova, Pa, 1986.

National Committee for Clinical Laboratory Standards, Preliminary evaluation of clinical chemistry methods, tentative guideline, NCCLS publication EP10-T, Villanova, Pa, 1989.

National Committee for Clinical Laboratory Standards, User comparison of methods using patients samples; proposed guideline, NCCLS publication EP9-P, Villanova, Pa.

National Committee for Clinical Laboratory Standards, User evaluation of precision performance of clinical chemistry devices, proposed guideline. NCCLS publication EP5-P, Villanova, Pa, 1982.

Tonks DB: A study of the accuracy and precision of clinical chemistry determination in 170 Canadian laboratories, Clin Chem 9:217, 1963.

Glossary

absorbance measure of monochromatic light that is absorbed by sample. Riciprocal of transmittance.

absorbance maxima peaks of an absorbance curve of a compound that show the highest absorbance.

absorbance minima peaks of an absorbance curve of a compound that show the lowest absorbance.

absorption light that will not pass through a substance.

abundance a measure of the number of ions with a given mass-to-charge ratio seen in a mass spectrum (see also intensity).

accuracy ability to determine the true or actual value of an analyte.

activity effective concentration of a solution ionic species that accounts for interactions with other ionic solutes in the solution.

activity coefficient measure of the degree with which an ionic species in solution interacts with other ionic species in the solution.

adsorption or liquid-solid chromatography LC technique that separates compounds based on their adsorption to an underivatized solid support.

affinity chromatography LC technique based on the specific and reversible interactions that occur between an immobilized molecule on a support and biologic molecules in the sample.

agaropectin sugar polymer similar to agarose except having many charged groups.

agarose sugar polymer, extracted from seaweed, containing few charges, used as a supporting medium for electrophoresis.

aggregation function of an activated platelet in which several platelets adhere to one another (adhesion) and then form a plug that closes the wound of a blood vessel.

alternating current (AC) type of current that periodically reverses polarity and is constantly changing in magnitude.

amidolytic assay chromogenic assay employing a synthetic substrate.

ammeter electronic device that measures current flow; it must be connected in the circuit to be tested using a series arrangement.

ampere (A) unit of measure for current; when 1 coulomb passes a point in circuit during 1 second.

amperometry controlled-potential technique in which current is measured at a fixed applied potential.

ampholyte trade name for a mixture of substances with a range of isoelectric points that have high buffering capacities at their isoelectric points.

amphoteric capable of being positively or negatively charged, depending on the pH.

amplification production of a large output signal by a small input signal.

amplitude refers to the peak value of the voltage in a sinusoidal waveform.

analog device component that produces an electrical signal that has continuous values.

analytic steps in actual test performance. Includes all related functions, (i.e., quality control and maintenance).

angle of detection angle at which scattered light is measured in nephelometry.

anion ion with a net negative charge.

anode electrode or pole of a battery (electrochemical cell) that has a positive charge (electron deficient) and thus attracts negatively charged ions (ions).

antibody immunuglobulin with specificity for a specific ligand such as a hapten or antigen.

antigen molecule capable of triggering an immune response, thus stimulating the production of antibodies.

astigmatism control on an oscilloscope that adjusts all parts of the sweep to ensure they are in focus at the same time.

atomic absorption photometry ground stated atoms absorb light of specific wavelength that is measured.

atomic mass unit (amu) unit of mass equal to $\frac{1}{16}$ the mass of the atom of oxygen of mass number 16.

atomization further disintegration beyond nebulization of liquid solution into microscopic droplets.

atomizer-burner assembly apparatus in which test solution, gas, and oxidant are mixed, and solution is broken into fine droplets for introduction into flame for burning.

autodilute instrument's ability to correct for an analyte concentration falling outside a predetermined assay range. This is usually accomplished by sampling and adding half of the required sample volume for a given test.

automation means of mechanizing the steps in a process or procedure.

autoradiography the separation of radioactive substances visualized by development on x-ray film.

backup analytic system or method that is kept operational and available in case the normal system becomes inoperable.

bandpass range of wavelengths between which points the transmittance is one-half the peak transmittance.

bar codes group of bars of various widths and shades that are used to encode information.

base peak ion with the greatest abundance (intensity) in a mass spectrum.

batch group of samples that are treated identically.

batch analysis specimens in the same analytic run are analyzed for the same test or combination of tests.

batch analyzer analytic instrument designed to operate more efficiently when processing a large number of samples at one time. The samples may require only a single test or multiple tests to be performed on each.

beam splitter device placed in light path between monochromator and sample to split, or redirect beams of light to both sample and reference pathways.

becquerel (Bq) Systeme Internationale d'Unites; (SI) unit of radioactivity corresponding to a decay rate of 1/sec (1 Bq = sec^{-1} = 2.70 × 10^{-9} Ci).

Beer's law statement of direct proportion of absorbance to concentration.

bi-directional interface two-way communication between a host computer system and an interfaced analyzer.

binary coded packs pouch made of a clear plastic film that contains prepackaged reagents (as used on the DuPont ACA). The reagent pack, which also serves as a cuvette, is binary coded with the test name.

bioluminescence light emission resulting from an enzyme catalyzed–reaction.

blaze angle specific angle used to cut grooves on grating surface for the best efficiency at the blaze wavelength.

blaze wavelength specific wavelength for which the angle of reflectance from the groove face and angle of diffraction from the grating are identical.

bleeder resistor resistor that is connected in parallel to a capacitor to discharge it to ground when the circuit/ instrument is turned off.

bleeding time test assay performed on the forearm of the patient by making uniform cuts and measuring the time to stop bleeding.

boiling point temperature at which the vapor pressure above a solution equals the atmospheric pressure.

bonded-phase gas chromatography technique in gas chromatography that uses a stationary phase that is chemically bonded to the support material.

Bouger-Lambert law statement of direct proportion of light path length to absorbance.

break even point volume of tests (or length of time) required for revenues to equal expenses.

breaker-mixer mechanical component of the DuPont ACA that breaks the reagent compartments of a binary coded pack and agitates the pack to mix the specimen, diluent, and reagents.

calibration procedure used to adjust a method or system to give a target value. For analytic instruments this usually involves the use of a liquid standard that is analyzed and then the instrument/method is adjusted accordingly.

CAP College of American Pathologists. Organization that inspects clinical laboratories and provides a quality control program for clinical laboratory testing.

capacitance (C) ability of a device to store electrical energy in an electrostatic field; measured in farads.

capacitive reactance (Xc) opposition of a capacitor to a change in current; measured in ohms.

capacitor device made by separating two conductors with an insulating material (dielectric) that when charged will oppose a change in voltage. Its function is to store electrical energy for release at a later time. When charged, it blocks DC and passes AC.

capacity factor (k′) fundamental measure of compound retention where $k = (t_r - t_o)/t_r$.

carrier free adjective describing a radionuclide free of its stable isotopes.

carrier gas term used to describe the mobile phase in gas chromatography.

carryover undesired transfer of sample or reagent material from one position to another, which reduces the integrity of the result.

cathode the electrode that has a net negative charge and thus attracts positively charged ions (cations).

cathode ray tube (CRT) in electronics a readout device that is often referred to as an oscilloscope.

cation ion with a net positive charge.

cell potential quantitative measure of the energy of an electrochemical cell; the difference in electron energy between two electrodes.

cellulose acetate acetylated cellulose fibers pressed into sheets; used as a supporting medium.

centrifugal analyzer instrument that uses centrifugal force to combine sample aliquot and reagents and a spinning rotor to pass the reaction mixture through a detector.

charge quantity of electricity (I) that reflects the total current (I) during a given time (t): $Q = It$.

chassis ground connection (ground) made between the metal chassis and the earth; used to neutralize any potential that may accumulate on the chassis because of improper grounding or if it is used as an inherent part of the instrument's circuit.

cheater plug adaptor device used to convert a three-prong plug to a two-prong plug.

chemical interference altered emission or absorption caused by interfering cations of anions that react or bind with atoms of interest.

chemical ionization (CI) mode of ionization wherein sample molecules are ionized by an ionized reagent gas in the ion source of a mass spectrometer.

chemiluminescence process of generating photons of light via a chemical reaction.

chip term that refers to an integrated circuit.

chopper mechanical device that breaks a continuous beam of light into a pulsating signal.

chromatogram plot of detector response vs elution time or volume on a chromatographic system.

chromatography separation technique based on the different interactions of sample compounds with two phases: a mobile phase and a stationary phase, as the compounds travel through a supporting medium.

chromogenic substrate substrate that produces a colored product when catalyzed by an enzyme.

chromogenic substrate molecule, which in the presence of a specific preformed enzyme, undergoes a chemical change, producing a colored endpoint.

circuit breaker electronic device used to protect power lines from experiencing an overload.

circuit, anticoincident circuit used in the pulse-height analyzer of a radioactive particle counter for setting window width (see window). It transmits a pulse arriving at its input from the lower discriminator only if there is no pulse arriving from the upper discriminator at the same time.

circuit, coincident a circuit used in a liquid scintillation counter to eliminate the electronic noise. It determines if a pulse from one photomultiplier tube is accompanied by a corresponding pulse from the other within the allowed time interval (see coincidence resolving tune).

circuit, summation circuit used in a liquid scintillation counter to sum all coincident pulses to improve counting efficiency

for low-energy beta-particle emitters.

clearing (supports) making the supports more transparent for densitometry.

CLIA '67 Clinical Laboratory Improvement Act of 1967. Legislation that regulates laboratories engaged in interstate testing and/or receiving Medicare funds.

CLIA '88 Clinical Laboratory Amendments of 1988. When finalized, legislation that will regulate all laboratories performing tests on human specimens.

closed reagent system analytic device that is not capable of using user-prepared reagents or reagents from another vendor.

closed tube sampling ability to aspirate sample from a tube (frequently the original collection tube) without having to remove the stopper.

clot endpoint final stage of a coagulation reaction measured by physical means.

clot signature recording of clot formation during the entire reaction.

coimmobilization technique where reagents such as urease and glucose oxidase are bonded to a nylon coil that feeds into an electrode chamber. As a specimen passes over the nylon coil, a reaction is catalyzed.

coagulation system interrelated series of enzymatic reactions that function to form a fibrin clot in blood.

coincidence photopeak photopeak resulting from the emission of two photons from one radionuclide within the resolving time of a radioactivity detector.

coincidence resolving time time interval within which the output pulses from each photomultiplier tube of a liquid scintillation counter have to arrive at the coincident circuit to be counted.

colligative properties four properties (boiling point, freezing point, vapor pressure, and osmotic pressure) that can be measured and are related to each other and to the osmolality of the solution.

collimating lens convergent lens, either transmitting or reflecting, that collects light rays and focuses them into an organized beam of parallel light.

colloid osmometry (oncometry) measurement of the contribution of macromolecules to the osmotic pressure of a solution.

colloid osmotic pressure (oncotic pressure) the contribution of serum proteins to the serum osmolality (in clinical laboratory terms).

colloid molecules with a mass of 30,000 daltons or greater.

colorimeter any instrument that measures colored light produced a fixed monochromator (i.e., glass filter).

colorimetric sensor sensor that is sensitive to carbon dioxide and is able to change color with increasing levels produced.

comparison of signal tracing/ waveform method approach to troubleshooting an electronic instrument that entails measuring the input voltage of the malfunctioning instrument (where a correct voltage or waveform can be found compared with the manufacturer's values) and then proceeding through the circuits, measuring the voltages and waveforms until the problem is found.

competitive binding protein (CPB) technique based on competition between a highly specific protein, its ligand, and the same ligand that has been tagged as a tracer.

competitive immunoassay immunoassay technique where the analyte in the patient sample competes with labeled analyte for a limited number of binding sites on an antibody/ binding protein.

Compton effect or scattering one process of interactions of photons with matter by which a photon loses only a portion of its energy through collisions with electrons.

computerization electronic processing of data.

concurrent calibration ability of an analyzer to perform a calibration while it is simultaneously analyzing patient samples.

conductance (G) ability of a material to support current flow: the reciprocal of resistance.

conductivity the readiness of a solution to conduct an electrical current; in an ionic solution, the sum of the product of the charge concentrations and charge mobilities.

conductivity detector measures the ability of the mobile phase to conduct a current when placed in an electrical field and is dependent on the number of ions or ionic compounds present in the mobile phase.

conductor any material (usually a metal) that conducts electricity through the transfer of orbital electrons; it is made up of materials that have three or fewer valence electrons.

continuous flow pumps reagents through the analyzer at all times while in operation, introducing samples at regular intervals.

continuous flow analyzer instrument that constantly pumps reagents and samples through its tubings and coils, forming a continuous stream.

continuum source background correction incorporates a white light source for broad

background absorption to be absorbed by this continuous emission of white light.

convection (bulk flow). Mass or bulk movement of one part of a solution relative to the rest, usually because of density differences.

conventional theory of current flow explanation of current based on the Franklinian theory in which current in an external circuit is thought to flow from the positive pole of a battery to its negative pole.

coulomb measure of charge equal to 6.24×10^{18} electrons.

coulometry technique in which the charge required to completely reduce a sample is measured.

counter-Emf voltage that is created by a chemical or magnetic effect that opposes the voltage applied to the circuit and its corresponding current flow.

counterion ion present that is of opposite charge to the one being considered.

crystalloid uncharged particles with a mass of less than 30,000 daltons.

curie (Ci) unit of radioactivity. One curie is defined as an activity of sample decaying at a rate of 3.7×10^{10} disintegrations/second (d/s).

current (I) rate at which a charge moves through a conductor (1 ampere = 1 coulomb/second); refers to the flow of electrons.

curve fitting mathematic analysis of the platelet histogram made by Coulter instruments to determine a platelet count from platelet "raw data" (partial counting of platelet-sized particles).

cutoff level level where a significant amount of false positives are likely to occur due to a lack of sensitivity.

cuvette absorption cell, or holding container of reaction constituents placed in light path of photometer for absorption.

d'Arsonval (moving coil) movement interaction of an induced electromagnetic field in coiled wire positioned between the two poles of a permanent magnet when a current flows through the coil.

d'Arsonval meter current-carrying meter that is based on the d'Arsonval principle.

data system computer-based system used to control the operation of a mass spectrometer and to process the data generated by the spectrometer.

dead volume amount of sample that is not consumed but must be present for proper analyzer sampling.

decay constant constant unique to each radioactive nuclide (see nuclide), representing the proportion of the atoms in a sample of that radionuclide undergoing decay in unit time.

decay factor fraction of radionuclides remaining after a time, *t*.

densitometer spectrophotometer that measures absorbances along a sheet or slab of material.

densitometry procedure for quantitating and recording an electrophoretic pattern.

derivatization technique used to convert a compound into another form to increase its volatility, thermolability, and/or detectability.

desorption chemical ionization technique of ionizing sample molecules by desorbing them from a solid surface and ionizing them with a reagent gas, which itself is ionized.

detector component of a mass spectrometer that collects and quantifies the ions produced and sorted by the ion source and mass analyzer of the system.

dew point temperature at which the molecules of solvent in the vapor phase, at constant pressure, will condense to form a liquid.

dichroid mirror one type of beam splitter, consisting of a half-silvered mirror, to redirect half of the original beam of light into a second pathway.

dielectric insulating (nonconducting) medium between two plates of a capacitor.

diffraction deviation in direction of a light beam as it passes by the edge of an opaque body.

diffusion remixing of separated substances in a solution because of molecular movement.

digital device component that produces an electrical signal that is converted to a binary system.

diode electronic component that allows current passage in only one direction.

direct current (DC) current that flows in only one direction; current neither changes polarity nor magnitude over a period of time.

direct probe analysis technique of ionizing sample molecules by introducing solid samples directly into the ion source. Often used with compounds that are difficult to derivatize or highly polar.

disc electrophoresis electrophoresis procedure in which ions are made to "stack" between solutions of different ions and then are electrophoresed normally in a support medium.

discrete processing a test in an individual test receptacle.

discrete analyzer analyzer that compartmentalizes each sample reaction in an individual cuvette or similar optical device.

discriminator circuit electronic device that can separate different sizes of electrical impulses.

dispersion orderly scattering of white light into its full spectrum of colors.

double beam in space design of a double beam photometer with two separate beams of light (sample and reference), two separate detectors, and possibly two separate monochromators.

double beam in time design of a double beam photometer with two separate beams of light (sample and reference) split and reconverged without duplication of detectors or monochromators.

double-focus mass spectrometer mass spectrometer using both magnetic field and electostatic field mass analyzers to increase resolution of ions.

downloading transferring information from a host computer to an interfaced analyzer.

downtime time that an instrument is not operational for patient testing because of maintenance or troubleshooting.

DRGs Diagnostic Related Groups. Procedures that are grouped by diagnosis, used for reimbursement purposes for Medicare.

dry multilayer film immunoassay technique that uses a test module composed of a polyester film base coated with an antibody bound to fluorescent-labeled analyte (immune complex) immobilized in an agarose matrix.

dynode component of the photomultiplier tube that is responsible for amplifying the electrical signal.

earth ground point of zero potential because of the fact that the earth has a tremendous accumulation of charge and thus has an infinite capacity to neutralize them.

effective mobility mobility of an ion reduced by its having a reduced average charge.

electric shock unpleasant sensation and sometimes fatal condition that occurs when an electrical current is conducted through human tissue. The severity of the condition depends on the amount of current, the part of the body involved, and the duration of contact.

electrical ground conducting material connected to the earth.

electro-osmosis tendency of a solution to move relative to a stationary substance when an electric field is applied.

electroblotting electrophoretic transfer of substances onto a sheet of material by binding or adsorption.

electrochemical cell two metal electrodes of different charge that develop a potential difference (voltage) when connected together.

electrochemical detector (LC/ EC) detects a wide range of compounds that can undergo electrochemical reactions (i.e., oxidation or deduction).

electrochemistry source of electricity produced chemically by the insertion of two dissimilar metals into a conducting solution called an electrolyte.

electrodes substances in contact with a conductor that are connected to a source of an electric field; the parts of the electrophoresis electrical circuit in contact with the electrophoresis solution.

electrolyte low molecular weight salts (ions) that are present throughout the electrophoresis solution.

electromagnetic radiation (EMR) spectrum full range of radiating energy waves, from high energy cosmic rays to low energy radio waves.

electromagnetism source of electricity produced by the relative motion of a conductor within a magnetic field.

electromotive force (EMF) force that causes electricity to flow when there is a difference in potential between two points. The unit of measurement is the volt.

electron capture one mode of radioactive decay in which the neutron-poor nuclides decay by capturing electrons from orbits closest to the nucleus to transform a proton to a neutron orbital vacancy created by the electron capture is filled by the electron from a higher orbit, resulting in emission of characteristic x-rays.

electron capture detector component of a gas chromatograph based on the principle that large organic molecules, particularly halogens, attract electrons and thus form negatively charged ions.

electron impact ionization ionization of sample molecules by striking them with a beam of electrons.

electron multiplier type of mass spectrometer detector in which a cascade of electrons is produced by ions striking its primary surface or dynode.

electron theory of current flow explanation of current based on the atomic theory in which current is carried by electrons that flow from the negative pole of a battery to the positive pole.

electron volt (eV) basic unit of energy commonly used in radiation, defined as the amount of energy acquired by an electron when it is accelerated through an electrical potential of 1 volt.

electrophoresis movement of charge particles (compounds) in an electrical field.

electrophoretogram pattern of separated compounds that is developed after electrophoresis.

electrostatic field force exerted between the charged plates and the atoms in the dielectric of a capacitor.

electrostatic or static electricity source of electricity produced when certain materials are rubbed together, thus transferring electrons by friction from one to the other.

emax maximum possible energy equivalent to the total energy available from the nuclear decay by beta-particle emission.

emission flame photometry ground state atoms absorb energy in flame and on moving to cooler part of flame, release (emit) this energy as specific wavelength of light that is measured.

emission spectrum specific light energy emission at characteristic wavelengths for specific atoms or molecules emitted from a light emitting diode that is reflected from a sensor to a photodiode, producing a voltage signal proportional to the intensity of the reflected light.

entrance slit small opening for entering beam of white light into monochromator housing.

enzyme-linked immunosorbent assay (ELISA) heterogeneous immunoassay that uses an enzyme-labeled tracer and an antibody immobilized on a solid phase.

enzyme multiplied immunoassay technique (EMIT) homogeneous enzyme immunoassay in which a low molecular weight ligand is attached to an enzyme whose activity is inhibited when the conjugate is bound to antibody. This inhibition is relieved when unlabeled ligand (in the patient sample) competes for sites on the antibody.

exciter lamp source of white light in a photometer.

exit slit small opening for exiting beam of monochromatic light out of monochromator housing.

exited state unstable condition of atom that has absorbed energy causing electrons to move from one orbiting shell to another.

extender board device used to connect a printed circuit board to the instrument to make the electronic components of the circuit board more accessible for electrical measurements.

farad (F) unit of measure of capacitance; when 1 coulomb raises the potential by 1 volt.

fast atom bombardment ionization of sample molecules by bombardment with a beam of fast-moving atoms supplied by a fast-atom gun.

fast-blowing fuse standard fuse that has a short lag time before the filament melts; it will "blow" very quickly with any increase in current beyond its rating.

Fatigue gradual decrease in the output voltage of a photocell because of its continued exposure to radiant energy.

feedback circuit when part of the output of an amplifier is returned to the input side to achieve some desirable effect.

fibrinolytic system interrelated series of enzymatic reactions that function to break down or lyse fibrinogen, fibrin, or formed blood clots.

fibrometer electromechanical instrument designed to measure to clot endpoint.

field desorption ionization ionization of samples in the solid state by exposure to a high-intensity electrostatic field. The sample molecule's ions are then desorbed from the probe containing them and mass analyzed.

field effect transistor semiconductor amplifier that consists of two types, N-channel and P-channel, which provide a high input impedance.

filter device that selectively passes certain colors or wavelengths of light and will block others.

filter network electronic circuit that converts pulsating direct current to smooth direct current.

fixed costs costs that are independent of the volume of tests performed (e.g., overhead costs).

flame ionization detector (FID) component of a gas chromatograph based on the principle that combustion of organic compounds produces ionic fragmentation and free electrons; ions and electrons between two oppositely charged electrodes will conduct a current.

flame protometric detector (FPD) used mainly for detecting phosphorus- and sulfur-containing compounds that emit light at 526 and 394 nm.

flexible access ability of an analyzer to perform one or more samples for several different analytes.

fluor substance that emits light when exposed to radiation.

fluorescence emission of light from an excited singlet state that has resulted from light absorption.

fluorescence detector measures the ability of compounds to fluoresce or to absorb and reemit light at a given set of wavelengths.

fluorescence polarization degree to which fluorescence intensity is greater in one plane than it is in another.

fluorescence polarization immunoassay (FPIA) homogeneous immunoassay technique based on the amount of polarized fluorescent light detected when the fluorophore label is excited with polarized light.

fluorogenic enzyme-linked immunosorbent assay (ELISA) technique that uses a fluorescent tag.

fluorogenic substrate nonfluorescent molecule that becomes fluorescent when modified by an enzymatic process.

fluorometer instrument capable of measuring fluorescence that uses filters for isolation of excitation and emission bands.

fluorophore molecule that is capable of reemitting absorbed light as fluorescence.

focus control on an oscilloscope that adjusts the sharpness of the signal.

fragment ion ion resulting from the rupture of intramolecular bonds when a neutral parent molecule is impacted by a suitable energy source.

freezing point temperature at which the liquid phase and the solid or crystalline phase of a solution exist at equilibrium.

freezing point depression osmometry measurement of the particle concentration (osmolality) of a solution by measurement of freezing point depression.

frequency (f) number of cycles/second of rotation for a generator, motor, or other circuit. The unit of measurement is the hertz.

frictional coefficient measure of the resistance a particle offers to movement through a solvent.

front surface fluorometer detector that measures fluorescence light that has been reflected from the surface. A specific excitation wavelength is selected by the user of a filter. The light is then reflected off the surface of a dichroic mirror onto the surface of the reaction vessel. Light emitted from the reaction vessel is selected by the use of the dichroic mirror and an emission filter.

front surface fluorometry analytic technique that measures the amount of fluorescence produced on the front surface of a tab, glass fiber matrix, or reaction vessel.

full-scale deflection when the meter movement deflects to the highest digit of a given range on a meter.

full-wave bridge rectifier solid-state electronic component with a circuit configuration of four semiconductor diodes that rectifies AC voltage to pulsating DC voltage by full-wave rectification. It converts an AC input signal to DC voltage.

full-wave rectifier circuit configuration composed of two diodes of correct polarity so as to rectify both half-cycles of an AC voltage signal.

fuse electronic device used to prevent excessive current from being drawn should a breakdown occur in an electronic instrument or a piece of electronic equipment.

gain the degree of amplification of a signal; the control used to adjust the amplification of a readout device.

galvanometer device capable of detecting very small amounts of current.

gas chromatography (GC) chromatographic technique in which the mobile phase is a gas.

gas chromatography/mass spectrometry (GC/MS) analytic system that combines a gas chromatograph with a mass spectrometer.

gas-liquid chromatography (GLC) GC technique that uses a liquid stationary phase coated onto a solid support.

gas-solid chromatography (GSC) GC technique that uses the same solid material as both the support and stationary phase.

Geiger-Müller counter gas-filled detector measuring radiation in the region where all radiation produces the same current flow regardless of energy of radiation or the number of primary ion pairs produced by radiation.

gel network of strands of polymer chains that are tangled together so they trap a large volume of solvent between them.

gradient elution technique in which compounds are eluted by changing the column conditions (i.e., solvent composition), with time.

graphite furnace graphite tube used for flameless sampling in atomic absorption into which injected solution is vaporized.

graticule grid pattern shown on the face of an oscilloscope.

grating device that employs refraction and diffraction to linearly disperse white light into its color spectrum.

ground state stable condition of atom whose electrons are in their normal orbiting shell positions.

ground common voltage reference point of a circuit; often the negative side of the power source.

growth index or value measurement of microbial metabolism given a numeric value.

half-cell one of two dissimilar metal electrodes that develops a positive or negative charge.

half-life ($t_{1/2}$) time required for a given number of radionuclides in the sample to decrease to one half its original value.

half-wave rectifier circuit configuration composed of one diode and therefore can only rectify one of the half-cycles of an AC voltage signal.

hapten a molecule of low molecular weight that itself is not antigenic in vivo, but can react with an antibody(s) in vitro.

headspace analysis injection technique used for compounds that are naturally volatile but are present in a solution that also contains nonvolatile or interfering components.

heat of condensation heat produced when water molecules in the gaseous phase above a liquid condense to re-form a liquid.

heat of fusion heat released from a solution during transition from the liquid to the solid phase (i.e., during formation of ice crystals).

height equivalent of a theoretic plate (H or HETP) length of a column needed to generate one theoretic plate.

henry (H) unit of measure for inductance; when 1 ampere/second induces 1 volt in a coil.

hertz (Hz) unit of measure for frequency; 1 hertz equals 1 cycle/second.

heterogeneous technique immunoassay technique that requires an analytic step to physically separate the bound from the free fraction.

high performance liquid chromatography (HPLC) LC method that uses small, uniform, and rigid support materials, typically 3 to 10 μm in diameter.

high-pressure mixing method of forming gradients by mixing solvents after they pass through the pumps.

histogram one dimensional display of "cell analysis" distribution. Analysis or measured values are shown on the X axis, and concentration is shown on the Y axis.

hollow cathode lamp special lamp for atomic absorption photometers that has cathode plate (filament) coated with metal to be tested, which emits light of a specific wavelength directed at solution containing metal.

homogeneous technique immunoassay technique that does not require the physical separation of the bound fraction from the free fraction.

horizontal electrophoresis electrophoresis on a horizontal support medium.

horizontal position control on an oscilloscope that moves the trace/waveshape left or right across the CRT screen.

human transportation system system that uses humans to move patients or specimens from one place to another.

hydrodynamic focus narrowing of one fluid (sample) stream by an outer (sheath) fluid brought about by a symmetric decrease in the cross-sectional area of the channel containing the fluids. The sample stream is narrowed and focused to pass through the center of the sensing zone for single cell analysis.

icons symbols that are displayed on a CRT or video display unit (VDU) that indicate the current activity of an analyzer.

immunofixation a procedure in which the antibody reacts with antigen and is fixed on the surface rather than diffusing through support medium.

immunometrix (NXT) technology technology based on the principle that the fluorescence intensity of a solution is proportional to the concentration of the fluorophore.

impedance (Z) total opposition to the flow of alternating current that results from the combined effect of resistance and reactance; measured in ohms.

immunoelectrophoresis group of procedures in which electrophoretic separation and immunologic reactions are used.

incident light beam of light entering a cuvette.

indicator electrode electrode, (e.g., Ag/AgCl), whose potential varies as the concentration of reactants and products change in solution. This potential is governed by the Nernst equation.

inductance (L) property of an electric circuit that opposes any change in current flow caused by the counter EMF generated in a coil; the unit of measure is the henry.

induction conversion of mechanical energy into electrical energy by the relative motion of a conductor with respect to a magnetic field.

inductive reactance (X_L) opposition to a changing current that results from inductance; measured in ohms.

inductor (choke or coil) device (coil) made by wrapping turns of a conductor around an air core or a soft iron core that opposes any change in current. It stores electromagnetic energy to be released at a later time.

Infrared detection source of infrared light used to measure a specific by-product of microbial growth.

inlet portion of a mass spectrometer that allows entry of sample molecules into the spectrometer. The inlet may be part of an interface that mates the spectrometer to another system (e.g., a gas chromatograph or liquid chromatograph).

inlet splitters (splitless or direction injection) approaches that influence injections by applying a narrow plug of sample to the column without causing excessive broadening of the resulting peaks in the chromatogram.

inner filter effect process whereby emitted light is absorbed before leaving the

solution. Usually caused by nonfluorescent solutes.

insulator material, or a combination of materials, having an atomic structure that provides very few electrons; it is composed of materials having seven or eight valence electrons.

integrated circuit miniaturized functional circuit incorporated into a tiny piece of silicon; often referred to as a "chip."

integrator device that can determine the area under a curve by measuring a change in some parameter in intervals over time or distance and then summing them to produce a total.

intensity measure of the number of ions with a given mass-to-charge ratio seen in a mass spectrum (see **abundance**).

inter system crossing when electron spins become unpaired and the triplet state results.

interference filter dielectric spacer of low refractive index sandwiched between semitransparent silver films and sharp cut-off filters to eliminate diffuse order spectral effects.

internal standard element of known concentration used in flame photometer as reference to compare with tested elements for true signal responses of elements.

ion source part of a mass spectrometer where ionization (and fragmentation) of simple molecules occurs.

ion trap detector combined ion source and mass analyzer. Such a combination accomplishes ionization (fragmentation, when it occurs) and mass analysis within the one device.

ion-exchange chromatography (IEC) LC technique that separates compounds based on their different extents of adsorption onto a support containing fixed charges on its surface.

ion-pair chromatography (IPC) LC technique that uses a reversed-phase or normal-phase column along with an ion-pairing agent in the mobile phase.

ion-photon conversion process wherein ion impacts result in the production of photons. The photons are then measured in a photomultiplier whose output signal is proportional to the number of impacting ions.

ion-selective electrode indicator electrode used in potentiometry that responds to specific ions in solution.

ion charged particles with a mass of less than 30,000 daltons.

ion source region of mass spectrometer where ionization and fragmentation of sample molecules occurs.

ionic strength (u) one half the sum of the concentration (C_i) multiplied by the square of the charge (Z_i) for each ionic species in solution: $u = \frac{1}{2}$ sum $C_i Z_i^2$.

ionization interference alteration of light emission or absorption because of altered flame temperature.

ionized state unstable condition of atom in which one or more electrons have been thrown out of their orbits around nucleus and do not return to their positions.

ionophore neutral carrier molecule incorporated into an ion-selective electrode to detect a specific ion.

isobar nuclides with the same atomic mass number but different atomic number.

isocratic elution elution of compounds using a constant mobile phase composition.

isoelectric having a net charge of zero.

isoelectric focusing electrophoresis procedure in which ions are made to line up in order of their isoionic pHs.

isoelectric point pH at which the net charge on a molecule (protein) is zero.

isotacophoresis ordering and concentration of substances of intermediate effective mobilities between an ion of high effective mobility and one of much lower effective mobility followed by their migration at a uniform velocity.

isothermal elution elution of compounds using a constant temperature.

isotope nuclides with the same atomic number but a different atomic mass number.

isotopic abundance amounts of isotopes present for a given element.

isozymes (isoenzymes) multiple forms of an enzyme that catalyze the same reaction.

JCAHO Joint Commission for Accreditation of Healthcare Organizations. Agency that inspects and accredits healthcare institutions receiving Medicare funds.

jet separator device for interfacing a gas chromatograph to a mass spectrometer. It concentrates sample while removing carrier gas and allows the transition from a high pressure condition to one of high vacuum.

joule heating heating of a conductor by the passage of an electrical current.

LUC (Large Unstained Cells) term used (by Technicon) in white cell analysis to describe large white cells that do not stain for peroxidase.

label atom or molecule attached to a substrate that is capable of generating a signal for monitoring.

lag time time between

introduction of the sample and production of first result.

laminar flow burner specially designed burner that creates a long ribbon of flame to expose more surface area of burning solution.

laminar flow two liquids traveling together down a long channel with the particles in the fluids traveling in parallel lines to one another. These two distinct fluids do not mix as long as the velocities differ and no turbulence is introduced into the system.

LASER Light Amplification by Stimulated Emission of Radiation; very intense, highly collimated light source often used in nephelometers.

leaking voltage accumulation of charge on the chassis of an instrument caused by the chassis being inadequately grounded.

least squares method method of performing linear regression analysis and obtaining estimates of the slope, intercept, and correlation coefficient.

light emitting diode (LED) solid-state digital readout device consisting of a seven-segmented display or small dot diodes.

light scattering interaction of light with particles that cause the light to be bent away from its original path.

linear regression technique for comparing two variables to assess the degree to which their relationship can be described by a straight line. Often used to compare results obtained by one method/instrument with another method/instrument.

linearity extent to which a range over the response (e.g., absorbance) is directly proportional to concentration.

liquid chromatography (LC) chromatographic technique in

which the mobile phase is a liquid.

liquid-liquid junction potential potential that develops at the interface between two nonidentical solutions because of differences in ion mobilities and concentrations.

low-performance liquid chromatography or column chromatography LC method that uses large, nonrigid support materials.

low-pressure mixing method of forming gradients in which solvents are mixed before the pumps.

luciferin/luciferase enzyme used in microbial assays to detect the presence of bacterial or yeast adenosine triphosphate (ATP).

magnetic sector mass spectrometer mass spectrometer whose mass analyzer is based on a magnetic field that deflects ions to a varying extent depending on their mass-to-charge ratios.

mass selective detection detection of only selected ions in a molecule's mass spectrum. The ions selected are those most characteristic of the molecule. They may serve in place of that molecule's complete spectrum for purposes of identification, quantitation, or sensitivity enhancement (see **selected ion monitoring**).

mass-to-charge ratio (m/z) ratio of an ion's mass to atomic mass units to the units of charge possessed by the ion.

matrix interference physical differences in viscosities of standards and samples cause different responses in instruments.

membrane separator type of gc/ms interface that allows organic molecules to diffuse across a selectively permeable membrane while restricting the passage of carrier gas into the ion source of the mass spectrometer.

metal oxide semiconductor field effect transistor (MOSFET) semiconductor amplifier that has a gate insulated from the channel by a film of metal oxide and thus has an extremely high impedance.

mho unit of measure for conductance.

microparticle enzyme immunoassay (MEIA) technique that uses a submicron particle coated with antibody specific for the analyte that is being tested.

minimal inhibitory concentration (MIC) minimal concentration of an antimicrobial agent that inhibits bacterial growth.

mobile phase The solvent used to elute sample components from a chromatographic column.

mobility how far a particular ion will move under standard conditions of electrophoresis.

mode of acquisition way in which a capital equipment asset can be acquired (e.g., reagent rental).

modulation electronic means of chopping a light beam into a pulsating signal.

module component of an analyzer that performs the testing and may be replaced in its entirety with minimal analyzer downtime.

molality concentration of a solution expressed as moles of solute/kilogram of solvent.

molar absorptivity absorbance of 1 g/L of a substance (1 M) measured in a 1 cm light path at a specific wavelength.

molecular ion sample molecule that has become ionized without fragmentation. This ion, when seen in the mass spectrum, yields important information (the molecular weight of the parent molecule).

molecular marker term applied to molecular weight products found circulating in blood that are generated on activation of enzymatic reactions in the hemostasis systems or released from activated cells.

molecular sieving filtration of a solution of substances of difference sizes so that the biggest molecules move the slowest.

monochromator any device that disperses white light into its spectrum of colors.

multiple ion detection (MID) form of selective ion monitoring as employed by ion trap mass spectrometers.

multiprobe concept of one instrument having the capability of performing different endpoint readings on one machine, (e.g., clotting, chromogenic, and ELISA).

mutual excitation result of photons emitted by excited sodium atoms, which in turn excite potassium atoms.

mutual inductance linking of two coils by the magnetic field that surrounds one of the coils. The coil that generates the magnetic field and thus induces a current is called the primary coil; the coil that receives the induced current is called the secondary coil.

nebulization disintegration of liquid solution into small, intermedite size droplets.

nephelometer specially designed spectrophotometer with a fixed or variable angle of detection for measuring light scatter by particles.

nephelometry technique that measures the amount of light scattered by particles suspended in a solution.

Nernst equation expression that relates the cell potential to the standard cell potential and the activities of reactants and products in the electrochemical cell.

neutrino nuclear particle with no mass or electrical charge emitted during a nuclear decay process. It virtually does not interact with matter.

nitrogen-phosphorus detector component of a gas chromatograph based on the principle that the release of ions from an alkaline metal (rubidium) is increased in the presence of compounds containing nitrogen or phosphorus.

nominal wavelength specific wavelength at the peak transmittance.

noncompetitive immunoassay an immunoassay technique where analyte in a patient sample does not compete for antibody binding sites with labeled analyte.

normal-phase liquid chromatography (NPLC) type of partition chromatography that uses a polar stationary phase.

nucleon collective term for protons and neutrons in the nucleus.

nuclide nucleus with a particular atomic number and atomic mass number.

number of theoretic plates (N) measure of the efficiency or width of sample peaks on a chromatographic system.

off-line incubation incubation of a test independent of the measurement system.

Ohm's law in an electrical circuit; current is directly proportional to the voltage between the ends of the conductor and inversely proportional to the resistance.

ohmmeter electronic device that is configured to measure resistance; it has its own internal power supply, thus components that are being measured with this device must be disconnected from their power source.

oil diffusion pump high-vacuum pump in which oil is vaporized by heating and used to entrap gas molecules diffusing from a region to which the pump is connected.

open-reagent system ability of an analyzer to use reagents or assays from vendors other than the manufacturer of the system.

open-split interface gc/ms interface in which the gc effluent passes across a small gap between the exit and of the gc column, and a restrictor line is connected to the ion source of the ms.

opened circuit refers to a circuit in which the path for current flow has been broken.

operational amplifier solid state electronic component consisting of a multistage amplifier system contained within one small unit or package.

orthagonal term used by Unipath to describe the angle of scatter analysis in their instruments. Orthagonal means right angle or 90 degrees.

oscilloscope readout device used for viewing electrical waveforms; measuring voltage, amplitude, and frequency; determines phase relationships between signals.

osmolal gap difference between the measured and calculated osmolality.

osmolality number of moles of particles of solute/kg of water.

osmometry measurement of the osmolality of a solution.

osmotic pressure hydrostatic pressure required to stop the diffusion of a solvent through a semipermeable membrane from a region of low solute concentration to a region of high solute concentration.

paper chromatography paper used as both the support and the stationary phase for thin layer chromatography.

parallax optical illusion that makes an object appear displaced when viewed from an angle.

parallel circuit circuit that contains two or more paths for current flow that is supplied by a single power supply.

partition or liquid-liquid chromatography LC method that separates compounds based on their ability to partition between a liquid mobile phase and a liquid or bonded stationary phase coated on a solid support.

payback period period of time after instrument acquisition required for revenues to equal costs.

peak voltage (current) maximum amplitude of a changing voltage or current.

peak-to-peak voltage measured value of a sine wave from peak-positive voltage to peak negative voltage.

Peltier effect phenomenon whereby when an electrical current is passed through a junction of two metals of dissimilar properties; one metal will heat and the other will cool.

period time for completion of one cycle.

phosphorescence emission of light from an excited triplet state that has resulted from light absorption.

photochopper one type of beam splitter, consisting of a rotating wheel with holes and a silvered surface to allow the beam of light to both pass through and be reflected.

photocurrent electric current produced by light.

photoelectric effect one process by which the photon interacts directly with one of the orbital electrons in matter to transfer the entire photon energy to the electron, resulting in ionization and excitation of the matter.

photoelectricity source of electricity produced by the emission of electrons from photosensitive materials.

photometer any instrument that measures light.

photomultiplier tube (PMT) photosensitive detector capable of internal amplification of the electronic signal using electronic devices known as dynodes.

photons discrete packets of light energy.

photoresistor (photoconductor) semiconductor transducer that converts changes in radiant energy into changes of resistance/conductance.

photovoltaic cell photosensitive device that converts light energy into voltage; often is affected by a phenomenon called electronic "fatigue."

piezoelectricity source of electricity produced by the mechanical compression, stretching, and twisting of certain crystals.

Planck's constant proportionality constant for interrelationship between energy and frequency of light.

pneumatic tube system mechanical, air-driven system that moves specimens from one place to another.

polarity term that refers to the negative or positive direction of a current or voltage; also refers to points in a circuit as being relatively positive or negative with respect to each other.

polarography voltammetry performed at a dropping mercury working electrode.

polyacrylamide polymer of acrylamide and usually some cross-linking derivative.

postanalytic steps taken after test results are obtained.

postcolumn derivatization technique in which compounds leaving the column are combined with a reagent that converts them into a more easily detected form.

potentiometer (POT) three-terminal variable resistor used to select a potential for application to a subsequent circuit.

potentiometry technique where the potential difference between two electrodes is measured under equilibrium conditions.

power (P) time rate of doing work. The unit of measurement is the watt.

power supply electronic device that can produce an assortment of AC and DC voltage levels, a source of direct current, and a means of regulating voltage levels at specific circuit locations. They characteristically consist of five stages: transformer, rectifier, filter, voltage regulator, and voltage divider.

preanalytic steps taken before actual test performance. Begins with the actual test request and proceeds through specimen preparation.

precolumn derivatization technique in which sample components are derivatized before they are injected onto a column.

pre-mix burner apparatus in which test solution, gas, and oxidant are mixed and nebulized before atomization into flame.

precision degree to which multiple measurements result in similar values.

primary tube tube or collection container in which the specimen was initially placed.

primary tube sampling ability to aspirate sample from the original tube in which it was obtained.

prism device that nonlinearly refracts white light through it and spreads light into a full range of colors.

proboscis positive-displacement pump in the metering tower of a Kodak Ektachem analyzer that aspirates aliquots of specimens and dispenses uniform volumes of specimens onto reagent slides.

proportional counter gas-filled detector measuring radiation in the region where the number of primary ion pairs produced or energy deposited by radiation is proportional to the magnitude of the current flow.

pulsating direct current type of current that has a fixed polarity but its magnitude varies over time.

pulsating DC (ripple) voltage that is initially generated during rectification of an AC signal to a DC signal. Although the current is unidirectional, the voltage is not maintained at a constant level.

quadrupole mass analyzer that separates ions based on their movement through a field established by combined DC and RF voltages applied to four rods in a rectangular configuration.

qualifier ions or peak qualifiers ions that are used to confirm the identification of a compound using selected ion monitoring (SIM).

quencher molecule that results in a decrease in fluorescence when present with the fluorophore.

quenching process that causes a decrease in fluorescence.

radial partition immunoassay (RPIA) immunoassay technique in which antibody is immobilized on a glass filter paper; both competitive and noncompetitive assays can be used.

radiation absorbed dose (rad) measure of local energy deposition/unit mass of material irradiated. One rad is equal to 100 ergs of absorbed energy/gram of absorber.

radiative energy attenuation (REA) technique based on the principle that the measured intensity of a solution containing a fluorophore is related to the absorbance properties of the solution.

radioimmunoassay (RIA) immunoassay technique that uses a radioactive isotope as a tracer.

Raleigh scatter reflection of light at different angles by particles suspended in a solution. This scattering occurs when the wavelength of light is greater than the size of the particles.

raman scatter scattered light that results from the interaction to light with solutes and is slightly higher in wavelength than the exciting light.

random access ability to process a sample independently of the other samples.

random access analyzer analyzer thay may be programmed to perform individual assays or test panels without the need for an operator to intervene.

range term that refers to the full scale deflection of a recording device of recorder or other readout system that is equal to the input voltage.

ratio-recording photometer photometer in which detector response to the readout device is a ratio of sample to reference absorbance signals.

reactance (X) opposition to alternating current that results from capacitance reactance or inductance reactance (the effective resistance to current flow in an AC circuit caused by the presence of capacitance and/or inductance) measured in ohms.

reactor electronic device (capacitor, inductor) that can store and return power in a circuit; it does not dissipate electrical energy in the form of heat.

readout device device that measures an electrical signal, such as a change in current, voltage, or resistance that has been generated by the instrument's detector, and then converts it into a presentable format.

reagent layer layer of an Ektachem slide that contains the reactants and/or indicator dye.

rearrangement ion ion formed by combination of two individual ions during the ionization process in an ion source.

rectification process of converting AC voltage to DC voltage.

rectifier electronic circuit that converts alternating current into unidirectional or direct current.

reference blank solution of all reaction constituents except test solute used to adjust photometer to 100% T, or 0 A.

reference electrode electrode with a stable half-cell potential against which the relative potential of the working electrode is measured.

reflectance photometry bouncing of an optical beam through a fixed medium off a shiny surface to a light-detecting device.

reflection light that is totally deflected by the surface of a substance.

reflectometer instrument that measures the amount of light.

refraction bending of incident light after it passes obliquely from one medium to another of different density.

refractive index ratio of the speed of light in two different mediums, where the reference medium is air.

refractivity relative ability of a substance to bend light.

refractometer instrument that measures the refractive index of solutions.

relay electromagnetic switch that operates on the principle of induction.

reservoir solution between the electrodes and the supporting medium.

resistance (R) refers to the opposition of current flow.

resistance-measurement/ continuity method approach to troubleshooting an electronic instrument that involves comparing resistance measurements made on the malfunctioning instrument with the resistance data supplied by the manufacturer.

resolution (R$_s$) measure of the separation between two peaks based on the difference in their retention and their baseline widths.

resolution ability of the monochromator to distinguish test compound's true absorbance peak(s) from adjacent, interfering absorbances; primarily a function of bandpass.

retardation factor (R$_f$) distance a compound travels from its point of application to the distance traveled by the mobile phase (solvent) in the same amount of time.

retention time (t$_r$) time it takes a retained compound to elute from a chromatographic system.

retention volume (V$_r$) volume it takes a retained compound to elute from a chromatographic system.

reversed-phase liquid chromatography (RPLC) type of partition chromatography that uses a nonpolar stationary phase.

rheostat two-terminal variable resistor used to vary current within a circuit.

robotic system mechanical, computerized system used to transport specimens from one place to another.

rocket bullet-shaped streak of protein made by electrophoresing antigen proteins into gel containing antibody.

roentgen (R) unit of x-rays or gamma rays representing the quantity of ionization produced by photon radiation in a given sample of air. One roentgen equals that quantity of photon radiation capable of producing one electrostatic unit of ions of either sign in 0.001293 g of air.

roentgen equivalent, man (rem) dose of any ionizing radiation that causes the same amount of biologic injury to human tissue as 1 rad of x-ray, gamma ray, or beta-particle radiation. In the case of x-ray, gamma, or beta radiation, rems are equal to the absorbed dose in rads; in the case of alpha radiation, however, the dose in rems equals the dose in rads multiplied by 20, because only 0.05 rad of alpha radiation is needed to produce the same biological effect as 1 rad of x-ray gamma-ray, or beta particle radiation.

root-mean-square (RMS) voltage amount of AC voltage or current that has the same heating effect as an equal amount of DC voltage. The RMS voltage is equal to 0.707 times the peak voltage.

salt bridge device that allows ionic movement between compartments of an electrochemical cell to maintain electrical contact and at the same time prevents mixing of the separate solutions. Sample molecules are able to transit the gap and enter the restrictor, which, at the same time, limits carrier gas flow into the ion source.

sandwich (immunometric) assay assay in which the analyte in the patient sample binds to an antibody that has been covalently linked to a solid-phase support. A labeled antibody is added that reacts with a second antigenic site on the analyte, thus forming a complex know as a "sandwich."

scattergram two-dimensional display of cell measurements. One measurement is shown on the X axis and the second on the Y axis with the display appearing as dots/clusters.

scintillation term that refers to light flashes ($sec^{-1} = 2.7 \times 10^9$ Ci).

Seebeck effect phenomenon whereby when strips of two metals of dissimilar properties are joined, the temperature of the junction increases when passage of an electrical current through the junction is stopped.

selected ion monitoring (SIM) monitoring of only selected ions in a sample molecule's mass spectrum (see **mass selective detection**).

selective instrument instrument capable of performing multiple tests on any sample but only those tests that are programmed.

self-absorption type of concentration quenching in which the fluorophore absorbs exciting light excessively and results in a loss of linear response with concentration.

self-inductance back EMF generated in a coil caused by the AC current that generates an expanding and collapsing magnetic field around the coil.

semiconductor substance that does not conduct electricity as well as metal but is considerably better than an insulator. It is often referred to as a "solid-state" device and is composed of materials that have four valence electrons.

semiconductor diode solid state device that primarily functions to convert AC current to DC current. A special type called a zener diode serves as a voltage regulator.

sensitivity (meter) amount of current required to deflect a meter movement full-scale.

sensitivity lowest value that can be reliably detected without a false positive result.

separation factor (α) measure of the separation between two peaks based on the ratio of their capacity factors.

sequential analyzer each sample in a batch enters the analytic process one after another with each respective result emerging in the same order as specimens are processed.

sequential immunoassay technique where unlabeled analyte (patient sample) is first mixed with excess antibody, incubated, and then followed by addition of labeled analyte.

series circuit circuit that contains only one possible pathway for current flow.

sheath fluid liquid stream filling a channel (outer layer) and surrounding a second liquid stream (inner layer-sample stream).

shelf-life length of time a reagent can remain on the shelf, unopened, without deterioration.

short term that refers to a path of zero resistance.

shorted circuit path that has zero resistance for current flow.

size exclusion chromatography (SEC) LC technique that separates molecules based on their different degrees of exclusion from the pores of the support material.

slab gel electrophoresis electrophoresis on a supporting medium that is a gel-shaped like a sheet or slab.

slide metering block device that transfers an Ektachem reagent slide from the slide supply to the proboscis and finally to its respective incubator.

slow-blowing fuse special type of fuse that has a high lag time before the filament melts; it will not blow immediately if there is a sudden rise in current.

sodium dodecylsulfate (SDS) detergent used in protein electrophoresis; a very effective protein denaturant or unfolding agent.

specific activity activity of the radionuclide/unit mass of the radioactive sample expressed as Ci/μg, μCi/μ/mol.

specific ionization number of ion pairs produced/unit path length of ionizing radiation.

specificity ability to measure only the analyte requested.

specimen oriented analyzer analyzer that performs all of the requested tests on a specimen before sampling commences on another specimen.

specimen processing prepares a specimen for the testing process. Can include such procedures as mixing and configuration.

spectral interference Background emission or absorption by extraneous elements or compounds.

spectral scan recording of absorbances of test sample by scanning through multiple wavelengths.

spectral slit width all of the wavelengths that the exit slit will allow to be transmitted.

spectrofluorometer instrument capable of measuring fluorescence that uses monochromators for isolation of excitation and emission wavelengths.

spectrophotometer any instrument that measures monochromatic light produced by an adjustable monochromator (i.e., prism or grating).

spreading layer uppermost layer of an Ektachem slide that uniformly disperses specimens across the entire surface area of the slide while trapping interfering particles.

sputtering inert gas ions in hollow cathode lamp collide with the cathode plate and dislodge individual metal atoms from the surface.

stability length of time a reagent or sample remains viable.

stacking making ions line up in order of their effective mobilities.

staining making separated bands of zones of material visible, usually by making them adsorb (bind) a dye.

standard cell potential electrochemical cell potential measured under standard state conditions.

stat analyzer analytic instrument designed to provide the shortest lag time between sample introduction and result availability.

stationary phase chemical layer that is coated or covalently attached to the support material in a column.

step-down transformer transformer in which the primary voltage is larger than the secondary voltage.

step-up transformer transformer in which the secondary voltage is larger than the primary voltage.

stray light extraneous light of higher order spectra, or room light, that has entered the instrument.

strong mobile phase solvent that quickly elutes sample components from a column.

submarine electrophoresis electrophoresis on a supporting medium that is submerged in the electrophoresis solution.

substitution of parts/modules-symptom method approach to troubleshooting that consists of substituting a spare part, usually a plug-in module, based on the symptoms displayed by the malfunctioning instrument.

supercooling rapid cooling of a solution to a temperature below its freezing point, as in freezing point depression osmometry.

supporting media insoluble inert framework through which electrophoresis occurs but that stops convection.

sweep flow fluid used to prevent recirculation of cells into the sensing zone by flowing (sweeping) past the exit from the aperture and sweeping away the counted cells.

sweep frequency number of times the oscilloscope beam moves from the left side to the right side of the graticule.

sweep time time required for the beam of an oscilloscope to move from the left side to the right side of the graticule.

switch device used to turn current "on" or "off" or redirect current flow.

synthetic substrate assay test based on a specific enzyme-substrate reaction in which the natural substrate is replaced by a synthetic version of the natural substrate.

tandem access programming mode where an operator prioritizes the assays to be run in a manner that maximizes throughput.

temperature programming elution technique in which the temperature of the chromatographic system is varied with the time.

test menu number of procedures that can be performed on the analytic system.

test mix variety of analytes that a laboratory performs.

thermal conductivity detector component of a gas chromatograph that is based on the principle that differences in the rate of heat conduction exist between pure carrier gas and the carrier with a sample mixture.

thermistor electronic temperature-sensing device made of semiconductor metals used in freezing point depression osmometry.

thermochemistry source of electricity produced when the junction of two dissimilar metals is heated.

thermocouple two strips of dissimilar metals joined together at one end and attached to a voltmeter at their separate ends.

thin layer chromatography (TLC) flat beds or planar supports used in liquid chromatography.

threshold concentration at which the presence or absence of drug/metabolite is flagged or shown to be greater or less than a level where a significant amount of false positives is likely.

throughput measure of the speed of an analytic system. It is usually described in terms of the number of tests that are performed in a fixed period of time.

time base generator associated circuit of the oscilloscope that applies a sawtooth voltage signal to the horizontal deflection plate. This signal causes the electron beam to move at a constant rate across the screen, and then rapidly returns it to the starting position where it begins another sweep across the screen.

time-resolved fluorescence spectroscopy technique that is capable of measuring fluorescence decay from a fluorophore after light from the excitation source and possibly from background; fluorescence is no longer present.

time/cm control on an oscilloscope that in conjunction with a calibration control selects a calibrated time/cm along the horizontal grid of the CRT.

top-to-top fluorescence process of measuring fluorescence by directing light of a specific wavelength to a dichroic mirror which then becomes reflected onto the upper surface of a reaction vessel (cup/tab). This reaction vessel subsequently emits light in the form of fluorescence that can pass through the dichroic mirror. A specific wavelength is selected by the use of an emission filter.

total consumption burner apparatus into which test solution is drawn directly into the base of the flame, at which point gas and oxidant are also introduced.

tracer any moiety that can be tagged to a molecule to produce a signal to monitor a reaction.

transducer electronic device that detects one form of energy and converts it to another form.

transformer device that transfers electrical energy from one coil to another by mutual induction.

transistor solid-state device that used primarily for amplification.

transmission ability of a substance to permit light to travel through it.

transmitted light beam of light exiting a cuvette.

transmutation radioactive decay process that results in a change in nuclear constitution, such as electron capture decay.

% transmittance percent of transmitted light exiting sample to incident light entering sample.

turbidimetry technique that measures the decreased amount of transmitted light through a solution as a result of light scatter by particles.

turbo-molecular pump high-vacuum pump operating on the principle of gas evacuation by means of high-velocity rotating vanes.

Tyndall light scattered light measured at an angle of 90 degrees.

turbonephelometry technique used by the TDx to detect radiant energy emitted by the light scattering from particles suspended in solution.

unidirectional interface interface in which information is only sent in one direction (e.g., from the instrument to the computer).

uploading information (e.g., test results) sent from the analytic system to the laboratory information system or other device.

user-defined parameter any assay parameter or calibration parameter that may differ from what the manufacturer has established or recommends.

user-friendliness subjective assessment of the ease with which an instrument is capable of being operated by a user.

UV/Vis absorbance detector measures the ability of compounds to absorb light at one or more wavelengths in the ultraviolet or visible range.

vapor pressure (dew point) depression osmometry measurement of the osmolality of a solution by measurement of vapor pressure depression.

vapor pressure pressure exerted by the vapor, or gaseous, phase of a solvent when in equilibrium with the liquid state of the same solvent.

variable costs costs that depend on the volume of tests performed (e.g., reagent costs).

Venturi action flow of liquid through capillary tube caused by negative pressure at the nonimmursed end of the tube as gas rushes by the open tip.

vertical electrophoresis electrophoresis on a vertical (upright) support medium.

vertical position control on an oscilloscope that moves the trace/waveshape up or down on the screen of the CRT.

void time (t$_o$) time it takes the mobile phase or a nonretained compound to elute from a chromatographic system.

void volume (V$_o$) volume required for the mobile phase or a nonretained compound to elute from a chromatographic system.

volt (V or E) unit of measure for an EMF or potential. The EMF present when 1 ampere flows through a resistance of 1 ohm. One volt = 1 joule/coulomb.

volt-ohm-milliammeter (VOM) d'Arsonval meter configured to measure current, voltage, and resistance.

Volt. The unit of electrostatic potential.

voltage divider circuit suitable for supplying two or more voltages from one voltage source.

voltage drop voltage measured across a resistive device.

voltage measurement method approach to troubleshooting that entails the measuring of voltages at a test point and subsequently compares them with the values given in the manufacturer's maintenance manual.

voltage regulator electronic component that provides a supply of constant DC current.

voltammetry technique whereby current is measured as a function of applied potential.

voltmeter electronic device that measures voltage; it must be connected in parallel across the two points where the potential difference is to be measured.

volts/cm control on an oscilloscope that adjusts the amplitude of the signal applied to the vertical deflection plates.

walk-away capability ability to program an instrument, then leave the instrument to perform other tasks.

watt (W) unit of measure for electrical power; 1 watt of power is consumed when 1 volt causes 1 ampere to flow.

wave amplitude height of an energy wave.

wave frequency number of energy waves through space/second.

wavelength distance between two successive crests of energy waves.

wavelength drive motorized attachment to monochromator drive shaft to provide automatic spectral scanning of multiple wavelengths with the test sample.

wavelength shifter secondary scintillator added to scintillation liquid for shifting the wavelength of light emitted by the primary scintillator for more efficient detection by the photocathodes of photomultiplier tubes in liquid scintillation counting.

weak mobile phase solvent that slowly elutes sample components from a column.

wheatstone bridge circuit electronic circuit composed of two fixed resistors in parallel that are in series with a variable resistor and resistive device of unknown resistance. When the bridge is balanced, the value of the unknown resistance is equal to the value of the variable resistor setting.

window voltage limit set by the upper-level and lower-level discriminators of the pulse-height analyzer of a radioactive particle counter for differential counting.

workflow manner in which laboratory processes work.

workload number of tests generated by a laboratory in a given period of time.

workload recording methods system to document laboratory workload in terms of test volume and personnel requirements and attempts to quantify personnel productivity.

Zeeman effect background correction uses magnetic fields to differentiate true absorption (affected) from background absorption (unaffected).

zener diode semiconductor device designed to carry a specific amount of current when reversed-biased at a given voltage. Generally used to regulate voltage.

zero adjustment control used to set the recorder pen to baseline.

Index